AF342266

Allergy Frontiers: Clinical Manifestations

Volume 3

Ruby Pawankar • Stephen T. Holgate
Lanny J. Rosenwasser
Editors

Allergy Frontiers:
Clinical Manifestations

Volume 3

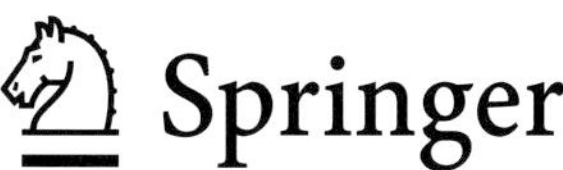 Springer

Ruby Pawankar, M.D., Ph.D.
Nippon Medical School
1-1-5 Sendagi, Bunkyo-ku
Tokyo
Japan

Lanny J. Rosenwasser, M.D.
Childrens Mercy Hospital and Clinic
UMKC School of Medicine
2401 Gillham Road
Kansas City, MO 64108
USA

Stephen T. Holgate, M.D., Ph.D.
University of Southampton
Southampton General Hospital
Tremona Road
Southampton
UK

ISBN: 978-4-431-88316-6   Springer Tokyo Berlin Heidelberg New York
e-ISBN: 978-4-431-88317-3
DOI: 10.1007/978-4-431-88317-3

Library of Congress Control Number: PCN applied for

Springer is a part of Springer Science+Business Media
springer.com

Foreword

When I entered the field of allergy in the early 1970s, the standard textbook was a few hundred pages, and the specialty was so compact that texts were often authored entirely by a single individual and were never larger than one volume. Compare this with *Allergy Frontiers: Epigenetics, Allergens, and Risk Factors*, the present six-volume text with well over 150 contributors from throughout the world. This book captures the explosive growth of our specialty since the single-author textbooks referred to above.

The unprecedented format of this work lies in its meticulous attention to detail yet comprehensive scope. For example, great detail is seen in manuscripts dealing with topics such as "Exosomes, naturally occurring minimal antigen presenting units" and "Neuropeptide S receptor 1 (NPSR1), an asthma susceptibility gene." The scope is exemplified by the unique approach to disease entities normally dealt with in a single chapter in most texts. For example, anaphylaxis, a topic usually confined to one chapter in most textbooks, is given five chapters in *Allergy Frontiers*. This approach allows the text to employ multiple contributors for a single topic, giving the reader the advantage of being introduced to more than one viewpoint regarding a single disease.

This broad scope is further illustrated in the way this text deals with the more frequently encountered disorder, asthma. There are no fewer than 26 chapters dealing with various aspects of this disease. Previously, to obtain such a comprehensive approach to a single condition, one would have had to purchase a text devoted solely to that disease state.

In addition, the volume includes titles which to my knowledge have never been presented in an allergy text before. These include topics such as "NKT ligand conjugated immunotherapy," "Hypersensitivity reactions to nano medicines: causative factors and optimization," and "An environmental systems biology approach to the study of asthma."

It is not hard to see that this textbook is unique, offering the reader a means of obtaining a detailed review of a single highly focused subject, such as the neuropeptide S receptor, while also providing the ability to access a panoramic and remarkably in-depth view of a broader subject, such as asthma. Clearly it is intended primarily for the serious student of allergy and immunology, but can also serve as a resource text for those with an interest in medicine in general.

I find it most reassuring that even though we have surpassed the stage of the one-volume, single-author texts, because of the wonderful complexity of our specialty and its broadening scope that has evolved over the years, the reader can still obtain an all-inclusive and comprehensive review of allergy in a single source. It should become part of the canon of our specialty.

Phil Lieberman, M.D.

Foreword

When I started immunology under Professor Kimishige Ishizaka in the early 1950s, allergy was a mere group of odd syndromes of almost unknown etiology. An immunological origin was only suspected but not proven. The term "atopy," originally from the Greek word *à-topòs*, represents the oddness of allergic diseases. I would call this era "stage 1," or the primitive era of allergology.

Even in the 1950s, there was some doubt as to whether the antibody that causes an allergic reaction was really an antibody, and was thus called a "reagin," and allergens were known as peculiar substances that caused allergy, differentiating them from other known antigens.

It was only in 1965 that reagin was proven to be an antibody having a light chain and a unique heavy chain, which was designated as IgE in 1967 with international consensus. The discovery of IgE opened up an entirely new era in the field of allergology, and the mechanisms of the immediate type of allergic reaction was soon evaluated and described. At that point in time we believed that the nature of allergic diseases was a mere IgE-mediated inflammation, and that these could soon be cured by studying the IgE and the various mediators that induced the inflammation. This era I would like to call "stage 2," or the classic era.

The classic belief that allergic diseases would be explained by a mere allergen-IgE antibody reaction did not last long. People were dismayed by the complexity and diversity of allergic diseases that could not be explained by mere IgE-mediated inflammation. Scientists soon realized that the mechanisms involved in allergic diseases were far more complex and that they extended beyond the conventional idea of a pure IgE-mediated inflammation. A variety of cells and their products (cytokines/chemokines and other inflammatory molecules) have been found to interact in a more complex manner; they create a network of reactions via their receptors to produce various forms of inflammatory changes that could never be categorized as a single entity of inflammation. This opened a new era, which I would like to call the modern age of allergology or "stage 3."

The modern era stage 3 coincided with the discovery that similar kinds of cytokines and cells are involved in the regulation of IgE production. When immunologists investigated the cell types and cytokines that regulate IgE production, they found that two types of helper T cells, distinguishable by the profile of cytokines they produce, play important regulatory roles in not only IgE production but also in regulating allergic inflammation. The advancement of modern molecular technologies has enabled detailed analyses of molecules and genes involved in this extremely complex regulatory mechanism. Hence, there are a number of important discoveries in this area, which are still of major interest to allergologists, as can be seen in the six volumes of this book.

We realize that allergology has rapidly progressed during the last century, but mechanisms of allergic diseases are far more complex than we had expected. New discoveries have created new questions, and new facts have reminded us of old concepts. For example, the genetic disposition of allergic diseases was suspected even in the earlier, primitive era but is still only partially proven on a molecular basis. Even the molecular mechanisms of allergic inflammation continue to be a matter of debate and there is no single answer to explain the phenomenon. There is little doubt that the etiology of allergic diseases is far more varied and complex than we had expected. An immunological origin is not the only mechanism, and there are more unknown origins of similar reactions. Although therapeutic means have also progressed, we remain far from our goal to cure and prevent allergic diseases.

We have to admit that while we have more knowledge of the many intricate mechanisms that are involved in the various forms of allergic disease, we are still at the primitive stage of allergology in this respect. We are undoubtedly proceeding into a new stage, stage 4, that may be called the postmodern age of allergology and hope this era will bring us closer to finding a true solution for the enigma of allergy and allergic diseases.

We are happy that at this turning point the editors, Ruby Pawankar, Stephen Holgate, and Lanny Rosenwasser, are able to bring out such a comprehensive book which summarizes the most current knowledge on allergic diseases, from epidemiology to mechanisms, the impact of environmental and genetic factors on allergy and asthma, clinical aspects, recent therapeutic and preventive strategies, as well as future perspectives. This comprehensive knowledge is a valuable resource and will give young investigators and clinicians new insights into modern allergology which is an ever-growing field.

Tomio Tada, M.D., Ph.D., D.Med.Sci.

Foreword

Allergic diseases represent one of the major health problems in most modern societies. The increase in prevalence over the last decades is dramatic. The reasons for this increase are only partly known. While in former times allergy was regarded as a disease of the rich industrialized countries only, it has become clear that all over the world, even in marginal societies and in all geographic areas—north and south of the equator—allergy is a major global health problem.

The complexity and the interdisciplinary character of allergology, being the science of allergic diseases, needs a concert of clinical disciplines (internal medicine, dermatology, pediatrics, pulmonology, otolaryngology, occupational medicine, etc.), basic sciences (immunology, molecular biology, botany, zoology, ecology), epidemiology, economics and social sciences, and psychology and psychosomatics, just to name a few. It is obvious that an undertaking like this book series must involve a multitude of authors; indeed, the wide spectrum of disciplines relevant to allergy is reflected by the excellent group of experts serving as authors who come from all over the world and from various fields of medicine and other sciences in a pooling of geographic, scientific, theoretical, and practical clinical diversity.

The first volume concentrates on the basics of etiology, namely, the causes of the many allergic diseases with epigenetics, allergens and risk factors. Here, the reader will find up-to-date information on the nature, distribution, and chemical structure of allergenic molecules, the genetic and epigenetic phenomena underlying the susceptibility of certain individuals to develop allergic diseases, and the manifold risk factors from the environment playing the role of modulators, both in enhancing and preventing the development of allergic reactions.

In times when economics plays an increasing role in medicine, it is important to reflect on this aspect and gather the available data which—as I modestly assume—may be yet rather scarce. The big effort needed to undertake well-controlled studies to establish the socio-economic burden of the various allergic diseases is still mainly ahead of us. The Global Allergy and Asthma European Network (GA2LEN), a group of centers of excellence in the European Union, will start an initiative regarding this topic this year.

In volume 2, the pathomechanisms of various allergic diseases and their classification are given, including such important special aspects as allergy and the bone marrow, allergy and the nervous system, and allergy and mucosal immunology.

Volume 3 deals with manifold clinical manifestations, from allergic rhinitis to drug allergy and allergic bronchopulmonary aspergillosis, as well as including other allergic reactions such as lactose and fructose intolerances.

Volume 4 deals with the practical aspects of diagnosis and differential diagnosis of allergic diseases and also reflects educational programs on asthma.

Volume 5 deals with therapy and prevention of allergies, including pharmacotherapy, as well as allergen-specific immunotherapy with novel aspects and special considerations for different groups such as children, the elderly, and pregnant women.

Volume 6 concludes the series with future perspectives, presenting a whole spectrum of exciting new approaches in allergy research possibly leading to new strategies in diagnosis, therapy, and prevention of allergic diseases.

The editors have accomplished an enormous task to first select and then motivate the many prominent authors. They and the authors have to be congratulated. The editors are masters in the field and come from different disciplines. Ruby Pawankar, from Asia, is one of the leaders in allergy who has contributed to the understanding of the cellular and immune mechanisms of allergic airway disease, in particular upper airway disease. Stephen Holgate, from the United Kingdom, has contributed enormously to the understanding of the pathophysiology of allergic airway reactions beyond the mere immune deviation, and focuses on the function of the epithelial barrier. He and Lanny Rosenwasser, who is from the United States, have contributed immensely to the elucidation of genetic factors in the susceptibility to allergy. All three editors are members of the Collegium Internationale Allergologicum (CIA) and serve on the Board of Directors of the World Allergy Organization (WAO).

I have had the pleasure of knowing them for many years and have cooperated with them at various levels in the endeavor to promote and advance clinical care, research, and education in allergy. Together with Lanny Rosenwasser as co-editor-in-chief, we have just started the new *WAO Journal* (electronic only), where the global representation in allergy research and education will be reflected on a continuous basis.

Finally, Springer, the publisher, has to be congratulated on their courage and enthusiasm with which they have launched this endeavor. Springer has a lot of experience in allergy—I think back to the series *New Trends in Allergy*, started in 1985, as well as to my own book *Allergy in Practice,* to the *Handbook of Atopic Eczema* and many other excellent publications.

I wish this book and the whole series of *Allergy Frontiers* complete success! It should be on the shelves of every physician or researcher who is interested in allergy, clinical immunology, or related fields.

Johannes Ring, M.D., Ph.D.

Preface

Allergic diseases are increasing in prevalence worldwide, in industrialized as well as industrializing countries, affecting from 10%–50% of the global population with a marked impact on the quality of life of patients and with substantial costs. Thus, allergy can be rightfully considered an epidemic of the twenty-first century, a global public health problem, and a socioeconomic burden. With the projected increase in the world's population, especially in the rapidly growing economies, it is predicted to worsen as this century moves forward.

Allergies are also becoming more complex. Patients frequently have multiple allergic disorders that involve multiple allergens and a combination of organs through which allergic diseases manifest. Thus exposure to aeroallergens or ingested allergens frequently gives rise to a combination of upper and lower airways disease, whereas direct contact or ingestion leads to atopic dermatitis with or without food allergy. Food allergy, allergic drug responses and anaphylaxis are often severe and can be life-threatening. However, even the less severe allergic diseases can have a major adverse effect on the health of hundreds of millions of patients and diminish quality of life and work productivity. The need of the hour to combat these issues is to promote a better understanding of the science of allergy and clinical immunology through research, training and dissemination of information and evidence-based better practice parameters.

Allergy Frontiers is a comprehensive series comprising six volumes, with each volume dedicated to a specific aspect of allergic disease to reflect the multidisciplinary character of the field and to capture the explosive growth of this specialty. The series summarizes the latest information about allergic diseases, ranging from epidemiology to the mechanisms and environmental and genetic factors that influence the development of allergy; clinical aspects of allergic diseases; recent therapeutic and preventive strategies; and future perspectives. The chapters of individual volumes in the series highlight the roles of eosinophils, mast cells, lymphocytes, dendritic cells, epithelial cells, neutrophils and T cells, adhesion molecules, and cytokines/chemokines in the pathomechanisms of allergic diseases. Some specific new features are the impact of infection and innate immunity on allergy, and mucosal immunology of the various target organs and allergies, and the impact of the nervous system on allergies. The most recent, emerging therapeutic strategies are discussed, including allergen-specific immunotherapy and anti-IgE treatment, while also covering future perspectives from immunostimulatory DNA-based therapies to probiotics and nanomedicine.

A unique feature of the series is that a single topic is addressed by multiple contributors from various fields and regions of the world, giving the reader the advantage of being introduced to more than one point of view and being provided with comprehensive knowledge about a single disease. The reader thus obtains a detailed review of a single, highly focused topic and at the same time has access to a panoramic, in-depth view of a broader subject such as asthma.

The chapters attest to the multidisciplinary character of component parts of the series: environmental, genetics, molecular, and cellular biology; allergy; otolaryngology; pulmonology; dermatology; and others. Representing a collection of state-of-the-art reviews by world-renowned scientists from the United Kingdom and other parts of Europe, North America, South America, Australia, Japan, and South Africa, the volumes in this comprehensive, up-to-date series contain more than 150 chapters covering virtually all aspects of basic and clinical allergy. The publication of this extensive collection of reviews is being brought out within a span of two years and with the greatest precision to keep it as updated as possible. This six-volume series will be followed up by yearly updates on the cutting-edge advances in any specific aspect of allergy.

The editors would like to sincerely thank all the authors for having agreed to contribute and who, despite their busy schedules, contributed to this monumental work. We also thank the editorial staff of Springer Japan for their assistance in the preparation of this series. We hope that the series will serve as a valuable information tool for scientists and as a practical guide for clinicians and residents working and/or interested in the field of allergy, asthma, and immunology.

Ruby Pawankar, Stephen Holgate, and Lanny Rosenwasser

Contents

Contributors

Eitan Amir
Department of Medical Oncology, Christie Hospital NHS Trust,
Manchester, M20 4BX, UK

Paraya Assanasen
The Department of Otorhinolaryngology, Faculty of Medicine, Siriraj Hospital,
Mahidol University, Bangkok, Thailand

James N. Baraniuk
Division of Rheumatology, Immunology and Allergy, Georgetown University,
Washington DC, USA

Stephan C. Bischoff
Department of Nutritional Medicine and Immunology, University of Hohenheim,
Stuttgart, Germany

Sergio Bonini
II University of Naples and Institute of Neurobiology and Molecular Medicine,
National Research Council (INMM-CNR), Rome, Italy

Stefano Bonini
Department of Ophthalmology, University of Rome "Campus Bio-Medico",
Via Alvaro del Portillo, 21 - 00128 Rome, Italy

Christopher Brightling
Institute for Lung Health, Department of Infection, Inflammation and Immunity,
University of Leicester, Leicester, UK

Robert K. Bush
Professor, Department of Medicine, Section of Allergy/Immunology,
Pulmonary and Critical Care Medicine, University of Wisconsin, Madison,
WI, USA; Chief of Allergy, Wm. S. Middleton VA Hospital, Madison, WI, USA;
K4/910 CSC, Box 9988, 600 Highland Avenue, Madison, WI 53792, USA

Lawrence Du Buske
Brigham and Women's Hospital, Harvard Medical School, 75 Francis Street,
Boston, MA 02115, USA

Kai-Håkon Carlsen
Voksentoppen, Ullveien 14, NO 0791 Oslo, Norway

Thomas B. Casale
Professor, Department of Medicine, Chief, Allergy/Immunology,
Creighton University, Division of Allergy/Immunology Suite 5850, Omaha,
NE 68131, USA

Kazuyuki Chibana
Division of Pulmonary, Allergy and Critical Care Medicine, University of
Pittsburgh, Pittsburgh, PA, USA

Diana S. Church
Infection, Inflammation and Repair Research Division, School of Medicine,
University of Southampton, UK

Martin K. Church
Infection, Inflammation and Repair Research Division, School of Medicine,
University of Southampton, UK;
South Block 825, Southampton General Hospital, Southampton, SO16 6YD, UK

Marco Coassin
Department of Ophthalmology, University of Rome "Campus Bio-Medico",
Via Alvaro del Portillo, 21 - 00128 Rome, Italy

Lauren Cohn
Section of Pulmonary and Critical Care Medicine, Yale University School of
Medicine, PO Box 208057, New Haven, CT 06520, USA

Chris Corrigan
Professor of Asthma, Allergy and Respiratory Science, King's College London
School of Medicine, Department of Asthma, Allergy and Respiratory Science
and MRC and Asthma UK Centre for Allergic Mechanisms of Asthma,
5th Floor, Tower Wing, Guy's Hospital, London, SE1 9RT, UK

James H. Day
Professor and Head, Division of Allergy and Immunology, Department of
Medicine, Queen's University, Kingston, ON, Canada

Pascal Demoly
Exploration des Allergies – Maladies Respiratoires et INSERM, Hôpital Arnaud
de Villeneuve, University Hospital of Montpellier, 34295 Montpellier, France

Anne K. Ellis
Assistant Professor, Division of Allergy and Immunology, Department
of Medicine and Department of Microbiology and Immunology, Queen's
University Kingston, ON Canada

Eugenia Galdi
Allergy and Immunology Unit, Fondazione "Salvatore Maugeri",
Institute of Research and Care, Scientific Institute of Pavia, Italy

Deborah A. Gentile
Allegheny General Hospital, Division of Allergy, Asthma and Immunology,
Pittsburgh, PA, USA

Tari Haahtela
Professor of Clinical Allergology, Skin and Allergy Hospital,
Helsinki University Central Hospital, PO Box 160, 00029 HUS, Finland

Daniel L. Hamilos
Massachusetts General Hospital and Harvard Medical School, Boston,
Massachusetts, USA

Peter J. Helms
Department of Child Health, University of Aberdeen, Royal Aberdeen
Children's Hospital, Aberdeen, AB25 2ZG, UK

Fay Hollins
Institute for Lung Health, Department of Infection, Inflammation and Immunity,
University of Leicester, Leicester, UK

Pramod S. Kelkar
Allergy and Asthma Care, PA, 12000 Elm Creek Blvd, #200, Maple Grove,
MN 55369, USA

Kevin J. Kelly
Joyce C. Hall Distinguished Professor of Pediatrics, Chairman – Department
of Pediatrics, Children's Mercy Hospitals & Clinics, Associate Dean – University
of Missouri Kansas City School of Medicine, Kansas City, Missouri

Brian T. Kelly
University of Missouri, Kansas City School of Medicine, Kansas City, Missouri

Stephen F. Kemp
Division of Clinical Immunology and Allergy, Department of Medicine,
The University of Mississippi Medical Center, Jackson, MS 39216, USA

Alan P. Knutsen
Pediatrics Research Institute, St. Louis University Health Sciences,
3662 Park Avenue, St. Louis, MO 63110, USA

Krzysztof Kowal
Medical University of Bialystok, Sklodowskiej-Curie 24a, 15-276 Bialystok,
Poland

Viswanath P. Kurup
Department of Pediatrics, Medical College of Wisconsin, Asthma and Allergy
Center, 9000 West Wisconsin Avenue, Suite 408, Milwaukee, WI 53226, USA

Richard F. Lockey
Division of Allergy and Immunology, Department of Internal Medicine,
University of South Florida College of Medicine and The James A. Haley
Veterans Administration Hospital, 13000 Bruce B. Downs Blvd. (111D),
Tampa, FL 33612, USA

James I. McGill
Infection, Inflammation and Repair Research Division, School of Medicine,
University of Southampton, UK

Samantha Jean Merck
Division of Rheumatology, Immunology and Allergy, Georgetown University,
Washington DC, USA

Gianna Moscato
Allergy and Immunology Unit, Fondazione "Salvatore Maugeri",
Institute of Research and Care, Scientific Institute of Pavia, Italy

Robert M. Naclerio
The Section of Otolaryngology-Head and Neck Surgery, The Pritzker School
of Medicine, The University of Chicago, 5841 S. Maryland Ave., MC 1035,
Chicago, IL 60637, USA

Ewa Nizankowska-Mogilnicka
Department of Medicine, Jagiellonian University School of Medicine,
Krakow, Poland

Nikolaos G. Papadopoulos
Allergy Research Center, 2nd Pediatric Clinic, University of Athens, Greece

Ruby Pawankar
Nippon Medical School, 1-1-5, Sendagi, Bunkyo-ku, Tokyo, Japan

César Picado
Department of Pneumology and Respiratory Allergy Hospital Clinic,
University of Barcelona, Villarroel 170, 08036, Barcelona, Spain

Werner J. Pichler
Division of Allergology, Clinic for Rheumatology and Clinical Immunology/
Allergology, Inselspital, University of Bern, CH-3010, Bern, Switzerland

Antonino Romano
Unità di Allergologia, Complesso Integrato Columbus, via G. Moscati,
31, I-00168 Rome, Italy;
IRCCS Oasi Maria S.S., Troina, Italy

Marek Sanak
Department of Medicine, Jagiellonian University School of Medicine,
Krakow, Poland

Glenis K. Scadding
Consultant Allergist and Rhinologist, Royal National TNE Hospital, London, UK

Christine A. Schad
Allegheny General Hospital, Division of Allergy, Asthma and Immunology,
Pittsburgh, PA, USA

Timothy J. Schaffner
Allegheny General Hospital, Division of Allergy, Asthma and Immunology,
Pittsburgh, PA, USA

Roberto Sgrulletta
Department of Ophthalmology, University of Rome "Campus Bio-Medico",
Via Alvaro del Portillo, 21 - 00128 Rome, Italy

Salman Siddiqui
Institute for Lung Health, Department of Infection, Inflammation and Immunity,
University of Leicester, Leicester, UK

David P. Skoner
Allegheny General Hospital, Division of Allergy, Asthma and Immunology,
Pittsburgh, PA, USA

Jeffrey R. Stokes
Associate Professor Department of Medicine, Program Director Allergy/
Immunology, Creighton University, Division of Allergy/Immunology,
Suite 5850, Omaha, NE 68131, USA

Andrzej Szczeklik
Department of Medicine, Jagiellonian University School of Medicine,
Krakow, Poland

Michael S. Tankersley
Department of Allergy/Immunology, Wilford Hall Medical Center,
59th MDOS/SGO5A, 2200 Bergquist Dr. Ste 1, Lackland AFB, TX 78236, USA

Ioanna M. Velissariou
Allergy Research Center, 2nd Pediatric Clinic, University of Athens, Greece

Jean-Baptiste Watelet
Department of Otorhinolaryngology and Head and Neck Surgery,
Ghent University Hospital, Belgium

Sally Wenzel
Division of Pulmonary, Allergy and Critical Care Medicine,
University of Pittsburgh, Pittsburgh, PA, USA

Kevin M. White
Department of Allergy/Immunology, Wilford Hall Medical Center,
59th MDOS/SGO5A, 2200 Bergquist Dr. Ste 1, Lackland AFB, TX 78236, USA

Peter J. Whorwell
Whorwell, University Hospitals of South Manchester, Education and Research Centre, Wythenshawe Hospital, Wythenshawe, Manchester, M23 9LT, UK

Paraskevi Xepapadaki
Allergy Research Center, 2nd Pediatric Clinic, University of Athens, Greece

Anna Zawodniak
Division of Allergology, Clinic for Rheumatology and Clinical Immunology/ Allergology, Inselspital, University of Bern, CH-3010, Bern, Switzerland

Allergic Rhinitis and Conjunctivitis: Update on Pathophysiology

Jean-Baptiste Watelet, James I. McGill, Ruby Pawankar,
Diana S. Church, and Martin K. Church

Introduction

Our understanding on the development and mechanism(s) of allergic diseases has changed dramatically over the last 20 years. In their review of the genetic and immunological basis of atopic responses in 1987 [1] Blumenthal and Amos wrote: "The genetic control of asthma is complex. The evidence suggests a gene or genes associated with and linked to the human leukocyte antigen system (HLA). The disease phenotype may also be regulated by genetically determined levels of IgE and the outcome of the balance between immune response and immunosuppression". The view that all allergic diseases could be explained by genetic predisposition of the immune system to produce specific IgE antibodies to common environmental allergens gave rise to a linear model of the progression of allergic diseases. This paradigm became known as the 'allergic march' [2] in which there is a common progression from atopic dermatitis to allergic asthma. This theory was supported by the publication of a clinical trial using the antihistamine, cetirizine, in infants aged 1–2 years who suffered from atopic dermatitis. The results indicated that 2 years treatment with cetirizine halved the number of children developing asthma in the groups who were sensitised to grass pollen or house dust mite [3]. Following this publication, it was suggested that many drugs available for the treatment of atopic disease have properties which might render them valuable in inhibiting the progression of the allergic march [4].

However, with the advent of genetic studies it has now become clear the linear model as defined by the allergic march is no longer tenable. Instead, we must consider all allergies as complex multi-compartment models in which we must consider not only genes which control IgE production but also genes which govern

J.B. Watelet
Department of Otorhinolaryngology and Head and Neck Surgery, Ghent University Hospital, Belgium

J.I. McGill, D.S. Church, and M.K. Church (✉)
Infection, Inflammation and Repair Research Division, South Block 825, Southampton General Hospital, Southampton SO16 6YD, UK
e-mail: mkc@soton.ac.uk

R. Pawankar
Nippon Medical School, 1-1-5, Sendagi, Bunkyo-ku, Tokyo, Japan

R. Pawankar et al. (eds.), *Allergy Frontiers: Clinical Manifestations*,
DOI: 10.1007/978-4-431-88317-3_1, © Springer 2009

other aspects of allergic disease. For example, adequate inhibition of the activity of serine proteases, both endogenous and exogenous, is necessary for maintenance of the integrity of the epithelium in allergy. Such an inhibitor is the lympho-epithelial Kazaltype-related inhibitor (LEKTI) encoded by the SPINK5 gene encodes [5]. Polymorphisms in this gene which lead to defective protein expression have been associated with both asthma and atopic dermatitis [5–7]. Another example is that of the DPP10 gene which encodes a member of the dipeptidyl peptidase family of proteins. Deficiency of these peptidases, which cleave the C-terminal portions of many pro-inflammatory cytokines, chemokines and leukotrienes, have been associated with asthma [8, 9]. The third example is that of ADAM33, a gene which is associated with remodelling of the lung in asthma [10]. This gene, which is restricted to mesenchymal cells where it is involved with the structural airway components, particularly causing smooth muscle hypertrophy, is associated with bronchial hyper-responsiveness and an accelerated decline in lung function [11, 12].

One of the factors in allergy that is still largely unanswered is why all individuals who are atopic i.e. have raised immunoglobulin E (IgE) levels and positive skin test reactions to one or more common allergens, do not express overt allergic disease. Even if they do so, this may be seen at one site and not another. In this context, the prevalence of atopy in the UK is around 40% and yet the prevalence of rhino-conjunctivitis and atopic eczema is only around 20% [13, 14].

Before focusing on their pathophysiology, it is pertinent to look briefly at the clinical presentation and epidemiology of allergic conjunctivitis and allergic rhinitis and ask whether they are separate conditions or different manifestations of the same condition as all allergies were originally considered to be in the past.

Allergic conjunctivitis comprises a family of conditions increasing in severity from seasonal allergic conjunctivitis (SAC) and perennial allergic conjunctivitis (PKC) to vernal keratoconjunctivitis (VKC) and atopic keratoconjunctivitis (AKC). The milder and the most common forms, seasonal and perennial allergic conjunctivitis, have symptoms of itch, tearing, mucus discharge and redness, which, while irritating, are not sight-threatening. In contrast, vernal keratoconjunctivitis and atopic keratoconjunctivitis have more severe signs and symptoms which may result in ocular morbidity and even sight loss [15].

In allergic rhinitis, patients present with nasal irritation, sneezing, rhinorrhoea, and nasal blockage, which may be either intermittent or persistent. There is usually a clear relationship with exposure to known allergens, most frequently pollens in intermittent allergic rhinitis and house dust mite or household pets in persistent allergic rhinitis. Even though the severe allergic rhinitis may cause significant morbidity, there are no reports of permanent damage to the nose resulting from it. Several reviews have considered the possibility of permanent tissue changes in nasal mucosa in patients with rhinitis [16]. A wide variety of histomorphological features have been reported to occur in all types of chronic inflammation of the upper airways: epithelial shedding or metaplasia, thickening of basement membrane, collagen deposition in the lamina propria. For many years, they were considered as technical artefacts in tissue sampling or preparation, but more recently more data have become available and analogies have been made with tissue remodelling in the lower respiratory tract [17]. However, the observed tissue changes in the nose are less extensive than those reported in asthma and none appear to be specific for allergic rhinitis (see section on tissue remodelling).

Epidemiological evidence indicates that allergic rhinitis and allergic conjunctivitis are not always co-expressed and have a different prevalence. In a recent study in adults [18] the prevalence of allergic rhinitis was found to be 44% while that of allergic conjunctivitis was only 16% while in a group of Danish children aged 5–15 years diagnosed with allergic rhinitis, only 30% had concomitant allergic conjunctivitis [19]. The difference in the prevalence of the two diseases suggests that there may be differences in their pathophysiology. To explore these possible differences between allergic conjunctivitis and allergic rhinitis we will review their pathophysiology by asking four main questions:

1. Is there any evidence of an abnormality in the conjunctival or nasal mucosa, which would allow increased allergen penetration?
2. What is known about the immunology of sensitisation in allergic conjunctivitis and allergic rhinitis?
3. What is the pattern of mediator release in the immediate allergic response and the development of allergic inflammation in allergic conjunctivitis and allergic rhinitis?
4. Is there any evidence for clinically relevant persistent inflammation or organ remodelling in allergic conjunctivitis and allergic rhinitis?

1. Is there any evidence of an abnormality in the conjunctival or nasal mucosa, which would allow increased allergen penetration?

The integrity of the epithelial barrier is paramount in defending the underlying tissues from both physical and chemical insults. Epithelial barrier function depends upon the integrity of the epithelium, which depends on epithelial cell adhesion, mediated by junctional and non-junctional cell adhesion molecules, and the cell cytoskeleton. The structural adhesion molecules are essential for the dynamic adhesion and interaction of epithelial cells, and changes in their expression or function may result in cell malfunction and, consequently, in altered epithelial permeability. In allergy, a reduction in the epithelial integrity of mucosal surfaces would allow allergen to penetrate more easily and activate the underlying mast cells, which store, manufacture and release the factors responsible for initiating the allergic cascade. Many of the major allergens contain both cysteine and serine proteases and are, therefore, capable of taking advantage of a weakened epithelial barrier. The major allergen of *Dermatophagoides pteronyssinus, Der p 1*, is able to increase epithelial permeability [20, 21] by proteolytic cleavage of occludin, therefore disrupting tight junctions, cleaving intercellular adhesion molecules [21–25] and causing structural damage to the epithelium [14, 16, 24, 26]. A normal mucosal epithelium would act as a protective barrier to these allergens making it difficult for them to penetrate. Thus, it is possible that in allergic disease the epithelium is weak thus allowing easier allergen penetration. There are precedents for this hypothesis in the skin where individuals genetically predisposed to atopic dermatitis have demonstrable epidermal barrier dysfunction [6, 27–29], in the intestine in ulcerative colitis [30] and Crohn's disease [31] and in the lung in asthma [32].

Allergic Conjunctivitis

In order to investigate possible abnormalities in the conjunctival epithelium, we have examined sections of conjunctival biopsies from SAC patients, whose seasonal symptoms correlate with environmental increases in grass pollens or other aeroallergens, indicating that their disease is allergen driven [33]. Out of season there are no symptoms and clinically the conjunctiva looks normal [34]. This seasonal nature makes it an ideal condition to compare epithelial biopsies from individuals with SAC not currently exposed ("out of season") with biopsies from "normal" non-atopic individuals and SAC patients currently exposed to allergen ("in season"). Bulbar conjunctival were processed into glycol methacrylate and sections of $2\,\mu m$ thickness cut for immunocytochemical and image analysis of the structural proteins of the epithelium [34].

E-cadherin and CD44 were selected as examples of inter-cellular adhesion molecules because of their known involvement in epithelial structure and repair. Normal expression and functional activity of E-cadherin are critical for the maintenance of tight junctions and normal epithelial barrier function [35], whilst CD44 is a widely distributed multi-functional trans-membrane protein involved in epithelial repair [36]. Its affinity for hyaluronic acid facilitates its role in cell–cell and cell–matrix adhesion [37]. The results showed that the area of immuno-staining for E-cadherin in biopsies from SAC patients "out of season" of $1.9 \pm 0.8\%$ of the epithelial area was significantly ($P < 0.0001$) lower than the $30.9 \pm 2.4\%$ observed in normal conjunctiva. Similarly, the area of immuno-staining for CD44 in biopsies from SAC patients "out of season" of $1.7 \pm 0.6\%$ was significantly lower ($P < 0.0001$) than the $29.3 \pm 4.1\%$ in normal conjunctiva [33] (Figs. 1 and 2).

Desmosomes are highly organized intercellular junctions that provide mechanical integrity to tissues by anchoring intermediate filaments to sites of strong adhesion. In patients with asthma or allergy, the relative length of columnar cell or basal cell desmosomes in nasal polyps is reduced compared with non-allergic, non-asthmatic patients. This has lead to the suggestion that there is a weakness in the desmosomes in asthma and allergic disease where epithelial shedding may play an important role in the pathophysiological process [38, 39]. Also, in atopic dermatitis, skin barrier function is compromised by the proteolytic degradation of corneodesmosomes joining the corneocytes together [29]. The median area of the epithelium showing immuno-staining for desmosomal proteins in biopsies from SAC patients "out of season" was less than 1% compared with 18% in the conjunctiva of normal individuals [33].

This study also found a loss of conjunctival epithelial intermediate filament proteins in SAC patients "out of season", expression of keratins K5/6, K7, K8, K13, K14, K18 and Pan K all being reduced compared with normal conjunctiva [33]. Keratin pairs expressed in epithelial cells are adapted to the structural and functional requirements of the epithelium. For example, keratins K1, K2, K3, K6, K9 and K17 are found in stratified epithelium, K14 and K9 in the basal cells of non-keratinizing stratified epithelium of mucosal surfaces, while K4 and K13 are markers of differentiating supra-basal cells [40]. The conjunctival epithelium contains K4, K5, K13, K14,

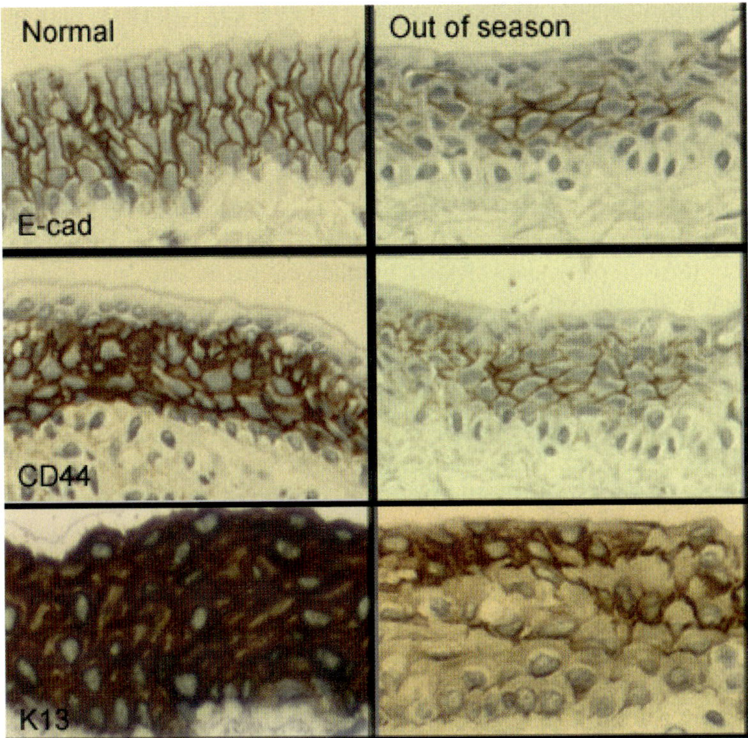

Fig. 1 Micrographs of sections of conjunctival epithelium demonstrating that the epithelium in SAC "out of season" is intact with no visible damage but has reduced expression of E-cadherin CD-44 and cytokeratin 13 compared with normal

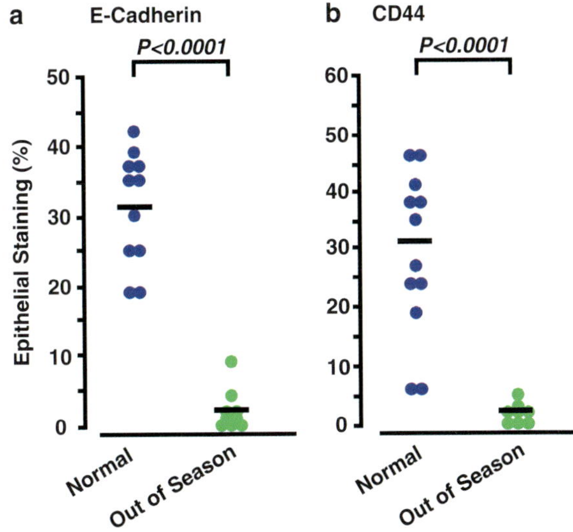

Fig. 2 The expression of E-cadherin and CD44 immunoreactivity in the conjunctival epithelium of SAC patients "out of season" and normal controls. Bars indicate mean values

K15, and K19, with little expression of K6, K10, K12, K16 or K17 [41–43]. Because these keratin intermediate filaments give strong mechanical support to the epithelium and help cells to retain their shape even under repeated episodes of stress [44], their loss of expression is likely to lead to an altered conjunctival epithelium barrier function and reduce the ability of the epithelium to resist allergen penetration.

The observation that proteinase-activated receptors-2 (PAR-2) is increased in the respiratory epithelium of patients with asthma [45] stimulated us to examine its distribution in the conjunctival epithelium. Activation of proteinase-activated receptors (PARs), particularly PAR-2 by allergen-derived enzymes may also be important in the epithelial response to allergen. PARs are a family of G protein-coupled receptors (GPCRs) which are widely distributed in the mammalian body, playing a variety of physiological and pathophysiological roles. They are members of the Gq/11 family of GPCRs, stimulation of which leads to the activation of the phospholipase Cβ and the consequential rise of intracellular calcium [46]. PAR-2, is of particular interest in allergy as it may be activated by both house dust mite derived proteinases and mast cell tryptase [47–49].

PAR-2 is considered to have primarily pro-inflammatory effects. In the epithelium, PAR-2 opens tight junctions, causes desquamation and produces cytokines, chemokines and growth factors. In addition it also promotes maturation, proliferation of fibroblasts in many tissues, including the conjunctiva [50, 51]. In the airways, they have been suggested to promote allergic inflammation by stimulating the release of GM-CSF from epithelial cells, a cytokine which promotes eosinophil survival and activation [52]. Its ability to stimulate neurons suggests its involvement in neurogenic inflammation and pain [49]. PAR-2 may also have anti-allergic and anti-inflammatory properties. In bronchial epithelial cells, it stimulates the release of the bronchodilator prostanoid, PGE_2 [46] while in sensitized rabbits, it increases the production of the anti-inflammatory cytokine, IL-10 [53].

To determine whether PAR-2 was expressed in the conjunctival epithelium and whether this expression was altered in seasonal allergic conjunct, sections were stained with a polyclonal antibody to PAR-2 (kindly supplied by MD Hollenberg [54]). In SAC "in season", the area of immunostaining for PAR-2 was 53.0 ± 4.1%, not significantly different from the 56.5 ± 3.3% seen in normal conjunctiva (P = 0.521). However, in SAC "out of season" the area of immunostaining for PAR-2 was only 8.8 ± 1.2%, significantly (P < 0.0001) lower than that seen in normal conjunctiva. Similar results were obtained using a monoclonal antibody, P2A, to PAR-2 (kindly supplied by A. Walls [55]), the correlation between the two antibodies being highly significant (P < 0.0001).

Allergic Rhinitis

Even in cases of no light microscopic evidence of epithelial disruption in perennial allergic rhinitis, electron microscopy reveals two characteristic features of epithelial damage in these patients in comparison with healthy controls, namely the presence of cytoplasmic vacuoles in the epithelial cells and a marked widening of the intercellular spaces at this site, both consistent with structural airway epithelial abnormalities and disease expression [56].

PARs are widely expressed in several tissues and involved in rhinitis and asthma [50, 56]. Strong immunoreactivity for messenger RNA and PAR-2 protein has been found in nasal mucosa of patients with allergic rhinitis as compared with normal nasal mucosa [57]. The increased expression of PAR 2 in epithelial cells and the increased number of eosinophils with PAR-2 suggest that this receptor could be a pivotal factor for sustaining nasal allergic inflammation [58]. Finally, in animal models, activation of PAR-2 receptor in trigeminal sensory neurons by trypsin and mast cell tryptase can trigger tachykinin-mediated phenomena such neurogenic inflammation in allergic and non-allergic rhinitis [59].

Recently, it has been suggested that the greater epithelial exfoliation between basal cells and the more superficial columnar ciliated and goblet cells should reflect a different attachment quality of these cells. No data are available about a constitutive dysregulation of desmosomes. However, it has been clearly established that cysteine proteinases from both house dust mite and pollen allergens can lead to cleavage of the tight junction adhesion protein occludin, suggesting that tight junctions may be opened by environmental proteinases [24, 60]. Cleavage of tight junctions involves proteolysis of the junction protein occludin but E-cadherin of adherence junctions is cleaved less extensively [61]. This effect can be blocked by inhibitors of serine and cysteine proteases [60].

Besides the destructive effect of exogenous proteinases, it has been shown that HLA-DR- and CD11c-positive dendritic cells can express claudin-1 and can penetrate beyond occludin in nasal epithelium of patients with but not without allergic rhinitis [62]. Finally, guinea-pig models suggest that the epithelial cell contact mediated by E-cadherin is loosened as a consequence of eosinophil infiltration [63].

Epithelial Changes

Epithelial changes are present in both allergic conjunctivitis and rhinitis, which are likely to facilitate allergen penetration. However, it would appear that they are different. For example, epithelial PAR-2 expression is elevated in allergic rhinitis but not in allergic conjunctivitis. Also, there is increasing evidence of structural changes in active allergic rhinitis, but whether these changes are a cause or a consequence of the disease is not clear.

In patients with seasonal allergic conjunctivitis, the observations that E-cadherin, CD44, desmosomes, keratins K5/6, K7, K8, K13, K14, K18 and PAR-2 are all reduced in the conjunctival epithelium of "out of season" indicates a basic epithelial abnormality in these individuals. The panel of down-regulated adhesion proteins is too large to implicate problems with individual molecules, but rather it reflects a possible underlying protease defence. A possible candidate for causing this is the SPINK5 gene, which encodes a serine protease inhibitor. Polymorphisms in this gene have been associated with allergic diseases, including allergic rhinitis [7, 64, 65].

2. What is known about the immunology of sensitisation in allergic conjunctivitis and allergic rhinitis?

During the sensitization phase of all allergic conditions, the generation of allergen specific IgE antibodies, driven by complex interactions between antigen presenting cells (APC) and T-lymphocytes, involves many mechanisms influenced by the genetic background, environmental circumstances, allergen exposure and other cofactors.

Allergic Conjunctivitis

There are few lymphoid dendritic cells in the conjunctiva of individuals who do not have allergic conjunctivitis. However, there is a large increase and change of phenotype in SAC. An analysis of the dendritic cell subsets in human and mouse conjunctiva indicates that the phenotype of these key antigen-presenting cells is unusual in the conjunctiva [66]. This is supported by the success of treating ocular allergy in murine models using IL-1 receptor antagonist and CpG oligonucleotides [67]. From these results, Ono and colleagues [66] hypothesize that the arrested activation of resident antigen-presenting cells in the conjunctiva of IL-1 receptor antagonist-treated mice inhibits the release of mast cell co-stimulatory factors thus inhibiting both mast cell activation and the late-phase response.

Another avenue of research has focused on the role of IL-10. While investigating the responsiveness of different mouse strains to ocular allergen challenge, Bundoc and Keane-Myers showed that IL-10 knockout mice were particularly sensitive to challenge, suggesting a role for regulatory T cells. From further studies they concluded that IL-10 confers protection by stabilizing mast cells against degranulation [68].

A linkage analysis in human subjects has shown that although some susceptibility loci are shared with other allergic diseases, there are unique genetic loci associated with SAC, such as the eotaxin-1 gene [66]. This is supported by observations that antagonism of CCR3, the receptor for eotaxin-1, is able to inhibit both the early phase response and late phase inflammation in the murine model of ocular allergy and neutralization of eotaxin-1 in situ by using the humanized anti-eotaxin-1 antibody (CAT-213) is able to inhibit the activation of human conjunctival mast cells [66].

Allergic Rhinitis

Dendritic cells, in the form of Langerhans' cells, are actively involved in the aetiology of allergic rhinitis, possibly playing an immunomodulatory role because of their ability to present allergen and to activate T-cells. Like lymphocytes and macrophages, Langerhans' cells have been shown to be present in large numbers in the nasal mucosa of allergic patients, when compared to non allergic patients or nasal polyp tissue [69] but also after allergen challenge [70]. Langerhans' cells are also significantly increased in numbers during pollen season [71]. In patients with grass pollen-sensitive seasonal rhinitis, significant increases in submucosal and epithelial CD1a + Langherhans' cells, but not CD68 + macrophages or CD20 + B cells have been observed during the pollen season [72]: this phenomenon is inhibited by corticosteroids. Finally, in seasonal allergic rhinitis, mononuclear phagocytes are found increased during season and after allergen challenge [73].

In genetically susceptible individuals, these antigen-presenting cells activate nasal inflammatory cells by instructing T cells to polarize into Th2 cells. Increased numbers of peripheral blood Th2 cells have been found in patients with allergic rhinitis when compared to non-allergic controls [74]. This leads also to a massive local production of IL-4, IL-5, IL-9 and IL-13 cytokines. These cytokines drive B cell switching to IgE (IL-4, IL-5), basophil/mast cell development (IL-4, IL-9), eosinophil accumulation (IL-5, IL-9), as well as mucus production (IL-9, IL-13). These target cells amplify the reaction through release of cytokines and growth factors that are acting on resident cells.

The role of T regulatory (Treg) cells has been pointed in allergic disorders including allergic rhinitis [75, 76]. Increased numbers of Treg cells have been observed in nasal biopsies from allergic rhinitis patients by some authors [77] particularly in those with persistent allergic rhinitis where they correlated with total serum IgE [78]. However, other workers have found decreased numbers [79].

Little comparative research has been performed which suggest great differences between the mechanisms of sensitisation in the eye and nose. It is known that priming of Treg within peripheral lymph nodes leads to the expression of selectin ligands, which facilitate migration into inflamed skin, while their activation within mesenteric lymph nodes leads to induction of the $\alpha_4\beta_7$ integrin, which is required for migration into mucosal tissues [80]. However, whether there are more subtle differences which allow differential migration into the eye and the nose is not yet known.

3. What is the pattern of mediator release in the immediate allergic response and the development of allergic inflammation in allergic conjunctivitis and allergic rhinitis?

The major early phase clinical manifestations of allergic conjunctivitis and rhinitis after allergen exposure are mediated through the activation of mast cells. This may be followed by an influx of neutrophils, basophils and eosinophils, the major source of cysteinyl-leukotrienes, which drive the late-phase response and initiate allergic inflammation. Cytokine generation from activated Th-2 lymphocytes further prolong allergic inflammation. Other mediators that are produced during late-phase responses include enzymes particularly matrix metallo-proteinases (MMPs) and chemokines.

Allergic Conjunctivitis

Allergen conjunctival challenge of "out of season" SAC sufferers causes the rapid development of all symptoms, viz. hyperaemia, chemosis, lacrimation and itching which are significantly increased at the first observation point at 10 min and maximal by 20–30 min [34, 81]. After this time, the symptoms reduce only partially before rising again at 6 h, the time of the late phase allergic response. In bulbar biopsies taken at 6 h after challenge, the median percentage lengths of blood vessels expressing E-selectin and ICAM-1 are greatly increased but there was no significant up-regulation of VCAM-1 at this time. A granulocytic infiltrate is also seen at this time [34].

Knowledge of both mediator levels and cell numbers allows us to formulate suggestions into the events occurring in the conjunctiva. First, the finding of histamine, tryptase and PGD_2 during the early phase response is entirely consistent with mast cell activation and degranulation, as this cell is the only one in the conjunctiva to contain large amounts of histamine and tryptase and be able to generate PGD_2. Second, the finding at 6 h of significant amounts of histamine in the absence of detectable amounts of tryptase and PGD_2 would suggest the basophil rather than the mast cell to be the source of the histamine at this time. This is supported by the influx of basophils at this time [34]. Third, no eosinophil derived eosinophil chemotactic protein (ECP) is present in the tear fluid during the early phase response, but it can be detected 6 h after challenge. This is consistent with the observation of increased numbers of eosinophils in both the epithelium and sub-epithelial tissues at this time.

While the role of mast cells in all forms of allergic disease is clear, eosinophilic inflammation only appears to be associated with the more severe forms. In a histological study by Anderson and colleagues [82], no mast cells or eosinophils were found in the conjunctival epithelium of normal subjects. Although mast cell numbers were increased, the lack of an increase in eosinophil numbers in the conjunctival lamina propria from subjects with SAC in season is consistent with the mild nature of the inflammation and the absence of sight threatening complications. The presence of large numbers of eosinophils in the lamina propria is characteristic of AKC and VKC, the migration of these cells into the epithelium and the finding of the cytotoxic eosinophil proteins in the tears of patients with VKC [83–85] strongly suggests that eosinophil recruitment and subsequent activation leads to the sight threatening damage in these conditions.

Allergic Rhinitis

The inflammatory response comprises typically of the early phase and late phase response. In the sensitized individual, upon re-exposure to allergens, crosslinking of bound IgE by allergen, mast cells degranulate to release inflammatory mediators like histamine, leukotrienes and prostaglandins. Mast cells are increased in the epithelial compartment of the nasal mucosa and can be easily activated upon re-exposure to the allergens. The late phase response is characterized by an inflammatory cellular influx composed of predominantly T lymphocytes, basophils and eosinophils. Recent studies have demonstrated the role of mast cells in the late phase response. Cytokines and chemokines like IL-4, IL-13 from T cells and mast cells [86–88] upregulate the expression of vascular cell adhesion molecule-1

(VCAM-1) on the endothelial cells facilitating the infiltration of eosinophils, T cells and basophils into the nasal mucosa. In addition, chemokines like RANTES, eotaxin, monocyte chemoattractant protein-4 and thymus and activation regulated chemokine (TARC) released from structural cells like epithelial cells serve as chemoattractants for eosinophils, basophils and T cells [89–92]. Granulocyte–macrophage colony stimulating factor (GM-CSF) released largely by epithelial cells and IL-5 from T cells and mast cells prolong the survival of the infiltrated eosinophils in the nasal mucosa [88]. Mast cells-epithelial cell interactions upregulate the production of GM-CSF, RANTES, TARC and eotaxin from nasal epithelial cells via histamine, tryptase, IL-4/IL-13 and TNF-α [89–92]. Eosinophils are major players in the late phase response releasing an array of proinflammatory mediators, such as cysteinyl leukotrienes, cationic proteins, eosinophil peroxidase, and major basic protein, as well as IL-3, IL-5, GM-CSF, and IL-13.

Nasal allergen provocation has proven to be an indispensable tool to investigate the pathophysiology of allergic rhinitis, allowing to differentiate early and late phase [86, 93] and to describe the time course of release for several inflammatory mediators [94].

After unilateral allergen challenge, an immediate and bilateral increase of histamine was demonstrated that can be assigned to a direct activation of mast cells after cross-linking of IgE by allergen [94, 95]. This is accompanied by a rapid swelling of the nasal turbinates (Fig. 3). This has been confirmed by the finding of

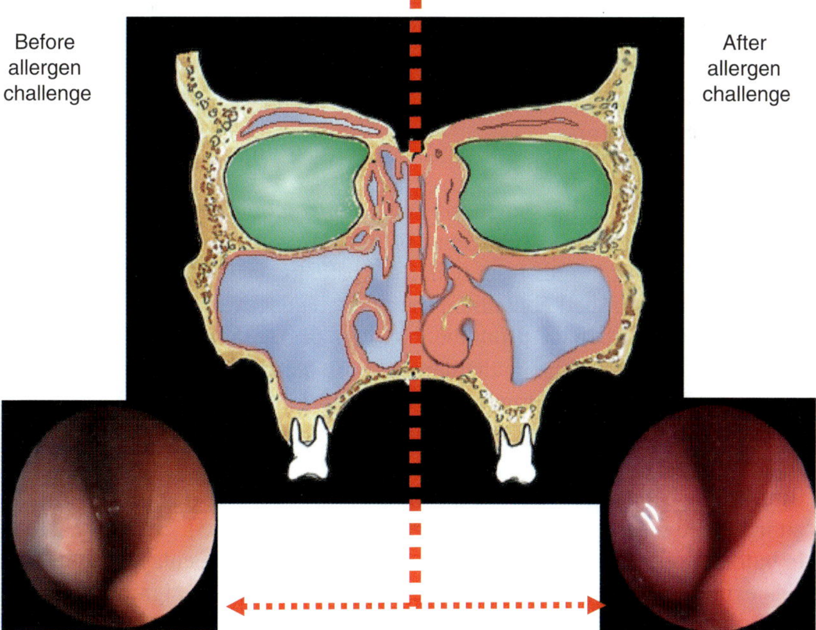

Fig. 3 The swelling of the nasal turbinates following allergen challenge

similar increases in tryptase [96, 97]. After a transient decease, histamine values rise again between 2 and 6h after allergen provocation, probably due to the activation of basophils that enter the nasal mucosa [98]. Sim and colleagues [99] found an increase of IL-1β and IL-5 in the early and late phases and a more delayed rise of GM-CSF and IL-6. IL-1Ra, a naturally occurring antagonist of IL-1β, is modestly increase after allergen provocation [98]. IL-8, produced by nasal epithelial cells and mast cells, has been found to be increased 5 min after challenge and during the late phase [100]. IL-4 release presented a peak at 5h after provocation [98].

The pattern of the early phase allergic response in the eye and nose seem similar. The primary difference appears to be the presence of an eosinophil dominated late phase response and allergic inflammation which is only present in the severe forms of allergic conjunctivitis such as AKC and VKC.

4. Is there any evidence for clinically relevant persistent inflammation or organ remodelling in allergic conjunctivitis and allergic rhinitis?

Over the past few years, the concepts of persistent inflammation and tissue remodelling have been widely discussed with relevance to allergic diseases. In asthma, there is a chronic eosinophilic infiltrate and clear structural alterations or remodelling, including epithelial fragility and thickening of the reticular basement membrane, increased airway smooth muscle mass, hypertrophy of mucus-secreting glands, increased vascularity, greater numbers of fibroblasts and increased deposition of collagen [12, 101, 102]. Persistent inflammation and tissue remodelling is also seen in the intestine in inflammatory bowel disease [103–105]. But is there any evidence for persistent inflammation or organ remodelling in allergic conjunctivitis and allergic rhinitis and, if so, is it clinically relevant?

Allergic Conjunctivitis

Patients with SAC have no symptoms and a macroscopically normal conjunctiva "out of season" when the pollen count is zero. Also, examination of 2 μm thick sections from bulbar biopsies from both SAC patients "out of season" and normals had a continuous stratified epithelium over the conjunctival surface with no areas of gross histological damage. Both the thickness of the epithelium, 46.1 ± 7.0 μm, and the mean cell area in the epithelium, 135.4 ± 6.2 μm², in SAC "out of season" were similar to those of the normal conjunctiva, 48.1 ± 3.3 μm and 133.5 ± 17.3 μm² respectively. This is in contrast to the findings in the pollen season when thickness of the epithelium, 72.6 ± 5.9 μm, and the mean cell area in the epithelium, 169.6 ± 14.0 μm², were both significantly increased. These increases were caused primarily by an increased mean cell volume rather than hyperplasia [33].

In bulbar biopsies from SAC patients, "out of season" percentage of total blood vessels expressing E-selectin, ICAM-1 and VCAM-1 was not significantly different from the percentages, 15%, 21% and 13% respectively, seen in normal controls

[106]. Also, there was a paucity of inflammatory cells, such as neutrophils, eosinophils, basophils, macrophages and CD3+, CD4+ and CD8+ T-cells [34]. Finally, SAC patients "out of season" and normal controls showed similar low levels of histamine, mast cell tryptase and eosinophil cationic protein [34, 81].

Taken together, these data strongly suggest that there is no remodelling nor persistent inflammation of the conjunctiva in SAC patients "out of season" when no symptoms are present.

Local IgE Production

IgE is the hallmark of allergic diseases. Ishizaka & Tomioka first described the presence of IgE receptors on mast cells and that these cells could be activated to degranulate upon crosslinking of the FcεRI-bound IgE with bivalent or multivalent antigen. Therefore, the expression of the high affinity IgE receptor (FcεRI) in mast cells and basophils is critical to the development of allergic diseases. The FcεRI is a tetrameric structure comprising of an α-subunit, a β subunit and two di-sulphide linked γ-subunits [28–30, 107–109] The extracellular portion of the FcεRIα chain contains the entire IgE-binding site [31, 32, 110, 111], and the β subunit is considered to be largely within the cell membrane, spanning it four times so that both the amino and carboxy termini are within the cytoplasm [33, 112]. The β and γ-subunits are known to be involved in signal transduction [34–36, 113–115]. Studies in FcεRIα chain-deficient mice have demonstrated the inability of these mice to exert allergen-induced anaphylaxis even with normal number of mast cells [37, 116]. Several lines of evidence indicate that mast cells or basophils must display the high affinity IgE receptors on their surface to be able to have significant IgE-antigen specific effector function. Mast cells in AR patients exhibit increased expression of the FcεRI. Moreover, IL-4 as well as IgE can upregulate the FcεRI expression in mast cells [20, 38, 39, 117–119]. This enhanced expression of the FcεRI in mast cells is also seen in asthmatics and is associated with increased mediator release [20, 21, 24, 117, 120, 121]. Furthermore, the FcεRI expression in NMC correlated well with the levels of serum IgE [20, 117]. These findings taken in concert with the observations of Pastorello et al. who demonstrated a strong positive correlation between the levels of serum IgE and clinical symptoms, in symptomatic patients with allergic rhinoconjunctivitis, suggest a very important role for mast cells in regulating ongoing allergic inflammation. Moreover, mast cells can induce IgE synthesis and several studies have demonstrated that local IgE synthesis occurs at sites of allergic inflammation [24, 41, 42, 121–123]. Putting together all these observations one can perceive a very important role for the mast cell in perpetuating allergic inflammation via the mast cell-IgE- FcεRI cascade [21, 120]. Such local IgE production and IgE-IgE network cascades are also relevant to allergic conjunctivitis.

Minimal Persistent Inflammation

The terminology, introduced in rhinitis in analogy to the persistent inflammation in asymptomatic asthmatic patients, refers to the evidence of mucosal inflammation despite the absence of clinical symptoms of the disease at the time inflammation. This potentially relates to the variability of the disease manifestations and to mechanisms of persistence and chronicity of inflammatory responses. As basis of this concept, a mild infiltration of eosinophils and neutrophils and the expression of ICAM-1 on nasal epithelial cells were found in rhinitis patients allergic to house dust mites in an asymptomatic period [100, 124]. The concept of minimal persistent inflammation is still actively debated in rhinitis.

Nasal Hyperresponsiveness

A hallmark of allergic rhinitis is hyperresponsiveness of symptomatic individuals to specific allergens (priming), and to nonspecific stimuli such as irritants, odors, etc.; The molecular mechanisms of hyperresponsiveness are not understood, but several inflammatory products appear to be playing a role. Activated inflammatory cells and inflammatory mediators may facilitate mucosal penetration by allergen and provide additional targets for antigen-specific stimulation. In symptomatic patients, hyperresponsiveness to nonspecific irritants may reflect interactions among inflammatory cellular influx, epithelial injury, and increased end-organ responsiveness caused by exposure to an antigen. Upregulation of the nasal nervous system can result in neural hyperresponsiveness, as well as in neurogenic inflammation. Neurotrophins, such as the nerve growth factor (NGF), are prime candidates as mediators of neural hyperresponsiveness. NGF mRNA is increased in nasal epithelium of patients with allergic rhinitis with high levels of NGF in serum and nasal fluids and this is further increased in nasal fluids after specific allergen challenge [48, 49, 125, 126]. Furthermore, mast cells in patients with allergic rhinitis express higher levels of very late antigen (VLA)-4 and 5 and mast cell–extracellular matrix interactions upregulate cytokine secretion from these cells [21, 120] suggesting that such a cascade may contribute to exacerbation of the condition.

Remodelling

A sustained inflammation and tissue remodelling is well established in the lower airways in asthma where they contribute significantly to the symptoms. However in upper airways, tissue damage seems to be more limited and overt remodelling questionable in allergic rhinitis.

Epithelial shedding is increased in the nasal passages of patients with allergic rhinitis [127], reflecting the poorer quality of attachment between the basal cells of

Fig. 4 Eosinophils in nasal mucosa (EG2 staining) From magnification ×200

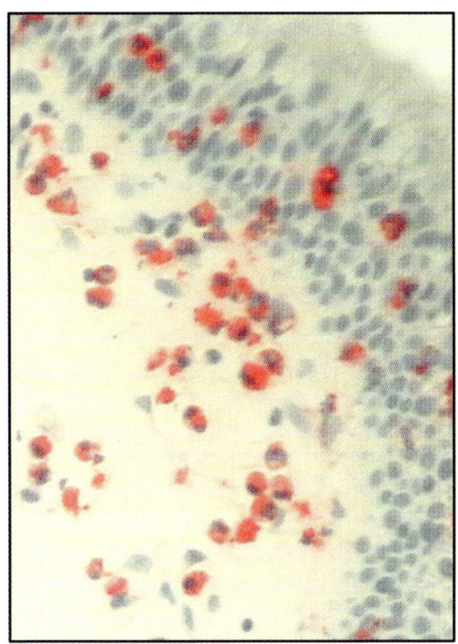

the epithelium and the basement membrane [128]. Epithelial shedding is attributed to the cytotoxic effects of inflammatory mediators such as major basic protein, eosinophilic cationic protein, eosinophil peroxidase and eosinophil peroxidase released from activated eosinophils [129]. In clinical disease occurring during the pollen season, the enhanced epithelial shedding is correlated to the clinical disease expression and the accumulation of eosinophils rather than mast cells at this site [130]. However, authors have found only a minor degree [131, 132] or no significant change in shedding or thickness of basement membrane of the nasal mucosa in individuals with perennial allergic rhinitis compared with controls [133].

In perennial rhinitis, while the number of goblet cells is unchanged in inferior turbinate [134], the number of sub-epithelial glands is increased in middle turbinate [135] and the superficial glands show compression or dilatation of acini and eosinophilic cell infiltration [136] (Fig. 4). Regarding the extracellular matrix, in comparison with non-allergic nasal mucosa, a change in the proportion of different collagens has been observed in perennial rhinitis, with increased amounts of collagen types I and III [137].

The participation of several growth factors has been explored. The participation of epidermal growth factor and its receptor has been suggested as an explanation for both the morphological changes and functional disorders such as mucus hypersecretion [138]. In addition, submucosal glands, nasal epithelium, and eosinophils constitute the major sources of nerve growth factor in nasal mucosa [139]. Finally, other factors like metalloproteinases such as MMP-9, required for eosinophil migration but also potential inductor of extracellular matrix damage, show a parallel release with ECP during the late-phase inflammatory response after nasal provocation with allergen [140, 141].

The bulk exudation of plasma into the airway tissue (vascular exudation) and lumen (mucosal exudation) occurring during allergic rhinitis is usually limited and reversible. Increased angiogenesis has also been suspected. Using staining techniques, Kirmaz and colleagues [142] demonstrated that vascular endothelial growth factor (VEGF) and CD34, already known as angiogenic markers, showed higher microvessel staining density in seasonal allergic rhinitis when compared to controls.

Other Factors

Besides tissue remodelling, other factors are suggested to influence the severity, persistence or the resolution of nasal inflammation during an allergic reaction. The effects of continuous triggering of the nasal mucosa by pathogens, irritants or outdoor pollutants are only poorly explored but more data are available about the role played by the nervous system [143]. In order to perform all its physiological functions, the nasal mucosa contains a complex nervous system including sensory, parasympathetic and sympathetic nerves. During allergen exposure, these structures are actively involved in occurrence of symptoms such as pruritus, sneezing, and mucus production. Furthermore, they are the key-players of the systemic interactions between the nose and lower respiratory tract [144]. During an allergic response, there is evidence of an exaggerated neural response and increased capacity for generation of neurogenic inflammation. Using immunohistology and computerized image analysis, nerve fibres in the epithelium, in the sub-epithelium, in the glandular and vascular regions were significantly increased in allergic rhinitis [145]. In these patients, epithelial nerve growth factor immunoreactivity is increased and nasal sensitivity is correlated with a nerve marker, protein gene product 9.5 (PGP 9.5). The nasal mucosa of patients with allergic rhinitis contains threefold higher amounts of substance P compared with that of healthy control subjects. This was seen particularly in patients with seasonal allergic rhinitis. When exposed to whole-nose provocation with capsaicin, plasma extravasation could be detected in subjects with perennial allergic rhinitis but not normals, an observation which may reflect the activity of an axonal reflex to sensorineural stimulation [146]. These factors have been suspected to influence the clinical severity of the disease.

While there is clear evidence in asthma and intestinal disease of clinically relevant structural remodelling which persists in the absence of periods of allergen challenge, there is no such evidence in either seasonal allergic conjunctivitis or allergic rhinitis "out of season" when no symptoms are present. However, there do appear to be functional changes in the nose which appear particularly during prolonged allergen exposure. Perhaps the most clinically relevant of these are the changes of sensory structure and function.

References

1. Blumenthal MN, Amos DB. Genetic and immunologic basis of atopic responses. Chest 1987;91:176S–84S.

2. Wahn U. What drives the allergic march? Allergy 2000;55:591–9.

3. ETAC Study Group. Allergic factors associated with the development of asthma and the influence of cetirizine in a double-blind, randomised, placebo-controlled trial: first results of ETAC. Early Treatment of the Atopic Child. Pediatr Allergy Immunol 1998;9:116–24.

4. Warner JO. Future aspects of pharmacological treatment to inhibit the allergic march. Pediatr Allergy Immunol 2001;12(Suppl 14):102–7.

5. Walley AJ, Chavanas S, Moffatt MF, Esnouf RM, Ubhi B, Lawrence R, et al. Gene polymorphism in Netherton and common atopic disease. Nat Genet 2001;29:175–8.

6. Kato A, Fukai K, Oiso N, Hosomi N, Murakami T, Ishii M. Association of SPINK5 gene polymorphisms with atopic dermatitis in the Japanese population. Br J Dermatol 2003;148:665–9.

7. Moffatt MF. SPINK5: a gene for atopic dermatitis and asthma. Clin Exp Allergy 2004;34:325–7.

8. Allen M, Heinzmann A, Noguchi E, Abecasis G, Broxholme J, Ponting CP, et al. Positional cloning of a novel gene influencing asthma from chromosome 2q14. Nat Genet 2003;35:258–63.

9. Lilly CM. Diversity of asthma: evolving concepts of pathophysiology and lessons from genetics. J Allergy Clin Immunol 2005;115:S526–S531.

10. Van Eerdewegh P., Little RD, Dupuis J, Del Mastro RG, Falls K, Simon J, et al. Association of the ADAM33 gene with asthma and bronchial hyperresponsiveness. Nature 25-7-2002;418:426–30.

11. Holgate ST, Yang Y, Haitchi HM, Powell RM, Holloway JW, Yoshisue H, et al. The genetics of asthma: ADAM33 as an example of a susceptibility gene. Proc Am Thorac Soc 2006;3:440–3.

12. Holgate ST, Davies DE, Powell RM, Howarth PH, Haitchi HM, Holloway JW. Local genetic and environmental factors in asthma disease pathogenesis: chronicity and persistence mechanisms. Eur Respir J 2007;29:793–803.

13. Cullinan P, Harris JM, Newman Taylor AJ, Jones M, Taylor P, Dave JR, et al. Can early infection explain the sibling effect in adult atopy? Eur Respir J 2003;22:956–61.

14. Arshad SH, Bateman B, Matthews SM. Primary prevention of asthma and atopy during childhood by allergen avoidance in infancy: a randomised controlled study. Thorax 2003;58:489–93.

15. McGill JI, Holgate ST, Church MK, Anderson DF, Bacon A. Allergic eye disease mechanisms. Br J Ophthalmol 1998;82:1203–14.

16. Salib RJ, Howarth PH. Remodelling of the upper airways in allergic rhinitis: is it a feature of the disease? Clin Exp Allergy 2003;33:1629–33.

17. Watelet JB, Van ZT, Gjomarkaj M, Canonica GW, Dahlen SE, Fokkens W, et al. Tissue remodelling in upper airways: where is the link with lower airway remodeling? Allergy 2006;61:1249–58.

18. Senol M, Ozcan A, Kandi B, Karaca S, Aki T, Bayram N. Incidence of atopic stigmata and prick test results in patients with asthma, allergic rhinitis and conjunctivitis. Asian Pac J Allergy Immunol 2006;24:105–9.

19. Gradman J, Wolthers OD. Allergic conjunctivitis in children with asthma, rhinitis and eczema in a secondary outpatient clinic. Pediatr Allergy Immunol 2006;17:524–6.

20. Herbert CA, Holgate ST, Robinson C, Thompson PJ, Stewart GA. Effect of mite allergen on permeability of bronchial mucosa. Lancet 3-11-1990;336:1132.

21. Herbert CA, King CM, Ring PC, Holgate ST, Stewart GA, Thompson PJ, et al. Augmentation of permeability in the bronchial epithelium by the house dust mite allergen Der p1. Am J Respir Cell Mol Biol 1995;12:369–78.

22. Stewart GA, Lake FR, Thompson PJ. Faecally derived hydrolytic enzymes from Dermatophagoides pteronyssinus: physicochemical characterisation of potential allergens. Int Arch Allergy Appl Immunol 1991;95:248–56.

23. Petersen A, Grobe K, Schramm G, Vieths S, Altmann F, Schlaak M, et al. Implications of the grass group I allergens on the sensitization and provocation process. Int Arch Allergy Immunol 1999;118:411–3.

24. Wan H, Winton HL, Soeller C, Tovey ER, Gruenert DC, Thompson PJ, et al. Der p 1 facilitates transepithelial allergen delivery by disruption of tight junctions. J Clin Invest 1999;104:123–33.
25. Widmer F, Hayes PJ, Whittaker RG, Kumar RK. Substrate preference profiles of proteases released by allergenic pollens. Clin Exp Allergy 2000;30:571–6.
26. Robinson C, Baker SF, Garrod DR. Peptidase allergens, occludin and claudins. Do their interactions facilitate the development of hypersensitivity reactions at mucosal surfaces? Clin Exp Allergy 2001;31:186–92.
27. Palmer CN, Irvine AD, Terron-Kwiatkowski A, Zhao Y, Liao H, Lee SP, et al. Common loss-of-function variants of the epidermal barrier protein filaggrin are a major predisposing factor for atopic dermatitis. Nat Genet 2006;38:441–6.
28. Weidinger S, Illig T, Baurecht H, Irvine AD, Rodriguez E, az-Lacava A, et al. Loss-of-function variations within the filaggrin gene predispose for atopic dermatitis with allergic sensitizations. J Allergy Clin Immunol 2006;118:214–9.
29. Cork MJ, Robinson DA, Vasilopoulos Y, Ferguson A, Moustafa M, MacGowan A, et al. New perspectives on epidermal barrier dysfunction in atopic dermatitis: gene-environment interactions. J Allergy Clin Immunol 2006;118:3–21.
30. Heller F, Florian P, Bojarski C, Richter J, Christ M, Hillenbrand B, et al. Interleukin-13 is the key effector Th2 cytokine in ulcerative colitis that affects epithelial tight junctions, apoptosis, and cell restitution. Gastroenterology 2005;129:550–64.
31. Zeissig S, Burgel N, Gunzel D, Richter J, Mankertz J, Wahnschaffe U, et al. Changes in expression and distribution of claudin 2, 5 and 8 lead to discontinuous tight junctions and barrier dysfunction in active Crohn's disease. Gut 2007;56:61–72.
32. Xaio C, Bedke M, Holgate ST, Davies DE, Puddicombe SM. Bronchial epithelial barrier integrity is altered in asthma but not normal subjects, independent of atopy. Am J Respir Crit Care Med. ATS Abstracts, San Francisco Meeting, A886. 2007. Ref Type: Abstract.
33. Hughes JL, Lackie PM, Wilson SJ, Church MK, McGill JI. Reduced structural proteins in the conjunctival epithelium in allergic eye disease. Allergy 2006;61:1268–74.
34. Bacon AS, Ahluwalia P, Irani AM, Schwartz LB, Holgate ST, Church MK, et al. Tear and conjunctival changes during the allergen-induced early- and late-phase responses. J Allergy Clin Immunol 2000;106:948–54.
35. Alattia JR, Tong KI, Takeichi M, Ikura M. Cadherins. Methods Mol Biol 2002;172:199–21.
36. Leir SH, Baker JE, Holgate ST, Lackie PM. Increased CD44 expression in human bronchial epithelial repair after damage or plating at low cell densities. Am J Physiol Lung Cell Mol Physiol 2000;278:L1129–L1137.
37. Miyake K, Underhill CB, Lesley J, Kincade PW. Hyaluronate can function as a cell adhesion molecule and CD44 participates in hyaluronate recognition. J Exp Med 1-7-1990;172:69–75.
38. Roche WR, Montefort S, Baker J, Holgate ST. Cell adhesion molecules and the bronchial epithelium. Am Rev Respir Dis 1993;148:S79–S82.
39. Shahana S, Jaunmuktane Z, Asplund MS, Roomans GM. Ultrastructural investigation of epithelial damage in asthmatic and non-asthmatic nasal polyps. Respir Med 2006;100:2018–28.
40. Pitz S, Moll R. Intermediate-filament expression in ocular tissue. Prog Retin Eye Res 2002;21:241–62.
41. Ryder MI, Weinreb RN. Cytokeratin patterns in corneal, limbal, and conjunctival epithelium. An immunofluorescence study with PKK-1, 8.12, 8.60, and 4.62 anticytokeratin antibodies. Invest Ophthalmol Vis Sci 1990;31:2230–4.
42. Kasper M, Moll R, Stosiek P, Karsten U. Patterns of cytokeratin and vimentin expression in the human eye. Histochemistry 1988;89:369–77.
43. Zhang M, Liu Z, Xie Y. The study on the expression of keratin proteins in pterygial epithelium. Yan Ke Xue Bao 2000;16:48–52.
44. Galou M, Gao J, Humbert J, Mericskay M, Li Z, Paulin D, et al. The importance of intermediate filaments in the adaptation of tissues to mechanical stress: evidence from gene knockout studies. Biol Cell 1997;89:85–97.

45. Knight DA, Lim S, Scaffidi AK, Roche N, Chung KF, Stewart GA, et al. Protease-activated receptors in human airways: upregulation of PAR-2 in respiratory epithelium from patients with asthma. J Allergy Clin Immunol 2001;108:797–803.
46. Kawabata A, Kawao N. Physiology and pathophysiology of proteinase-activated receptors (PARs): PARs in the respiratory system: cellular signaling and physiological/pathological roles. J Pharmacol Sci 2005;97:20–4.
47. Macfarlane SR, Seatter MJ, Kanke T, Hunter GD, Plevin R. Proteinase-activated receptors. Pharmacol Rev 2001;53:245–82.
48. Asokananthan N, Graham PT, Stewart DJ, Bakker AJ, Eidne KA, Thompson PJ, et al. House dust mite allergens induce proinflammatory cytokines from respiratory epithelial cells: the cysteine protease allergen, Der p 1, activates protease-activated receptor (PAR)-2 and inactivates PAR-1. J Immunol 15-10-2002;169:4572–8.
49. Hollenberg MD. Physiology and pathophysiology of proteinase-activated receptors (PARs): proteinases as hormone-like signal messengers: PARs and more. J Pharmacol Sci 2005;97:8–13.
50. Reed CE, Kita H. The role of protease activation of inflammation in allergic respiratory diseases. J Allergy Clin Immunol 2004;114:997–1008.
51. Asano-Kato N, Fukagawa K, Okada N, Dogru M, Tsubota K, Fujishima H. Tryptase increases proliferative activity of human conjunctival fibroblasts through protease-activated receptor-2. Invest Ophthalmol Vis Sci 2005;46:4622–6.
52. Vliagoftis H, Befus AD, Hollenberg MD, Moqbel R. Airway epithelial cells release eosinophil survival-promoting factors (GM-CSF) after stimulation of proteinase-activated receptor 2. J Allergy Clin Immunol 2001;107:679–85.
53. D'Agostino B, Roviezzo F, De PR, Terracciano S, De NM, Gallelli L, et al. Activation of protease-activated receptor-2 reduces airways inflammation in experimental allergic asthma. Clin Exp Allergy 2007;37:1436–43.
54. Vergnolle N, Hollenberg MD, Sharkey KA, Wallace JL. Characterization of the inflammatory response to proteinase-activated receptor-2 (PAR2)-activating peptides in the rat paw. Br J Pharmacol 1999;127:1083–90.
55. Aslam A, Buckley MG, Wilson SJ, Howarth PH, Hollenberg MD, Walls AF. Protease activated receptor-2 (PAR-2) expression is increased in the bronchial epithelium of asthmatics. Clin Exp Allergy 2002;32:1384; Clin Exp Allergy 32, 1384, 2002. Ref Type: Abstract.
56. Nagata H, Motosugi H, Sanai A, Suzuki H, Ohno K, Numata T, et al. Enhancement of submicroscopic damage of the nasal epithelium by topical allergen challenge in patients with perennial nasal allergy. Ann Otol Rhinol Laryngol 2001;110:236–42.
57. Lee HM, Kim HY, Kang HJ, Woo JS, Chae SW, Lee SH, et al. Up-regulation of protease-activated receptor 2 in allergic rhinitis. Ann Otol Rhinol Laryngol 2007;116:554–8.
58. Dinh QT, Cryer A, Trevisani M, Dinh S, Wu S, Cifuentes LB, et al. Gene and protein expression of protease-activated receptor 2 in structural and inflammatory cells in the nasal mucosa in seasonal allergic rhinitis. Clin Exp Allergy 2006;36:1039–48.
59. Dinh QT, Cryer A, Dinh S, Trevisani M, Georgiewa P, Chung F, et al. Protease-activated receptor 2 expression in trigeminal neurons innervating the rat nasal mucosa. Neuropeptides 2005;39:461–6.
60. Runswick S, Mitchell T, Davies P, Robinson C, Garrod DR. Pollen proteolytic enzymes degrade tight junctions. Respirology 2007;12:834–42.
61. Wan H, Winton HL, Soeller C, Taylor GW, Gruenert DC, Thompson PJ, et al. The transmembrane protein occludin of epithelial tight junctions is a functional target for serine peptidases from faecal pellets of Dermatophagoides pteronyssinus. Clin Exp Allergy 2001;31:279–94.
62. Takano K, Kojima T, Go M, Murata M, Ichimiya S, Himi T, et al. HLA-DR- and CD11c-positive dendritic cells penetrate beyond well-developed epithelial tight junctions in human nasal mucosa of allergic rhinitis. J Histochem Cytochem 2005;53:611–9.
63. Kobayashi N, Dezawa M, Nagata H, Yuasa S, Konno A. Immunohistochemical study of E-cadherin and ZO-1 in allergic nasal epithelium of the guinea pig. Int Arch Allergy Immunol 1998;116:196–205.

64. Benson M, Svensson PA, Adner M, Caren H, Carlsson B, Carlsson LM, et al. DNA micro-array analysis of chromosomal susceptibility regions to identify candidate genes for allergic disease: a pilot study. Acta Otolaryngol 2004;124:813–9.
65. Kusunoki T, Okafuji I, Yoshioka T, Saito M, Nishikomori R, Heike T, et al. SPINK5 polymorphism is associated with disease severity and food allergy in children with atopic dermatitis. J Allergy Clin Immunol 2005;115:636–8.
66. Ono SJ, Abelson MB. Allergic conjunctivitis: update on pathophysiology and prospects for future treatment. J Allergy Clin Immunol 2005;115:118–22.
67. Keane-Myers AM, Miyazaki D, Liu G, Dekaris I, Ono S, Dana MR. Prevention of allergic eye disease by treatment with IL-1 receptor antagonist. Invest Ophthalmol Vis Sci 1999;40:3041–6.
68. Bundoc VG, Keane-Myers A. IL-10 confers protection from mast cell degranulation in a mouse model of allergic conjunctivitis. Exp Eye Res 2007;85:575–9.
69. Fokkens WJ, Bruijnzeel-Koomen CA, Vroom TM, Rijntjes E, Hoefsmit EC, Mudde GC, et al. The Langerhans cell: an underestimated cell in atopic disease. Clin Exp Allergy 1990;20:627–38.
70. Godthelp T, Holm AF, Fokkens WJ, Doornenbal P, Mulder PG, Hoefsmit EC, et al. Dynamics of nasal eosinophils in response to a nonnatural allergen challenge in patients with allergic rhinitis and control subjects: a biopsy and brush study. J Allergy Clin Immunol 1996;97:800–11.
71. Fokkens WJ, Vroom TM, Rijntjes E, Mulder PG. Fluctuation of the number of CD-1(T6)-positive dendritic cells, presumably Langerhans cells, in the nasal mucosa of patients with an isolated grass-pollen allergy before, during, and after the grass-pollen season. J Allergy Clin Immunol 1989;84:39–43.
72. Till SJ, Jacobson MR, O'Brien F, Durham SR, Kleinjan A, Fokkens WJ, et al. Recruitment of CD1a + Langerhans cells to the nasal mucosa in seasonal allergic rhinitis and effects of topical corticosteroid therapy. Allergy 2001;56:126–31.
73. Bachert C, Behrendt H, Nosbusch K, Hauser U, Ganzer U. Possible role of macrophages in allergic rhinitis. Int Arch Allergy Appl Immunol 1991;94:244–5.
74. Francis JN, Lloyd CM, Sabroe I, Durham SR, Till SJ. T lymphocytes expressing CCR3 are increased in allergic rhinitis compared with non-allergic controls and following allergen immunotherapy. Allergy 2007;62:59–65.
75. Jutel M, Akdis M, Budak F, ebischer-Casaulta C, Wrzyszcz M, Blaser K, et al. IL-10 and TGF-beta cooperate in the regulatory T cell response to mucosal allergens in normal immunity and specific immunotherapy. Eur J Immunol 2003;33:1205–14.
76. Ling EM, Smith T, Nguyen XD, Pridgeon C, Dallman M, Arbery J, et al. Relation of CD4 + CD25 + regulatory T-cell suppression of allergen-driven T-cell activation to atopic status and expression of allergic disease. Lancet 21-2-2004;363:608–15.
77. Malmhall C, Bossios A, Pullerits T, Lotvall J. Effects of pollen and nasal glucocorticoid on FOXP3 +, GATA-3 + and T-bet + cells in allergic rhinitis. Allergy 2007;62:1007–13.
78. Lee JH, Yu HH, Wang LC, Yang YH, Lin YT, Chiang BL. The levels of CD4 + CD25 + regulatory T cells in paediatric patients with allergic rhinitis and bronchial asthma. Clin Exp Immunol 2007;148:53–63.
79. Xu G, Mou Z, Jiang H, Cheng L, Shi J, Xu R, et al. A possible role of CD4 + CD25 + T cells as well as transcription factor Foxp3 in the dysregulation of allergic rhinitis. Laryngoscope 2007;117:876–80.
80. Siewert C, Menning A, Dudda J, Siegmund K, Lauer U, Floess S, et al. Induction of organ-selective CD4 + regulatory T cell homing. Eur J Immunol 2007;37:978–89.
81. Ahluwalia P, Anderson DF, Wilson SJ, McGill JI, Church MK. Nedocromil sodium and levocabastine reduce the symptoms of conjunctival allergen challenge by different mechanisms. J Allergy Clin Immunol 2001;108:449–54.
82. Anderson DF, MacLeod JD, Baddeley SM, Bacon AS, McGill JI, Holgate ST, et al. Seasonal allergic conjunctivitis is accompanied by increased mast cell numbers in the absence of leucocyte infiltration. Clin Exp Allergy 1997;27:1060–6.

83. Trocme SD, Kephart GM, Allansmith MR, Bourne WM, Gleich GJ. Conjunctival deposition of eosinophil granule major basic protein in vernal keratoconjunctivitis and contact lens-associated giant papillary conjunctivitis. Am J Ophthalmol 15-7-1989;108:57–63.

84. Foster CS, Rice BA, Dutt JE. Immunopathology of atopic keratoconjunctivitis. Ophthalmology 1991;98:1190–6.

85. Trocme SD, Leiferman KM, George T, Bonini S, Foster CS, Smit EE, et al. Neutrophil and eosinophil participation in atopic and vernal keratoconjunctivitis. Curr Eye Res 2003;26:319–25.

86. Bradding P, Feather IH, Wilson S, et al. Immunolocalization of cytokines in the nasal mucosa of normal and perennial rhinitic subjects. J Immunol 1993;151:3853–65.

87. Pawankar R, Okuda M, Hasegawa S, et al. Interleukin-13 expression in the nasal mucosa of perennial allergic rhinitis. Am J Respir Critical Care Med 1995;152:2059–67.

88. Pawankar R, Ra C. Heterogeneity of mast cells and T cells in the nasal mucosa. J Allergy Clin Immunol 1996;98:249–62.

89. Pawankar R, Takizawa R, Saito H, et al. RANTES can regulate mast cell migration into the allergic nasal epithelium [abstract]. J Allergy Clin Immunol 2002;101:153.

90. Lilly CM, Nakamura H, Kesselman H, et al. Expression of eotaxin by human lung epithelial cells: induction by cytokines and inhibition by glucocorticoids. J Clin Invest 1997;99:1767–73.

91. Li L, Xia Y, Nguyen A, et al. Effects of Th2 cytokines on chemokine expression in the lung: IL-13 potently induces eotaxin expression by airway epithelial cells. J Immunol 1999;162:2477–87.

92. Sekiya T, Miyamasu M, Yamaguchi M, Pawankar R, et al. Inducible expression of a Th2-typeCCchemokine, thymus-and activation regulated chemokine (TARC) by human bronchial epithelial cells. J Immunol 2000;165:2205–13.

93. Naclerio RM, Proud D, Togias AG, Adkinson NF, Jr., Meyers DA, Kagey-Sobotka A, et al. Inflammatory mediators in late antigen-induced rhinitis. N Engl J Med 11-7-1985;313:65–70.

94. Naclerio RM, Meier HL, Kagey-Sobotka A, Adkinson NF, Jr., Meyers DA, Norman PS, et al. Mediator release after nasal airway challenge with allergen. Am Rev Respir Dis 1983;128:597–602.

95. Wagenmann M, Baroody FM, Cheng CC, Kagey-Sobotka A, Lichtenstein LM, Naclerio RM. Bilateral increases in histamine after unilateral nasal allergen challenge. Am J Respir Crit Care Med 1997;155:426–31.

96. Juliusson S, Holmberg K, Baumgarten CR, Olsson M, Enander I, Pipkorn U. Tryptase in nasal lavage fluid after local allergen challenge. Relationship to histamine levels and TAME-esterase activity. Allergy 1991;46:459–65.

97. Rasp G, Hochstrasser K. Tryptase in nasal fluid is a useful marker of allergic rhinitis. Allergy 1993;48:72–4.

98. Wagenmann M, Schumacher L, Bachert C. The time course of the bilateral release of cytokines and mediators after unilateral nasal allergen challenge. Allergy 2005;60:1132–8.

99. Sim TC, Grant JA, Hilsmeier KA, Fukuda Y, Alam R. Proinflammatory cytokines in nasal secretions of allergic subjects after antigen challenge. Am J Respir Crit Care Med 1994;149:339–44.

100. Bachert C, Hauser U, Prem B, Rudack C, Ganzer U. Proinflammatory cytokines in allergic rhinitis. Eur Arch Otorhinolaryngol 1995;252(Suppl 1):S44–S49.

101. Jeffery PK. Remodeling and inflammation of bronchi in asthma and chronic obstructive pulmonary disease. Proc Am Thorac Soc 2004;1:176–83.

102. An SS, Bai TR, Bates JH, Black JL, Brown RH, Brusasco V, et al. Airway smooth muscle dynamics: a common pathway of airway obstruction in asthma. Eur Respir J 2007;29:834–60.

103. Funayama Y, Sasaki I, Naito H, Fukushima K, Matsuno S, Masuda T. Remodeling of vascular wall in Crohn's disease. Dig Dis Sci 1999;44:2319–23.

104. Meijer MJ, Mieremet-Ooms MA, van der Zon AM, van DW, van Hogezand RA, Sier CF, et al. Increased mucosal matrix metalloproteinase-1, -2, -3 and -9 activity in patients with

inflammatory bowel disease and the relation with Crohn's disease phenotype. Dig Liver Dis 2007;39:733–9.

105. Brandtzaeg P. The changing immunological paradigm in coeliac disease. Immunol Lett 15-6-2006;105:127–39.

106. Bacon AS, McGill JI, Anderson DF, Baddeley S, Lightman SL, Holgate ST. Adhesion molecules and relationship to leukocyte levels in allergic eye disease. Invest Ophthalmol Vis Sci 1998;39:322–30.

107. Shimizu A, Tepler I, Benfey PN, Berenstein EH, Siriganian RP, Leder P. Human and rat mast cell high-affinity immunoglobulin E receptors: characterization of putative alpha-chain gene products. Proc Natl Acad Sci USA 1988;85:1907–11.

108. Kuster H, Zhang L, Brini AT, MacGlashan Jr DW, Kinet J-P. The gene and cDNA for the high affinity immunoglobulin E receptor β chain and expression of complete human receptor. J Biol Chem 1992;18:12782–87.

109. Kuster H, Thompson H, Kinet J-P. Characterization and expression of the gene for the human Fc receptor gamma subunit. Definition of a new gene family. J Biol Chem 1990;265:6448–52.

110. Blank U, Ra C, Kinet J-P. Characterization of truncated α chain products from human, rat and mouse high affinity receptor for immunoglobulin E. J Biol Chem 1991;266:2639–45.

111. Hakimi J, Seals C, Kondas JA, Pettine L, Danho W, Kochan JP. The α subunit of the human IgE receptor (FcεRI) is sufficient for high affinity IgE binding. J Biol Chem 1990;265:22079–85.

112. Kinet J-P, Blank U, Ra C, White K, Metzger H, Kochan J. Isolation and characterization of the β-subunit cDNAs coding for the of the high affinity receptor for immunoglobulin E. Proc Natl Acad Sci USA 1993;85:6483–7.

113. Benhamou M, Gutkind JS, Robbins KC, Siriganian RP. Tyrosine phosphorylation coupled to an IgE receptor mediated signal transduction and histamine release. Proc Natl Acad Sci USA 1990;87:5327–32.

114. Connelly PA, Farrell CA, Marenda JM, Conklyn MJ, Showell HJ. Tyrosine phosphorylation is an early signalling event common to Fc receptor crosslinking in human neutrophils and rat basophilic leukemia cells (RBL-2H3). Biochem Biophys Res Commun 1991;177:192–99.

115. Kawakami T, Inagaki N, Takei M, et al. Tyrosine phosphorylation is required for mast cell activation through FcεRI cross linking. J Immunol 1992;175:1285–92.

116. Dombrowicz D, Flamand V, Brigman KK, Koller BH, Kinet J-P. Abolition of anaphylaxis by targeted disruption of the high affinity immunoglobulin E receptor α chain gene. Cell 1993;75:969–76.

117. Pawankar R, Okuda M, Yssel H, et al. Nasal mast cells in perennial allergic rhinitis exhibit increased expression of the FcepsilonRI,CD40L, IL-4, and IL-13, and can induce IgE synthesis in B cells. J Clin Invest 1997;99:1492–99.

118. Yamaguchi M, Lantz CS, Oettgen HC, et al. IgE enhances mouse mast cell FcεRI expression in vitro and in vivo: evidence for a novel amplification mechanism in IgE-dependent reactions. J Exp Med 1997;185(4):663.

119. Saito H, Nakajima T, Tachimoto H. Upregulation of the FcεRIα by IgE molecules on human cultured mast cells and basophils. J Allergy Clin Immunol 1997;99(1): S103.

120. Pawankar R, Ra C. IgE-IgE receptor mast cells axis in allergy. Clin Exp Allergy 1998;28:6–11.

121. Pawankar R. Revisting the roles of mast cells and its relation to local IgE synthesis. Am J Rhinol 2001;14:309.

122. Durham SR, Gould HJ, Thienes CP, et al. Expression of epsilon germ-line gene transcripts and mRNA for the epsilon heavy chain of IgE in nasal B cells and the effects of topical corticosteroid. Eur J Immunol 1997;27(11):2899.

123. Pawankar R, Yamagishi S, Takizawa R, Yagi T. Local IgE synthesis: its functional significance and strategy for new therapy. J Rhinol 2000;39:69.

124. Ciprandi G, Buscaglia S, Pesce G, Pronzato C, Ricca V, Parmiani S, et al. Minimal persistent inflammation is present at mucosal level in patients with asymptomatic rhinitis and mite allergy. J Allergy Clin Immunol 1995;96:971–9.

125. Naito K, Takeda N, Yokoyama N, Ibata K, Ishihara M, Senoh Y, et al. The distribution of eosinophil cationic protein positive eosinophils in the nasal mucosa of the nasal allergy patients. Auris Nasus Larynx 1993;20:197–204.
126. Berger G, Bernheim J, Ophir D. Epithelial shedding of the inferior turbinate in perennial allergic and nonallergic rhinitis: a riddle to solve. Arch Otolaryngol Head Neck Surg 2007;133:78–82.
127. Gleich GJ, Flavahan NA, Fujisawa T, Vanhoutte PM. The eosinophil as a mediator of damage to respiratory epithelium: a model for bronchial hyperreactivity. J Allergy Clin Immunol 1988;81:776–81.
128. Amin K, Rinne J, Haahtela T, Simola M, Peterson CG, Roomans GM, et al. Inflammatory cell and epithelial characteristics of perennial allergic and nonallergic rhinitis with a symptom history of 1 to 3 years' duration. J Allergy Clin Immunol 2001;107:249–57.
129. Watanabe K, Kiuna C. Epithelial damage of nasal mucosa in nasal allergy. Ann Otol Rhinol Laryngol 1998;107:564–70.
130. Montero MP, Blanco E, Matta Campos JJ, Gonzalez EA, Guidos FG, Tinajeros Castaneda OA. Nasal remodeling in patient with perennial allergic rhinitis. Rev Alerg Mex 2003;50:79–82.
131. Chanez P, Vignola AM, Vic P, Guddo F, Bonsignore G, Godard P, et al. Comparison between nasal and bronchial inflammation in asthmatic and control subjects. Am J Respir Crit Care Med 1999;159:588–95.
132. Berger G, Marom Z, Ophir D. Goblet cell density of the inferior turbinates in patients with perennial allergic and nonallergic rhinitis. Am J Rhinol 1997;11:233–6.
133. Malekzadeh S, Hamburger MD, Whelan PJ, Biedlingmaier JF, Baraniuk JN. Density of middle turbinate subepithelial mucous glands in patients with chronic rhinosinusitis. Otolaryngol Head Neck Surg 2002;127:190–5.
134. Tos M, Morgensen C. Nasal glands in nasal allergy. Acta Otolaryngol 1977;83:498–504.
135. Sanai A, Nagata H, Konno A. Extensive interstitial collagen deposition on the basement membrane zone in allergic nasal mucosa. Acta Otolaryngol 1999;119:473–8.
136. Matovinovic E, Solberg O, Shusterman D. Epidermal growth factor receptor – but not histamine receptor – is upregulated in seasonal allergic rhinitis. Allergy 2003;58:472–5.
137. Wu X, Myers AC, Goldstone AC, Togias A, Sanico AM. Localization of nerve growth factor and its receptors in the human nasal mucosa. J Allergy Clin Immunol 2006;118:428–33.
138. van Toorenenbergen AW, Gerth van WR, Vermeulen AM. Allergen-induced matrix metalloproteinase-9 in nasal lavage fluid. Allergy 1999;54:293–4.
139. Kirmaz C, Ozbilgin K, Yuksel H, Bayrak P, Unlu H, Giray G, et al. Increased expression of angiogenic markers in patients with seasonal allergic rhinitis. Eur Cytokine Netw 2004;15:317–22.
140. Sarin S, Undem B, Sanico A, Togias A. The role of the nervous system in rhinitis. J Allergy Clin Immunol 2006;118:999–1016.
141. Pawankar R, Inflammatory mechanisms in allergic rhinitis. Curr Opin Allergy Clin Immunol. 2007;7(1):1–4.
142. Fontanari P, Zattara-Hartmann MC, Burnet H, Jammes Y. Nasal eupnoeic inhalation of cold, dry air increases airway resistance in asthmatic patients. Eur Respir J 1997;10:2250–4.
143. O'Hanlon S, Facer P, Simpson KD, Sandhu G, Saleh HA, Anand P. Neuronal markers in allergic rhinitis: expression and correlation with sensory testing. Laryngoscope 2007;117:1519–27.
144. Fang SY, Shen CL, Ohyama M. Distribution and quantity of neuroendocrine markers in allergic rhinitis. Acta Otolaryngol 1998;118:398–403.
145. Heppt W, Dinh QT, Cryer A, Zweng M, Noga O, Peiser C, et al. Phenotypic alteration of neuropeptide-containing nerve fibres in seasonal intermittent allergic rhinitis. Clin Exp Allergy 2004;34:1105–10.
146. Sanico AM, Philip G, Proud D, Naclerio RM, Togias A. Comparison of nasal mucosal responsiveness to neuronal stimulation in non-allergic and allergic rhinitis: effects of capsaicin nasal challenge. Clin Exp Allergy 1998;28:92–100.

Allergic Conjunctivitis: Update on Its Pathophysiology and Perspectives for Future Treatment

Stefano Bonini, Roberto Sgrulletta, Marco Coassin, and Sergio Bonini

Introduction

Allergic conjunctivitis is one of the most common syndromes that a general ophthalmologist is presented with, with a prevalence ranging from 5% to 22% in the general population [1, 2].

Ocular allergic diseases share some common eye symptoms and signs such as redness, itching, tearing and discharge. However, symptoms and signs represent the final clinical outcome of different pathophysiological mechanisms that are peculiar to different phenotypes of allergic eye disease [3, 4].

Four Forms of Allergic Conjunctivitis: A Clinical Simplification

Allergic eye disease, in fact, includes a spectrum of different clinical entities with variable presentation. The milder and the most common forms are seasonal allergic conjunctivitis (SAC) and perennial allergic conjunctivitis (PAC). Generally, SAC and PAC patients complain of symptoms such as itching, tearing, mucus discharge and redness, but these two forms are not sight threatening. On the contrary, more severe forms of ocular allergies, such as vernal keratoconjunctivitis (VKC) and atopic keratoconjunctivitis (AKC), can involve the cornea and may be sight threatening if not promptly diagnosed and adequately treated.

If three are the "classic" phenotypes of allergic conjunctivitis, two are the main pathological pathways usually considered as the basis of these forms: conjunctival

S. Bonini (✉), R. Sgrulletta, and M. Coassin
Department of Ophthalmology, University of Rome "Campus Bio-Medico", Via
Alvaro del Portillo, 21 - 00128 Rome, Italy,
e-mail: s.bonini@unicampus.it

Se. Bonini
II University of Naples and Institute of Neurobiology & Molecular Medicine,
National Research Council (INMM-CNR) - Rome, Italy

R. Pawankar et al. (eds.), *Allergy Frontiers: Clinical Manifestations*,
DOI: 10.1007/978-4-431-88317-3_2, © Springer 2009

mast cell activation and eosinophil recruitment into the ocular surface. Indeed, ophthalmologists know that such a plain classification and simplified pathophysiological description do not adequately account for the complexity of diagnostics and treatment in clinical settings [5]. Moreover, the biological mechanisms at the base of ocular allergy seem to be distinct from those involved in allergic diseases that affect other organs in the body. This complexity is attributable to the unique immunological characteristics of the anterior segment of the eye, and to the specific mechanisms by which the structural cells (i.e., epithelial cells and stromal fibroblasts) interact with the inflammatory cells infiltrating the conjunctiva.

Seasonal and Perennial Allergic Conjunctivitis

Seasonal allergic conjunctivitis (SAC) and perennial allergic conjunctivitis (PAC) account for 95% of the allergic eye diseases in the practice. These forms involve both eyes and occur seasonally (spring, fall) or perennially (year round), respectively, and do not induce severe ocular surface damage [6].

SAC (Hay fever conjunctivitis) is usually an acute or subacute disease that is characterized by peaks of self-limiting signs and symptoms (i.e., red eye, tearing, itching and mucous discharge), and is mostly due to pollens (e.g., grass, trees, ragweed) that appear during specific seasons.

PAC is less common than SAC and is related to animal dander, dust mites or other allergens that are present in the environment year-round. The symptoms are present all year with seasonal exacerbation depending on the individual sensitization. The hallmarks of this form are itching, redness and puffy eyes. Patients may also complain of tearing, mucous discharge, burning and swelling. However, no symptom or sign is specific to SAC and PAC [7, 8] and seasonal allergens may cause PAC as perennial allergens may be responsible for seasonal forms. Accordingly, the classification in the intermittent and persistent forms may result more appropriately than that in SAC or PAC.

Immunopathogenesis of SAC and PAC

Allergic inflammation of the conjunctiva is a type I hypersensitivity, an immediate reaction associated with IgE-mediated cell activation.

The first step of the process is sensitization: small (picograms) quantities of environmental allergens such as pollens, dust mite fecal particles, animal dander, and other proteins reach the conjunctival mucosa. Here, these particles are processed by Langerhans, dendritic or other antigen-presenting cells (APCs). Proteolitically cleaved antigens subsequently bind to the antigen-recognition site of the major histocompatibility complex (MHC) class II molecules. Carried by APCs, the antigens are then presented to native Th0 lymphocytes that express antigen-specific receptors and recognize the antigenic peptides. This process probably occurs at the local draining lymph nodes. Multiple contacts and cytokine exchanges between APC and T cells are necessary to induce a Th2-type reaction. The cytokines released by the type-2 helper T-lymphocytes (interleukin-3, IL-4, IL-5, IL-6, IL-13 and granulocyte-macrophage colony stimulate factor – GM-CSF) stimulate the production of IgE by B cells.

The second step of the pathophysiology of conjunctival allergy is the triggering, in the sensitized host, of the mast cells residing in the conjunctival mucosa and bearing specific IgE antibodies on the cell surface with the help of high affinity receptors. Exposure to environmental allergens in sensitized individuals causes the cross-linking of IgE at the mast cell membrane level, with subsequent cell degranulation and release of histamine, tryptase, prostaglandins and leukotrienes. These mediators trigger clinical manifestations of the acute phase of the disease (early phase). Mast cell degranulation, however, also induces activation of vascular endothelial cells, and thus expression of chemokine and adhesion molecules, such as: 'Regulated-upon-Activation Normal T-cell Expressed and Secreted' (RANTES), monocytes chemotactic protein-1 (MCP-1), intracellular adhesion molecule (ICAM-1), vascular cell adhesion molecule (VCAM) and p-Selectin and chemotactic factors (IL-8, eotaxin). These factors initiate the recruitment phase of activated inflammatory cells in the conjunctiva. The late-phase reaction to allergen stimulation occurs hours after allergen exposure and is characterized by the recurrence or prolongation of symptoms due to the infiltration of eosinophils, neutrophils and T lymphocytes into the mucosa (Fig. 1). The late-phase reaction plays a major role in the pathophysiology of the most severe forms of ocular allergic disorders [9–12].

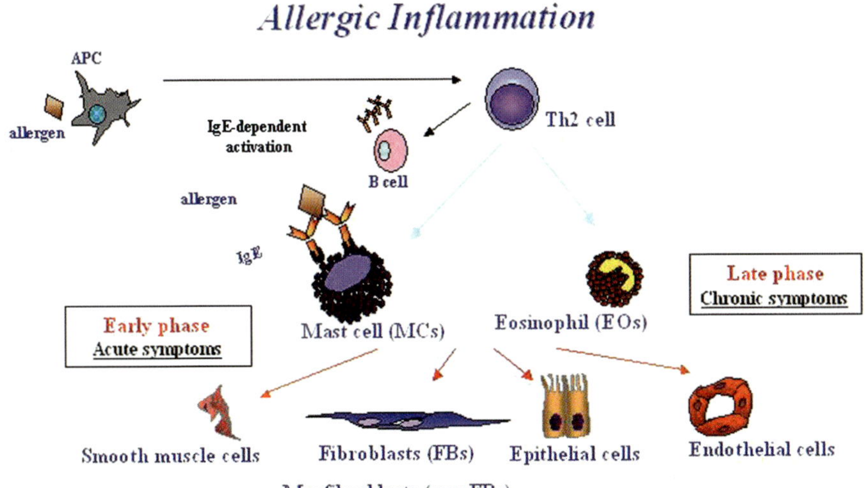

Fig. 1 The early and late phase of ocular allergic reactions

Vernal and Atopic Keratoconjunctivitis

Vernal keratoconjunctivitis (VKC) is a severe allergic disease of childhood with a higher prevalence in male subjects living in warm climates [13]. It is characterized by the presence of corneal epithelial and stromal lesions as well as of conjunctival proliferative changes (i.e., the giant papillae of the upper tarsal conjunctiva) and limbal abnormalities. Patients with VKC are usually, but not necessarily, sensitized to the most common allergens, such as grass, Parietaria and Dermatophygoides. It has been suggested that VKC represents a phenotypic model of overexpression of the cytokine gene cluster on chromosome 5q [14]. This chromosomal area includes genes that regulate the expression of IL-3, IL-4, IL-5 and GM-CSF. The up-regulation of these factors is critical in modulating Th2 prevalence, IgE production, as well as mast cell and eosinophil function.

Two clinical variants of VKC are usually described: the limbal and the tarsal forms. The hallmarks of these two pathologic entities are the giant papillae on the upper tarsal conjunctiva and the gelatinous limbal infiltrates, respectively [15]. Both forms of VKC are characterized by intense itching, tearing, mucous discharge and severe photophobia, that often force children to live virtually in the dark. The intense foreign body sensation is due to the conjunctival surface irregularity and the copious mucous secretion. The onset of ocular pain is indicative of cornea involvement, which can be present in the form of superficial punctate keratitis, epithelial erosions or ulcers and plaques. The different prevalence between genders, and its resolution with puberty, are features that have suggested a role of hormonal factors in the development of VKC [16].

Atopic keratoconjunctivitis (AKC) occurs more frequently in men aged 30–50 years [17]. A family history of allergies, asthma, urticaria or hay fever is often present. Typically, patients have atopic dermatitis or eczema from childhood, but develop ocular symptoms later in life. These symptoms are represented by an intense bilateral itching of the eyes and of the skin of the lids and periorbital areas. Tearing, burning, photophobia, blurred vision and a stringy, rope-like mucus discharge are also observed.

Tylosis and swollen eyelids with a scaly indurate appearance and meibomiam gland dysfunction with associated dry eye are the signs of atopic blepharitis. The conjunctiva can be hyperemic and edematous, and tarsal conjunctival papillae are commonly seen [18].

Immunopathogenesis of VKC and AKC

Vernal keratoconjunctivitis is traditionally thought to be an allergic disorder. The role of an IgE-mediated hypersensitivity in VKC is one of the essential pathogenic steps [19], supported by seasonal incidence, association with other allergic manifestations, increased number of conjunctival mast cells and eosinophils, high levels of total and specific IgE and others mediators in serum and tears [20] and the therapeutic response to mast cell stabilizers in mild cases of VKC [21, 22]. However, the fact that specific sensitization is not found in many patients, suggests that additional mechanisms, apart from a typical type I hypersensivity mechanism, contribute to the pathogenesis of conjunctival inflammation in VKC patients.

Role of Eosinophils in Chronic Ocular Allergy

Selective infiltration of eosinophils is one of the characteristics of all the forms of allergic conjunctival diseases [23]. In normal individuals, eosinophils are not found in the conjunctival epithelium, although a small number of these cells is present in the substantia propria of the conjunctiva [24]. On the contrary, eosinophils are markedly increased in the substantia propria and infiltrate the conjunctival epithelium in VKC [25]. Eosinophils in VKC are activated, as shown by the expression of eosinophil cationic [26, 27]. Activated eosinophils release cytotoxic proteins such as MBP-1, eosinophil peroxidase, eosinophil-derived neurotoxin and eosinophil cationic protein, and the concentration of these proteins is increased in the tear fluid of these individuals [28–31]. Proteolytic enzymes, cytotoxic proteins and oxygen radicals released by neutrophils contribute to the exacerbation of corneal damage [32, 33]. Corneal fibroblasts are stimulated by neutrophils and participate in collagen degradation, which leads to the subsequent corneal ulceration [33, 34]. This evidence suggests that the interactions between the immune cells and the corneal resident cells play a major role in the pathogenesis of corneal involvement in VKC. The infiltration and degranulation of eosinophils at the limbus are also responsible for the disruption of the corneal epithelium [32]. Moreover, the corneal plaque (also called shield ulcer), which develops in patients with severe VKC [35] is composed of debris derived from eosinophils and epithelial cells [36, 37]. Extravasation of immune cells is regulated by the chemokines expressed by vessels and other structural cells, such as fibroblasts and smooth muscle cells [38]. Although many bioactive substances, including complement C5a [39], leukotriene B4 [40, 41] and platelet activating factor (PAF) are able to induce local infiltration of eosinophils, other factors, in particular chemokines, may also activate different types of immune cells. Most chemokines belong to the CC or CXC sub-families [42–44], with only a few C and CX3C chemokines having been identified to date. In general, CC chemokines mostly induce the infiltration of eosinophils or lymphocytes, whereas, CXC chemokines mostly induce the infiltration of neutrophils or monocyte-macrophages [45]. Eosinophils express the CC receptors CCR1 and CCR3 on their surface. CCR1 docks several chemokines, that is, RANTES, macrophage inflammatory protein-1a (MIP-1a), monocyte chemoattractant protein (MCP-2) and MCP-3. CCR3 binds to RANTES, MCP-2, MCP-3 and eotaxin. For example, the chemokine RANTES induces the local infiltration of eosinophils through interaction with CCR1 and CCR3 [46, 47]. Indeed, the signalling mediated by CCR3 is more effective than the one mediated by CCR1 [42, 48, 49]. CCR3 is expressed by mast cells [50, 51] basophils [52, 53], Th2 lymphocytes [54] and eosinophils [51, 55, 56], but is not present in neutrophils [57]. One of the most potent eosinophil chemoattractant, the eotaxin, binds specially to CCR3 [58–61]. This small protein is synthesized by a number of different cell types, and is stimulated by interleukin-4 and interleukin-13, which are produced by T-helper type-2 lymphocytes [62].

Eotaxin and Corneal Involvement in Ocular Allergy

It is believed that VKC, like other allergic diseases, is a Th2-dominant condition [63, 64]. The cytokines produced by T helper type-2 lymphocytes are IL-4, IL-5, IL-10 and IL-13, and play a pivotal role in the pathogenesis of corneal damage in VKC.

It has been demonstrated that the stimulation of corneal fibroblasts by the Th2 cytokines IL-4 and IL-13 results in a marked release of eotaxin. In fact, corneal fibroblasts are the most significant source of this strong eosinophil chemoattractant, among the structural cells of the ocular surface [65]. The eosinophils present in the conjunctiva in VKC may release a substance that induces a breakdown of the barrier function of the corneal epithelium [66]. Corneal fibroblasts may then be exposed to different factors present in the tears of VKC patients, including TNF-a [67, 68], IL-4 [69] and IL-13. Moreover, the barrier function of the corneal epithelium is diminished in individuals with atopic dermatitis [70], which is often associated with VKC. Activated corneal fibroblasts and the subsequent release of eotaxin may induce a subsequent marked infiltration of eosinophils in the cornea. Breakdown of the barrier function of the corneal epithelium is thus probably a key event in the exacerbation of ocular allergic inflammation.

The Interactions Between Conjunctiva and Cornea in Ocular Allergy

Allergic inflammation begins in the conjunctiva, in which immune cells, such as, lymphocytes, mast cells and eosinophils are increased in number. These cells release Th2 cytokines (TNF-a, IL-4 and IL-13) that also stimulate the conjunctival fibroblasts to produce eotaxin. The chemotactic effect of this chemokine enhances eosinophil infiltration into the conjunctiva. The corneal epithelium is damaged by eosinophil-derived cytotoxic proteins, resulting in the impairment of its barrier function and consequent exposure of the corneal fibroblasts to the bioactive substances present in the tears. The corneal fibroblasts release eotaxin into the tear fluid in response to stimulation with TNF-a, IL-4 and IL-13. Allergic inflammation is then exacerbated as a result of eosinophils and other immune cells infiltrating the cornea and the conjunctiva, thus completing the cycle. Loss of the barrier function of the corneal epithelium and exposure of corneal fibroblasts to the bioactive substances in the tear film is likely to exacerbate the ocular allergy in additional ways, including induction of the release of other chemokines such as thymus- and activation-regulated chemokine (TARC or CCL17) and matrix metalloproteinase-2 (MMP-2) by corneal fibroblasts.

The giant papillae in VKC manifest a dense infiltration of eosinophils immediately beneath the denuded conjunctival epithelium, corresponding to the location of the Trantas' dots. Eosinophils thus probably migrate from the conjunctiva into the tear fluid and ocular discharge. Such migration may indicate that the concentration of eosinophil chemoattractant in tear fluid is greater than that in the conjunctiva. The release of RANTES and IL-8 by corneal fibroblasts is markedly stimulated by pro-inflammatory cytokines, such as TNF-a [46, 71]. The concentration of these cytokines is increased in the tears of individuals with a variety of ocular inflammatory conditions. These cytokines might contribute to ocular inflammatory reactions regardless of the causative factor [72, 73]. Increased concentrations of several pro-inflammatory cytokines and IL-4 (and possibly IL-13), on the other hand, may be a specific finding of VKC among ocular allergic diseases [66].

A Closer Look at the Cytokine Cascade in Ocular Allergy

Local infiltration of specific types of leukocytes is controlled by the interaction of these cells with adhesion molecules following the chemoattractive effects of chemokines. Adhesion molecules expressed on the surface of vascular endothelial cells facilitate the transmigration of immune cells. Among these adhesion molecules, intercellular adhesion molecule-1 (ICAM-1) and vascular cell adhesion molecule-1 (VCAM-1) play a prominent role [38]. ICAM-1 contributes to the local infiltration of the immune cells – including neutrophils, eosinophils and lymphocytes – during the inflammatory responses. VCAM-1 interacts with very late antigen-4 (VLA-4), which is expressed on the surface of eosinophils and lymphocytes. Inhibition of the VCAM-1–VLA-4 interaction thus suppresses eosinophil infiltration in allergic animals [74, 75]. ICAM-1 expression on human corneal epithelial cells is increased by stimulation of the cells with TNF-a in a concentration-dependent manner [76]. Furthermore, exposure of corneal fibroblasts to IL-4 or IL-13 in the presence of TNF-a induces a synergistic increase in the expression of VCAM-1 [77]. Corneal fibroblasts, but not corneal epithelial cells, up-regulate VCAM-1 expression in a synergistic manner in response to stimulation with TNF-a and either IL-4 or IL-13 [66]. These observations support the importance of the synergistic effects of these cytokines on corneal fibroblasts in the pathogenesis of VKC.

In addition to promoting eosinophil infiltration into the tissue, VCAM-1 induces the activation of these cells, increasing their survival [8, 78] superoxide generation [79], and leukotriene C4 secretion [80]. These effects of VCAM-1 may also contribute to the pathogenesis of allergic eye diseases.

The Th2 cytokines IL-4 and IL-13 are central mediators of allergic diseases [81, 82]. IL-4 and IL-13 regulate biological responses by binding to specific IL-4 receptors (IL-4Rs) expressed by a wide range of cell types, including T and B lymphocytes, monocytes, granulocytes, endothelial cells, epithelial cells and fibroblasts

[83–86]. The combination of TNF-a with either IL-4 or IL-13 induces the release of eotaxin and expression of VCAM-1 by corneal fibroblasts [66]. The IL-4Ra chain is the functional subunit of IL-4R complexes that mediates the activation of STAT6 [85, 87–90]. STAT (signal transducer and activator of transcription) proteins are intracellular signalling molecules that are activated on exposure of cells to various cytokines, growth factors or hormones. STAT6, one of the seven known mammalian members of the STAT family, is phosphorylated and activated in response to IL-4 or IL-13. Phosphorylated STAT6 molecules form dimers that translocate to the nucleus, where they activate transcription of target genes. The promoter of the eotaxin gene contains consensus-binding sites for STAT6 [91], suggesting that the effects of IL-4 and IL-13 on eotaxin expression in corneal fibroblasts might be mediated at the transcriptional level by the IL-4R-STAT6 signalling pathway. STAT6 knockout mice exhibit defects in various IL-4-mediated functions, such as induction of the expression of CD23 and major histocompatibility complex class II genes, Ig class switching to IgE, proliferation of B and T cells, and Th2 cell development, demonstrating the importance of STAT6 in IL-4 signalling [92, 93].

The Th1 and Th2 Paradigm in Ocular Allergy

Type-2 T helper lymphocytes (Th2) are thought to play a key role in the development of allergic disorders by producing regulatory and inflammatory cytokines such as, interleukin-4 (IL-4), IL-5 and IL-13. These cytokines have been found in tears and tissues of patients affected by VKC and AKC [94–98]. Although there is no doubt in the role played by Th2 cells in ocular allergy, a Th1 response has also been demonstrated [99]. In fact, it is not clear if the expression of the IFNγ – a Th1-type, proinflammatory cytokine – in chronic ocular allergic disorders is an attempt to down-regulate the Th2 response or a separate inflammatory pathway.

IFNγ, IL-4 and IL-13 may be produced and expressed together in ocular inflammatory allergic responses [99, 100]. Both VKC and AKC tears contain higher levels of IL-4 and IL-13 than normal tears [32]. IFNγ, increased in the tears of patients with corneal damage, significantly correlates with the corneal score, suggesting that the overproduction of this pro-inflammatory cytokine might be related to a worsening of the allergic inflammation. Conversely, in peripheral blood mononuclear cells of allergic patients, the frequency of the IL-4-producing T-cell is increased compared with that of healthy subjects, indicating that Th1 cells are only locally activated [101]. It has been proposed that Th1 cells protect against allergic disease by dampening the activity of Th2 lymphocytes. In fact, Th1 cells inhibit the proliferation and development of Th2 cells and IFNγ inhibits IgE synthesis [102–105]. IFNγ-secreting cells may be important in perpetuating chronic inflammation, since this cytokine up-regulates the expression and production of adhesion molecules, chemokines and co-stimulatory molecules by conjunctival [104] and corneal [105] epithelial cells [106].

IFNγ has been reported to up-regulate VCAM-1 expression on endothelial cells [107]. Ocular surface irritation due to external stimuli results in an immediate response from ocular surface conjunctival epithelial and endothelial cells, which includes the secretion of pro-inflammatory mediators at the site of injury. These pro-inflammatory mediators stimulate endothelial cell expression of adhesion molecules (e.g., VCAM-1), which are necessary for migration of immune cells to the ocular surface. In other words, IFNγ acts as a gatekeeper by inducing the expression of VCAM-1 to facilitate cellular extravasation into the injured tissue and enhancing the recruitment of immune cells [100]. In fact, the absence of IFNγ significantly reduces eosinophil migration into the conjunctiva. In conclusion, IFNγ may play an important role in ophthalmic Th2-type inflammation because it may control the capability of immune cells to gain entry into the extravascular tissue in both Th1 and Th2 response.

Both type 1 and type 2 cytokines are present in the tears during the active phase of severe SAC, VKC and AKC [108]. Even in SAC there is an increase of IL-1, IL-2, IL-4, IL-5, IL-6, IL-12, IL-13, IFNγ and MCP-1, suggesting that mast cells are not the only immune cells involved. There is a positive correlation between the percentages of tear-containing lymphocytes and IL-12 and IL-13 levels, whereas, no association is found with eosinophils [109]. This is surprising and suggests a possible general over-estimation of the role of eosinophils in ocular allergy. On the other hand, the conjunctival fibroblasts are receiving increasing attention for their potential contribution to the pathogenesis of allergic eye diseases. In fact, conjunctival fibroblasts constitutively produce IL-6, IL-8, MCP-1 and RANTES [108] and release eotaxin when stimulated with IL-4. The expression of CXC chemokines (IP-10, Mig) by conjunctival fibroblasts in response to pro-inflammatory cytokines, further supports a major role of these cells in the recruitment of T cells during chronic allergic eye disease [108].

Although SAC, VKC and AKC tears contain different levels of cytokines, these forms of conjunctivitis do not show a disease-specific Th1 or Th2 profile. Results of studies on tears reveal that allergic diseases differ predominantly in the quantity, rather than the quality, of cytokines present in tears as a result of complex interactions or mutual regulation.

Tissue Remodeling in Chronic Ocular Allergy

Fibroblasts and epithelial cells are not a simple target of ocular allergy, but play a pivotal role in the initiation and modulation of inflammation in the tissues by attracting and activating specific sets of immune cells [65, 110, 111]. In particular, conjunctival and corneal fibroblasts participate in the pathogenesis of ocular inflammation in severe forms of allergic keratoconjunctivitis, such as VKC [112], and they contribute to the formation of corneal ulcers inducing the degradation of collagen [33]. For this reason, nowadays, ocular fibroblasts represent a potential target for new therapeutic approaches to severe ocular allergy.

From a molecular point of view, corneal fibroblasts, stimulated by the combination of TNF-a and either IL-4 or IL-13, release TARC (CCL17) and the macrophage-derived chemokine (MDC or CCL22). These two CC chemokines are potent and selective chemoattractants for Th2 lymphocytes [113, 114], that express the corresponding receptor CCR4 on their surface [115, 116]. The local release of TARC and MDC contributes to the maintenance of allergic inflammation through the promotion of Th2 cell infiltration. This process is then amplified by the incoming inflammatory cells that cooperate with different mechanisms, to the Th2 response started by the tissue resident cells, that is, fibroblasts and epithelial cells.

The structure and functions of the corneal epithelium are regulated by the underlying basement membrane. Changes in the components of the basement membrane cause epithelial defects and corneal ulcers [117]. Type IV collagen and laminin are predominant components of the basement membrane of the corneal epithelium [118]. These two proteins are specifically degraded by MMP-2 and MMP-9. MMPs are released from various types of cells as latent proenzymes, which undergo proteolytic cleavage to generate the active form of each enzyme. The activities of MMPs are also down-regulated by tissue inhibitors of metalloproteinases (TIMPs).

The tears normally contain the pro forms of MMP-2 and MMP-9, but not the active forms. The presence of activated MMP-2 and MMP-9 in the tear fluid of VKC patients suggests that these proteins may induce degradation of the basement membrane, contributing to the formation of corneal ulcers. Corneal epithelial cells and fibroblasts are the probable source of lachrymal MMP-2 and MMP-9, because both these cell types constitutively express these MMPs and release them in response to stimulation by pro-inflammatory cytokines such as TNF-a and IL-1 [119]. The increased expression of MMP-2 and MMP-9 by resident cells of the cornea also prolongs reepithelialization of the cornea after injury [117].

Giant tarsal papillae and limbal Trantas dots are characteristic proliferative changes of the conjunctiva in VKC [15]. These lesions are mainly constituted by collagen types I and III and fibronectin, and are infiltrated by eosinophils, mast cells, Th2 lymphocytes and fibroblasts [120]. Conjunctival fibroblasts, balancing the synthesis and degradation of the extracellular matrix (ECM), control the metabolism of ECM proteins and proteoglycans and maintain the normal tissue structure. In vitro, Th2 cytokines IL-4 or IL-13 induce the proliferation of cultured conjunctival fibroblasts, increase the deposition of fibronectin and collagen types I and III by inhibiting the production of MMP-1 and stimulate their production of TIMP-1 [68]. An increased synthesis of collagen by the fibroblasts may lead to conjunctival hypertrophy and fibrosis in VKC.

Collagen and fibronectin not only provide structural support to cells, but also function as signalling molecules, playing key roles in allergic inflammation by regulating the activation of infiltrating immune cells. For instance, the interaction of eosinophils with the ECM facilitates their survival and activation, while the attachment of monocytes or macrophages to ECM stimulates their expression of IL-6 and TNF-a [121]. The ECM also serves as a reservoir for cytokines and growth factors: Transforming growth factor beta (TGF-b), basic fibroblast growth factor (bFGF) and the granulocyte-macrophage colony-stimulating factor (GMC-SF) bind with theECM components, and the ECM stabilizes or increases the local concentration of these growth factors.

IL-4 or IL-13 stimulate conjunctival fibroblasts to secrete ECM proteins such as collagen and fibronectin during allergy. In this way, fibroblasts increase the retention of inflammatory cytokines by the conjunctival stroma and further activate inflammatory cells. All these mechanisms induce subepithelial fibrosis and proliferation of capillaries that provide vascular support to the giant papillae in VKC. Ialin degeneration of conjunctival stroma and mucus metaplasia are also signs of chronic, severe ocular allergy [15].

The Emerging Role of the Innate Immune System, Toll-Like Receptors and Allergic Conjunctivitis

The innate immune system allows a fast and proper immune response to limit or completely destroy the invading pathogens [122]. Toll-like receptors (TLRs) play a crucial role by recognizing proteins or DNA/RNA sequences belonging to bacteria, protozoa, helminths, fungi and viruses [122]. Specific TLR activation, results in the production of pro-inflammatory mediators and cytokines, driving an antimicrobial host response [123].

TLRs are transmembrane type I glycoproteins characterized by an extracellular leucine-rich domain and a cytoplasm tail, homologous to the signal domain of the IL-1 receptor, which predominantly mediate the activation of mitogen-activated protein kinase and nuclear factor kappa B/activator protein-1 pathways and lead to cell activation and differentiation [123]. Eleven human TLRs have been characterized so far and classified according to their specific natural agonists: in general, TLR-2 and TLR-4 recognize bacterial products, whereas, TLR-3, TLR-7, TLR-8 and TLR-9 are principally designed to join nucleic acids [123]. A hallmark of the cell's response to the activation of innate immune systems is the release of TNF-[alpha], IL-1[beta] and IFN-[gamma] cytokines [123].

Innate/adaptive cross-talk has recently been demonstrated to be driven by TLR expression on APCs and structural cells of the ocular surface [124]. Ocular surface inflammation results from complex interactions between innate and adaptive responses. TLR expression has been found in the corneal and conjunctival epithelia, and this expression seems to be affected during bacterial/viral infections as well as in allergic conditions [124]. The presence of TLRs in the ocular epithelium may be relevant for defence mechanisms towards microbial agents in contact with the ocular surface. It has been hypothesized that commensal flora may be critical for the maintenance of epithelial mucosal homeostasis, by playing a paradoxically protective role after epithelial injury [124]. Moreover, changes in the commensal flora might influence the immune response in disease states. Certain micro-organisms may thus actually be important for protection against allergy [125].

Corneal epithelial cells express TLR-4 and co-stimulatory molecules (CD14, MD2), and stimulation by TLR-4 agonists results in pro-inflammatory cytokine and chemokine secretion [126]. Interestingly, the corneal epithelium does not normally respond to commensal flora, although this is commonly present in the tear film, as observed by the fact that patients suffering from bacterial conjunctivitis do not display corneal inflammation. The corneal epithelium appears to posses a unique way (intracellular localization) to modulate the functional activity of the highly expressed TLR-2 and TLR-4, and therefore to control unnecessary inflammation. In fact, corneal epithelial cells do not express TLR-2 and TLR-4 at the cell surface, failing to elicit immune response to ligands [127]. In a recent study, the role played by TLR-4/CD14/MD-2-expressingfibroblasts (activated keratocytes) in lipopoly-saccharide-induced inflammation associated with bacterial corneal ulceration, has been demonstrated [128]. In agreement with its role as a first line of defence, the healthy conjunctival epithelium expresses high levels of TLR-9, compared with the average expression of TLR-2 and TLR-4, whereas, the expression by the underside stroma is at similar levels [129]. This expression is modified in patients with VKC, as demonstrated by our group [124, 129]. Real-time evaluation of VKC conjunctiva showed a significant up-regulation of TLR-4 and down-regulation of TLR-9, with a slight reduction in TLR-2, compared with healthy conjunctiva. Confocal analysis showed that in VKC, stromal TLR-4 expression was mainly caused by fibroblasts, infiltrating eosinophils and mast cells. High levels of TLR-4 expression in VKC tissues is substantiated by previous reports correlating TLR-4 expression to the allergic phenotype.

The hypothesis that early life-specific activation of TLRs may contribute to a more balanced T helper type 1/2 response, avoiding over-activation of the T helper type 2 pathway, has been proposed [130, 131]. In line with this hypothesis, further studies on the role of commensal flora in influencing innate immunity in the eye, mainly during the early stages, may lead to a re-evaluation of the mechanisms that activate the adaptive immune responses after microbial ocular infections (Fig. 2). Finally, pharmacological activation and regulation of TLRs may also offer new therapeutic alternatives for the modulation of allergic and immune responses [132].

Treatment of Allergic Conjunctivitis

Preventive environmental measures are useful, but not sufficient for the complete control of signs and symptoms of allergic conjunctivitis. A change of climate, especially a move to high mountains during the critical months, avoiding exposure to non-specific triggering factors can provide significant relief to patients. Anyway, the pharmacological therapy in chronic subtypes is usually needed.

Vasocostrictors

The alpha-adrenergic agonists are used topically to control the conjunctival redness. They are non-specific and not pharmacologically active in the cascade of events that leads to the allergic reaction. Moreover, they may also cause side effects such as follicular conjunctivitis, lacrimal punctual occlusion and systemic hypertension, in view of their abuse by chronic allergy sufferers [133].

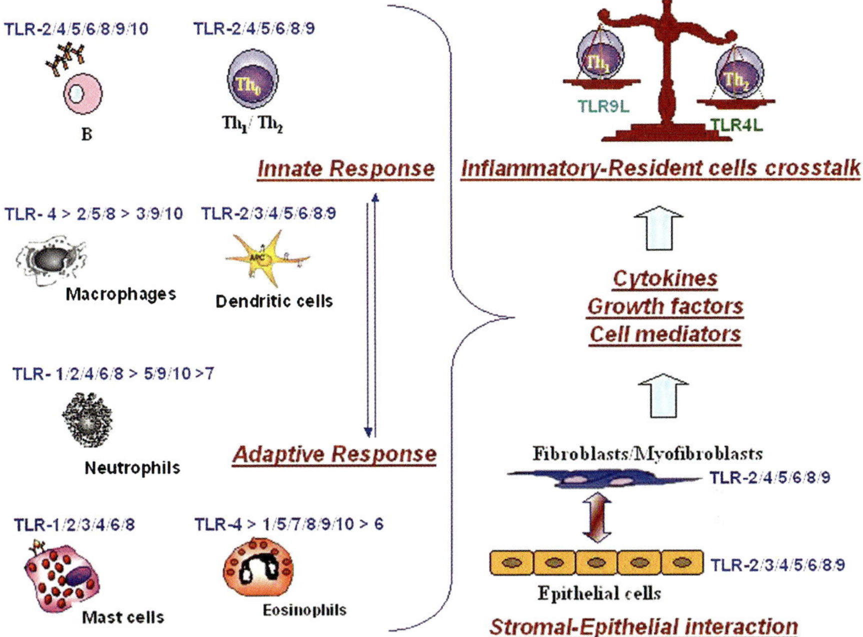

Fig. 2 TLR expression in inflammatory and resident cells. TLR are involved in the cross-talking between innate and adaptive immunity and between immune and resident cells during inflammatory reactions

Antihistamines

Antihistamines are the first line of treatment in ocular allergy, acting as H1-receptor competitive agonists. The new antihistamines have a longer duration of action (4–6 h) and are better tolerated. The second generation topical antihistamines (Cetrizine, Ebastine, Loratadine) offer the same efficacy of their predecessors, but with a low sedative effect and lack of anticholinergic activity. Moreover, for several of these new drugs an inflammatory effect beyond the antihistamine one is reported. In fact, these drugs attenuate the early phase and some features of the late phase of allergic ocular response, above all swelling and redness.

Levocabastine and Emedastine blocked IL-8 and IL-6 release from conjunctival epithelial cells and fibroblasts [134, 135].

Mozolastine is a new H-1 antihistamine with anti-inflammatory properties, developed for treatment of allergic conjunctivitis. Its high efficacy in relieving SAC and PAC is due to the inhibition of the production and release of histamine involved in the late phase of allergic response [136].

EV-131 is a new compound that binds free histamine, stabilizes mast cells, inhibits vascular adhesion molecule expression, and blocks neutrophil and eosinophil chemotaxis.

Finally Transilat, a drug used for keloid, shows potential application in the future in ocular allergic disease. In fact, its inhibitory action on mediator release by mast cells and basophils seems to stop collagen synthesis by fibroblasts.

Mast Cell Stabilizers

This class of drugs inhibits degranulation from mast cells by interrupting the cross-linking and activation of FceRI. All these membrane stabilizers act on the release of histamine and of mediators derived from the arachidonic acid cascade.

Cromolyn sodium was the first molecule studied. It partially inhibits cell degranulation and histamine release [137]. This preventive effect may explain the modest efficacy of these drugs in the clinical treatment of ongoing ocular allergy.

Nedocromil is more potent than cromolyn. It stabilizes conjunctival mast cells and possibly inhibits eosinophils. These drugs are approved for seasonal and perennial allergic conjunctivitis, even if Lodoxamide [138, 139] has been available for VKC.

In addition, it has been shown that N-acetyl aspartyl glutammic acid [139] and Pemirolast alleviate the signs of allergic conjunctivitis [140]. Dipeptide N-acetyl aspartyl glutammic acid 6% is used in Europe as topical eye drops in VKC and GPC because it inhibits leukotriene synthesis, histamine release by mast cells and complement derived anaphylatoxin production [141].

Dual-Action Anti-allergic Drugs

These drugs, at the same time, inhibit histamine release from mast cells and histamine binding to H1 receptors. The advantage is the rapid relief of symptoms given by immediate histamine receptor antagonism (which alleviates itching and redness) and the long-term benefits of mast cell stabilization.

Olapatadine is effective in perennial and seasonal conjunctivitis and allergic symptoms associated with contact lens wear [142]. Ketotifen inhibits release of mediators from mast cells, basophil and neutrophils. It also inhibits PAF production by neutrophils and eosinophil chemotaxis [143, 144].

Azelastine reduces ICAM-1 expression on conjunctival epithelium and inflammatory cell infiltration [145].

Epinastine is a new generation drug with no effect on muscarine receptors [146].

Nonsteroidal Anti-inflammatory Drugs

Ketorolac, a COX inhibitor, acts by blocking the synthesis of prostaglandins, particularly PGD2, which is known to produce significant and immediate allergic symptoms. However, its clinical efficacy seems inferior to olopatadine [147].

Corticosteroids

Corticosteroids should be the last choice in treating allergic diseases, although their use is sometimes unavoidable in VKC and AKC. In fact they may induce the development of cataracts, glaucoma, infections and corneal melting. Fluorometholone can reduce the signs and symptoms of VKC including tearing, discharge, conjunctival redness, papillary hypertrophy and Trantas dots [148].

Anti-leukotrienes

Oral Montelukast demonstrated its efficacy in a pilot study on patients affected by asthma and vernal conjunctivitis in reducing signs and symptoms of ocular allergy after 15 days of treatment [149].

Anti-IgE

Human IgE pentapeptide (HEPP), a synthetic antiallergic agent, which has been under investigation for many years, is thought to competitively block the binding of IgE to cell receptors [150].

Omalizumab, a human recombinant non-anaphylactogenic antibody, is directed against the receptor binding domain of IgE. This binding is specific to free IgE, so IgE is unable to interact with the FceRI on the cells, thereby preventing the antibody from attaching to the mast cell [151]. The use of omalizumab may represent an interesting, still not tested, option for the most severe forms of ocular allergy.

Adhesion Molecule Inhibitors

Adhesion molecule inhibitors may have a role in the treatment of chronic disease with a significant late-phase component, such as VKC or AKC. Natalizumab is a monoclonal antibody to α4-integrin that selectively blocks the VLA-4, which is critical for lymphocytes and eosinophil to adhere to endothelial cells before extravasation [11]. The reported potential side effects of these drugs seem to discourage their use, although, in very severe forms of ocular allergy.

Chemokine Inhibitors

Bertilimumab (CAT-213) is a human IgG4 monoclonal antibody against eotaxin-1, still under development. It is able to inhibit the activation of both the early and late phases of inflammation in murine models of ocular allergy [152].

Immunomodulators

Cyclosporin and Tacrolimus are effective treatments for VKC and AKC [153]. They block cell proliferation and inhibit histamine release from mast cells through the inhibition of calcineurin, a phosphate that plays a key role in the FceRI-mediated exocytosis of pre-formed mediators from mast cell. NFAT, a transcriptor regulator for the production of inflammatory cytokines, is regulated by calcineurin [154, 155]. Cyclosporin and Tacrolimus block the release of NFAT-mediated cytokines from T-lymphocytes and mast cells, reduce eosinophil infiltration and decrease cellular adhesion to the site of inflammation. However treatment with these drugs may be at risk of folliculitis, acne and herpes simplex [156].

References

1. Phipatanakul W. Allergic rhinoconjunctivitis:epidemiology. Immunol. Allergy Clin. North Am., 2005. 25(2): 263–281.
2. Weeke ER. Epidemiology of hay fever and perennial allergic rhinitis. Monogr. Allergy, 1987. 21: 1–20.
3. Foster CS. The pathophysiology of ocular allergy: current thinking. Allergy, 1995. 50(21 Suppl): 6–9; discussion 34–38.
4. Ehlers WH, Donshik PC. Allergic ocular disorders: a spectrum of diseases. Clao J., 1992. 18(2): 117–124.
5. MC Gill JI, Church MK, Anderson DF, Bacon A. Allergic eye disease mechabism. Br. J. Ophthalmol., 1998. 82: 1203–1214.
6. Bielory L. Allergic and immunology disorders of the eye. Part II: ocular allergy. J. Allergy Clin. Immunol., 2000. 106: 1019–1032.
7. Foster C. The pathophysiology of ocular allergy: current thinking. Allergy, 1995. 50: 6–9.
8. Dart JK, Monnickendan M, Prasad J. Perennial allergic conjunctivitis: definition, clinical characteristic and prevalance. A comparison with seasonal allergic conjunctivitis. Trans. Ophthalmol. Soc. UK, 1986. 105: 513–520.
9. Bonini S, Bucci MG et al. Allergen dose response and late symptoms in a human model of ocular allergy. J. Allergy Clin. Immunol., 1990. 86: 869–876.
10. Ono SJ. Allergic conjunctivitis: update on pathophysiology and prospects for future treatment. J. Allergy Clin. Immunol., 2005. 115: 118–122.
11. Ono SJ, Abelson MB. Allergic conjunctivitis: update on pathophysiology and prospects for future treatment. J. Allergy Clin. Immunol., 2005. 115: 118–122.
12. Bonini S, Bonini S, Bucci MG, Berruto A, Adriani E, Balsano F, Allansmith MR. Allergen dose response and late symptoms in a human model of ocular allergy. J. Allergy Clin. Immunol., 1990. 86: 869–876.
13. Bonini S, Bonini S, Lambiase A, Marchi S, Pasqualetti P, Zuccaro O, Rama P, Magrini L, Juhas T, Bucci MG. Vernal keratoconjunctivitis revisited: a case series of 195 patients with long-term follow up. Ophthalmology, 2000. 107(6): 1157–1163.
14. Bonini S, Bonini S, Lambiase A, Magrini L, Rumi C, Del Prete G, Schiavone M, Rotiroti G, Onorati P, Rutella S. Vernal keratoconjunctivitis: a model of 5q cytokine gene cluster disease. Int. Arch. Allergy Immunol., 1995. 107(1–3): 95–98.
15. Bonini S, Coassin M, Aronni S, Lambiase A. Vernal keratoconjunctivitis. Eye, 2004. 18(4): 345–351.
16. Bonini S, Lambiase A, Schiavone M, Centofanti M, Palma LA, Bonini S. Estrogen and progesteron receptors in vernal Keratoconjunctivitis. Ophthalmology, 1995. 102: 1374–1279.

17. Bonini S. Atopic keratoconjunctivitis. Allergy, 2004. 59(78 Suppl): 71–73.
18. Sarac O, Erdener U, Irkec M, Us D, Gungen Y. Tear exotin levels in giant papillary conjunctivitis associated with ocular prosthesis. Ocul. Immunol. Inflamm., 2003. 11: 223–230.
19. Allansmith MR. Vernal conjunctivitis. In: The Eye and Immunology, ed. C.V.M. Company, St. Louis, 1982. pp. 118–124.
20. Bonini S, Lambiase A, Sgrulletta R, Bonini S. Allergic chronic inflammation of the ocular surface in vernal keratoconjunctivitis. Curr. Opin. Allergy Clin. Immunol., 2003. 3(5): 381–387.
21. Bonini S, Pierdomenico R, Bonini S. Levocabastine eye drops in vernal conjunctivitis. Eur. J. Ophthalmol., 1995. 5(4): 283–284.
22. D'Angelo G, Lambiase A, Cortes M, Sgrulletta R, Pasqualetti R, Lamagna A, Bonini S. Preservative-free diclofenac sodium 0.1% for vernal keratoconjunctivitis. Graefes Arch. Clin. Exp. Ophthalmol., 2003. 241(3): 192–195.
23. Bonini S, Magrini A, Rotiroti G, Lambiase A, Tomassini M, Rumi C, Bonini S. The eosinophil and the eye. Allergy, 1997. 52(34 Suppl): 44–47.
24. Allansmith MR, Greiner JV, Baird RS. Number of inflammatory cells in normal conjunctiva. Am. J. Ophthalmol., 1978. 86: 250–259.
25. Allansmith MR, Baird RS, Greiner JV. Vernal conjunctivitis and contact lens-associated giant papillary conjunctivitis compared and contrasted. Am. J. Ophthalmol., 1979. 87: 545–555.
26. Di Gioacchino M, Cavallucci E, Di Sciascio MB, Di Stefano F, Verna N, Lobefalo L, Crudeli C, Volpe AR, Angelucci D, Cuccurullo F, Conti P. Increase in CD45R0 + cells and activated eosinophils in chronic allergic conjunctivitis. Immunobiology, 2000. 201: 541–551.
27. Tai PC, Spry CJF, Peterson C, Venge P, Olsson I. Monoclonal antibodies distinguish between storage and secreted form s of eosinophil cationic protein. Nature, 1984. 309: 182–184.
28. Trocme SD, Kephart GM, Allansmith MR, Bourne WM, Gleich GJ. Conjunctivasl deposition of eosinophil granule major basic protein in vernal keratoconjunctivitis and contact lens associated giant papillary conjunctivitis. Am. J. Ophthalmol., 1989. 108: 57–63.
29. Udell IJ, Gleich GJ, Allansmith MR, Ackerman SJ, Abelson MB. Eosinophil granule major basic protein and Charcot-Leyden crystal protein in human tears. Am. J. Ophthalmol., 1981. 92: 824–828.
30. Leonardi A, Borghesan F, Faggian D, Secchi AG, Plebani M. Eosinophil cationic protein in teras of normal subjects and patients affected by vernal keratoconjunctivitis. Allergy, 1995. 50: 610–613.
31. Montan PG, Van Hage-Hamsten M, Zetterstorm O. Sustained eosinophil cationic protein release into tears after a single high-dose conjunctival allergen challenge. Clin. Exp. Allergy, 1996. 26: 1125–1130.
32. Trocme SD, Hallaberg CK, Gill KS, Gleich GJ, Tyring SK, Brysk MM. Effects of eosinophil granule proteins on human corneal epithelial cell viability and morphology. Invest. Ophthalmol. Vis. Sci., 1997. 38: 593–599.
33. Li Q, Fukuda K, Lu Y, Nakamura Y, Chikama T, Kumagai N, Nishida T. Enhancement by neutrophils of collagen degradation by corneal fibroblast. J. Leukoc. Biol., 2003. 74: 412–419.
34. Trocme SD, Leiferman KM, George T, Bonini S, Foster CS, Smit EE, Sra SK, Grabowski LR, Dohlman CH. Neutrophil and eosinophil participation in atopic and vernal keratoconjunctivitis. Curr. Eye Res., 2003. 26(6): 319–325.
35. Cameron JA. Shield ulcers and plaques of the cornea in vernal keratoconjunctivitis. Ophthalmology, 1995. 102: 985–993.
36. Saitu T, Fukuchi T, Tazawa H, Sakaue F, Sawaguchi S, Iwata K. Histopathology of corneal plaque in vernal keratoconjunctivitis. Jpn. J. Ophthalmol. Soc., 1993. 97: 201–209.
37. Nakajima T, Matsumoto K, Suto H, Tanaka K, Ebisawa M, Tomita H, Yuki K, Katsunuma T, Akasawa A, Hashida R, Sugita Y, Ogawa H, Ra C, Saito H. Gene expression screening of humanamast cels and eosinophil using high-density oligonucleotide probe arrays: abundant expression of major basic protein in mast cells. Blood, 2001. 98: 1127–1134.
38. Rothenberg M. Eosinophilia. N. Engl. J. Med., 1998. 338: 1592–1600.

39. Fernandez HN, Henson PM, Otani A, Hugli TE. Chemotactic response to human C3a and C5a anaphylatoxins. Evaluation of C3a and C5a leukotaxis in vitro and under stimulated in vivo conditions. J. Immunol., 1978. 120: 109–115.

40. Goetzl EJ, Gorman RR. Chemotattic and chemokinetic stimulation of human eosinophil nad neutrophil polymorphonuclear leukocytes by 12-L-Hydroxy-5,8,10-heptadecatrienoic acid (HHT). J. Immunol., 1978. 120: 526–531.

41. Goetzl EJ. mediators of immediate hypersensitivityderived from arachidonic acid. N. Engl. J. Med., 1980. 303: 822–825.

42. Baggiolini M. Chemokines and leukocyte traffic. Nature, 1998. 392: 565–568.

43. Bazan JF, Bacon KB, Hardiman G, Wang W, Soo K, Rossi D, Greaves DR, Zlotkin A, Schall TJ. A new class of membrane vound-chemokine with a CX3C motif. Nature, 1997. 385: 640–644.

44. Dorner B, Muller S, Entshalden F, Schroder JM, Franke P, Kraft R, Friedl P, Clark-Lewis I, Kroczek RA. Purification, structural analysis, and function of natural ATAC, a cytokine secreted by CD8 + T cells. J. Biol. Chem., 1997. 272: 8817–8823.

45. Baggiolini M, Dewald B, Moser B. Human chemokines: an update. Annu. Rev. Immunol., 1997. 15: 675–705.

46. Teran LM, Noso N, Carroll M, Davies DE, Holgate S, Schroder JM. Eosinophil recruitment following allergen challenge is associated with the release of the chemokine RANTES into asthmatic airways. J. Immunol., 1996. 157: 1806–1812.

47. Venge J, Lampinen M, Hakansson L, Rak S, Venge P. Identification of IL-5 and RANTES as the major eosinophil chemoattractants in the asthmatic lung. J. Allergy Clin. Immunol., 1996. 97: 1110–1115.

48. Nagase H, Yamaguci M, Jibiki S, Yamada H, Ohta K, Kawasaki H, Yoshie O, Yamamoto K, Morita Y, Hirai K. Eosinophil chemotaxis by chemokines: a study by a simple photometric assay. Allergy, 1999. 54: 944–950.

49. Sabroe I, Hartnell A, Jopling LA, Bel S, Ponath PD, Pease IE, Collins PD, Williams TJ. Differential regulation of eosinophil chemokine signaling via CCR3 and non-CCR3 pathways. J. Immunol., 1999. 162: 2946–2955.

50. Ochi H, Hirani WM, Yuan Q, Friend DS, Austen KF, Boyce JA. T helper cell type 2 cytokine-mediated comitogenic responses and CCR3 expression during differentiation of human mast cells in vitro. J. Exp. Med., 1999. 190: 267–280.

51. Romagnani P, De Paulis A, Beltrame C, Annunziato F, Dente V, Maggi E, Romagnani S, Marone G. Tryptase-chymasedouble-positive human mast cells express the eotaxin receptor CCR3 and are attracted by CCR3-binding chemokines. Am. J. Pathol., 1999. 155: 1195–1204.

52. Forssmann U, Uguccioni M, Loetscher P, Dahinden CA, Langen H, Thelen M, Baggiolini M. Eotaxin-2, a novel CC chemokine that is selective for the chemokine receptor CCR3, and acts like eotaxin on human eosinophil and basophil leukocytes. J. Exp. Med., 1997. 185: 2171–2176.

53. Uguccioni M, Mackay CR, Ochensberger B, Loetscher P, Rhis S, LaRosa GJ, Rao P, Ponath PD, Baggiolini M, Dahinden CA. High expression of the chemokine receptor CCR3 in human blood basophils. Role in activation by eotaxin, MCP-4, and other chemokines. J. Clin. Invest., 1997. 100: 1137–1143.

54. Sallusto F, Mackay CR, Lanzavecchia A. Selective expression of the eotaxin receptor CCR3 by human T helper 2 cells. Science 1997. 277: 2005–2007.

55. Quackenbush EJ, Wershil BK, Aguirre V, Gutierrez-Ramos JC. Eotaxin modulates myelopoiesis and mast cell development from embryonic hematopoietic progenitors. Blood, 1998. 92: 1887–1897.

56. De Paulis A, Annunziato F, Di Gioia L, Romagnani S, Carfora M, Beltrame C, Marone G, Romagnani P. Expression of the chemokine receptor CCR3 on human mast cells. Int. Arch. Allergy Immunol., 2001. 124: 146–150.

57. Hochstetter R, Dobos G, Kimmig D, Dulkys Y, Kapp A, Elsner J. The CC chemokine receptor 3 CCR3 is functionally expressed on eosinophils but not on neutrophils. Eur. J Immunol., 2000. 30: 2759–2764.

58. Healt H, Qin S, Rao, Wu L, LaRosa G, Kassam N, Ponath PD, Mackay CR. Chemokine receptor usage by human eosinophils. The importance of CCR3 demonstrated using an antagonistic monoclonal antibody. J. Clin. Invest., 1997. 99: 178–184.

59. Kitaura M, Nakajima T, Imai T, Harada S, Combadiere C, Tiffany HL, Murphy PM, Yoshie O. Molecular cloning of human eotaxin, an eosinophil selective CC chemokin, an identification of a specific eosinophil eotaxin receptor, CC chemokine receptor 3. J. Biol. Chem., 1996. 271: 7725–7730.

60. Ponath PD, Qin S, Post TW, Wang J, Wu L, Gerrard NP, Newman W, Gerard C, Mackay CR. Molecular cloning characterization of a human eotaxin receptor expressed selectivity on eosinophils. J. Exp. Med., 1996. 183: 2437–2448.

61. Daugherty BL, Siciliano SJ, DeMartino JA, Malkowitz L, Sirotina A, Springer MS. Cloning, expression, and characterization of the human eosinophil eotaxin receptor. J. Exp. Med., 1996. 183: 2349–2354.

62. Conroy DM, Williams TJ. Eotaxin and the attraction of eosinophils to the asthmatic lung. Respir. Res., 2001. 2(3): 150–156.

63. Maggi E, Biswas P, Del Prete G, Parronchi P, Macchia D, Simonelli C, Emmi L, De Carli M, Tiri A, Ricci M et al., Accumulation of Th-2-like helper T cells in the conjunctiva of patients with vernal conjunctivitis. J. Immunol., 1991. 146: 1169–1174.

64. Leonardi A, DeFranchis G, Zancanaro F, Crivellari G, De Paoli M, Plebani M, Secchi AG. Identification of local Th2 and Th0 lymphocytes in vernal conjunctivitis by cytokine flow cytometry. Invest. Ophthalmol. Vis. Sci., 1999. 40: 3036–3040.

65. Kumagai N, Fukuda K, Ishimura Y, Nishida T. Synergistic induction of eotaxin expression in human keratocytes by TNF-a and IL-4 or IL-13. Invest. Ophthalmol. Vis. Sci., 2000. 41: 1448–1453.

66. Fukuda K, kumagai N, Fujitsu Y, Nishida T. Fibroblasts as local immune modulators in ocular allergic disease. Allergol. Int., 2006. 55(2): 121–129.

67. Leonardi A, Borghesan F, De Paoli M, Plebani M, Secchi AG. Procollagens and inflammatory cytokine concentrations in tarsal and limbal vernal keratoconjunctivitis. Exp. Eye Res., 1998. 67: 105–112.

68. Leonardi A, Brun P, Tavolato M, Plebani M, Abatangelo G, Secchi AG. Tumor necrosis factor-alpha (TNF-a) in seasonal allergic conjunctivitis and vernal keratoconjunctivitis. Eur. J. Ophthalmol., 2003. 16: 606–610.

69. Fujishima H, Takeuchi T, Shinozaki N, Saito I, Tsubota K. Measurement of IL-4 in tears of patients with seasonal allergic conjunctivitis and vernal keratoconjunctivitis. Clin. Exp. Immunol., 1995. 102: 395–398.

70. Yokoi K, Yokoi N, Kinoshita S. Impairment of ocular surface epithelium barrier function in patients with atopic dermatitis. Br. J. Ophthalmol., 1998. 82: 797–800.

71. Cubitt CL, Tang Q, Monteiro CA, Lausch RN, Oakes JE. IL-8 gene expression in cultures of human corneal epithelial cells and keratocytes. Invest. Ophthalmol. Vis. Sci., 1993. 34: 3199–3206.

72. Barton K, Monroy DC, Nava A, Pflugfelder SC. Inflammatory cytokines in the tears of patients with ocular rosacea. Ophthalmology, 1997. 104: 1868–1874.

73. Vesaluoma M, Teppo AM, Gronhagen-Riska C, Tervo T. Increased release of tumour necrosis factor-a in human tear fluid after excimer laser induced corneal wound. Br. J. Ophthalmol., 1997. 81: 145–149.

74. Nakajima H, Sano H, Nishimura T, Yoshida S, Iwamoto I. Role of vascular cell adhesion molecule 1/very late activation antigen 4 and intercellular adhesion molecule 1/lymphocyte function-associated antigen 1 interactions in antigen-induced eosinophil and T cell recruitment into the tissue. J. Exp. Med., 1994. 179: 1145–1154.

75. Ebihara N, Yokoyama T, Kimura T, Nakayasu K, Okumura K, Kanai A, Ra C. Anti VLA-4 monoclonal antibody inhibits eosinophil infiltration in allergic conjunctivitis model of guinea pig. Curr. Eye Res., 1999. 19: 20–25.

76. Kumagai N, Fukuda K, Fujitsu Y, Nishida T. Expression of functional ICAM-1 on cultured human keratocytes induced by tumor necrosis factor-alpha. Jpn. J. Ophthalmol., 2003. 47(2): 134–141.

77. Kumagai N, Fukuda K, Fujitsu Y, Nishida T. Synergistic effect of TNF-a and either IL-4 or IL-13 on VCAM-1 expression by cultured human corneal fibroblasts. Cornea, 2003. 22: 557–561.

78. Meerschaert J, Vrtis RF, Shikama Y, Sedgwick JB, Busse WW, Mosher DF. Engagement of a4b7 integrins by monoclonal antibodies or ligands enhances survival of human eosinophils in vitro. J. Immunol., 1999. 163: 6217–6227.

79. Nagata M, Sedgwick JB, Vrtis R, Busse WW. Endothelial cells upregulate eosinophil superoxide generation via VCAM-1 expression. Clin. Exp. Allergy, 1999. 29: 550–561.

80. Tsuruta R, Cobb RR, Mastrangelo M, Lazarides E, Cardarelli PM. Soluble vascular cell adhesion molecule (VCAM)-Fc fusion protein induces leukotriene C4 secretion in platelet-activating factor-stimulated eosinophils. J. Leukoc. Biol., 1999. 65: 71–79.

81. Wynn TA. IL-13 effector functions. Annu. Rev. Immunol., 2003. 21: 425–456.

82. Gauchat JF, Lebman DA, Coffman RL, Gascan H, de Vries JE. Structure and expression of germline e transcripts in human B cells induced by interleukin 4 to switch to IgE production. J. Exp. Med., 1990. 172: 463–473.

83. Vita, N, Lefort S, Laurent P, Caput D, Ferrara P. Characterization and comparison of the interleukin 13 receptor with the interleukin 4 receptor on several cell types. J. Biol. Chem., 1995. 270: 3512–3517.

84. Schnyder B, Lugli S, Feng N, Etter H, Lutz RA, Ryffel B, Sugamura K, Wunderli-Allenspach H, Moser R. Interleukin-4 (IL-4) and IL-13 bind to a shared heterodimeric complex on endothelial cells mediating vascular cell adhesion molecule-1 induction in the absence of the common g chain. Blood, 1996. 87: 4286–4295.

85. Doucet C, Brouty-Boye D, Pottin-Clemenceau C, Jasmin C, Canonica GW, Azzarone B. IL-4 and IL-13 specifically increase adhesion molecule and inflammatory cytokine expression in human lung fibroblasts. Int. Immunol., 1998. 10: 1421–1433.

86. Van der Velden VHJ, Naber BAE, Wierenga-Wolf AF, Debets R, Savelkoul HFJ, Overbeek SE, Hoogsteden HC, Versnel MA. Interleukin 4 receptors on human bronchial epithelial cells. An in vivo and in vitro analysis of expression and function. Cytokine, 1998. 10: 803–813.

87. Lai SY, Molden J, Liu KD, Puck JM, White MD, Goldsmith MA. Interleukin-4-specific signal transduction events are driven by homotypic interactions of the interleukin-4 receptor a subunit. EMBO J., 1996. 15: 4506–4514.

88. Fujiwara H, Hanissian SH, Tsytsykova A, Geha RS. Homodimerization of the human interleukin 4 receptor a chain induces Ce germline transcripts in B cells in the absence of the interleukin 2 receptor g chain. Proc. Natl. Acad. Sci. USA, 1997. 94: 5866–5871.

89. Reichel M, Nelson BH, Greenberg PD, Rothman PB. The IL-4 receptor a-chain cytoplasmic domain is sufficient for activation of JAK-1 and STAT6 and the induction of IL-4-specific gene expression. J. Immunol., 1997. 158: 5860–5867.

90. Harada N, Higuchi K, Wakao H, Hamasaki N, Izuhara K. Identification of the critical portions of the human IL-4 receptor a chain for activation of STAT6. Biochem. Biophys. Res. Commun., 1998. 246: 675–680.

91. Matsukura S, Stellato C, Plitt JR, Bickel C, Miura K, Georas SN, Casolaro V, Schleimer RP. Activation of eotaxin gene transcription by NF-k B and STAT6 in human airway epithelial cells. J. Immunol., 1999. 163: 6876–6883.

92. Kaplan MH, Schindler U, Smiley ST, Grusby MJ. Stat6 is required for mediating responses to IL-4 and for the development of Th2 cells. Immunity, 1996. 4: 313–319.

93. Takeda K, Tanaka T, Shi W, Matsumoto M, Minami M, Kashiwamura S, Nakanishi K, Yoshida N, Kishimoto T, Akira S. Essential role of Stat6 in IL-4 signalling. Nature 1996. 380: 627–630.

94. Abu El-Asrar AM, Struyf S, AL-Kharashi SA, Missotten L, Van Damme J, Geboes K. Chemokines in the limbal form of vernal keratoconjunctivitis. Br. J. Ophthalmol., 2000. 84: 1360–1366.

95. Abu El-Asrar AM, Struyf S, AL-Kharashi SA, Missotten L, Van Damme J, Geboes K. The T-lymphocyte chemoattractant Mig is Higly expressed in vernal keratoconjunctivitis. Am. J. Ophthalmol., 2003. 136: 853–860.

96. Fujitsu Y, Fukuda K, Kimura K, Seki K, Kumagai N, Nishida T. Protection of human conjunctival fibroblasts from No indiced apoptosis by interleukin-4 or interleukin-13. Invest. Ophthalmol. Vis. Sci., 2005. 46: 797–802.

97. Leonardi A, Borghesan F, DePaoli M, Plebani M, Secchi AG. Tear and serum soluble leukocyte activation markers in conjunctival allergic diseases. Am. J. Ophthalmol., 2000. 129: 151–158.

98. Trocme SD, Aldave AJ. The eye and the eosinophil. Surv. Ophthalmol., 1994. 39: 241–252.

99. Leonardi A, Fregona IA, Plebani M, Secchi AG, Calder VL. Th1- and Th2-type cytokines in chronic ocular allergy. Graefes Arch. Clin. Exp. Ophthalmol., 2006. 244(10): 1240–1245.

100. Stern ME, Siemasko KF, Niederkorn JY. The Th1/Th2 paradigm in ocular allergy. Curr. Opin. Allergy Clin. Immunol., 2005. 5(5): 446–450.

101. Matsura N, Uchio E, Nakazawa M, Yago T, Matsumoto S, Ohno S, Minami M. Predominance of infiltrating IL-4producing T cells in conjunctiva of patients with allergic conjunctival disease. Curr. Eye Res., 2004. 29: 235–243.

102. Abbas A, Murphy KM, Sher A. Functional diversity of helper T lymphocytes. Nature 1996. 383: 787–793.

103. Coffman R, Seymour BW, Lebman DA, Hiraki DD, Christiansen JA, Shrader B, Cherwinski HM, Savelkoul HF, Finkelman FD, Bond MW. The role of helper T cell products in mouse B cell differentiation and isotype regulation. Immunol. Rev., 1988. 102 5–28.

104. Larche' M, Robinson DS, Kay AB. The role of T lymphocytes in the pathogenesis of asthma. J. Allergy Clin. Immunol., 2003. 111: 450–463.

105. Zhan H, Towler HM, Calder VL. The immunomodulatory role of human conjunctival epithelial cells. Invest. Ophthalmol. Vis. Sci., 2003. 44: 3906–3910.

106. Parr M, Parr EL. Interferon-gamma up-regulates intracellular adhesion molecule-1 and vascular cell adhesion molecule-1 and recruits lymphocytes into the vagina of immune mice challenged with herpes simplex virus-2. Immunology, 2000. 99: 540–545.

107. Parr M, Parr EL. Immunity to vaginal herpes simplex virus-2 infection in B-cell knockout mice. Immunology, 2000. 101(1): 126–131.

108. Leonardi A, Curnow SJ, Zhan H, Calder VL. Multiple cytokines in human tear specimens in seasonal and chronic allergic eye disease and in conjunctival fibroblast cultures. Clin. Exp. Allergy, 2006. 36(6): 777–784.

109. Trocme SD, Hallberg CK, Gill KS, Gleich GJ, Tyring SK, Brysk MM. Effects of eosinophil granule proteins on human corneal epithelial cell viability and morphology. Invest. Ophthalmol. Vis. Sci., 1997. 38(3): 593–599.

110. Teran LM, Mochizuki M, Bartels J, Valencia EL, Nakajima T, Hirai K, Schroeder JM. Th1- and Th2-type cytokines regulate the expression and production of eotaxin and RANTES by human lung fibroblasts. Am. J. Respir. Cell Mol. Biol., 1999. 20: 777–786.

111. Smith RS, Smith TJ, Blieden TM, Phipps RP. Fibroblasts as sentinel cells. Synthesis of chemokines and regulation of inflammation. Am. J. Pathol., 1997. 151: 317–322.

112. Kumagai N, Fukuda K, Fujitsu Y, Yamamoto K, Nishida T. Role of structural cells of the cornea and conjunctiva in the pathogenesis of vernal keratoconjunctivitis. Prog. Retin. Eye Res., 2006. 25(2): 165–187.

113. Imai T, Baba M, Nishimura M, Kakizaki M, Takagi S, Yoshie O. The T cell-directed CC chemokine TARC is a highly specific biological ligand for CC chemokine receptor 4. J. Biol. Chem., 1997. 272: 15036–15042.

114. Imai T, Chantry D, Raport CJ, Wood CL, Nishimura M, Godiska R, Yoshie O, Gray PW. Macrophage-derived chemokine is a functional ligand for the CC chemokine receptor 4. J. Biol. Chem., 1998. 273: 1764–1768.

115. Sallusto F, Lenig D, Mackay CR, Lanzavecchia A. Flexible programs of chemokine receptor expression on human polarized T helper 1 and 2 lymphocytes. J. Exp. Med., 1998. 187: 875–883.

116. Bonecchi R, Bianchi G, Bordignon PP, D'Ambrosio D, Lang R, Borsatti A, Sozzani S, Allavena P, Gray PA, Mantovani A, Sinigaglia F. Differential expression of chemokine

receptors and chemotactic responsiveness of type 1 T helper cells (Th1s) and Th2s. J. Exp. Med., 1998. 187: 129–134.

117. Fini ME, Parks WC, Rinehart WB, Girard MT, Matsubara M, Cook JR, West-Mays JA, Sadow PM, Burgeson RE, Jeffrey JJ, Raizman MB, Krueger RR, Zieske JD. Role of matrix metalloproteinases in failure to re-epithelialize after corneal injury. Am. J. Pathol., 1996. 149: 1287–1302.

118. Fukuda K, Chikama T, Nakamura M, Nishida T. Differential distribution of subchains of the basement membrane components type IV collagen and laminin among the amniotic membrane, cornea, and conjunctiva. Cornea, 1999. 18: 73–79.

119. Ryan ME, Ramamurthy NS, Sorsa T, Golub LM. MMP-mediated events in diabetes. Ann. NY Acad. Sci., 1999. 878: 311–334.

120. Leonardi A, Abatangelo G, Cortivo R, Secchi AG. Collagen types I and III in giant papillae of vernal keratoconjunctivitis. Br. J. Ophthalmol., 1995. 79: 482–485.

121. Vaday GG, Franitza S, Schor H, Hecht I, Brill A, Cahalon L, Hershkoviz R, Lider O. Combinatorial signals by inflammatory cytokines and chemokines mediate leukocyte interactions with extracellular matrix. J. Leukoc. Biol., 2001. 69: 885–892.

122. Medzhitov R, Janeway C. Jr. Innate immune recognition: mechanisms and pathways. Immunol. Rev., 2000. 173: 89–97.

123. Beutler B. Inferences, questions and possibilities in Toll-like receptor signalling. Nature, 2004. 430(6996): 257–263.

124. Micera A, Stampachiacchiere B, Aronni S, Dos Santos MS, Lambiase A. Toll-like receptors and the eye. Curr. Opin. Allergy Clin. Immunol., 2005. 5(5): 451–458.

125. Elson CO, Cong Y. Understanding immune-microbial homeostasis in intestine. Immunol. Res., 2002. 26(1–3): 87–94.

126. Song PI, Abraham TA, Park Y, Zivony AS, Harten B, Edelhauser HF, Ward SL, Armstrong CA, Ansel JC. The expression of functional LPS receptor proteins CD14 and toll-like receptor 4 in human corneal cells. Invest. Ophthalmol. Vis. Sci., 2001. 42(12): 2867–2877.

127. Ueta M, Nochi T, Jang MH, Park EJ, Igarashi O, Hino A, Kawasaki S, Shikina T, Hiroi T, Kinoshita S, Kiyono K. Intracellularly expressed TLR2s and TLR4s contribution to an immunosilent environment at the ocular mucosal epithelium. J. Immunol., 2004. 173(5): 3337–3347.

128. Kumagai N, Fukuda K, Fujitsu Y, Lu Y, Chikamoto N, Nishida T. Lipopolysaccharide-induced expression of intercellular adhesion molecule-1 and chemokines in cultured human corneal fibroblasts. Invest. Ophthalmol. Vis. Sci., 2005. 46(1): 114–120.

129. Bonini S, Micera A, Iovieno A, Lambiase A, Bonini S. Expression of Toll-like receptors in healthy and allergic conjunctiva. Ophthalmology, 2005. 112(9): 1528; discussion 1548–1549.

130. Miyazaki D, Liu G, Clark L, Ono SJ. Prevention of acute allergic conjunctivitis and late-phase inflammation with immunostimulatory DNA sequences. Invest. Ophthalmol. Vis. Sci., 2000. 41(12): 3850–3855.

131. Lawton JA, Ghosh P. Novel therapeutic strategies based on toll-like receptor signaling. Curr. Opin. Chem. Biol., 2003. 7(4): 446–451.

132. Bellou A, Schaub B, Ting L, Finn PW. Toll receptors modulate allergic responses:interaction with dendritic cells, T cells and mast cells. Curr. Opin. Allergy Clin. Immunol., 2003 3(6): 487–494.

133. Abelson MB, Schaefer K, Wun PJ. Antihistamines and anthistamine\vasocostrictors combinations. In: Allergic Diseases of the Eye, ed. W.S. Co., Philadelphia, PA, 2001. pp. 206–214.

134. Yanni JM, Sharif NA, Gamache DA, Miller ST, Weimer LK, Spellman JM. A current appreciation of sites for pharmacological intervention in allergic conjunctivitis. Acta Ophthalmol., 1999. 77: 33–37.

135. Leonardi A, DeFranchis G, DePaoli M, Fregona IA, Plebani M, Secchi AG, 2002. Curr. Eye Res., 2002. 25: 189–196.

136. Bielory L, Lien KW, Bigelsen S. Efficacy and tolerability of newer anthistamines in the treatment of allergic conjunctivis. Drugs, 2005. 65: 215–228.
137. Yanni JM, Miller ST, Gamache DA, Spellman JM, Xu S, Sherif NA. Comparative effects of topical ocular anti-allergy drugs on human conjunctival mast cells. Ann. Allergy Asthma Immunol., 1997. 79: 541–545.
138. Cerqueti PM, Ricca V, Tosca MA, Buscaglia S, Ciprandi G. Lodoxamide treatment of allergic conjunctivitis. Int. Arch. Allergy Immunol., 1994. 105: 185–189.
139. Gunduz K, Ucakhan O, Budan K, Eryilmaz T, Ozkan M. Efficacy of lodoxamide 0.1% versus N-Acetyl aspartyl glutamic acid 6% ophthalmic solutions in patients with Vernal Keratoconjunctivitis. Ophthalmic Res., 1996. 28: 80–87.
140. Abelson MB, Berdy GJ, Mundrof T, Amadahl LD, Graves AL. Pemirolast study group. Pemirolast potassium 0.1% ophthalmic solution is an effective treatment for allergic conjunctivitis: a pooled analysis of two prospective, randomized, double-masked, placebo-controled, phase III studies. J. Ocul. Pharmacol. Ther., 2002. 18: 475–488.
141. Denis D, Bloch-Michel E, Verin P, Sebastiani A, Tazartes M, Helleboid L, Di Giovanni A, Lecorvec M. Treatment of common ocular allergic disorders; a comparison of lodoxamide and NAAGA. Br. J. Ophthalmol., 1998. 82(10): 1135–1138.
142. Abelson MB. A review of Olopatadine for the treatment of ocular allergy. Expert. Opin. Pharmacother., 2004. 5: 1979–1994.
143. Abelson MB, Ferzola NJ, McWirther CL Crampton HJ. Efficacy and safety of single- and multiple-dose ketotifen fumarate 0.025% ophthalmic solution in a pediatric population. Pediatr. Allergy Immunol., 2004. 15(6): 551–557.
144. Crampton HJ. A comparison of the relative clinical efficacy of a single dose of ketotifen fumarate 0.025% ophthalmic solution versus placebo in inhibiting the signs and symptoms of allergic rhinoconjunctivitis as induced by the conjunctival allergen challenge model. Clin. Ther., 2002. 24(11): 1800–1808.
145. Ciprandi G, Buscaglia S, Catrullo A, Pesce G, Fiorino M, Montagna P, Bagnasco M, canonica GW. Azelastine eye drops reduce and prevent conjunctival reaction and exert anti-allergic activity. Clin. Exp. Allergy, 1997. 27: 182–191.
146. Fraunfelder FW. Epinastine hydrochloride for atopic disease. Drugs Today, 2004. 40: 677–683.
147. Deschenes J, Discepola M, Abelson MB. Comparative evaluation of olopatadine solution (0.1%) versus ketorolac ophthalmic solution (0.5%) using the provocative antigen challenge model. Acta Ophthalmol. Scand., 1999. 77: 47–52.
148. Tabbara KF, al-Kharashi SA. Efficacy of nedocromil 2% versus fluorometholone 0.1%: a randomised, double masked trial comparing the effects on severe vernal keratoconjunctivitis. Br. J. Ophthalmol., 1999. 83(2): 180–184.
149. Lambiase A, Bonini S, Rasi G, Coassin M, Bruscolini A, Bonini S. Montelukast, a leukotriene receptor antagonist, in vernal keratoconjunctivitis associated with asthma. Arch. Ophthalmol., 2003. 121: 615–620.
150. Kalpaxis JG, Thayer TO. Double-blind trial of pentigetide ophthalmic solution, 0.5%, compared with cromolyn sodium, 4%, ophthalmic solution for allergic conjunctivitis. Ann. Allergy 1991. 66: 393–398.
151. Babu KS, Arshad SH, Holgate ST. Omalizumab, a novel anti-IgE therapy in allergic disorders. Expert. Opin. Biol. Ther., 2001. 1: 1049–1058.
152. Soler M. Omalizumab, a monoclonal antibody against IgEfor the treatment of allergic diseases. Int. J. Clin. Pract., 2001. 55(7): 480–483.
153. Ito F, Toyota N, Sakai H et al. FK506 and Cyclosporin A inhibit stem cell factor-dependent cell proliferation\survival, while inducing upregulation of c-kit expression in cells of mast cells line MC\9. Arch. Dermatol. Res., 1999. 291: 275–283.
154. Ito F, Toyota F, Sakai H, Takahashi H, Izuka H. FK506 and cyclosporin A inhibit stem cell factor-dependent cell proliferation/survival, while inducing upregulation of c-kit expression in cells of the mast cell line MC/9. Arch. Dermatol. Res., 1999. 291(5): 275–283.

155. Toyota N, Hashimoto Y, Matsuo S, Kitamura Y, Izuka H. Effects of FK506 and cyclosporin A on proliferation, histamine release and phenotype of murine mast cells. Arch. Dermatol. Res., 1996. 288(8): 474–480.
156. Matsuda S, Koyasu S. Mechanism of action of cyclosporin. Immunopharmacology, 2000. 47: 119–125.

Non-allergic Rhinitis

Glenis K. Scadding

Introduction

Rhinitis implies inflammation of the lining of the nose and is characterized by nasal running, itching, sneezing and blocking. Rhinitis can be categorized as in the ARIA document (Fig. 1), as allergic, infectious or arising from a multiplicity of other causes [1]. In practice some 80% of childhood rhinitis is allergic, but only one-third of adult rhinitis falls into this category [2].

Non-allergic rhinitis encompasses a variety of conditions in which there is no evidence of a systemic IgE-mediated inflammatory mechanism. Significantly less research has been undertaken in this area compared with allergic rhinitis and disease mechanisms are largely unknown. However there appears to be a division into inflammatory eosinophil – rich, non-allergic rhinitis (e.g., non-allergic rhinitis with eosinophilia syndrome, NARES and aspirin hypersensitivity) and non-inflammatory forms. The diagnosis is based on the exclusion of an allergic cause, with subsequent elimination of other known causes of rhinitis, leaving a proportion of up to 60%, that is, 36% [3] of all rhinitis sufferers, with an unknown disease pathway, called "idiopathic rhinitis". The terminology "vasomotor rhinitis" has been used to describe this condition because of the hyper-responsiveness of the nasal mucosa to various stimuli, but this must be abandoned, because vascular changes are not implicated and similar hyper-responsiveness also occurs in allergic rhinitis and in non-allergic rhinitis with eosinophilia (NARES). Most patients with idiopathic rhinitis are adult, female, and have persistent symptoms. Itching is usually absent, but hyposmia may occur.

In clinical practice mixed forms of rhinitis such as allergy plus infection or allergy together with non-inflammatory rhinitis are also found.

G.K. Scadding (✉)
Consultant Allergist and Rhinologist, Royal National TNE Hospital, London, UK
e-mail: g.scadding@ucl.ac.uk

R. Pawankar et al. (eds.), *Allergy Frontiers: Clinical Manifestations*,
DOI: 10.1007/978-4-431-88317-3_3, © Springer 2009

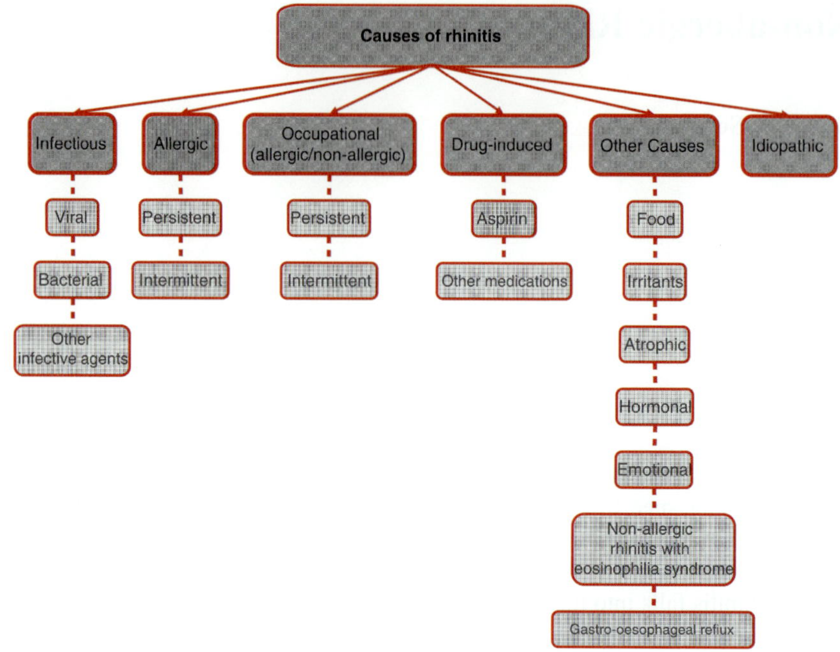

Fig. 1 ARIA classification of rhinitis

Local Allergic Rhinitis

In allergic rhinitis the immediate reaction results from mast cell degranulation, and mediator release is rapid and obvious. The late-phase reaction involves inflammation, with eosinophils predominant. This may be less obvious, as the major symptom is nasal blockage with decreased olfaction and hyper-reactivity of the mucosa, sometimes misdiagnosed as "vasomotor" rhinitis.

Allergic rhinitis is distinguished by the production of IgE against various allergens. The diagnosis rests upon an appropriate history, with confirmation of allergen sensitivity by related skin prick tests or serum-specific IgE.

Some studies indicate that in some skin prick test – negative rhinitis patients allergen – specific IgE is involved, but remains localised in the nasal mucosa. Powe [3] has reviewed the evidence for this, which falls into four categories (Table 1), and has coined a name "entopy". Although not yet generally accepted, the response of such patients to allergen avoidance and topical corticosteroid and the transient existence of a similar phenomenon in children in the early phase of allergic rhinitis (Scadding GK, 1996), suggest that it is a valid concept. To absolutely confirm or refute an allergy diagnosis in a skin prick test – negative patient, therefore – either measurement of IgE in nasal secretions or a positive nasal allergen challenge test is necessary (Fig. 2).

Table 1 Evidence for local IgE in the nose

1. Detection of allergen-specific IgE in nasal secretions [66]
2. Allergen provocation leading to rhinitis symptoms or to associated physiological changes [67, 68]
3. Immunohistology demonstrating mast cells and tryptase [69, 70], or local IgE heavy chain, IL-4, IL-13 [71–73]
4. Binding of specific allergen to non-atopic nasal mucosa [74]

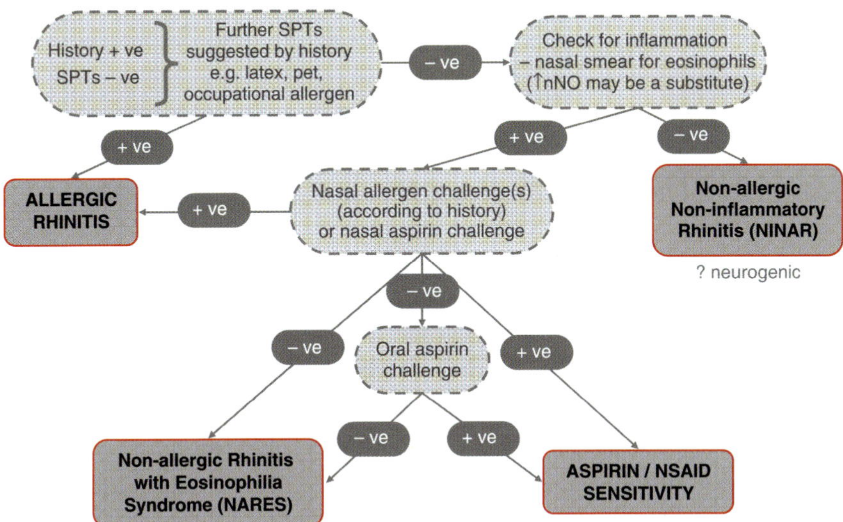

Fig. 2 Further investigation of rhinitis

Non-allergic Non-infectious Eosinophilic Rhinitis (NARES)

NARES was first described by Jacobs [4]. It occurs in roughly a third of patients (mostly adult women) with non-allergic rhinitis. It is characterized by perennial symptoms with paroxysmal episodes when nasal eosinophilia up to 25% can be detected, although some authors quote 5% as sufficient for this diagnosis [5]. The symptoms are sneezing, itching and nasal blockage, rhinorrhoea and occasional hyposmia. The precipitating factors are often nonspecific irritants, weather changes or strong odors. Paediatric NARES has been reported [6], but it is uncertain whether the negative skin prick tests are a permanent feature of the children described or whether they have had local IgE production as a stage in the development of allergic rhinitis.

NARES may be the result of local IgE production, as nasal challenges are abnormal in 50% of patients and mast cells and IgE positive cells can be demonstrated in the nasal epithelium. Approximately 50% of patients suffer from bronchial hyperreactivity and develop asthma and nasal polyposis later in life, sometimes together with Aspirin/NSAID intolerance. NARES may be the early stage of aspirin intolerance, which is associated with nasal polyposis and asthma (Samter's triad) and characterized by intense eosinophilia and high tissue IL-5 levels, but no IL-4 elevation [7]. Polyclonal IgE may be found locally in high levels in polyp tissues, probably related to Staphylococcal stimulation of non-antigen specific T cell receptors [8]. Hyper-reactivity of the nasal mucosa is common.

Nasal eosinophilia denotes a good response to nasal steroids. Responsiveness to antihistamines, cromones and montelukast have also been noted [9–11].

Blood eosinophilia non-allergic rhinitis syndrome (BENARES) is an associated disorder with high levels of blood eosinophils in conjunction with the features of NARES [5]. This disorder is thought to account for 4% of those with non-allergic rhinitis.

Basophilic/Metachromatic Nasal Disease

Nasal mastocytosis/Basophilic/Metachromatic nasal disease requires a histological diagnosis [2]. The condition is characterized by mast cell infiltration (more than 2,000 per cm) without nasal eosinophilia. Patients present with rhinorrhoea and nasal congestion without associated pruritis or sneezing. The aetiology is unknown.

Infectious Rhinitis

Viruses

Rhinovirus [12], influenza and para-influenza viruses are the most common causes of the common cold that affects millions of people each year. Children average 6–8 viral colds per year; however, these usually resolve within 7–10 days [13]. Sinusitis can be seen on CT scans taken during the common cold, and these changes persist for about 6 weeks [14, 15]. Nasal secretions may be purulent, but this does not necessarily imply bacterial superinfection. Oedema of the nasal mucosa can lead to occlusion of the sinuses at the osteomeatal complex causing sinusitis, which produces facial pain and/or eustachian tube dysfunction, and 0.5–2% of the viral upper airway infections progress to an acute bacterial form. This can also occasionally occur de novo.

Bacteria

Acute bacterial infections produce nasal obstruction, facial pain and crusting, often together with fever [16]. Acute rhinosinusitis can progress to a chronic form, which is thought to affect around 15% of the US population. It remarkably affects the quality of life, school and workplace attendance and performance. Streptococcus pneumoniae, Haemophilus influenzae and Moraxella Catarrhalis, Staphylococcus Aureus and occasionally anaerobic bacteria can be involved. Most of these bacteria have outer layers of carbohydrate, which enables them to resist the clearance mechanisms [17]. There is evidence of a bacterial biofilm formation in chronic rhinosinusitis, summarized recently [18].

Patients suffering from a primary mucociliary defect are particularly prone to upper respiratory tract infections [19].

Fungi and Other Opportunistic Infections

Fungi are found in all noses as they are present in respired air, but do not usually elicit untoward effects.

However moulds and fungi can be involved in both infective and allergic processes in the nose and sinuses.

Immunodeficient patients, such as those affected by HIV, can suffer fungal, mycobacterial and other opportunistic infections. There may be a co-existent allergic component, as the gp120 HIV coat protein stimulates the IgE production [20, 21].

Allergic fungal sinusitis, for which there are strict diagnostic criteria [22], is rare in temperate climates. The concept that all forms of chronic rhinosinusitis have an underlying fungal aetiology has been proposed, but clinical and microarray evidence suggests [23, 24] that eosinophilic mucus rhinosinusitis is a separate entity. Controlled trials of antifungal douching have proved negative in chronic rhinosinusitis [25, 26].

Occupational Rhinitis

This is characterized by sneezing, nasal discharge and/or congestion in response to airborne substances in the workplace [27]. It is a poorly researched area despite the fact that many occupations are involved, with new reports of problems appearing regularly [28–31]. Two forms are recognized. For one, high molecular weight agents in the urine and saliva of laboratory animals (guinea pigs, rats, mice, rabbits), in vegetable products, grains (flour) in mites and moulds (antibiotics), spores and enzymes act as allergens inducing a Type 1 mediated reaction. This allergic occupational rhinitis usually precedes or is coincidental with occupational asthma.

There is also a non-allergic form in which low molecular weight substances such as isocyanates, pine resins and acid anhydrides can act either as haptens or can operate through non-IgE mediated mechanisms. Triggering factors such as smoke, formaldehyde, cold air, ammonia, sulphur dioxide, glues and solvents are irritants and can act as adjuvants by damaging the nasal epithelium and inciting inflammatory mediator production.

The diagnosis is based on specific provocation tests [32]. Symptoms improve with avoidance, although if the exposure has been greater than a few months, long-term inhaled corticosteroids may be necessary for intractable asthma. Occupational airway disorders are a common cause of work absence and job loss [33].

Rhinitis in the Elderly

This has not been explored in detail. Changes in the nose because of aging include structural, hormonal, mucosal, olfactory and neural effects. The effects of polypharmacy may contribute to congestion and dryness [34].

There is however a characteristic clinical picture of an elderly male patient with persistent clear rhinorrhoea without other nasal symptoms. Patients often complain of the classical drip on the tip of the nose. Previously treatment with testosterone was helpful, but now ipratropium bromide nasal spray, an anti-cholinergic, is used with benefit in many patients. Autonomic dysfunction with parasympathetic overactivity is the probable pathomechanism for this form of rhinitis, but may also be relevant to idiopathic rhinitis in other patients, including those with chronic fatigue syndrome [35–37].

Gustatory or Food Related Rhinitis

There are multiple mechanisms accounting for rhinitis occurring after food or alcohol ingestion. IgE-mediated food allergy does not usually cause isolated rhinitis, but can be seen associated with gastrointestinal, dermatologic or systemic reactions.

Spicy foods cause rhinorrhoea probably via their capsaicin content, which stimulates sensory nerve fibres. Other possible aetiologies include vagally mediated mechanisms and nasal vasodilatation.

Additives and preservatives such as sulphites can predominantly provoke rhinitis symptoms in patients with pre-existing nasal hyper-reactivity, predominantly in those with aspirin hypersensitivity [38, 39]. The mechanism is unknown, but may involve non-IgE-mediated mast cell degranulation.

Drug-Induced Rhinitis

Due to Known Pharmacological Action

Beta blockers, ACE inhibitors and chlorpromazine can cause a congestive form of rhinitis, which depends on the pharmacological vasodilator action of these drugs. Rhinitis medicamentosa [40] consists of chronic nasal blockage because of a rebound effect following the chronic use of nasal alpha-adrenoceptor antagonists (vasoconstrictors) such as Xylometazoline or Oxymetazoline. Cocaine abuse can trigger rhinorrhoea, reduced olfaction and septal perforation via intense vasoconstriction.

Due to Idiosyncratic Hypersensitivity

Aspirin and NSAIDs are common triggers of rhinitis, asthma and nasal polyps. The mechanism is complex, but is thought to involve mast cell degranulation, not via IgE, excessive leukotriene production (because aspirin and NSAIDs inhibit cyclooxygenase 1 and in some patients leukotriene C4 synthase is raised by a gene promoter), upregulation of leukotriene receptors, and downregulation of prostaglandin production and E2 receptors [41–43]. Eosinophilia is usually present in nasal secretions and sometimes in blood.

The diagnosis is made by aspirin challenge [44], which can be nasal, bronchial or oral. In respiratory tract lysine aspirin, the only truly soluble form of aspirin is employed at gradually increasing concentrations until a positive response occurs. If a nasal challenge is negative then an oral challenge must follow.

Aspirin desensitization, either oral or topical has been shown to reduce symptoms and improve progress including the need for hospitalisation in asthma and for surgical treatment of polyps [45, 46].

Treatment is with topical nasal corticosteroids [16]. Leukotriene antagonists may also be beneficial in some patients with aspirin sensitivity [11]. Most aspirin sensitive individuals can tolerate Cox-2 inhibitors, but the initial dose must be given under observation [47].

Hormonal Rhinitis

Nasal congestion occurs in conjunction with the rise in serum oestrogens that occur at ovulation in the normal menstrual cycle [48]. High circulating levels of oestrogen may be associated with rhinitis symptoms.

In the last trimester of pregnancy nasal blockage or congestion are physiological with rhinitis symptoms paralleling oestrogen levels. Some 10–30% of pregnancies are complicated by rhinitis, but symptoms are severe in few of these [49, 50]. Hormonal rhinitis can also occur during puberty, and from the use of contraceptive pills and hormone-replacement therapies. Oestradiol and progesterone increase the expression of H1 receptors on human nasal epithelial cells and on microvascular endothelial cells. Other possible mechanisms that may increase nasal congestion and obstruction during pregnancy are an increase in the circulating plasma volume and progesterone-induced smooth muscle relaxation. Increased nasal mucus gland hyperactivity also occurs.

The evidence linking hypothyroidism and acromegaly with rhinitis is weaker although there are reports of chronic nasal obstruction [51]. Acromegaly causes turbinate hypertrophy and hypothyroidism can lead to mixed oedematous deposits in the turbinates and elsewhere in the upper respiratory tract, sufficient to cause sleep apnoea [52].

Atrophic Rhinitis

This is not only seen commonly in under-developed countries with poor hygiene, but also occurs following radical nasal tissue removal [52]. Atrophy of the nasal mucosa gives rise to symptoms of dryness, crusting, paradoxical congestion, a foul odour in the nose and colonisation by Klebsiella Pneumoniae Ozaenae. Squamous metaplasia, mucosal atrophy and chronic inflammatory cell infiltrate are seen on microscopic examination and the atrophy can gradually involve the underlying bone of the conchae [53]. A reduction in surfactant production may be relevant [54, 55].

The prevalence of primary atrophic rhinitis is decreased with the use of antibiotics, but it can be found occasionally in the elderly. Atrophic rhinitis can also occur secondary to trauma, radiation, chronic granulomatous disease and possibly autoimmune disorders such a Sjogren's syndrome and anti-phospholipid syndrome. In some cases treatment with ciprofloxacin for several weeks combined with nasal douching has proved helpful [56].

Non-infectious Non-allergic Non-eosinophilic Rhinitis (Idiopathic Rhinitis, NINAR)

Non-eosinophilic, non-allergic rhinitis is characterized by chronic nasal symptoms, which are not immunological or infectious in aetiology. It is the most common form of non-allergic rhinitis, comprising 61% of one study. It is a diagnosis of exclusion, so other causes of rhinitis must be ruled out (Fig. 1). The aetiology is unknown, but inflammation is not seen on biopsies of nasal mucosa [57]. Mast cell activation through a non-immunologic pathway may contribute to symptoms. Other possibilities include various forms of neural dysfunction [58] (Fig. 3).

This perennial form of rhinitis was previously called "vasomotor", but is now more appropriately termed "idiopathic". Eye involvement is rare. The condition usually develops in middle-aged persons and has an unfavourable course compared to allergic rhinitis. Symptoms result from dose-dependent upper airways, hyper-responsiveness to physical and chemical agents (cold air, spicy foods, alcohol, formaldehyde, high humidity, tobacco smoke, fumes etc.). In some, the balance between the sympathetic and parasympathetic nervous systems appears to be skewed towards a parasympathetic hyperactivity.

As there is no evidence of inflammation, routine rhinitis therapies such as corticosteroids and antihistamines are not often helpful, with the possible exception of intranasal azelastine [59]. If watery rhinorrhoea predominates then intranasal cholinergic antagonists such as ipratropium bromide are helpful, but need to be used several times a day [60]. Ipratropium is also useful for rhinorrhoea associated with skier's nose [61], upper respiratory tract infections in children and adults [62, 63] and allergic rhinitis in children [62].

The most interesting development in the therapy of NINAR is the use of capsaicin to affect c-fibre receptors in the nasal lining. Repeated administration of capsaicin, the extract from hot chilli peppers, given as five treatments on a single day at 1 h intervals after local anaesthesia, leads to a significant and long-term reduction of symptoms in patients with idiopathic rhinitis [64]. However this

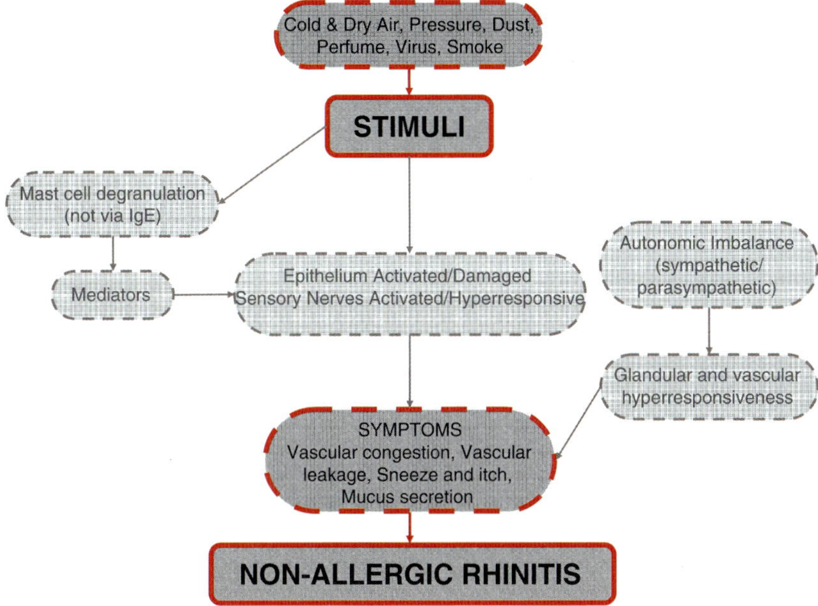

Fig. 3 Possible mechanisms of non-allergic rhinitis

extract is not widely available in forms suited to human use and as such treatment is found only in a few specialist centres. Although placebo-controlled studies are scarce and participants have not been adequately characterized, it is possible that abnormal nociceptor nerve endings play a role in the generation of the symptoms of NINAR. Alternatively, NINAR may represent a condition of increased perceptual acuity to irritants and environmental changes. This problem may also benefit from the defunctionalization of nociceptors. These concepts are further dealt with in the following chapter by James Baraniuk.

Rhinitis as Part of a Systemic Condition

In the differential diagnosis of a patient with rhinitis the following should also be considered.

Primary Defect in Mucus

In cystic fibrosis, the increased viscosity and tenacity of the mucus affects muco-ciliary clearance and limits sinus drainage favouring a susceptibility to infection.

Bacterial biofilms are thought to occur in the sinuses. These are protected by an alginate covering that increases their antibiotic resistance and also their resistance to normal immunological defence mechanisms. In these biofilms bacteria and quorum-sensing can act together to alter their phenotype. Nasal polyposis may occur. In children nasal polyps are very rare, so if any are found, investigations for cystic fibrosis should be conducted.

Primary Ciliary Dyskinesia

This includes a spectrum of syndromes. Kartagener's syndrome is an autosomal recessive genetic defect associated usually with dextrocardia or situs inversus. It consists of structural and functional abnormalities of the cilia, which facilitate chronic sinusitis, otitis and bronchiectasis. Young's syndrome is characterized by thickening of the mucus, possibly associated with an intrinsic ciliary defect. Mucociliary clearance is impaired, again predisposing to chronic infections and obstructive azoospermia on account of the obstruction of the epididymis.

Nitric oxide levels in the normal sinuses are sufficiently high to be toxic to viruses, bacteria, fungi and tumour cells. Nitric oxide levels are low in the upper and lower respiratory tract in patients with primary ciliary dyskinesia. Decreased levels of inducible nitric oxide synthase (iNOS), the enzyme responsible for nitric oxide production in response to inflammation, have been found in the nasal epithelium in primary ciliary dyskinesia and may be the most significant underlying abnormality. The finding of an NO level above 250 ppb in nasal air excludes the diagnosis of Primary cilliary dyskinesia (PCD) with 95% sensitivity.

Immunological Causes

Chronic inflammation in underlying rheumatological systemic disorders such as Systemic lupus crythematosus (SLE) and rheumatoid arthritis can also affect the nose and give rise to nasal obstruction. Antibody deficiency and acquired immune deficiency are predisposed to infective rhinitis. Churg-Strauss syndrome is an antineutrophilic cytoplasmic antibody (ANCA)-positive eosinophilic vasculitis causing polypoidal sinusitis, asthma and eosinophilia, sometimes accompanied by neurological symptoms.

Granulomatous Diseases

Wegener's disease and sarcoidosis can affect the upper as well as the lower airways. Presentation is with external swelling and high crusting in the nose with a highly inflamed mucosa, which bleeds on contact and forms strictures. Septal perforation and collapse of the nasal bridge can occur. Rhinoscleroma is a rare granulomatous disease associated with Klebsiella Rhinosclerematis. This condition includes crusting discharge and nodule formation, causing nasal obstruction.

Malignancy

A bloody or purulent unilateral discharge or increasing nasal blockage in an adult can indicate malignancy. Tumours from the maxillary sinus can invade the nasal mucosa in the later stages. In this case anosmia, pain and otalgia can occur in addition to bleeding.

Structural Abnormalities

Nasal septal deviation may block the flow of air, leading to unilateral obstruction. Compensatory hypertrophy of the opposite inferior turbinate usually occurs. When severe secretions pass posteriorly leading to post-nasal dripping, which can be a symptom of many forms of rhinitis, the other anatomical conditions include enlarged nasal turbinates, dysfunctional nasal valve, tumours and, usually in children, adenoidal hypertrophy. These conditions account for approximately 5–10% of chronic nasal disorders. Complications include sinusitis, snoring, sleep apnoea and fatigue.

Differential Diagnosis

CSF Rhinorrhoea

This usually occurs following trauma or as a complication of surgery. However the onset may be very delayed. The leak usually occurs in the morning on bending forwards and is frequently unilateral. If the nasal fluid tests are positive for beta-transferrin this is diagnostic of CSF (cerebrospinal fluid).

Nasal Polyps

These are present in 4% of the population, but are not always symptomatic when very small. The commonest symptom is probably hyposmia, others include nasal obstruction, rhinorrhoea and snoring. Polyps are pale, gelatinous outgrowths of the nasal mucosa. They are found in association with inflammatory non-allergic rhinitis. IgE-mediated allergy detectable by skin prick tests does not appear to contribute to polyp production. However, recent demonstrations of high levels of local IgE and of non-specific T-cell stimulation by staphylococcal toxins may be of greater relevance [8].

Management

Diagnosis

A careful history, with attention to major symptoms, their timing and relationship to place, occupation, irritants, allergen exposure and so on, should be noted. The nose should be examined for any structural factors such as septal deviation, perforations, nasal polyps, crusting or tumours. The nasendoscope is ideal for examination of the nose, sinus orifices and post-nasal space.

In any patient with persistent rhinitis the lower respiratory tract should also be evaluated by history, examination and functional testing, such as peak flow or spirometry.

Specific IgE should be tested in all patients, bearing in mind that in 15% of the population false positive skin prick tests occur. Thus only those skin prick tests that are relevant to the history should be taken into account. Nasal challenge with allergen or aspirin may be needed as the final arbiter (Fig. 1). Nasal smear eosinophilia is useful in determining an inflammatory form of rhinitis and predicts a response to corticosteroids.

Elevated levels of nasal nitric oxide (nNO) are thought to reflect the presence of inflammation, but false negative results are possible, as severe mucosal oedema can obstruct the osteomeatal complex and reduce the contribution from sinus NO [65].

Treatment

Specific treatment of any underlying cause, for example, hypothyroidism or drug-induced rhinitis, should be undertaken as a first measure. Occupational exposures are particularly relevant, as the rhinitis may progress to asthma unless the patient is removed from contact with the occupational allergen rapidly.

Inflammatory non-allergic rhinitis can be treated with medications used in allergic rhinitis, but the doses used often need to be increased. Specific desensitization to aspirin is an additional possibility.

Non-inflammatory disorders can be divided by mechanism into hormonal; sympathetic dysfunction (including anti-hypertensive adrenergic drug therapy); cholinergic rhinitis; and nociceptive syndromes with hyperalgesia and other features (e.g., the non-allergic rhinitis of chronic fatigue syndrome). Therapy should be based on the most probable pathophysiological mechanism. Reports of responsiveness of non-inflammatory rhinitis to standard anti-allergic therapy after prolonged use exist, however, the phenomenon of mixed rhinitis and local IgE may confound the issue.

Special Considerations

Hormonal rhinitis of pregnancy is usually treated with mild measures such as nasal saline. Decongestants should be avoided in the first trimester of pregnancy as they have been associated with gastroschisis in the newborn. In pre-existing rhinitis during pregnancy the least bioavailable topical corticosteroids are an option as are the non-sedating antihistamines, which have been in longest use, for example, Cetirizine and Loratadine.

Rhinitis Medicamentosa is difficult to treat. A brief course of oral corticosteroid with maintenance topical corticosteroid and the withdrawal of the decongestant from one nostril initially, progressing to both nostrils after a week, can be tried. The patient often needs emotional support plus subsequent investigation of factors leading to use of decongestants in the first place.

Surgery

Most authors feel that surgical therapy should only be considered for those patients who fail to obtain symptomatic relief with medical treatment. Surgical procedures in non-allergic, non-infectious rhinitis, mainly aim at modifying the size of the inferior turbinate or removing nasal polyps. The duration and effectiveness varies from 6 months to several years.

Conclusion

Non-allergic rhinitis comprises a variety of conditions, many of which are poorly understood. The initial aim with any patient is to establish a cause wherever possible, failing that, identify whether the rhinitis is inflammatory or not, as this decision guides treatment. Further careful research is needed, with the first step being abandonment of the outmoded and dysfunctional terminology of "vasomotor rhinitis". Investigation into the very accessible upper airway may also help to elucidate the various pathologies underlying the terminology "asthma", as it is already apparent that allergic rhinitis has a counterpart in allergic asthma and intrinsic asthma with NARES and nasal polyposis.

References

1. Bousquet J, Van Cauwenberge P, Khaltaev N. Aria Workshop Group; World Health Organization. Allergic rhinitis and its impact on asthma. J Allergy Clin Immunol. 2001 Nov;108(5 Suppl):S147–334. Review.
2. Temprano J, Dykewicz M. Nonallergic Rhinitis. In Rakel and Bope. Conn's Current Therapy 2005, pp. 236–40. Elsevier. 2005.
3. Powe DG, Jones NS. Local mucosal immunoglobulin E production: does allergy exist in non-allergic rhinitis? Clin Exp Allergy. 2006 Nov;36(11):1367–72.
4. Jacobs RL, Freedman PM, Boswell RN. Nonallergic rhinitis with eosinophilia (NARES syndrome). Clinical and immunologic presentation. J Allergy Clin Immunol. 1981 Apr;67(4): 253–62.

 5. Settipane GA, Klein DE. Non allergic rhinitis: demography of eosinophils in nasal smear, blood total eosinophil counts and IgE levels. N Engl Reg Allergy Proc. 1985;6(4):363–6.
 6. Rupp GH, Friedman RA. Eosinophilic nonallergic rhinitis in children. Pediatrics. 1982 Sep;70(3):437–9.
 7. Varga EM, Jacobson MR, Masuyama K, Rak S, Till SJ, Darby Y, Hamid Q, Lund V, Scadding GK, Durham SR. Inflammatory cell populations and cytokine mRNA expression in the nasal mucosa in aspirin-sensitive rhinitis. Eur Respir J. 1999 Sep;14(3):610–5.
 8. Bachert C, Gevaert P, Zhang N, van Zele T, Perez-Novo C. Role of staphylococcal superantigens in airway disease. Chem Immunol Allergy. 2007;93:214–36.
 9. Nelson BL, Jacobs RL. Response of nonallergic rhinitis with eosinophilia (NARES) syndrome to 4% cromolyn sodium nasal solution. J Allergy Clin Immunol. 1982 Aug; 70(2):125–8.
10. Swierczyńska M, Strek P, Składzień J, Nizankowska-Mogilnicka E, Szczeklik A. Nonallergic rhinitis with eosinophilia syndrome: state of knowledge. Otolaryngol Pol. 2003;57(1): 81–4.
11. Ragab S, Parikh A, Darby YC, Scadding GK. An open audit of montelukast, a leukotriene receptor antagonist, in nasal polyposis associated with asthma. Clin Exp Allergy. 2001 Sept;31(9):1385–91.
12. Pitkaranta A, Puhakka T, Makela MJ, Ruuskanen O, Carpen O, Vaheri A. Detection of rhinovirus RNA in middle turbinate of patients with common colds by in situ hybridization. J Med Virol. 2003 June;70(2):319–23.
13. Wald ER, Guerva N, Byers C. Upper respiratory tract infections in young children: duration and frequency of complications. Paediatrics. 1991;87:129–33.
14. Turner BW, Cail WS, Hendley JO, Hayden FG, Doyle WJ, Sorrentino JV, Gwaltney JM Jr. Physiologic abnormalities in the paranasal sinuses during experimental rhinovirus colds. J Allergy Clin Immunol. 1992 Sept;90(3 Pt 2):474–8.
15. Berg O, Carenfelt C, Rystedt G, Anggard A. Occurrence of asymptomatic sinusitis in common cold and other acute ENT infections. Rhinology. 1986;24:223–5.
16. Fokkens WF, Lund VJ, Mullol J et al. European Position paper on Chronic rhinosinusitis and nasal polyposis. Rhinology. 2007;supplement 20.
17. Nelson AL, Roche AM, Gould JM, Chim K, Ratner AJ, Weiser JN. Capsule enhances pneumococcal colonization by limiting mucus-mediated clearance. Infect Immun. 2007 Jan;75(1):83–90. Epub 2006 Nov 6.
18. Harvey RJ, Lund VJ. Biofilms and chronic rhinosinusitis: systematic review of evidence, current concepts and directions for research. Rhinology. 2007 Mar;45(1):3–13.
19. Scadding GK, Caulfield H. Paediatric Chronic Rhinosinusitis. In Scott Brown (ed). Otorhinolaryngology Hodder Arworld, London 2007. Hodder Arnold, London
20. Patella V, Florio G, Petraroli A, Marone G. HIV-1 gp120 induces IL-4 and IL-13 release from human Fc epsilon RI+ cells through interaction with the VH3 region of IgE. J Immunol. 2000 Jan 15;164(2):589–95.
21. Marone G, Florio G, Triggiani M, Petraroli A, de Paulis A. Mechanisms of IgE elevation in HIV-1 infection. Crit Rev Immunol. 2000;20(6):477–96.
22. Schubert MS. Allergic fungal sinusitis. Otolaryngol Clin North Am. 2004 Apr;37(2):301–26.
23. Ferguson BJ. Eosinophilic mucin rhinosinusitis: a distinct clinicopathological entity. Laryngoscope. 2000 May;110(5 Pt 1):799–813.
24. Orlandi RR, Thibeault SL, Ferguson BJ. Microarray analysis of allergic fungal sinusitis and eosinophilic mucin rhinosinusitis. Otolaryngol Head Neck Surg. 2007 May;136(5):707–13.
25. Weschta M, Rimek D, Formanek M, Polzehl D, Podbielski A, Riechelmann H. Topical antifungal treatment of chronic rhinosinusitis with nasal polyps: a randomized, double-blind clinical trial. J Allergy Clin Immunol. 2004 June;113(6):1122–8.
26. Ebbens FA, Scadding GK, Badia L, Hellings PW, Jorissen M, Mullol J, Cardesin A, Bachert C, van Zele TP, Dijkgraaf MG, Lund V, Fokkens WJ. Amphotericin B nasal lavages: not a solution for patients with chronic rhinosinusitis. J Allergy Clin Immunol. 2006 Nov;118(5):1149–56.

27. Garnier R, Villa A, Chataigner D. Occupational rhinitis Rev Mal Respir. 2007 Feb;24(2): 205–20.
28. Aguwa EN, Okeke TA, Asuzu MC. The prevalence of occupational asthma and rhinitis among woodworkers in south-eastern Nigeria. Tanzan Health Res Bull. 2007 Jan;9(1):52–5. Rhinology. 2007 Mar;45(1):40–6.
29. Di Stefano F, Di Giampaolo L, Verna N, Di Gioacchino M. Respiratory allergy in agriculture. Allerg Immunol (Paris). 2007 Mar;39(3):89–100.
30. Klusackova P, Lebedova J, Pelclova D, Salandova J, Senholdova Z et al. Occupational asthma and rhinitis in workers from a lasamide production line. Scand J Work Environ Health. 2007 Feb;33(1):74–8.
31. de Fátima Maçãira E, Algranti E, Medina Coeli Mendonça E, Antônio Bussacos M. Rhinitis and asthma symptoms in non-domestic cleaners from the Sao Paulo metropolitan area, Brazil. Occup Environ Med. 2007 July;64(7):446–53. Epub 2007 Feb 15.
32. Airaksinen L, Tuomi T, Vanhanen M, Voutilainen R, Toskala E. Use of nasal provocation test in the diagnostics of occupational rhinitis. Rhinology. 2007 Mar;45(1):3–13.
33. Peters J, Pickvance S, Wilford J, Macdonald E, Blank L. Predictors of delayed return to work or job loss with respiratory ill-health: a systematic review. J Occup Rehabil. 2007 June;17(2):317–26. Epub 2007 Feb 13.
34. Sahin-Yilmaz AA, Corey JP. Rhinitis in the elderly. Clin Allergy Immunol. 2007;19:209–19.
35. Vayisoglu Y, Ozcan C, Pekdemir H et al. Autonomic nervous system evaluation using heart rate variability parameters in vasomotor rhinitis patients. J Otolaryngol. 2006 Oct;35(5):338–42.
36. Elsheikh MN, Badran HM. Dysautonomia rhinitis: associated otolaryngologic manifestations and characterization based on autonomic function tests. Acta Otolaryngol. 2006 Dec;126(11):1206–12.
37. Baraniuk JN, Ho Le U. The nonallergic rhinitis of chronic fatigue syndrome. Clin Allergy Immunol. 2007;19:427–47.
38. Drouet M, Sabbah A, Le Sellin J, Bonneau JC, Fourrier E. Fernand Widal syndrome and sulfite intolerance. Therapeutic problems in general and ORL problems in particular. Allerg Immunol (Paris). 1990 Mar;22(3):90–6.
39. Vally H, Thompson PJ. Allergic and asthmatic reactions to alcoholic drinks. Addict Biol. 2003 Mar;8(1):3–11.
40. Scadding GK. Rhinitis medicamentosa. Clin Exp Allergy. 1995 May;25(5):391–4.
41. Stevenson DD, Szczeklik A. Clinical and pathologic perspectives on aspirin sensitivity and asthma. J Allergy Clin Immunol. 2006 Oct;118(4):773–86; quiz 787–8. Epub 2006 Sep 1.
42. Mastalerz L, Sanak M, Gawlewicz-Mroczka A, Cmiel A, Gielicz A, Szczeklik. Prostaglandin E2 systemic production in asthma patients with and without aspirin hypersensitivity. Thorax. 2007 June 21. Epub ahead of print.
43. Kim SH, Kim YK, Park HW, Jee YK, Kim SH, Bahn JW, Chang YS, Kim SH, Ye YM, Shin ES, Lee JE, Park HS, Min KU. Association between polymorphisms in prostanoid receptor genes and aspirin-intolerant asthma. Pharmacogenet Genomics. 2007 Apr;17(4):295–304.
44. Nizankowska-Mogilnicka E, Bochenek G, Mastalerz L, Swierczynska M, Picado C, Scadding G, Kowalski ML, Setkowicz M, Ring J, Brockow K, Bachert C, Wohrl S, Dahlen B, Szczeklik A. EAACI/GA2LEN guideline: aspirin provocation tests for diagnosis of aspirin hypersensitivity. Allergy. 2007 May 22. Epub ahead of print.
45. Macy E, Bernstein JA, Castells MC, Gawchik SM, Lee TH, Settipane RA, Simon RA, Wald J, Woessner KM. Aspirin desensitization joint task force aspirin challenge and desensitization for aspirin-exacerbated respiratory disease: a practice paper. Ann Allergy Asthma Immunol. 2007 Feb;98(2):172–4.
46. Page NA, Schroeder WS. Rapid desensitization protocols for patients with cardiovascular disease and aspirin hypersensitivity in an era of dual antiplatelet therapy. Ann Pharmacother. 2007 Jan;41(1):61–7. Epub 2007 Jan 2. Review.
47. Roll A, Wuthrich B, Schmid-Grendelmeier P, Hofbauer G, Ballmer-Weber BK. Tolerance to celecoxib in patients with a history of adverse reactions to nonsteroidal anti-inflammatory drugs. Swiss Med Wkly. 2006 Oct 28;136(43–44):684–90.

48. Philpott CM, El-Alami M, Murty GE. The effect of the steroid sex hormones on the nasal airway during the normal menstrual cycle. Clin Otolaryngol Allied Sci. 2004 Apr;29(2):138–42.
49. Ellegard EK, Karlsson NG, Ellegard LH. Rhinitis in the menstrual cycle, pregnancy, and some endocrine disorders. Clin Allergy Immunol. 2007;19:305–21.
50. Shushan S, Sadan O, Lurie S, Evron S, Golan A, Roth Y. Pregnancy-associated rhinitis. Am J Perinatol. 2006 Oct;23(7):431–3. Epub 2006 Sep 25.
51. Jeevanan J, Gendeh BS, Satpal S. Hashimoto's thyroiditis: a rare cause for rhinosinusitis. Med J Malaysia. 2004 Aug;59(3):428–30.
52. Mehrotra R, Singhal J, Kawatra M, Gupta SC, Singh M. Pre and post-treatment histopathological changes in atrophic rhinitis. Indian J Pathol Microbiol. 2005 July;48(3):310–3.
53. Sayed RH, Abou-Elhamd KE, Makhlouf MM. Light and electron microscopic study of primary atrophic rhinitis mucosa. Am J Rhinol. 2006 Sept–Oct;20(5):540–4.
54. Schlosser RJ. Surfactant and its role in chronic sinusitis. Ann Otol Rhinol Laryngol Suppl. 2006 Sep;196:40–4.
55. Garcia GJ, Bailie NA, Martins DA, Kimbell JS. Atrophic rhinitis: A CFD study of air conditioning in the nasal cavity. J Appl Physiol. 2007 June 14;E-pub.
56. Krzeska-Malinowska I, Held-Ziolkowska M, Januszek G. Successes and failures of ozena's medical treatment. Otolaryngol Pol. 2006;60(6):845–8.
57. van Rijswijk JB, Blom HM, Fokkens WJ. Idiopathic rhinitis, the ongoing quest. Allergy. 2005 Dec;60(12):1471–81.
58. Sanico A, Togias A. Noninfectious, nonallergic rhinitis (NINAR): considerations on possible mechanisms. Am J Rhinol. 1998 Jan–Feb;12(1):65–72.
59. Lee C, Corren J. Review of azelastine nasal spray in the treatment of allergic and non-allergic rhinitis. Expert Opin Pharmacother. 2007 Apr;8(5):701–9.
60. Georgitis JW, Banov C, Boggs PB, Dockhorn R, Grossman J, Tinkelman D, Roszko P, Wood C. Ipratropium bromide nasal spray in non-allergic rhinitis: efficacy, nasal cytological response and patient evaluation on quality of life. Clin Exp Allergy. 1994 Nov;24(11):1049–55.
61. Bonadonna P, Senna G, Zanon P, Cocco G, Dorizzi R, Gani F, Landi M, Restuccia M, Feliciello A, Passalacqua G. Cold-induced rhinitis in skiers – clinical aspects and treatment with ipratropium bromide nasal spray: a randomized controlled trial. Am J Rhinol. 2001 Sept–Oct;15(5):297–301.
62. Kim KT, Kerwin E, Landwehr L, Bernstein JA, Bruner D, Harris D, Drda K, Wanger J, Wood CC. Pediatric Atrovent Nasal Spray Study Group. Use of 0.06% ipratropium bromide nasal spray in children aged 2 to 5 years with rhinorrhea due to a common cold or allergies. Ann Allergy Asthma Immunol. 2005 Jan;94(1):73–9.
63. Eccles R, Pedersen A, Regberg D, Tulento H, Borum P, Stjarne P. Efficacy and safety of topical combinations of ipratropium and xylometazoline for the treatment of symptoms of runny nose and nasal congestion associated with acute upper respiratory tract infection. Am J Rhinol. 2007 Jan–Feb;21(1):40–5.
64. Blom HM, Van Rijswijk JB, Garrelds IM, Mulder PG, Timmermans T, Gerth van Wijk R. Intranasal capsaicin is efficacious in non-allergic, non-infectious perennial rhinitis. A placebo-controlled study. Clin Exp Allergy. 1997 July;27(7):796–801.
65. Scadding GK, Lund VJ. Investigative Rhinology. Taylor & Francis, London. 2004.
66. Huggins K, Brostoff J. Local production of specific IgE antibodies in allergic rhinitis patients with negative skin tests. Lancet. 1975;2:148.
67. Carney A, Powe D, Huskisson R, Jones N. Atypical nasal challenges results in patients with idiopathic rhinitis: more evidence for the existence of 'local allergy'. Con Exp Allergy. 2002;32:1436–40.
68. Wedback A, Enbom H, Ericksson N et al. Seasonal non-allergic rhinitis (SNAR) – a new disease entity? A clinical and immunological comparison between SNAR, seasonal allergic rhinitis and persistent non-allergic rhinitis. Rhinology. 2005;43:86–92.
69. Powe DG, Huskisson R, Carncy A et al. Evidence for an inflammatory pathophysiology in idiopathic rhinitis. Clin Exp Allergy. 2001;31:864–72.

70. Berger G, Goldberg A, Ophir D. The inferior turbinate mast cell population of patients with perennial allergic and nonallergic rhinitis. Am J Rhinol. 1997;11:63–6.

71. Humbert M, Durham SR, Ying S et al. IL-4 and IL-5 mRNA and protein in bronchial biopsies from patients with atopic and nonatopic asthma: evidence against 'intrinsic' asthma being distinct immunopathologic entity. Am J Resp Crit Care Med. 1996;154:1497–504.

72. Humbert M, Durham SR, Kimmitt P et al. Elevated expression of messenger ribonucleic acid encoding IL-13 in the bronchial mucosa of atopic and nonatopic subjects with asthma. J Allergy Clin Immunol. 1997;99:657–65.

73. Ying S, Humbert M, Meng Q et al. Local expression of epsilon germline gene transcripts and RNA for the epsilon heavy chain of IgE in the bronchial mucosa in atonic and nonatopic asthma. J Allergy Clin Immunol. 2001;107:686–92.

74. Powe DG, Mason M, Jagger C et al. 'Entopy': localised mucosal allergic disease in the absence of systemic responses for atopy. Clin Exp Allergy. 2003;33:1374–9.

Nasal Polyposis: A Model of Chronic Airways Inflammation

César Picado

Introduction

Nasal polyps (NP) are abnormal lesions that result from the prolapse of the mucosa lining the nose and sinuses. Nasal polyps can be bilateral or unilateral [1] (Figs. 1 and 2). Bilateral nasal polyposis (NP) usually coexists with a chronic hyperplastic inflammatory process of the nose and sinus (chronic rhinosinusitis), but the converse is not true, since only about 20% of the patients with chronic rhinosinusitis develop nasal polyps (Fig. 3). Accumulated evidence supports the concept that chronic rhinosinusitis with NP, and chronic rhinosinusitis without NP, are two different entities rather than different stages of one single disease [2]. NP usually originate from the paranasal sinuses, most often from the anterior ethmoid complex. Bilateral NP and chronic rhinosinusitis may also develop in patients with cystic fibrosis [1].

The most frequent unilateral polyp is the so-called antrochoanal polyp that usually originates from the mucosa of the maxillary sinus, growing through the ostium into the middle meatus and protruding posteriorly to the choana and nasopharynx [3].

This chapter will mostly concentrate on nasal polyps that are usually found in both sides of the nose and those not related to the presence of cystic fibrosis.

Epidemiology

In the general population the prevalence of NP ranges from 0.5% to 4.3%. NP are rare in children, if found, cystic fibrosis or cilia dyskinesis syndrome should be excluded. A strong male predominance is found in adults who have NP. Figures vary from series to series, but the ratio is between two and four to one. The prevalence of NP is increased in patients with asthma. Asthmatic patients have a twofold higher risk of having NP than non-asthmatic subjects. NP is more common in patients

C. Picado (✉)
Department of Pneumology and Respiratory Allergy Hospital Clinic, University of Barcelona, Vilarroel 170, 08036, Barcelona, Spain
e-mail: cpicado@ub.edu

R. Pawankar et al. (eds.), *Allergy Frontiers: Clinical Manifestations,*
DOI: 10.1007/978-4-431-88317-3_4, © Springer 2009

Fig. 1 Endoscopic view showing a nasal polyp. The most common bilateral polyps are semi-transparent nasal lesions that arise from the mucosa of the nasal cavity

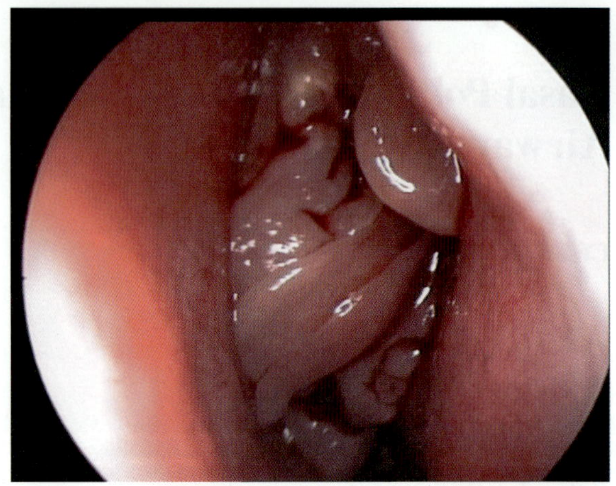

Fig. 2 Aspect of a removed nasal polyp shown in Fig. 1

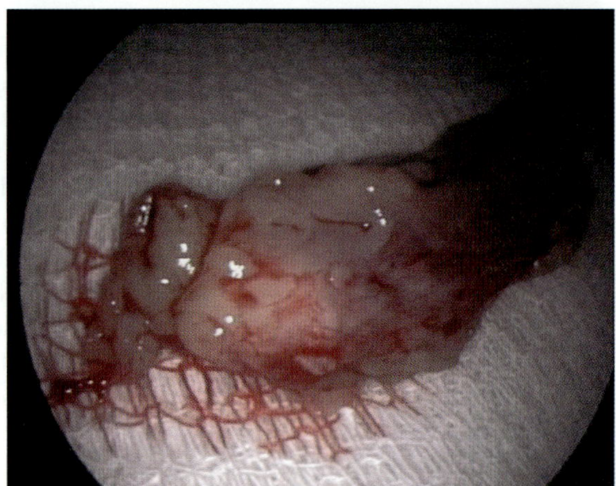

Fig. 3 A coronal section of a CT scan shows diffuse opacification of the ethmoid air cells, complete opacification of the left maxillary sinus and partial opacification of the right maxillary sinus, with sinus mucosal thickening. Bilateral nasal polyps are always associated with chronic hyperplastic rhinosinusitis

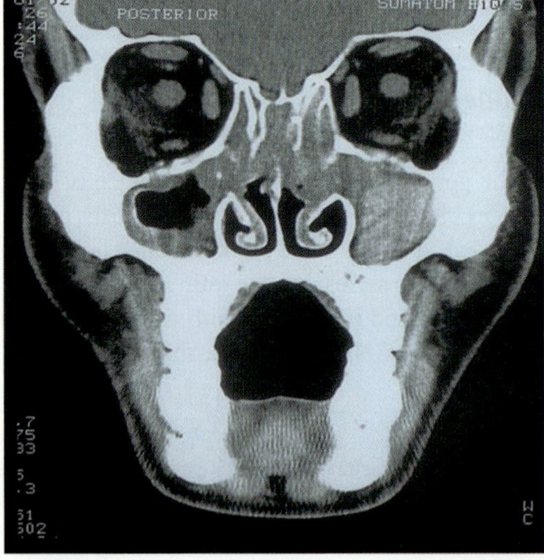

with non-allergic asthma (13%) compared with those with allergic asthma (5%) [4]. In patients with aspirin intolerance and asthma, NP are very frequent. On CT scans, more that 95% of these patients have extensive abnormalities of sinus mucosa and NP are found by endoscopy in more than 80% of the patients [5]. The coexistence of NP, asthma and aspirin intolerance is referred to as the "aspirin triad" [5].

Clinical Manifestations

Almost all patients with bilateral nasal polyposis have nasal obstruction to some degree. Other concomitant symptoms are nasal discharge and hyposmia or anosmia. The increased production of mucus often results in complaints of post-nasal drip. If the mucus is infected, then it may become green; however, the presence of abundant eosinophils may also cause a nasal secretion with a yellow green colour. Pain around the face is present occasionally [1]. In some patients, massive polyposis can alter the craniofacial structure and cause hypertelorism. Polyps rarely produce bone erosion, but it may be present following surgery and if the patient develops a mucocele.

Histopathology

Classification

According to Hellquist [6], NP can be classified in four histopathological groups: (1) Oedematous, eosinophilic (so-called allergic) nasal polyp, which is the most common (85–90%). The oedematous polyp is morphologically characterized by oedema, global cell hyperplasia of the epithelium and thickening of the basement membrane and of numerous leukocytes, predominantly eosinophils. (2) Ductal type. This histological type is a rare variant that presents with pronounced hyperplasia of the seromucinous glands, but otherwise shows many similarities with the oedematous type of polyp. (3) Fibrous or fibroinflammatory. This variant is also rare and characterized by the presence of a chronic inflammatory process and metaplastic changes of the overlying epithelium, and (4) Polyps with atypical stroma. This histological type is very rare and has to be distinguished from a genuine neoplasm by a careful histological examination.

Characteristics of the Inflammatory Process

Nasal polyps are characterized by a massive tissue oedema, resulting from the leakage of plasma proteins through widened endothelial junctions.

The cellular component comprises a variety of cells including eosinophils, mast cells, lymphocytes, neutrophils and plasma cells. In the majority of NP, eosinophils constitute more than 50% of the cell population [7, 8] (Fig. 3). Most eosinophils are activated with prolonged survival [9]. Eosinophilic influx is higher in polyps from patients with asthma than in non-asthmatic patients. This difference in eosinophil influx is even more marked in aspirin-intolerant asthmatics. Eosinophils seem to be attracted mainly by the release of interleukin-5 (IL-5), which is most probably produced by CD + Th2 lymphocytes [10–13]. Eosinophils also release IL-5, so they can extend their own lifespan in an autocrine fashion. Moreover, the epithelium may also contribute to attract and activate eosinophils by releasing various eosinophil chemoattractant mediators such as RANTES (regulated upon activation, normal T-cell expressed and secreted), eotaxina and GM-CSF [13–15]. Not only can epithelial cells attract eosinophils to the polyps, they can also increase their lifespan [14, 15]. When incubating peripheral blood eosinophils with a human nasal polyp epithelium cell-conditioned medium, eosinophil survival increases significantly as a result of the inhibition of apoptosis. This effect is almost completely blocked by the anti-GM-CSF antibody, indicating that this cytokine is the most important eosinophil survival enhancer released by the epithelial cells. Other cytokines with a less relevant role are interleukin 8 (IL-8) and tumor necrosis factor alpha (TNF-α) [14, 15].

Eosinophils have to emigrate from the blood vessels through the endothelium and then travel across the polyp stroma to infiltrate the polyp tissue. Extravasation takes place by the combined action of various cytokines such as interleukin-1β (IL-1β) and TNF-α. Chemokines such as RANTES and eotaxin are most probably responsible for the movement of eosinophils into the stroma of the polyp [13, 16].

Although the number of mast cells appears not to be increased in nasal polyps with respect to healthy nasal mucosa, the fact that they appear to be degranulated and the increased levels of tryptase found in NP, suggest that they are more activated than those present in healthy nasal mucosa [17] (Fig. 4).

Lymphocytes are usually detected infiltrating the stroma, sometimes organized in kinds of lymphatic follicles. Among lymphocytes, the most predominant nasal polyp-predominant cell population consists of T cells with the CD8 + phenotype, which out numbers CD4 + T cells [7, 18, 19]. Most of them are HLA-DR +, CD69 +, CD45RO +, CD45RA cells. These activated memory T cells also are characterized

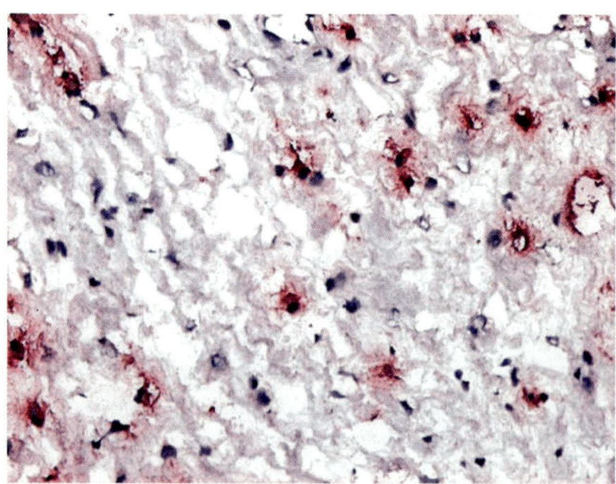

Fig. 4 Eosinophils infiltrating a nasal polyp (marked with an antibody against BMK-13). The histological picture of most polyps is dominated by the presence of abundant eosinophils. The eosinophilia varies from polyp to polyp and from one part of the polyp to another. Treatment with corticosteroids causes a dramatic decrease in eosinophil numbers (original magnification × 400)

by showing a low degree of anti-CD95-induced apoptosis. The lymphocytes that infiltrate nasal polyps produce both IL-5 and interferon gamma a finding that suggests that they are composed of a mixed pattern of TH1/TH2 cells [20].

Plasma cell numbers are usually high in NP compared to healthy nasal mucosa. Plasma cells are found in all tissue layers especially around the submucous glands. The increased number of plasma cells is associated with an elevated local production of immunoglobulines.

Inflammatory Mediators

A variety of chemical mediators and proteins with different pro-inflammatory activities have been described in NP. According to Hoffman and Wasserman these mediators can be classified into four groups [21]: (1) substances with vasoactive function: histamine, platelet activating factor (PAF), eicosanoids (prostaglandins, leukotrienes) and vascular endothelial growth factor (VEGF); (2) substances influencing cell migration: eicosanoids (prostaglandins and leukotrienes), interleukins, chemokines and adhesion molecules (selectins, integrins); (3) substances acting on the extracellular matrix: transforming growth factor (TGF), tumor necrosis factor (TNF) and mucins; and (4) mediators affecting cell growth, differentiation and proliferation: granulocyte-macrophage colony-stimulating factor (GM-CSF), transforming growth factor (TGF), TNF and interleukins.

Histamine, Tryptase and PAF

Increased levels of histamine and tryptase have been found in NP, a finding which suggests that mast cells and basophils are activated in the inflamed NP tissue [22] (Fig. 5).

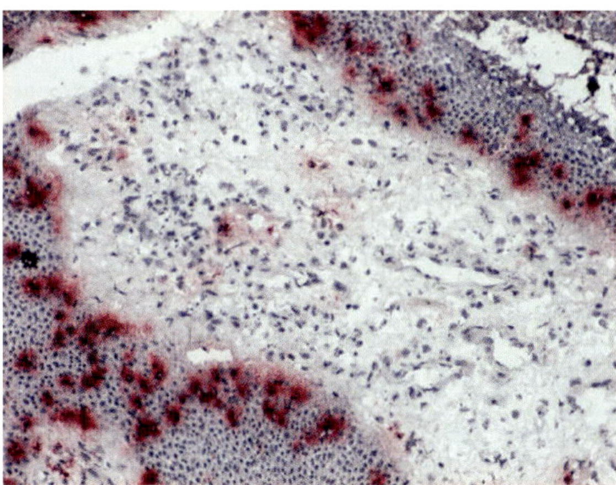

Fig. 5 Numerous mast cells are usually found in NP releasing tryptase (staining with antitryptase). Increased levels of histamine and tryptase are found in NP, a finding that suggests that mast cells and basophils are activated in the inflamed tissue of NP (original magnification × 400)

It has been reported that NP cells produce PAF and its level increases further upon stimulation with pro-inflammatory substances. PAF levels in nasal polyps correlate with eosinophil numbers and are higher in aspirin-sensitive asthmatics compared to aspirin-tolerant subjects [23]. There are no comparative studies of PAF production between NP and healthy nasal mucosa.

Arachidonic Acid Metabolites

5-lipoxygenase pathway. Arachidonic acid (AA) is a component of the lipid bilayer in both cellular and nuclear membranes. The enzyme cytosolic phospholipase A_2 ($cPLA_2$) generates AA from the lipid cell membranes. AA is used as a substrate to generate leukotrienes (LT), prostaglandins (PG) and lipoxins (LX) [24].

Arachidonic acid can be converted into leukotriene A_4 (LTA_4). LTA_4 can be released from the cell or converted into either LTB4 by a leukotriene A4 hydrolase or LTC4 by a LTC4 synthase (LTC4s). Outside the cell LTC4 is rapidly hydrolysed to LTD4 and then LTE4; these three LT are collectively referred to as cysteinyl leukotrienes (Cys-LT). Two receptors exist that can bind Cys-LT: Cys-LT-1 and Cys-LT-2 [24]. Most enzymes involved in the release of Cys-LT are expressed at high levels in NP, particularly in NP from patients with aspirin intolerance [25]. In addition, the Cys-LT-1 receptor is also up-regulated in the NP tissue of aspirin-sensitive asthmatics [26]. The increased activity of the 5-LO pathway results in an increased production of Cys-LT in the nose of patients with NP. Production is even higher in the NP of patients with aspirin intolerance [24]. The direct relationship of the elevated activity of the enzymes in the LO pathway and the increased production of Cys-LT in patients with NP is sustained by the observation that polypectomy, and the subsequent reduction in the amount of inflamed nasal tissue, is accompanied by a parallel decrease in the levels of Cys-LT in urine [27]. Cells that are capable of producing Cys-LT in the NP include mast cell, basophils and eosinophils.

Cyclooxygenase pathway. Prostaglandin G/H synthase, also known as cyclooxygenase (Cox), catalyses the conversion of AA into prostaglandins. At least two isoforms of Cox have been identified, Cox-1 and Cox-2. Cox-1 is a constitutive enzyme present in most mammalian cells. In contrast, measurable Cox-2 gene expression normally occurs in only a few cell types, but its expression can be induced in many, if not all cells, by a variety of stimuli, including cytokines, growth factors and mitogens. Based on the unique expression pattern of the two isoforms, it is thought that Cox-2 is the immediate gene involved in modulating inflammation. In contrast, Cox-1 functions as a housekeeping gene for maintaining the homeostasis of cells. PGs that are generated through Cox activities act locally as important micro-environmental hormones mediating autocrine and/or paracrine functions [24].

In contrast to the presence of an activated Cys-LT pathway, Cox-2 appears to be down-regulated in NP, an alteration that is even stronger in patients with aspirin intolerance [25, 28, 29]. The deficient regulation of Cox-2 is most probably responsible for the remarkable reduction in the capacity of NP to produce PGE_2 [25]. In line with the alteration in Cox-2 regulation, the production of PGE_2 is even more altered in the NP of aspirin-intolerant patients than their aspirin-tolerant counterparts [25]. Because it is commonly accepted that under the conditions of inflammation Cox-2 is up-regulated and as a result PGE_2 production increases, the unexpected down-regulation of Cox-2 and diminished production of PGE_2 detected in NP is an intriguing finding, the origin of which remains to be elucidated [24]. Interestingly, the alteration of the Cox-2 pathway appears to be a specific abnormality of idiopathic inflammatory nasal polyps, frequently associated with asthma, with or without aspirin intolerance. In NP associated with other pathologies such as cystic fibrosis, it has been shown that Cox-2 is up-regulated and the production of PGE_2 in the airways markedly increased [30]. Further work is needed to examine why Cox-2 is down-regulated in NP and to clarify the role of this anomaly in the development of NP.

Mucins

The gel-like properties of mucus secretions depend primarily on the content of high molecular weight glycoproteins named mucins (MUC). Mucus gel is formed on the surface of mucosa when the secreted mucins absorb water. On hydration of mucins, their volume increases by several hundred times in a few seconds [31].

Mucins are synthesized and secreted by epithelial globet cells and mucus cells of the submucosal glands. Nineteen human mucin genes have been identified and subdivided into secreted and membrane-tethered mucins. MUC2, MUC5AC, MUC5B, MUC6-MUC9 and MUC19 are secreted mucins, while MC1, MUC3, MUC4, MUC11-MUC13, MUC17, MUX18 and MUC20 are membrane-tethered mucins. Other mucin genes (MUC15, MUC16) have not been fully characterized [31].

Although all mucins appear to contribute to the mucociliary defence of airways against pathogens and toxins, different roles have been described depending on whether they are secreted or membrane-tethered. Secreted mucins such as MUC2, MUC5A, MUC5B and MUC6 seem to be directly involved in mucus formation, while membrane-bound mucins such as MUC1 and MUC4 modulate cell–cell and cell-extracellular matrix interactions and participate in cellular signalling.

MUC1, MUC2, MUC4, MUC5AC, MUC5B, MUCC7, MUC8 and MUC13 are normally expressed in the human respiratory tract, but only MUC5AC and MUC5B are major components of human airway secretions. MUC2 and MUC5AC are produced by epithelial globet cells, whereas mucous cells in submucosal glands express MUC5B (Fig. 6). The remaining respiratory mucins, both secreted and membrane-tethered, do not have such a well-defined distribution pattern, and are found at the epithelial and glandular level. Only MUC7, together with MUC5B, is exclusively expressed in the submucosal glands [31].

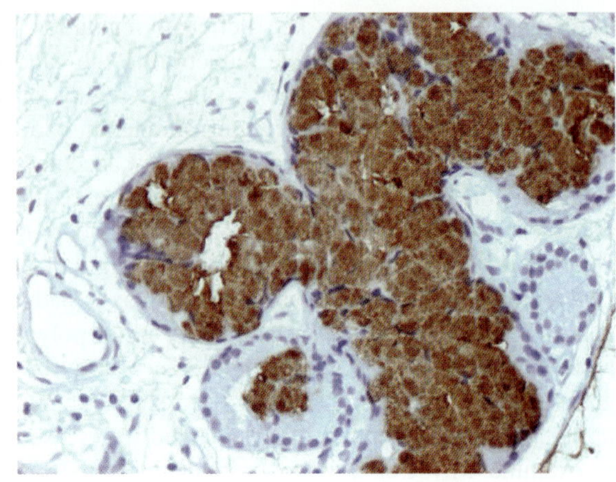

Fig. 6 Immunohistochemistry of mucin expression in a nasal polyp. The microscopic preparation shows the positive immunohistochemistry of MUC5B, which is mainly expressed in glandular mucous cells (original magnification × 400)

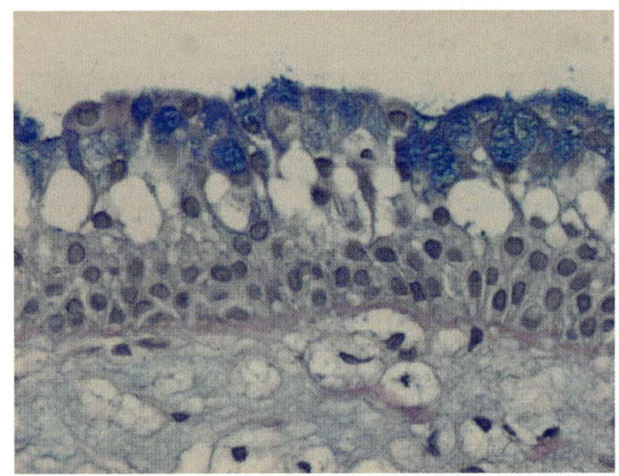

Fig. 7 Globet cell hyperplasia is a common finding in NP. In this microscopic examination, globet cells (staining with Alcian Blue-Periodic acid Schiff) can be seen in the epithelium of NP (original magnification × 400)

The pattern of expression of mucins in NP is characterized by a decreased expression of MUC5AC and an increased expression of MUC1, MUC2, MUC4 and MUC8 [32].

During the development of nasal polyps, activation of some mucins together with the hyperplasia of globet cells may result in a qualitative as well as a quantitative alteration of mucus secretion in nasal polyps (Fig. 7).

Cytokines

Several recent studies have demonstrated that IL-4, IL-5, IL-6, IL-8, GM-CSF, eotaxin and interferon gamma (IFN-γ) are expressed higher in nasal polyps than in nasal mucosa [12].

The increased production of IL-5 and eotaxin contributes to an increase in the number of eosinophils in NP [10, 33]. T cells, mast cells and eosinophils are the cellular source of these cytokines [10, 33]. By releasing IL-5, eosinophils may create an autocrine loop for their activation and survival within the NP tissue. In addition, IL-4 may play a role in increasing eosinophil influx by enhancing vascular cell adhesion molecule (VCAM-1) expression in NP vessels [16]. The NP tissue also expresses more GM-CSF than nasal mucosa, a finding that may contribute to increase the survival of eosinophils by inhibiting programmed cell death (apoptosis). All in all, the increased eosinophil numbers in NP result from the combined action of various cytokines produced by a variety of inflammatory and structural cells.

Low levels of transforming growth factor-β1 have been found in NP relative to nasal mucosa. Since TGF-β1 is an essential regulator of cell proliferation, its low presence might somehow contribute to NP development [34].

The chemokines eotaxin and RANTES have been postulated to be involved in the recruitment and activation of eosinophils to certain inflamed tissues, characterized by the presence of abundant eosinophils, such as NP. Eotaxin has been reported to be significantly elevated in both allergic and non-allergic NP with respect to healthy nasal mucosa. In addition, the tissue eosinophilia level is significantly correlated with eotaxin levels, a finding that suggests that eotaxin is involved in the eosinophil infiltration frequently detected in NP [33]. The relevance of RANTES in tissue eosinophilia is controversial, with some studies showing increased levels of expression in NP [13], while others do not find such a difference in RANTES expression [11].

Remodelling in Nasal Polyps

Microscopic examination of NP revealed a number of findings that characterized the process called remodelling that typically includes respiratory epithelium with areas of damage and squamous metaplasia, thickening of the basal membrane underneath the damaged epithelium, globet cell hyperplasia and subepithelial fibrosis. These observations had similarities, but also some differences in the observations of the airways of asthmatics.

Myofibroblasts are considered to be activated phenotypes of fibroblasts, with the capacity to produce large amounts of extracellular matrix molecules, such as collagens and fibronectin. Myofibroblasts are not present in healthy nasal mucosa, but are usually found underneath the thickened basal membrane in NP. It has been hypothesized that myofibroblasts that are more abundant in the pedicle than in the central parts of NP may be involved in the growth of nasal polyps, by inducing the production of extracellular matrix molecules [35].

Proteolitic enzymes called matrix metalloproteinases (MMP) regulate the amount and composition of the extracellular matrix, and tissue inhibitors (TIMPs) regulate the biological activity of MMP. The relationship between MMP and TIMPs is thought to be critical in regulating tissue remodelling. An increase in MMP-7 and MMP-9 expression has been demonstrated in NP [36, 37]. The tissue inhibitor of metalloproteinase-1 has also been found to be significantly increased in NP compared to nasal mucosa [37].

Recently, the protective of destructive function of MMPs and TIMPs was evaluated in eosinophilic and non-eosinophlic NP by comparing MMP-8/TIMP-1 and MMP-9/TIMP-1 levels. Significantly increased levels of MMP-8/TIMP-1 and MMP-9/TIMP-1 were found in non-eosinophilic NP relative to both eosinophlic NP and nasal mucosa. Moreover, MMP-8/TIMP-1 and MMP-9/TIMP-1 levels were also found to be higher in patients who did not require re-operation in comparison with re-operated patients. These results suggested that the proteolytic spectrum differed in NP according to the presence of eosinophils. In addition, the enhanced expression of MMP-8 and MMP-9 was associated with a better clinical outcome, and thus these results suggested that these MMPs had a protective role, at least, in non-eosinophilic NP [38].

Pathogenesis

The etiology of chronic rhinosinusitis with and without NP is a matter of debate. Based on the study of the bioelectric properties of polyps, Bernstein has suggested a theory on the pathogenesis of nasal polyps [39]. In Bernstein's theory, inflammatory changes first occur in the lateral nasal wall or sinus mucosa as a result of viral or bacterial infections or secondary to turbulent airflow. In most cases, polyps originate from the contact areas of the middle meatus, especially in the narrow clefts of the anterior ethmoid region where the turbulent airflow arises, particularly when the area narrows further as a result of mucosal inflammation. Ulceration of the submucosa can occur with re-epithelialization and new gland formation. During this process, a polyp can form because the inflammatory process affects the bioelectric integrity of the sodium channels at the luminal surface of the respiratory epithelial cell. This response increases sodium absorption, leading to water retention and polyp formation.

The mucosal surface of the nose is continuously exposed to allergens and microorganisms including fungi and bacteria. A recently proposed theory speculates that a non-allergic eosinophilic reaction to fungi might be involved in chronic recurrent nasal polyposis [40]. According to this theory antifungal therapy could be the solution to this usually difficult-to-treat inflammatory process. Although the preliminary results of an open study using antifungal agents appears to demonstrate the validity of the proposal [41], well-designed, placebo-controlled studies could not find any significant effects, either clinical or radiological, in patients treated with an antifungal antibiotics compared to the placebo [42].

Staphylococcus aureus (*SA*) is the most common organism isolated from the mucus adjacent to bilateral nasal polyposis. SA produces enterotoxins, which show superantigen activity that significantly modifies the functions of T and B cells. Superantigens can stimulate TH2 responses directly. This results in the excessive production of TH2 cytokines, such as IL-5, which in turn activate eosinophil inflammation in the upper airways. B-cell stimulation also results in the production of specific immunoglobulin E (IgE) antibodies to SA enterotoxins that can be found within the nasal mucosa tissue. IgE levels against enterotoxins correlate with the intensity of the inflammatory process underlying chronic rhinosinustis with NP. All these findings have been used to support the hypothesis that the inflammatory response triggered by SA may contribute to the development of chronic eosinophilic rhinosinustis with chronic NP [43, 44]. Many questions, however, remain to be clarified, to clearly demonstrate that SA antigens and IgE antibodies are responsible for the development of the chronic eosinophilic inflammatory process present in patients with NP.

Conclusion

Nasal polyps are benign tumours that usually occur in association with chronic rhinosinusitis. A variety of inflammatory mediators including cytokines, chemokines, mucines, prostaglandins, leukotrienes and matrix metalloproteinases, contribute to the inflammatory and remodelling process that takes place in the nasal mucosa. The pathogenesis of nasal polyposis is still an enigma; however, the molecular biology of the disease is beginning to unravel.

References

1. Fokkens W, Lund V, Bachert C, et al. EAACI position paper on rhinosinusitis and nasal polyps executive summary. Allergy 2005;60:583–601.
2. Pawankar R, Novaka M. Inflammatory mechanisms and remodelling in chronic rhinosinusitis and nasal polyps. Cur Allergy Asthma Rep 2007;7:202–208.
3. Maldonado M, Martinez A, Alobid I, Mullol J. The antrochoanal polyp. Rhinology 2004;43:178–182.
4. Settipane GA. Epidemiology of nasal polyps. Allergy Asthma Proc 1996;17:231–236.
5. Kowalski M. Rhinosinusitis and nasal polyposis in aspirin sensitive and aspirin tolerant patients: are they different? Thorax 2000;55(Suppl 2):s84–s86.
6. Hellquist HB. Histopathology. In: Settipane GA Ed. Nasal polyps: epidemiology, pathogenesis and treatment. Oceanside, Providence, RI, pp. 31–39.
7. Stoop AE, Hameleers DM, van Run PE, et al. Lymphocytes and non-lymphoid cells in the nasal mucosa of patients with nasal polyps and healthy subjects. J Allergy Clin Immunol 1989;84:734–741.
8. Fokkens WJ, Holm AF, Rijntjes E, et al. Characterization and quantification of cellular infiltrates in nasal mucosa of patients with grass pollen allergy, non-allergic patients with nasal polyps and controls. Int Arch Allergy Appl Immunol 1990;93:66–72.
9. Simon HU, Yousefi S, Schranz C, Schapowal A, Bachert C, Blaser K. Direct demonstration of delayed eosinophil apoptosis as a mechanism causing tissue eosinophilia. J Immunol 1998;158:3902–3908.
10. Bachert C, Wagenmann M, Huaser U, et al. IL-5 synthesis is upregulated in human nasal polyps. J Allergy Clin Immunol 1997;99:837–842.
11. Bachert C, Wagenmann M, Rudack C, Hopken K, Hillebrandt M, Wang D, van Cauwenberge P. The role of cytokines in infectious sinusitis and nasal polyposis. Allergy 1998;53:2–13.

12. Lee CH, Rhee CS, Min YG. Cytokine gene expression in nasal polyps. Ann Otol Rhinol Laryngol 1998;107:665–670.
13. Lee CH, Le KS, Rhee CS, Lee SO, Min YG. Distribution of RANTES and interleukin-5 in allergic nasal mucosa and nasal polyps. Ann Otol Rhinol Laryngol 1999;108:594–598.
14. Mullol J, Xaubet A, Gaya A, et al. Cytokine gene expression and release from epithelial cells. A comparison study between healthy nasal mucosa and nasal polyps. Clin Exp Allergy 1995;25:607–615.
15. Xaubet A, Mullol J, Loez E, et al. Comparison of the role of nasal polyps and normal nasal mucosa epithelial cells on in vitro eosinophil survival. Mediation by GM-CSF and inhibition by dexamethasone. Clin Exp Allergy 1994;24:307–317.
16. Im GJ, Hwang CS, Jung HH. Quantitative expression levels of regulated on activation Tcell expressed and secreted and eotaxin transcripts in toluene diisozyanate-induced allergic rats. Acta Otolaryngol 2005;125:370–377.
17. Min YG, Kim YJ, Yun YS. Distribution of eosinophilic granule proteins in nasal mucosa of atopic patients with nasal polyposis. ORL 1996;58:82–86.
18. Bernstein JM, Ballow M, Rich G, Allen C, Swanson M, Dmochowski J. Lymphocyte sub-populations and cytokines in nasal polyps: is there a local immune system in the nasal polyp ? Otolaryngol Head Neck Surg 2004;130:526–535.
19. Morinaka S, Nakamura H. Inflammatory cells in nasal mucosa and nasal polyps. Auris Nasus Larynx 2000;27:59–64.
20. Sanchez Segura A, Brieva JA, Rodriguez C. T lymphocytes that infiltrate nasal polyps have a specialized phenotype and produce mixed TH1/TH2 pattern of cytokines. J Allergy Clin Immunol 1998;102:953–960.
21. Hoffman HA, Wasserman SI. Chemical mediators in polyps. In: Settipane GA Ed. Nasal polyps: epidemiology, pathogenesis and treatment. Oceanside. Providence, RI, pp. 41–47.
22. Di Lorenzo G, Drago A, Esposito Pelliteri M, et al. Measurement of inflammatory mediators of mast cells and eosinophils in native nasal lavage fluid in nasal polyposis. Int Arch Allergy Immunol 2001;125:164–175.
23. Furukawa M, Ogura M, Tsutsumi T, Ssuji H, Yamashita T. Presence of platelet-activating factor in nasal polyps and eosinophils. Acta Otolaryngol 2002;122:872–876.
24. Picado C. Mechanisms of aspirin sensitivity. Curr Allergy Asthma Rep 2006;6:198–202.
25. Perez Novo CA, Watelet JB, Claeys C, Van Cauwenberge P, Bachert C. Prostaglandin, leuko-triene, and lipoxin balance in chronic rhinosinusitis with and without nasal polyps. J Allergy Clin Immunol 2006;115:1189–1196.
26. Sousa AR, Perikh A, Scadding G, Corrigan CJ, Lee TH. Leukotriene-receptor expres-sion on nasal mucosal inflammatory cells in aspirin-sensitive rhinosinusitis. N Engl J Med 2002;347:1493–1499.
27. Higashi N, Taniguchi M, Mita H, et al. Clinical features of asthmatic patients with increased urinary leukotriene E4 excretion (hyperleukotrienuria): Involvement of chronic hyperplastic rhinosinusitis with nasal polyposis. J Allergy Clin Immunol 2004;113:277–283.
28. Picado C, Fernandez-Morata JC, Juan M, et al. Cyclooxygenase-2 mRNA is down-regulated in nasal polyps from aspirin-sensitive asthmatics. Am J Respir Crit Care Med 1999;160:291–296.
29. Pujols L, Mullol J, Alobid I, Roca-Ferrer J, Xaubet A, Picado C. Dynamics of Cox-2 in nasal mucosa and nasal polyps from aspirin-tolerant and aspirin-intolerant patients with asthma. J Allergy Clin Immunol 2004;114:814–819.
30. Roca-Ferrer J, Pujols L, Gartner S, et al. Up-regulation of Cox-1 and Cox-2 in nasal polyps in cystic fibrosis. Thorax 2006;61:592–596.
31. Martinez-Anton A, Roca-Ferrer J, Mullol J, et al. Mucin gene expresión in rhinitis sindromes. Curr Allergy Asthma Rep 2006;6:189–197.
32. Martinez-Anton A, de Bolos C, Garrido M, et al. Mucin genes have different expresión pat-terns in healthy and diseased upper airway mucosa. Clin Exp Allergy 2006;36:448–457.
33. Shin SH, Park JY, Jeon CH, Choi JK, Lee SH. Quantitative analysis of eotaxin and RANTES messenger RNA in nasal polyps: association of tissue and nasal eosinophils. Laryngoscope 2000;110:1353–1357.

34. Hirschberg A, Jokuti A, Darvas Z, Almay K, Repassy G, Falus A. The pathogenesis of nasal polyposis by immunoglobulin E and interleukin-5 is completed by transforming growth factor-β1. Laryncoscope 2003;113:120–124.
35. Wang QP, Escudier E, Roudot-Thoraval F, et al. Myofibroblast accumulation induced by transforming growth factor-beta is involved in the pathogenesis of nasal polyps. Laryngoscope 1997;107:926–931.
36. Lechapt-Zalcman E, Coste A, d'Ortho MP, et al. Increased expression of matrix metalloproteinase-9 in nasal polyps. J Pathol 2001;193:223–241.
37. Watelet JB, Bachert C, Claeys C, van Cauwenberge P. Matrix metalloproteinases MMP-7,MMP-9 and their tissue inhibitor TIMP-1 expression in chronic sinusitis vs nasal polyps. Allergy 2004;59:54–60.
38. Kostomo K, Tervahartrada T, Sorsa T, Richardson M, Toskale E. Metalloproteinase function in chronic rhinosinustis with nasal polyposis. Laryngoscope 2007;117:638–643.
39. Bernstein JM, Gorfien J, Noble B, Yankaskas JR. Nasal polypsosis: immunohistochemistry and bioelectrical findings (a hypothesis for the development of nasal polyps). J Allergy Clin Immunol 1997;99:165–175.
40. Ponikau JU, Sherris DA, Kita H, Kern EB. Intranasal antifungal treatment in 51 patients with chronic rhinosinusitis. J Allergy Clin Immunol 2002;110:862–866.
41. Ponikau JU, Sherris DA, Kephart GM, Adolphson C, Kita H. The role of ubiquitous airbone fungi in chronic rhinosinusitis. Clin Rev Allergy Immunol 2006;30:187–194.
42. Ebbens FA, Scadding GG, Badia L, et al. Amphotericin B nasal lavages: not as solution for patients with chronic rhinosinusitis. J Allergy Clin Immunol 2006;118:1149–1156.
43. Bachert C, van Zele T, Gevaert P, De Schrijver L, Van Cauwenberge P. Superantigens and nasal polyps. Curr Allergy Asthma Rep 2003;3:523–531.
44. Bernstein JM, Kansal R. Superantigen hypothesis for the early development of chronic hyperplastic sinusitis with massive nasal polyposis. Cur Opin Otolaryngol Head Neck Surg 2005;13:39–44.

The Nonallergic Rhinitis of Chronic Fatigue Syndrome

James N. Baraniuk and Samantha Jean Merck

Introduction

Chronic fatigue syndrome (CFS) has had a series of case designation criteria that have evolved since the 1980s [1–3]. It shares many characteristics with myalgic encephalopathy (ME) and may represent the same condition. Diagnosis varies from country to country, but shares several themes with the Center for Disease Control and Prevention (CDC) guidelines. The 1994 criteria of Fukuda et al. focus on the combination of disabling fatigue plus at least four of the eight minor elements (Table 1). The fatigue often has a sudden onset and may develop after motor vehicle accidents, physiological life stressors or as a lingering fatigue following many types of viral, parasitic and bacterial diseases. The fatigue must last for at least 6 months and cause significant disability with a decrement in work productivity and strain on the ability to perform daily activities. Medically related fatigue is considered when chronic illnesses such as untreated thyroid, diabetes, other endocrinopathies, cerebrovascular, cancer, autoimmune and other inflammatory conditions or depression are present. Fatigue without four of the minor elements is called chronic idiopathic fatigue.

The ancillary symptoms must also have been present for at least 6 months [1–3]. Five of these symptoms are related to nociception: sore throat, sore lymph nodes, sore muscles (myalgia), sore joints without swelling or redness (arthralgia) and new onset headaches. The other three are "cognitive" or "higher functions" such as periods of marked difficulty in concentrating, choosing the right work, the perception of short-term memory loss ("brain fog"), sleep disturbances and exertional exhaustion. The latter is one of the stronger ancillary predictors, and can be readily identified when subjects perform exercise that is more than their usual daily

J.N. Baraniuk and S.J. Merck
Division of Rheumatology, Immunology and Allergy, Georgetown University,
Washington DC, USA

J.N. Baraniuk(✉)
Room B-105, Lower Level Kober-Cogan Building, 3800 Reservoir Road, NW,
Washington DC 20007–2197, USA
e-mail: baraniuj@georgetown.edu

R. Pawankar et al. (eds.), *Allergy Frontiers: Clinical Manifestations*,
DOI: 10.1007/978-4-431-88317-3_5, © Springer 2009

Table 1 1994 Fukuda criteria for CFS [4–7] and American College of Rheumatology criteria for FM [12–14]

Chronic fatigue syndrome (CFS)	Fibromyalgia (FM)
Severe, disabling fatigue for 6 months[a] PLUS at least four of the following: Nociception: 1. New onset headaches 2. Sore throat 3. Sore lymph nodes (cervical and axillary regions) 4. Myalgia 5. Arthralgia Neurocognitive: 6. "Brain fog" with slow thinking, difficulty with arithmetic or choosing the correct word, short-term memory changes 7. Sleep dysfunction, and[b] 8. Exertional exhaustion	Pain in four quadrants for at least 3 months that has no other explanation and affects the: – Left and right sides – Above and below the waist, and – Axial skeleton (neck, thoracic and lower back, costochondritis) Tenderness to manual thumb pressure of ~4 kg at 11 or more of 18 symmetrical tender points at the occiput, lower lateral cervical muscles, supraspinatus, trapezius, anterior 2nd rib, lateral epicondyle, gluteus maximus, greater trochanter, and medial knee fat pad

[a]Fatigue may be assessed by questionnaires such as the Multidimensional Fatigue Inventory [28] and disability or poor quality of life by the Medical Outcomes Survey Short Form 36 (SF-36) [29, 30]
[b]Abnormal sleep studies or appropriate questionnaires

exertion. This effort is sufficient to induce a relapse of their condition with extreme exhaustion that may send the subjects to bed for several days with severe fatigue, disordered neurocognitive functions, systemic pain and tenderness. These criteria were first selected by consensus after a statistical review of a large number of cases, and have subsequently been validated in epidemiological studies [2–4].

The Rhinitis of CFS

The majority of CFS subjects complain of refractory rhinitis (74 ± 3%; range 66–80%) [5–7]. They would have often seen multiple allergists, otolaryngologists and other specialists seeking an explanation for their rhinopathy. They average seven visits per year to subspecialists for their myriad complaints. They often try many over-the-counter and herbal remedies, nasal glucocorticoids and azelastine, and would have had sinus surgeries without relief of the sensations of nasal fullness, congestion and discharge. Often they feel as bad or worse after nasal or sinus surgery as before. If they have positive allergy skin tests, they are commonly considered to have severe refractory allergic rhinitis. Their atopic condition will respond to the usual therapies, but they will be left with the remainder of their extensive list of problems. If skin tests are negative, then they are likely to be labelled as having "vasomotor rhinitis". However, this term is no longer appropriate to use as a grab-bag for "all other types of nonallergic rhinitis" since there are no precise criteria for its diagnosis, and no vascular or efferent motor mechanisms.

In contrast to other chronic idiopathic nonallergic rhinitis syndromes, the potential mechanisms of CFS may offer insights that distinguish this subset of nonallergic rhinitis subjects. Clues may also accrue from the coexistence of fibromyalgia (FM) [8], posttraumatic fatigue syndrome, irritable bowel, irritable bladder, irritable vagina (vulvodynia) [9], and other nonspecific "functional" disorders that share mechanisms of neural dysregulation and hyperalgesia in mucosal and other organs without specific physical signs or laboratory abnormalities [10]. As a rule of thumb, if you are considering whether to order a third CT or MRI scan for vague complaints when the previous ones have recently been normal, then you should stop and consider CFS/FM in the differential diagnosis.

Fibromyalgia

FM is a condition of systemic dysesthesia and autonomic dysfunction. It is defined for research purposes using the American College of Rheumatology case designation criteria. These depend on pain and tenderness lasting for at least 3 months that have no other explanation (Table 1) [11]. The symptom of pain must affect all four quadrants of the body and the axial skeleton. The sign of hyperalgesia, or tenderness, is pain elicited by pressure. The standard research criteria is to induce pain by pressing with one's thumb over the "tender points" (formerly trigger points) until the thumb nail blanches (about 4 kg of pressure) [11]. The subject must complain of pain at ≥11 of 18 of these traditional points. There is no magic to the tender point sites, since digital or mechanical pressure applied to the patient's thumb nails and other random spots is sufficient to identify the nociceptive deep pressure–induced hyperalgesia [12]. In fact, randomized delivery of different deep tissue pressures in a double-blind pain testing paradigm is far superior for detecting hyperalgesia, since the elements of anxiety and predictability of the next pressure to be applied are limited [13]. Tenderness can also be detected by the average pressure causing pain when a strain gauge (dolorimeter) is applied to the 18 tender points [6]. Studies such as these indicate faulty intrinsic spinal cord mechanisms of hyperalgesia in FM.

FM subjects have larger flare responses to intradermal injections of capsaicin, indicating hyperactivity of transient receptor potential vanilloid 1 (TRPV1) ion channel-bearing nociceptive neurons, with an increase in their release of calcitonin gene-related peptide (CGRP) that is responsible for the vasodilation and flare [14–16]. It is unclear if this represents peripheral sensitization with an increased sensitivity of Type C nerve endings to peripheral mediators or central sensitization with dysregulated spinal cord regulation of peripheral nociceptive afferent signalling to dorsal horn substantia gelatinosa interneurons and secondary, ascending pain neurons. These ascending nociceptive signals may not be "gated" or blocked by the usual opioid and other spinal cord inhibitory interneuron circuits. Descending brainstem to the spinal cord inhibitory, antinociceptive aminergic (norepinephrine, dopamine, serotonin) neurons may also be dysfunctional and fail to block the dorsal horn nociceptive transmission pathways. Since FM and CFS are present in many subjects, it is highly likely that an analogous type of trigeminal nerve dysfunction plays a role in nasal pathophysiology. Analogous neural dysfunction in visceral, mucosal organs and myofascial sheaths may also explain irritable syndromes of the airways, gastrointestinal, genitourinary and musculoskeletal systems.

Clinical Investigation

As an allergist in a joint Allergy and Rheumatology tertiary care clinic specializing in FM, one of us (JNB) received many referrals for allergy evaluations of FM subjects. About one quarter of CFS subjects met the formal FM criteria, although nearly three quarters had ≥11 tender points indicating hyperalgesia (Table 2) [6].

The majority of CFS subjects complained of "sinus" problems. They had more facial tenderness over the sinus regions than healthy controls or acute sinusitis subjects when tested by dolorimetry [17]. CFS subjects had higher **Rhinitis Scores**, and about half had positive allergy skin tests [6]. However, they did not have the typical symptoms of histamine-induced itch, sneeze, watery rhinorrhea or eosinophilia. Therefore, allergic rhinitis and atopy were unlikely to explain the diverse sets of symptoms. Instead, a pattern emerged of nasal sensitivity to irritant substances leading to sensations of congestion ± rhinorrhea.

CFS subjects had significantly more complaints in a review of systems than the controls (Table 2) [6]. About half of the CFS group self-reported greater sensations

Table 2 CFS and other symptom complexes in mucosal and somatic organs in 138 healthy control and 125 CFS subjects [2]. Mean ± SEM (n)

Questionnaires and subsets of questionnaire items	Items (n)	Control	CFS
Fibromyalgia (American College of Rheumatology criteria)		0% (57)	28.7% (66)*
Widespread pain		0% (57)	52% (66)*
Manual tender point count	18	7.1 ± 0.9 (46)	12.3 ± 0.9 (36)*
Dolorimetry tender point count	18	3.7 ± 0.5 (105)	9.0 ± 0.7 (65)**
Dolorimetry pain threshold (kg)	–	7.41 ± 2.51 (105)	5.12 ± 0.31 (65)**
Rhinitis Score	40	7.43 ± 0.76	15.97 ± 0.82*
Irritant Rhinitis Score	72	8.95 ± 0.83	15.75 ± 0.99*
Tobacco Score	88	10.33 ± 1.13	24.12 ± 1.71*
Self-report of "Sinusitis"	1	29.2% (106)	69.2% (65)**
Systemic Complaints	52	7.9 ± 0.8 (106)	25.6 ± 1.3 (65)**
– Neurocognitive system	4	0.59 ± 0.10	3.10 ± 0.16*
– Ear, nose and throat system	6	0.62 ± 0.09	2.50 ± 0.16*
– "Dyspnea"/pulmonary system	9	0.36 ± 0.07	2.33 ± 0.19*
– Gastrointestinal system	8	0.52 ± 0.12	3.05 ± 0.24*
– Bladder system	5	0.99 ± 0.08	2.15 ± 0.14*
– Musculoskeletal system	10	0.94 ± 0.13	4.79 ± 0.21*
– Irritable Bowel Syndrome	8	5.8%	44.0%*

Significant ANOVA followed by two-tailed unpaired student's t-test: *$p < 0.0001$; **$p < 10^{-6}$

Table 3 Psychometric comparison of control and CFS populations (mean ± SEM [number analyzed])

Questionnaire	Control (n)	CFS (n)
Minnesota Heart Score	11.5 ± 1.7 (102)	8.1 ± 2.3 (63)
Beck Depression Index	6.3 ± 0.7 (104)	13.6 ± 1.0 (62)[***]
State-Trait Anger Expression Inventory	32.2 ± 1.3 (68)	40.8 ± 1.8 (48)[**]
McGill Pain Score	1.2 ± 0.3 (62)	4.8 ± 1.5 (20)[**]
McGill Present Pain Index	0.94 ± 0.24 (31)	2.64 ±0.28 (11)[***]
McGill Visual Analog Scale	1.05 ± 0.34 (31)	5.05 ± 0.68 (10)[***]
McGill Total Pain Score	2.63 ± 0.71 (62)	16.15 ± 2.33 (20)[***]
McGill Affective Score	0.47 ± 0.18 (62)	3.75 ± 0.68 (20)[***]
McGill Sensory Score	2.6 ± 1.0 (31)	14.9 ± 2.2 (11)[***]
Multidimensional fatigue inventory	(n = 66)	(n = 23)
– General fatigue	9.49 ± 0.54	15.48 ± 0.85[***]
– Physical fatigue	8.1 ± 0.5	12.7 ± 0.9[***]
– Reduced activity	8.3 ± 0.5	11.7 ± 0.9[**]
– Reduced motivation	8.0 ± 0.4	11.4 ± 0.9[**]
– Mental fatigue	9.0 ± 0.6	13.3 ± 1.0[**]
SF-36	(n = 102)	(n = 65)
– Physical function	61.3 ± 3.4	41.9 ± 3.5[**]
– Social function	52.0 ± 3.9	38.8 ± 3.9[*]
– Role functioning physical	44.2 ± 4.6	16.5 ± 3.6[**]
– Role functioning emotional	50.5 ± 4.6	39.1 ±5.1
– Mental health	56.7 ± 2.7	50.5 ± 3.1
– Energy/vitality	38.3 ± 2.9	24.0 ± 2.6[**]
– Bodily pain	50.1 ± 3.8	30.9 ± 3.2[**]
– General health perception	49.4 ± 3.2	29.7 ± 2.8[**]

[*]Unpaired two-tailed student's t-tests, unconstrained

of congestion and nasal discharge to tobacco smoke [18] and other irritants [19] than control subjects. CFS/FM subjects had greater hyperalgesia (lower pain thresholds) and higher prevalence of irritable bowel syndrome, bladder symptoms and dyspnea [20]. CFS subjects also had significantly more affective complaints including anxiety, anger, pain and disability, with reduced quality of life (SF-36) (Table 3).

Potential theories to explain the symptom complex of CFS have included atopy, inflammation, viral infection, autonomic and nociceptive nerve dysfunction. Investigations of these mechanisms are described below.

Atopy in CFS

The hypothesis that atopy was more prevalent and causative in CFS [6] began when positive allergy skin tests were found in 50% of 24 [21] and 55% of 28 [22] CFS subjects. These rates were higher than the 20–30% that had been published a decade earlier [23]. CFS subjects complained of skin rashes, urticaria, rhinitis, asthma and drug and food reactions. Each condition was regarded as "atopic" even though there were no other confirmatory or provocation tests to evaluate IgE-mediated mechanisms. CFS subject complaints were lumped together, leading early authors to conclude that 83–90% of CFS subjects were "atopic". However, many of their complaints could be equally well explained as nonallergic syndromes, such as, maculopapular skin rashes, inappropriate self-reported descriptions of "hives" without pruritus, nonallergic rhinitis, vocal cord dysfunction, dyspnea without asthma, non-IgE drug idiosyncratic or expected pharmacological reactions and food intolerances [24]. IgE was not compared between the CFS and local control population. The long differential diagnosis of inflammatory eosinophilic, chronic nonallergic rhinosinusitis, and neutrophilic chronic infectious rhinosinusitis were not investigated. Noninflammatory rhinitides related to hormonal, neural, sympathetic, parasympathetic (cholinergic rhinitis [25]) and nociceptive ("vasomotor rhinitis", idiopathic rhinitis) neural dysfunction [26] were not investigated. As early as 1992, Metzger's group had proposed that nonallergic rhinitis was the most likely diagnosis [5]. This finding was largely ignored as investigators stampeded to the TH2 lymphocyte dysfunction hypothesis of CFS pathology.

If TH2–IgE mechanisms were responsible for CFS rhinitis, then it was reasonable to expect that typical antiallergy therapies would improve the condition. This expectation was false. Both antihistamines (terfenadine) [22] and topical nasal glucocorticoids [27] had no benefit from the presumed "allergic rhinitis" of CFS. This implied that TH2–IgE–mast cell–eosinophil pathways did not contribute to either CFS or its associated rhinitic syndrome.

Atopy was investigated further by assessing the constellation of symptoms in CFS, allergic rhinitis and control groups, and their rates of positive allergy skin tests and elevated IgE levels. CFS and healthy control subjects retrospectively scored the severities of 30 skin, eye and airway symptoms over the previous 6 months using an Airway Symptoms Severity Questionnaire [2, 28, 29]. The severity of each symptom was scored as none (score = 0), trivial (1), mild (2), moderate (3) or severe (4). This questionnaire was validated by prospectively assessing changes in symptoms prior to, during and after periods of seasonal allergic rhinitis, and following the emergency room treatment of acute asthma. The score for "trivial" complaints was justified statistically to prevent a "floor" effect between "none" and "mild" that was scored by subjects who had minimal symptoms that were not persistent or disabling enough to be considered "mild". There was no ceiling effect, since the category of "extremely severe" was not statistically valid by Cronbach's α testing. A score of 13 for the nose, sinus and throat questions was defined as an "abnormal" or "positive" ***Rhinitis Score***. This score exceeded the 95th percentile for a negative control group ($n = 79$) who had no allergic rhinitis, sinusitis, FM or CFS and who were recruited for a separate protocol where rhinitis and skin testing status were not used as inclusion or exclusion criteria.

Allergy Skin Test Results. Skin testing was positive for at least two allergens plus histamine in 39% of 92 CFS, 50% of 139 healthy control, and 100% of the allergic rhinitis subjects ($n = 27$). Rates for CFS and normal groups were not significantly different (Chi^2).

Rhinitis Classification. **Rhinitis Scores** < and ≥ 13, and positive or negative allergy skin tests were used to classify CFS and control subjects into different subsets of rhinitis [6]. (1) Nonallergic rhinitis (***NAR***) was defined by negative allergy skin

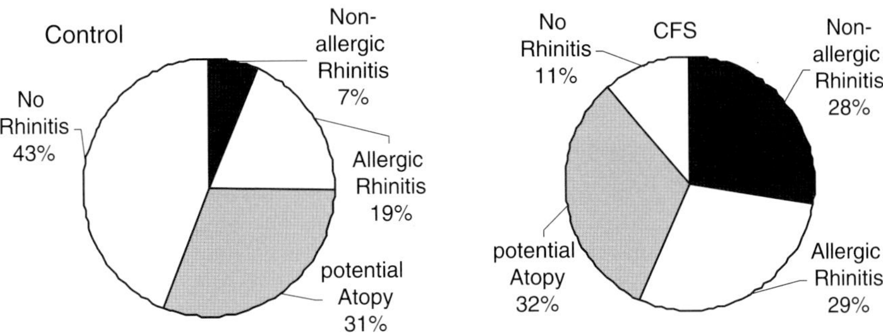

Fig. 1 Comparison of rhinitis types in control and CFS groups. There were significantly more subjects with negative **Rhinitis Scores** (**No Rhinitis** and **potential Atopy**) in the Control group. In contrast, the high **Rhinitis Scores** found in the CFS group lead to higher prevalences of **Nonallergic** and **Allergic Rhinitis**

tests with a positive histamine response plus a positive **Rhinitis Score** of ≥ 13. (2) Allergic rhinitis (**AR**) had positive allergy skin tests with positive **Rhinitis Scores**. (3) Potential atopy (**potAt**) subjects had positive allergy skin tests with negative **Rhinitis Scores**. The **potAt** designation implied allergen sensitization without significant nasal symptoms. (4) The no Rhinitis group (**noRh**) had negative allergy skin tests and **Rhinitis Scores**. The distributions of these groups were compared between CFS and healthy control (HC) groups (Fig. 1). Subjects were not aware that the purpose of the investigation was to assess rhinitis. The significantly higher RhSc in the CFS population generated higher percentages of NAR and AR subjects compared to the control group. However, there were no differences in the frequencies of the positive allergy skin tests. Stratification by serum IgE concentrations also showed no significant differences between normal and CFS subsets [30].

In a multivariate analysis, a positive **Rhinitis Score** was more predictive of CFS ($p < 0.000001$) than a positive allergy skin test result (not significant). The absence of a relationship between CFS and allergy skin test results [6] combined with similar distributions of IgE concentrations [30] in CFS and control populations confirmed that atopy was not more frequent in CFS. Stratification by Rhinitis Score and allergy skin test status did not generate any differences between CFS and control subgroups. The hypothesis that atopy was responsible for CFS [21, 31] was not supported by these data.

Mucosal Inflammation

An alternative hypothesis was that CFS rhinitis was the result of airway inflammation. The hypothesis was derived from the original cardinal features of CFS that resembled those of an infectious illness (e.g., sore throat, fatigue, sensation of fever, myalgias) [32]. Chronic viral infections by Epstein-Barr virus (EBV) [32] were suggested because of the similarity of CFS to prolonged infectious mononucleosis.

Early studies found high titres of antibodies to EBV in CFS [32]. Later studies showed that antibody titres for EBV, human herpes virus 6 (HHV-6), cytomegalovirus (CMV), varicella, enteroviruses and retroviruses lacked sensitivity and specificity for CFS [33, 34]. Elevated titers to numerous ubiquitous infectious agents weakened the hypothesis that any single virus provoked CFS. In addition, high viral titres have been reported in subjects living under high stress conditions such as the caregivers to Alzheimer patients [35, 36]. This suggested that chronic physiological stressors may modulate immune responses in a wide variety of situations. Finally, chronic viral and immune aberrations have been postulated to cause CFS, but not the overlapping illnesses of fibromyalgia, somatoform disorders, irritable bowel syndrome, migraine headaches, interstitial cystitis and neurally mediated hypotension that are common in the CFS population.

If active infections or inflammation were responsible for CFS rhinitis, then changes in vascular, glandular and cellular biomarkers should occur. Nasal lavage fluid was assessed in CFS, active allergic rhinitis, cystic fibrosis, rhinovirus infections and healthy control subjects [37]. Allergic rhinitis subjects had significantly higher total protein, IgG (vascular permeability), 7F10-mucin (submucosal gland serous cell mucin), eosinophil cationic protein (ECP) and neutrophil elastase than healthy control and CFS groups [37, 38]. Cystic fibrosis patients with chronic infectious rhinosinusitis had significantly higher 7F10-mucin, Alcian Blue positive acidic mucin (submucosal gland mucous cells) and elastase. In a separate study, healthy students were inoculated with *Rhinovirus Hanks* [39]. Vascular exudation of albumin and IgG was increased fourfold to sevenfold on Days 3 and 4, followed by fourfold increases in secretory IgA (sIgA). Gel phase acid mucins and IL-8 levels were increased twofold. These values were significantly different from the noninfected healthy control and CFS groups. CFS did have a trend towards mucous hypersecretion and mucosal friability (increased free hemoglobin in nasal lavage fluid) compared to healthy control subjects [40, 41]. Cytokine levels were measured, to implicate inflammatory mechanisms in CFS. However, there were no differences from control values in the baseline nasal lavage fluid concentrations for tumor necrosis factor-α (TNF-α), interleukin-8 (IL-8) or nerve growth factor (NGF) [42]. In contrast, the positive control of acute sinusitis had significantly higher total protein, TNF-α and IL-8. Concentrations for active allergic rhinitis were equivalent to healthy controls and CFS subjects, possibly because of the ongoing allergically triggered secretion of copious volumes of plasma and glandular mucus components that diluted these mediators in the active disease. Overall, these data reduced the likelihood that allergic rhinitis, eosinophilic nonallergic rhinosinusitis, chronic infectious sinusitis, humoral or other immunodeficiencies contributed to CFS rhinitis.

Dysautonomia in CFS

CFS and FM subjects have a significant autonomic dysfunction. This has been demonstrated by heart rate variability [43], neurally mediated hypotension on tilt table testing [44], and impaired sympathetic responses to stressors such as exercise, muscle contraction, noise and other stimuli [45]. These data generated the hypothesis that dysautonomia with a blunted sympathetic response to stressors and generalized elevation in parasympathetic influences contributed to CFS and FM pathophysiology.

Dysautonomia has been identified in irritable bowel syndrome (IBS) and migraine headaches [46, 47]. These syndromes have increased prevalences in CFS and FM. Migraine headaches have baseline sympathetic hypofunction and instability of sympathetic responses [48, 49]. Nociceptive nerve axon responses with the release of CGRP are also implicated in the migraines.

Intestinal smooth muscle dysmotility in irritable bowel syndrome is generalized to smooth muscle dysmotility throughout the entire body. This includes the bladder, lungs, and oesophagus [50–52]. Numerous studies have shown that IBS is characterized by increased visceral nociception [53]. However, the crampy pain may be due to a distinct central activation of pain pathways, while the diarrhea/constipation component appears to be the result of dysmotility mediated by the dopaminergic regulatory systems of the intrinsic intestinal submucosal and myenteric plexuses. A similar relationship exists between oesophageal motor tone and visceral nociception. Oesophageal spasm ("nutcracker oesophagus") can cause noncardiac chest pain that must be carefully distinguished from coronary artery disease and atypical angina. It is not known if there is intrinsic dysfunction of vascular smooth muscle in nasal arterial or arteriovenous vessels in CFS.

Adrenal function. CFS and FM subjects have blunted morning cortisol surges that are compatible with tertiary adrenal insufficiency, and are reminiscent of the findings in atypical seasonal depression in the winter, dysthymia and less common chronic fatigue states [54]. These changes are opposite to those seen in me ancholic depression, which are characterized by increased stress system activity [55]. Adrenal insufficiency occurs in response to exercise in FM, since cortisol levels fall paradoxically rather than rise in response to physical exertion [56]. This postexercise adrenal insufficiency, as well as the decreased sympathetic response to exercise could be responsible for the severe post-exertional fatigue that these syndromes. It is possible that these disturbances are surrogate markers of a central nervous system dysfunction in the dopaminergic mesocorticolimbic system or the reticular activating system [54].

Sympathetic Nervous System Responses to Isometric Handgrip. Isometric hand grip contraction is a simple, well-understood method to stimulate systemic sympathetic reflexes. Strong sympathetic discharge causes vasoconstriction of all tissue vascular beds including the nasal arteriovenous anastomoses and venous sinusoids [57]. In an initial pilot study, six control and five CFS subjects contracted a hand dynamometer to maximum strength [58]. After a 30 min rest period, they sat relaxed for a 5 min "sham" contraction with the dynamometer in their hands. Vital signs and acoustic rhinometry variables of the minimum cross-sectional area of the anterior nasal valve (Amin) and airspace volume of the anterior 8 cm of the nasal cavity were averaged for the sham period [59]. Subjects then contracted the dynamometer at 30% of maximum strength for as long as possible (1.5–2.5 min, no difference between CFS and control subjects). The final "peak" measurements were taken before each subject reached exhaustion, and the incremental differences from the average for the "sham" period were calculated. In preliminary studies, both the minimum cross-sectional area and the nasal cavity volumes were significantly increased in the control subjects, but the incremental changes were not significant in CFS (Fig. 2). The control subjects had significantly increased diastolic and systolic blood pressures, but not heart rates (Fig. 3). Only systolic blood pressure was significantly increased in CFS. These data are consistent with decreased sympathetic function in CFS. Alternative sites for reflex dysfunction following isometric forearm muscle contraction include defective sensing of contracted muscle length, ischemia or acidosis; spinal cord or brain stem coordination of sympathetic outflow, efferent postganglionic norepinephrine or neuropeptide Y (NPY) vasoconstrictor release; insensitivity of α-adrenergic receptors or absent signal transduction in arterial smooth muscle leading to reduced sympathetic vasoconstriction. Multiple other molecular targets are conceivable.

Systemic parasympathetic dysfunction may contribute to CFS pathophysiology based on heart rate variability studies [43], increased cholinergic reactivity in the subset of "runners" with excessive cholinergic reflex rhinorrhea [25], and increased vasoactive intestinal peptide-immunoreactive, non-cholinergic neurons described in idiopathic rhinitis [60].

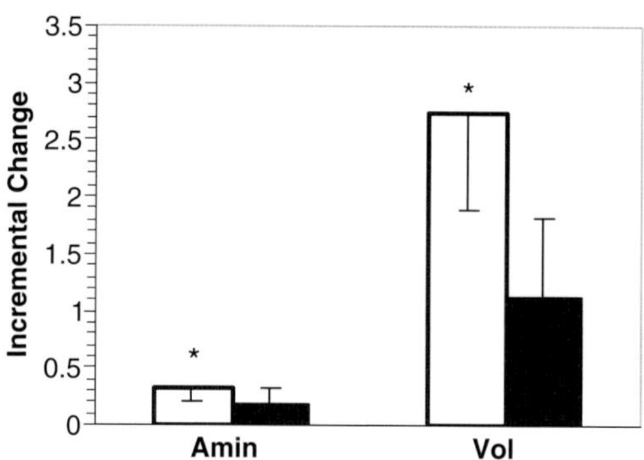

Fig. 2 Acoustic rhinometry in isometric handgrips. The incremental changes in Amin and airspace volume (Vol) are shown between an isometric hand grip at 30% of maximum and a relaxed "sham contraction". Changes were significant ($^*p < 0.05$) for control subjects (white bars) but not CFS subjects (black bars)

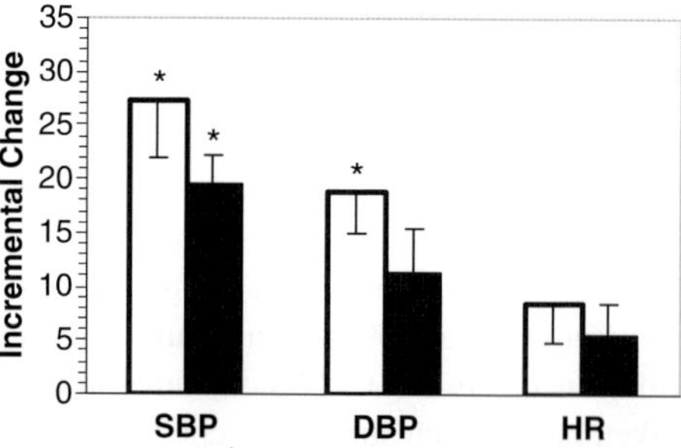

Fig. 3 Vital signs in isometric hand grips. The incremental change between isometric and sham hand grip contractions are shown for systolic (SBP) and diastolic (DBP) blood pressure and heart rate (HR) for control (white bars) and CFS (black bars) groups. The asterixes indicate $p < 0.01$ for the incremental changes

Nociceptive Dysfunction in CFS Rhinitis

The studies of baseline nasal lavage fluid cited above demonstrated that there were limited differences between healthy control and CFS subjects, but very significant differences from the inflammatory syndromes of allergic rhinitis, cystic fibrosis and viral infections. Nociceptive nerve function was assessed by hypertonic saline provocation. Hypertonic saline (HTS) mimics the effects of capsaicin, and is desensitized by capsaicin pretreatment [61]. In allergic, nonallergic, and post-viral asthma and rhinitis, HTS causes exaggerated effects or mucosal hyperresponsiveness [62]. HTS may lead to nociceptive nerve depolarization by acting on chloride ion channels to directly depolarize nociceptive nerves; or by osmotically drawing water out of epithelial cells causing them to shrink and so activate transient receptor potential ion channels or adjacent chemosensitive/mechanicothermal C-fibers [63]. Dry powders such as mannose, the high osmolarity induced by the sudden release of pollen components upon hydration on the nasal mucosa and inhaled irritants on particulate material may activate additional mechanisms [64, 65]. Irritant hyperresponsiveness occurs in both allergic and nonallergic subjects [61, 62], with glandular exocytosis being stimulated by potential nociceptive nerve axon response mechanisms [66]. Other mucosal irritants may activate additional mechanisms that remain to be determined.

Unilateral Hypertonic Saline (HTS) Nasal Provocations. Unilateral HTS provocations were performed in CFS subjects [59, 66]. Sensations and secretions were assessed from both the ipsilateral challenged nostril and the contralateral nostril [67].

Pain. HTS caused an immediate, intense, but short-lived (up to 20 s) burning (Fig. 4) that was followed by a more prolonged dose-dependent paresthetic, dull ache. These two sensations may be analogous to the First and Second Pain mediated by Type Aδ and C nociceptive fibers, respectively [68]. Pain Intensity ($p = 0.01$ by ANCOVA) and Duration ($p = 0.008$) were significantly higher in CFS than control subjects, indicating nociceptive dysfunction in CFS.

Nasal Blockage. Self-reported sensations of blockage were higher in CFS ($p < 0.000001$) than controls after the first normal saline provocation (Fig. 5). The control subjects had a significant HTS dose response with increasing obstruction. In contrast, the CFS response was significantly blunted. This suggested that CFS subjects could not effectively detect or report changes in blockage compared to the

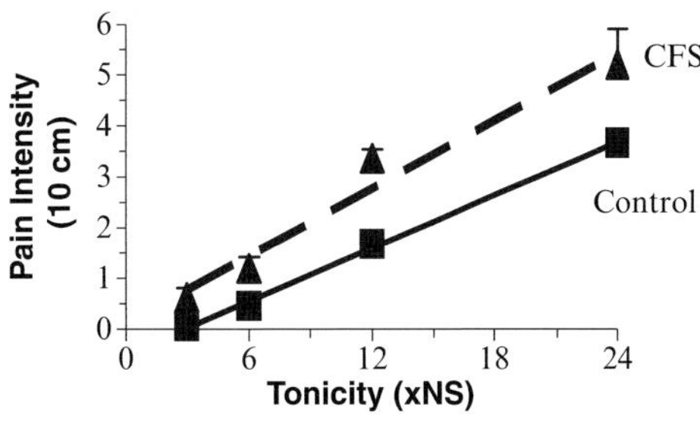

Fig. 4 Pain intensity after unilateral HTS. CFS (solid triangles, dashed line, $n = 10$) had significantly greater pain intensity (first pain) than control subjects (solid squares, solid line, n = 29) ($p = 0.01$)

Fig. 5 Nasal blockage after unilateral HTS. The CFS group had a significantly greater sensation of nasal blockage after challenge with 0.9% (normal) saline. The control group had a dose dependent increase in blockage, while there was no significant change in the CFS group

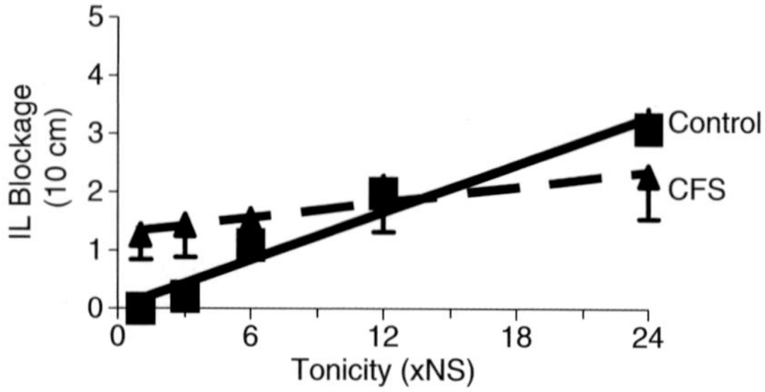

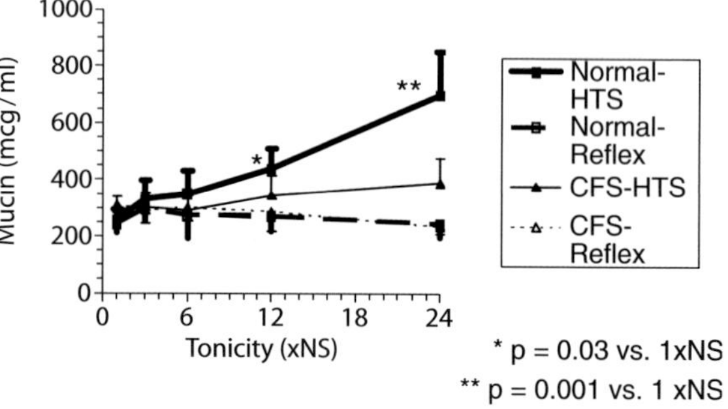

Fig. 6 Nasal lavage mucin after unilateral HTS. The normal control subjects had an HTS dose dependent increase in mucin secretion (heavy solid line). They had no significant contralateral reflex (dashed line). The CFS subjects had no ipsilateral (thin solid line) or contral-ateral (dotted line) secretion

controls. The sensation of nasal obstruction did not change on the contralateral side for either group.

Rhinorrhea. The weight of the nasal lavage fluid increased in an HTS dose-dependent fashion in control subjects. However, there was almost a net loss of fluid in the CFS subjects. This suggested absorption of lavage fluid by the mucosa.

A neutral mucin ("7F10-mucin") (Fig. 6) and the submucosal gland serous cell markers, urea and lysozyme (not shown), were secreted in an HTS dose-dependent fashion in normal subjects, but only on the ipsilateral side. There was no contralateral reflex secretion. In the CFS group at the baseline, urea was significantly elevated in the CFS group compared to controls, while mucin was the same as in controls. HTS did not cause ipsilateral or contralateral secretion of either urea or mucin in CFS. These data indicated that submucosal gland exocytosis was highly disrupted in CFS.

There were no changes in albumin or IgG during HTS provocations at these levels of induced pain. This indicated that the direct effect of HTS or nociceptive axon responses did not increase plasma exudation in either normal or CFS subjects.

The unilateral nature of these responses suggested that HTS-stimulated noci-ceptive nerves caused pain in the central nervous system, and were extensively branched around glands in the nasal mucosa. These branches presumably released neuropeptides that stimulated glandular exocytosis (Fig. 7). There was no change in vascular permeability suggesting that superficial post-capillary venules were not innervated by these HTS-sensitive neurons. Central cholinergic reflexes were not

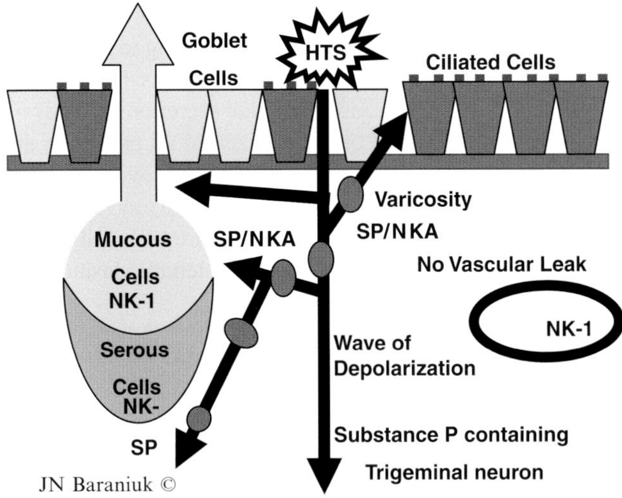

Fig. 7 Neurogenic axon response to hypertonic saline (HTS) nasal provocation. HTS lead to depolarization of a subset of substance P (SP) – containing trigeminal neurons. The wave of depolarization spreads throughout the highly branched, dendritic neuronal processes in the mucosa. Varicosities that contain SP and probably other neurotransmitters are activated and release these near glands. SP and/or neurokinin A (NKA) act on neurokinin-1 receptors (NK1) that are most dense on glands to induce glandular exocytosis. Unlike animal models or much higher doses of HTS, the superficial vessels do not appear to be significantly activated. There is no plasma extravasation as part of the nociceptive nerve axon response under these conditions *in vivo* (Used with permission of the copyright holder *JN Baraniuk©*)

recruited since there was no contralateral secretion. The significant differences in CFS suggested an increase in Type C nociceptive neuron sensitivity to HTS, with more intense and prolonged pain sensations. However, unilateral glandular secretion did not occur, suggesting that the axon response mechanism was defective in CFS. This was likely chronic, since there was elevation of glandular protein markers at the baseline compared to the control subjects. Further pharmacological investigations are required to localize the specific defects associated with CFS nerve dysfunction.

Conclusion

These data indicate that CFS subjects have neural dysfunction that affects their cognitive, pain, nasal and other mucosal organs. Perhaps the adage, "It's all in your head," applies [69], but only because that is where most of the body's neurons and nasal passages are located. Functional differences were demonstrated between the nonallergic rhinitis of CFS and nasal function and dysfunction in healthy controls, allergic rhinitis, sinusitis, virus-infected and cystic fibrosis subjects. The nasal nociceptive nerves conveyed sensations leading to increased perceptions of nasal pain, blockage and discharge after hypertonic saline nasal provocation. However, mucosal axon responses and glandular secretion were dysfunctional in CFS. Although these studies cannot be generalized to all groups of noninfectious, nonallergic, noninflammatory persistent rhinitis, they provide a strong indication that functional defects in nociceptive nerve function, axon responses and potentially other mechanisms may be identifiable in future, carefully phenotyped and clinical subsets of patients studied in a rigorous, systematic fashion.

Acknowledgements Supported by US Public Health Service Awards RO1 AI42403, RO1 ES053820, M01-RR13297, and P50 DC000214 to Dr. Baraniuk, and a Glaxo research grant to Ms. Merck.

References

1. Fukuda K, Straus SE, Hickie I, Sharpe MC, Dobbins JG, Komaroff A. The International Chronic Fatigue Syndrome Study Group. The chronic fatigue syndrome: a comprehensive approach to its definition and study. Ann Intern Med 1994; 121:953–959.
2. Reeves WC, Lloyd A, Vernon SD, Klimas N, Jason LA, Bleijenberg G, Evengard B, White PD, Nisenbaum R, Unger ER. International Chronic Fatigue Syndrome Study Group. Identification of ambiguities in the 1994 chronic fatigue syndrome research case definition and recommendations for resolution. BMC Health Serv Res 2003; 3:25.
3. Reeves WC, Wagner D, Nisenbaum R, Jones JF, Gurbaxani B, Solomon L, Papanicolaou DA, Unger ER, Vernon SD, Heim C. Chronic fatigue syndrome - a clinically empirical approach to its definition and study. BMC Med 2005; 3:19
4. Taylor RR, Jason LA. Chronic fatigue, abuse-related traumatization, and psychiatric disorders in a community-based sample. Soc Sci Med 2002; 55:247–256.
5. Cleveland CH, Jr., Fisher RH, Brestel EP, Esinhart JD, Metzger WJ. Chronic rhinitis: an under-recognized association with fibromyalgia. Allergy Proc 1992. Sept–Oct 1993; 13:263–267.
6. Baraniuk JN, Clauw DJ, Gaumond E. Rhinitis symptoms in chronic fatigue syndrome. Ann Allergy Asthma Immunol 1998; 81:359–365.
7. Baraniuk JN, Clauw D, Yuta A, Ali M, Gaumond E, Upadhyayula N, Fujita K, Shimizu T. Nasal secretion analysis in allergic rhinitis, cystic fibrosis, and nonallergic fibromyalgia/chronic fatigue syndrome subjects. Am J Rhinol 1998; 12:435–440.
8. White KP, Speechley M, Harth M, Ostbye T. Co-existence of chronic fatigue syndrome with fibromyalgia syndrome in the general population. A controlled study. Scand J Rheumatol 2000; 29:44–51.
9. Baraniuk JN. Neurogenic inflammation. In: Leppert PC, Turned ML, eds. Vulvodynia: Toward Understanding a Pain Syndrome. Proceedings from the workshop April 14–15, 2003, supported by the National Institute of Child Health and Human Development (NICHD), the Office of Research on Women's Health, and the Office of Rare Diseases. pp. 16–18, 2004. http://www.nichd.nih.gov/publications/pubs/final_vulvodynia_report.pdf
10. Baraniuk JN. CFS and overlapping conditions. CFS Res Rev 2004; 6–9.
11. Wolfe F, Smythe HA, Yunus MB, Bennett RM, Bombardier C, Goldenberg DL, Tugwell P, Campbell SM, Abeles M, Clark P, et al. The American College of Rheumatology 1990 Criteria for the Classification of Fibromyalgia. Report of the Multicenter Criteria Committee. Arthritis Rheum 1990; 33:160–172.

12. Petzke F, Ambrose K, Gracely RH, Clauw DJ. What do tender points measure? Arthritis Rheum 1999; 42:S342, abstr.

13. Gracely RH, Geisser ME, Giesecke T, Grant MA, Petzke F, Williams DA, Clauw DJ. Pain catastrophizing and neural responses to pain among persons with fibromyalgia. Brain 2004; 127:835–843.

14. Littlejohn GO. Balanced treatments for fibromyalgia. Arthritis Rheum 2004; 50:2725–2729.

15. Caterina MJ. Vanilloid receptors take a TRP beyond the sensory afferent. Pain 2003; 105:5–9.

16. Weidner C, Klede M, Rukwied R, Lischetzki G, Neisius U, Skov PS, Petersen LJ, Schmelz M. Acute effects of substance P and calcitonin gene-related peptide in human skin: a microdialysis study. J Invest Dermatol 2000; 115:1015–1020.

17. Naranch K, Park Y-J, Repka-Ramirez SM, Velarde A, Clauw D, Baraniuk JN. A tender sinus does not always mean sinusitis. Otolaryngol Head Neck Surg 2002; 127:387–397.

18. Baraniuk, JN, Naranch K, Maibach H, Clauw D. Tobacco sensitivity in Chronic Fatigue Syndrome. J CFS 2000; 7:33–52.

19. Baraniuk, JN, Naranch K, Maibach H, Clauw D. Irritant rhinitis in allergic, nonallergic, control and Chronic Fatigue Syndrome populations. J CFS 2000; 7:3–31.

20. Naranch K, Singer A, Gaumond E, Khine A, Velarde A, Clauw D, Baraniuk JN. Dyspnea in fibromyalgia (FM) and chronic fatigue syndrome (CFS). Am J Respir Crit Care Med 1999; 103:A763.

21. Straus SE, Dale JK, Wright R, Metcalfe DD. Allergy and chronic fatigue syndrome. J Allergy Clin Immunol 1988; 81:791–794.

22. Steinberg P, McNutt BE, Marshall P, Schenck C, Lurie N, Pheley A, Peterson PK. Double-blind placebo-controlled study of efficacy of oral terfenadine in the treatment of chronic fatigue syndrome. J Allergy Clin Immunol 1996; 97:119–126.

23. Gergen PJ, Turkeltaub PC, Kovar MG. The prevalence of allergic skin test reactivity to eight common aeroallergens in the U.S. population: results from the second National Health and Nutrition Examination Survey. J Allergy Clin Immunol 1987; 80:669.

24. Middleton E, Reed CE, Ellis EF, Adkinson NF, Yunginger JW, Busse WW. Allergy Principles and Practice. 4th edition. Mosby, St. Louis, MO, 1993.

25. Stjarne P, Lundblad L, Lundberg JM, Anggard A. Capsaicin and nicotine sensitive afferent neurones and nasal secretion in healthy human volunteers and in patients with vasomotor rhinitis. Br J Pharmacol 1989; 96:693–701.

26. Mygind N, Naclerio RM, eds. Allergic and Nonallergic Rhinitis. WB Saunders, Philadelphia, PA, 1993.

27. Kakumanu SS, Mende CN, Lehman EB, Hughes K, Craig TJ. Effect of topical nasal corticosteroids on patients with chronic fatigue syndrome and rhinitis. J Am Osteopath Assoc 2003; 103:423–427.

28. Wasserfallen JB, Gold K, Schulman KA, Baraniuk JN. Development and validation of a rhinoconjunctivitis and asthma symptom score for use as an outcome measure in clinical trials. J Allergy Clin Immunol 1997; 100:16–22.

29. Wasserfallen JB, Gold K, Schulman KA, Baraniuk JN. Item responsiveness of a rhinitis and asthma symptom score during a pollen season. J Asthma 1999; 36:459–465.

30. Repka-Ramirez MS, Naranch K, Park Y-J, Velarde A, Clauw D, Baraniuk JN. IgE levels are the same in Chronic Fatigue Syndrome (CFS) and control subjects when stratified by allergy skin test results and rhinitis types. Annals Allergy Asthma Immunol 2001; 87:218–221.

31. Manu P, Lane TJ, Matthews DA. The pathophysiology of chronic fatigue syndrome; confirmations, contradictions, and conjectures. Int J Psychiatry Med 1992; 22:397–408.

32. Wray BB, Gaughf C, Chandler FW, Berry SS, Latham JE, Wood L, DuRant RH. Detection of Epstein-Barr virus and cytomegalovirus in patients with chronic fatigue. Ann Allergy 1993; 71:223–226.

33. Straus SE. Studies of herpesvirus infection in chronic fatigue syndrome. Ciba Found Symp 1993; 173:132–197.

34. Anonymous. Inability of retroviral tests to identify persons with chronic fatigue syndrome, 1992. MMWR 1993; 42:189–190.
35. Schulz R, Visintainer P, Williamson GM. Psychiatric and physical morbidity effects of caregiving. J Gerontol 1990; 45:181–191.
36. Glaser R, MacCallum RC, Laskowski BF, Malarkey WB, Sheridan JF, Kiecolt-Glaser JK. Evidence for a shift in the Th-1 to Th-2 cytokine response associated with chronic stress and aging. J Gerontol A Biol Sci Med Sci 2001; 56:M477–M482.
37. Baraniuk JN, Clauw D, Yuta A, Ali M, Gaumond E, Upadhyayula N, Fujita K, Shimizu T. Nasal secretion analysis in allergic rhinitis, cystic fibrosis, and nonallergic fibromyalgia/ chronic fatigue syndrome subjects. Am J Rhinol 1998; 12:435–440.
38. Yuta A, Ali M, Sabol M, Gaumond E, Baraniuk JN. Mucoglycoprotein hypersecretion in allergic rhinitis and cystic fibrosis. Am J Physiol 1997; 273 (Lung Cell Mol Physiol 17):L1203–L1207.
39. Yuta A, van Deusen M, Gaumond E, Ali M, Baraniuk JN, Doyle W, Cohen S, Skoner D. Rhinovirus infection induces mucus hypersecretion. Am J Physiol 1998; 274 (Lung Cell Mol Physiol 18):L1017–L1023.
40. Naranch K, Repka-Ramirez SM, Park Y-J, Velarde A, Finnegan R, Murray J, Pheiffer A, Hwang E, D Clauw, MD, JN Baraniuk. Differences in baseline nasal secretions between Chronic Fatigue Syndrome (CFS) and control subjects. J CFS 2002; 10:3–15.
41. Park Y-J, Repka-Ramirez SM, Naranch K, Velarde A, Clauw D, Baraniuk JN. Nasal lavage concentrations of free hemoglobin as a marker of microepistaxis during nasal provocation testing. Allergy 2002; 57:329–335.
42. Repka-Ramirez MS, Naranch K, Park Y-J, Clauw D, Baraniuk JN. Cytokines in nasal lavage fluids from acute sinusitis, allergic rhinitis, and Chronic Fatigue Syndrome subjects. Allergy Asthma Proc 2002; 23:185–190.
43. Stein PK, Domitrovich PP, Ambrose K, Lyden A, Fine M, Gracely RH, Clauw DJ. Sex effects on heart rate variability in fibromyalgia and Gulf War illness. Arthritis Rheum 2004; 51:700–708.
44. Rowe PC, Bou-Holaigah I, Kan JS, Calkins H. Is neurally mediated hypotension an unrecognised cause of chronic fatigue? Lancet 1995; 345:623–624.
45. Qiao ZG, Vaerøy H, Mørkrid L. Electrodermal and microcirculatory activity in patients with fibromyalgia during baseline, acoustic stimulation and cold pressor tests. J Rheumatol 1991. Sept 1993; 18:1383–1389.
46. Lynn R, Friedman L. Irritable bowel syndrome. N Engl J Med 1993; 329:1940–1945.
47. Buzzi M, Bonamini M, Cerbo R. The anatomy and biochemistry of headache. Funct Neurol 1993; 8:395–402.
48. Pogacnik T, Sega S, Pecnik B, Kiauta T. Autonomic function testing in patients with migraine. Headache 1993; 33:545–550.
49. Appel S, Kuritzky A, Zahavi I, Zigelman M, Akselrod S. Evidence for instability of the autonomic nervous system in patients with migraine headache. Headache 1992; 32:10–17.
50. White AM, Stevens WH, Upton AR, et al. Airway responsiveness to inhaled methacholine in patients with irritable bowel syndrome. Gastroenterology 1991; 100:68–74.
51. Whorwell PJ, Clouter C, Smith CL. Oesophageal motility in the irritable bowel syndrome. Br Med J 1981; 282:1101–1102.
52. Whorwell PJ, Lupton EW, Erduran D, et al. Bladder smooth muscle dysfunction in patients with irritable bowel syndrome. Gut 1986; 27:1014–1017.
53. Adam V. Visceral Perception. Understanding Internal Cognition. Plenum, New York, 1998. pp. 1–232.
54. Chrousos GP, Gold PW. The concepts of stress and stress system disorders. Overview of physical and behavioral homeostasis. JAMA 1992; 267:1244–1252.
55. Griep EN, Boersma JW, de Kloet ER. Altered reactivity of the hypothalamic-pituitary-adrenal axis in the primary fibromyalgia syndrome. J Rheumatol 1993; 20:469–474.

56. van Denderen JC, Boersma JW, Zeinstra P, et al. Physiological effects of exhaustive physical exercise in primary fibromyalgia syndrome (PFS): is PFS a disorder of neuroendocrine reactivity? Scand J Rheumatol 1993; 21:35–37.

57. Wilde AD, Cook JA, Jones AS. The nasal response to isometric exercise in non-eosinophilic intrinsic rhinitis. Clin Otolaryngol 1996; 21:84–86.

58. Park Y-J, Naranch K, Repka-Ramirez SM, Clauw D, Baraniuk JN. Sympathetic dysfunction demonstrated by isometric handgrip responses in CFS. American Association for Chronic Fatigue Syndrome. Seattle, WA (oral presentation), Jan 2001.

59. Baraniuk JN, Ali M, Naranch K. Hypertonic saline nasal provocation and acoustic rhinometry. Clin Exp Allergy 2002; 32:543–550.

60. Kurian SS, Blank MA, Sheppard MN. Vasoactive intestinal polypeptide (VIP) in vasomotor rhinitis. Clin Biochem 1983; 11:425–427.

61. Togias A, Lykens K, Kagey-Sobotka A, Eggleston PA, Proud D, Lichtenstein LM, Naclerio RM. Studies on the relationships between sensitivity to cold, dry air, hyperosmolar solutions, and histamine in the adult nose. Am Rev Respir Dis 1990; 141:1428–1433.

62. Sanico AM, Philip G, Proud D, Naclerio RM, Togias A. Comparison of nasal mucosal responsiveness to neuronal stimulation in non-allergic and allergic rhinitis: effects of capsaicin nasal challenge. Clin Exp Allergy 1998; 28:92–100.

63. Liedtke W, Tobin DM, Bargmann CL, Friedman JM. Mammalian TRPV4 (VR-OAC) directs behavioral responses to osmotic and mechanical stimuli in Caenorhabditis elegans. PNAS 2003; 100:14531–14536.

64. Baraniuk JN, Bolick M, Esch R, Buckley CE. Quantification of pollen solute release using pollen grain column chromatography. Allergy 1992; 47:411–417.

65. Peterson B, Saxon A. Global increases in allergic respiratory disease: the possible role of diesel exhaust particles. Ann Allergy Asthma Immunol 1996; 77:263–268.

66. Baraniuk JN, Petrie KN, Le U, Tai C-F, Park Y-J, Yuta A, Ali M, VandenBussche CJ, Nelson B. Neuropathology in rhinosinusitis. Am J Respir Crit Care Med 2005; 171:5–11.

67. Baraniuk JN, Ali M, Yuta A, Fang SY, Naranch K. Hypertonic saline nasal provocation stimulates nociceptive nerves, substance P release, and glandular mucous exocytosis in normal humans. Am J Respir Crit Care Med 1999; 160:655–662.

68. Dray A, Urban L, Dickenson A. Pharmacology of chronic pain. TiPS 1994; 15:190–197.

69. Raine R, Carter S, Sensky T, Black N. General practitioners' perceptions of chronic fatigue syndrome and beliefs about its management, compared with irritable bowel syndrome: qualitative study. BMJ 2004; 328:1354–1357.

Epigenetics Chapter: The Role of Allergy in Chronic Rhinosinusitis

Daniel L. Hamilos

The central question "What is the role of allergy in chronic rhinosinusitis (CRS)?" has several facets. Rather than being amenable to a single answer, the research in this field has asked a series of questions addressing components of the relationship. First, "Does underlying allergic disease contribute to the development of CRS?" Although there are no prospective studies examining this relationship, this question has been addressed in terms of studies showing a relationship between allergic rhinitis and sinus mucosal abnormalities and studies of the incidence of acute bacterial rhinosinmusitis in allergic rhinitis versus nonallergic controls. Second, "Is CRS more severe in patients with underlying allergies?" This question has been addressed in cross-sectional studies examining the extent of sinus mucosal disease in allergic versus nonallergic CRS patients. Third, "Is systemic IgE-mediated allergy a feature of CRS pathology?" This question has been addressed in studies examining differences in CRS tissue pathology in allergic versus nonallergic CRS patients. Fourth, "Is there a special role for local IgE medicated allergy in CRS pathogenesis?" This question has been addressed in studies that have searched for local IgE production to staphylococcal exotoxins and fungal allergens. Fifth, "Is there a different role for allergy in CRS/ NP compared to CRS?" This question has been addressed in cross-sectional studies of systemic IgE-mediated allergy in these two conditions as well as studies showing a differential role for local IgE-mediated allergy in CRS/NP patients. Sixth, "Does allergic status impact results of sinus surgery?" This question has been addressed in prospective studies of the outcomes of endoscopic sinus surgery. Finally, "Is there a special role for non-IgE fungal allergen-driven eosinophil accumulation in CRS?" This question has been examined in studies of systemic immune hyperresponsiveness to particular fungal allergens, particularly Alt a1 and direct histopathologic studies of CRS mucus samples.

The clinical and basic research studies that have addressed these questions will be discussed followed by a proposed unifying concept of the role of allergy in CRS pathogenesis.

D.L. Hamilos (✉)

Massachusetts General Hospital and Harvard Medical School, Boston, Massachusetts, USA

R. Pawankar et al. (eds.), *Allergy Frontiers: Clinical Manifestations,*

DOI: 10.1007/978-4-431-88317-3_6, © Springer 2009

Does Underlying Allergic Disease Contribute to the Development of CRS?

Prevalence of IgE-Mediated Allergy in Patients with CRS

Systemic IgE-mediated allergy is sufficiently prevalent in CRS that is warrants consideration in the underlying disease pathogenesis. Based on several studies, the prevalence of allergy in patients with CRS ranges from 60–84% [1–3]. A more precise breakdown reveals that perennial allergies are more prevalent than pollen allergies [2–4]. In Asero and Bottazzi's study, 68 patients with NP were compared with 1,128 patients with respiratory allergy. The prevalence of allergy in NP versus respiratory allergy group was as follows: any positive skin prick test 63% versus 100%; seasonal allergy 38.2% versus 84%; perennial mold or mite allergy 44.1% versus 16%, and dust mite 17.6% versus 14%.

Prevalence of Sinus Mucosal Disease in Patients with Perennial Allergic Rhinitis

In a study comparing the prevalence of sinusitis in patients with perennial allergic rhinitis versus normal controls, Berrettini et al. [5] found a prevalence of 67.5% in 40 patients with perennial allergic rhinitis versus 33.4% in 30 nonallergic controls. This difference was statistically significant. Sinusitis was defined by sinus CT scan or rhinoscopy. Thirty-six of the 40 patients with perennial allergic rhinitis also had positive endoscopic findings.

Support from Animal Studies

Studies by Naclerio and colleagues investigated the role of allergic inflammation in augmenting the severity of acute bacterial rhinosinusitis. They showed that sensitization to ovalbumin (Ova) followed by intranasal Ova challenge increased the bacterial counts and the number of neutrophil clusters following intranasal inoculation with *Streptococcus pneumoniae* [6]. This augmentation was shown, using passive transfer of Ova-specific polarized Th1 or Th2 cells, to be dependent on Th2 cells without augmentation of infection from Th1 cells alone [7]. Furthermore, sensitization to Ova without intranasal Ova exposure did not augment the severity of bacterial infection or neutrophil infiltration. These studies certainly lend support to the concept that allergic inflammation may augment the severity of secondary acute bacterial infection. A logical extension of this concept is that allergen exposure might contribute to the severity of chronic infection as is seen in a subset of CRS patients.

Is CRS More Severe in Patients with Underlying Allergies?

Some studies have shown a relationship between atopic status and extent of sinus disease on sinus CT scan. Newman et al. [8] evaluated group of patients who presented to the emergency room for complaints of sinusitis. All patients underwent a sinus CT scan, blood testing for IgE-mediated allergies and measurement of blood eosinophil count. A correlation was found between extent of disease on sinus CT and specific IgE antibodies and extent of eosinophilia but not total serum IgE levels. In contrast, Baroody et al. found a correlation between extent of sinus mucosal thickening and total serum IgE but not allergen-specific IgE levels [9]. Ramadan et al. [10] studied a group of 42 adult patients with CRS who had not undergone previous sinus surgery. All patients were evaluated for allergy with modified RAST tests, and sinus CT scans were scored by the Lund and Mackay scoring system [11]. The prevalence of allergy was 40%. The sinus CT scores were higher in the allergic group. It is not clear from this study whether any of the patients had nasal polyps. In the study of Robinson [12], in which the prevalence of allergy was 30%, allergic CRS patients had a higher sinus CT score by the Lund-McKay scoring system than nonallergic patients (14 ±1.6 versus 12 +1.4, $P = 0.05$), however patients with nasal polyps also had higher sinus CT scores. Similarly, Banerji et al. [13] found that the sinus CT Lund/McKay scores were higher in patients with nasal polyps than in CRSsNP, whereas allergic status was not associated with higher sinus CT scores.

In summary, some but not all studies have shown an association between allergic status and extent of mucosal disease on sinus CT. In contrast, a more consistent association has been found between higher sinus CT scores and the presence of nasal polyps.

Is Systemic IgE-Mediated Allergy a Feature of CRS Pathology?

Mucosal Inflammatory Features of Allergic Versus Nonallergic CRS

In a well-done study, Suzuki et al. [14] studied a group of patients with CRS and perennial allergies and another group of CRS patients who were nonallergic. Some of the patients also had nasal polyps. All patients were assessed for allergies by (1) nasal smear for eosinophils, (2) intradermal skin test or RAST tests and (3) intranasal provocation test. Allergic subjects had ≥2 of 3 criteria. Aspirates of paranasal sinus secretions were obtained after carefully suctioning away nasal mucus using a Yamik sinus catheter. The secretions from allergic CRS showed statistically higher levels of eosinophils, activated EG2-positive eosinophils, lower levels of neutrophils and increased levels of IL-5 suggesting that the allergic status was associated with the sinus mucosal inflammation. Increased numbers of eosinophils and activated eosinophils were also found in ethmoid mucosae from the allergic CRS subjects. A higher level of cysteinyl leukotrienes was also found in the aspirates from allergic CRS. It is unclear how the presence of nasal polyps affected the results of this study.

It is possible that the difference in effusion eosinophils in the Suzuki study may have been due to the use of nasal smear for eosinophils as a criteria for allergic status. However, similar findings of higher percentage of eosinophils allergic CRS versus nonallergic CRS was reported by Demoly et al. [15], although increased eosinophil numbers were actually found in both the allergic and nonallergic group. In contrast, other studies of CRS have found no significant differences in the extent of eosinophil tissue infiltration in allergic versus nonallergic subjects. This includes studies of CRSsNP [16] and CRScNP [17].

Concordance Between Local T Cell Cytokine Profile and Systemic Allergic Phenotype

Whatever the underlying cause of CRS, aeroallergen sensitivity has an imprint on the nasal and sinus mucosa. This is been demonstrated in mucosal samples from the anterior ethmoid sinuses in non-polypoid CRS [16] and in nasal polyps [17, 18]. The presence of inhalant allergies by skin testing was associated with an increase in Th2 cytokines IL-4, IL-5 and IL-13 in these tissues. By comparison, the profile of cytokines found in patients who had negative allergy skin tests consisted of increased IL-5 and IL-13 without an increase in IL-4. In nasal polyps, the profile further included an increase in IFN-γ [18]. The studies suggest that there is a concordance between the systemic allergic phenotype (in the skin or blood) and the local phenotype (in the sinuses). They further argue in favor of a modified Th1/Th2 cytokine profile in nonallergic patients. As discussed below, other investigators have suggested that there is a disconcordance between local and systemic allergic phenotype, at least in nasal polyps.

Does Nasal Allergen Exposure Lead to Mucosal Changes in the Paranasal Sinuses?

A couple of studies have assessed whether intranasal allergen challenges affected sinus mucosal changes in patients with CRS who had no prior history of surgery. The most comprehensive of these was the study of Pelikan and Pelikan-Filipek [19]. In this study, intranasal allergen challenges were applied by means of a saturated wad of cotton wool, and responses were assessed hourly for 12 h and then again at 24 and 48 h. Although skin testing was performed in the study and most patients were allergic, the results of the nasal provocation tests were not presented in a way that would allow a direct comparison of skin test results with results of the nasal provocation or the maxillary sinus changes. Overall, 29 of 37 nasal provocation tests were positive. Strong positive nasal responses were associated with positive ipsilateral maxillary sinus responses with greater than 3 mm of mucosal thickening. Likewise, negative nasal responses were associated with negative ipsilateral maxillary sinus responses. Nearly all of the maxillary sinus responses resolved within 48 h following nasal allergen challenge. Positive maxillary sinus responses were accompanied by symptoms of maxillary sinus pressure, acute headache and, occasionally, otalgia. Some patients experienced only isolated late nasal allergic responses, and these were also associated with positive maxillary sinus responses. Control nasal challenges with phosphate buffered saline (PBS) elicited minor variations in maxillary mucosal thickening always <2 mm. A control group of nonallergic patients also had negative maxillary sinus responses. This study did not directly determine whether the maxillary sinus changes were inflammatory or simply due to obstruction of drainage from the maxillary sinus, but it certainly points to a strong relationship between sinus mucosal changes and acute allergen exposure.

Is There a Special Role for Local IgE-Mediated Allergy (in the Absence of Systemic IgE-Mediated Allergy) in CRS Pathogenesis?

The studies reviewed below summarize the evidence for discordance versus concordance between local and systemic allergic phenotype in CRS. In these studies, local refers to IgE mediated allergy in the sinus mucosa whereas systemic refers to IgE-mediated allergy measured in the skin or blood. Figure 1 summarizes the contrasting proposals for concordant versus discordant allergic phenotype in CRS pathogenesis.

Evidence for Discordant Allergic Phenotype

The most compelling argument for discordant allergic phenotype is the direct demonstration of a local specific IgE production in CRS tissues, particularly in nasal polyps, in the absence of systemic allergy to exotoxins from *Staphylococcus aureus* [20]. It has been suggested that this local staphylococcal superantigen-driven IgE response is a factor in NP pathogenesis, since local production of staphylococcal superantigen-specific IgE production has been found in NP tissue but not in sinus tissue from patients with CRSsNP [20]. Recent studies by Humbert et al. have confirmed a similar local IgE switching mechanism in the lungs of patients with intrinsic asthma [21], although in this study the antigenic stimulus was not investigated.

It is not clear why the allergic response to colonizing staphylococcal superantigens should remain local rather than systemic, but most patients with these antibodies were found to have undetectable antibodies in their serum [20]. Also, it

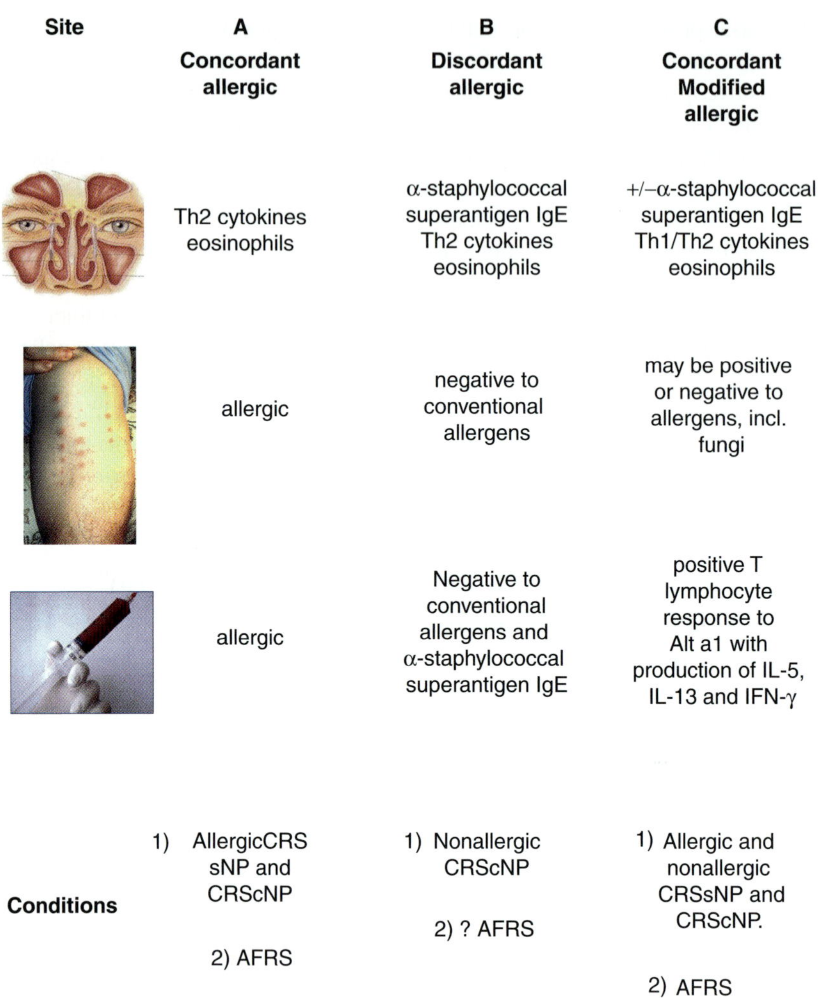

Fig. 1 Contrasting proposals for allergen involvement in the pathogenesis of CRS: concordant versus discordant allergic phenotypes

remains unknown the extent to which local IgE-mediated responses actually drive local eosinophilic inflammation. The extent to which anti-IgE treatment would affect mucosal eosinophilic inflammation in nonallergic CRS has not been studied.

Evidence for Concordant Allergic Phenotype

The most direct evidence for concordant allergic phenotype in CRS comes from the immunopathologic studies of patients with "allergic" CRSsNP or "allergic"

CRScNP discussed above. Further evidence comes from studies demonstrating that peripheral blood lymphocytes of "nonallergic" CRS patients can be stimulated *in vitro* with certain fungal antigens to produce a modified Th1/Th2 cytokine profile consisting of IL-5, IL-13 and IFN-γ [22]. This suggests that in "nonallergic" CRS patients a similar modified Th1/Th2 profile is seen locally and also systemically.

Significance of Mucosal Infiltration with Eosinophils

Mucosal infiltration with eosinophils has been found in both allergic and nonallergic patients with CRS and nasal polyps. In fact, mucosal eosinophil numbers are slightly but not significantly greater in nonallergic compared to allergic patients [16, 17]. Mucosal eosinophils are also higher in patients with associated asthma regardless of atopic status [23]. Overall, Bhattacharyya et al. found some level of eosinophilic infiltration and 82% of CRS cases versus none of five control patients undergoing endoscopic orbital decompression [24]. The highest levels of tissue eosinophils have been found in nasal polyps from patients with aspirin sensitivity regardless of atopic status [25]. The studies therefore confirm that eosinophils in CRS mucosal tissue do not correlate with systemic allergic phenotype and suggest that their presence may be dependent on local allergic mechanisms, modified responses to allergens that partially mimic classic allergy, or nonallergic local eosinophil-promoting mechanisms.

Along with the extent of tissue eosinophils, certain other features of allergic inflammation have been found to be independent of the systemic allergic phenotype in CRScNP, including local production of IL-13, epithelial expression of RANTES and eotaxin and endothelial VCAM-1 staining [26].

Is There a Special Role for Non-IgE Allergen-Driven Eosinophil Accumulation in CRS?

This discussion will be hypothetical drawing in part on studies of other conditions associated with tissue eosinophils. If we accept that allergy is synonymous with IgE-mediated disease caused by a Th2-driven disease process, a "modified allergy" can be defined as a condition mimicking allergy but lacking one or more central components of allergic inflammation. In my view, this is consonant with what has traditionally been regarded as "nonallergic" CRSsNP and "nonallergic" CRScNP. The term "modified allergy" further avoids the pitfall of suggesting that nonallergic disease is completely independent of allergy. By this definition, a modified allergy would have the phenotypic characteristics of allergic CRS (increased local eosi-nophils, increased local T lymphocytes) while lacking local IgE production and possibly certain Th2 cytokines. This would certainly apply to "nonallergic" CRS, "nonallergic" nasal polyps and "nonallergic" asthma. Bacterial colonization may be a factor in the development of this phenotype, since even classic atopic dermatitis looks phenotypically different in its chronic phase with increased skin eosinophils but a mixed Th1/Th2 cytokine profile lacking in IL-4 and instead having increased IL-12 and IFN-γ levels [27].

The T lymphocyte response is likely the critical factor in the modified allergic phenotpye. Classic allergic inflammation is purely Th2-lymphocyte driven. However, in the setting of chronic inflammation the phenotype may be "modified" to a mixed Th1/Th2 phenotype. There could be a combination of antigen-specific Th1 and Th2 cell clones involved in this response or perhaps an antigen-specific Th1/Th2 clone, but this remains unstudied. Other factors may modify classic allergic inflammation in this setting, including influences from bacterial and perhaps fungal colonization and, possibly genetic polymorphisms that promote tissue eosinophilia. An example of this is the gain of function polymorphism in epithelial eotaxin-3 expression that has been found in eosinophilic esophagitis. This condition is associated with increased local T lymphocytes and IL-5 production and may be seen in the absence of IgE-mediated food allergy [28].

Is There a Different Role for Allergy in CRS/NP Compared to CRS?

This question has been addressed mainly in studies of local anti-staphylococcal IgE production in CRS/NP as already described. Less information is available on the allergic profile of patients with CRS versus CRS/NP.

In the author's case series of 100 patients [3], the prevalence of allergy in CRSsNP versus CRScNP was as follows: pollen allergy 32.7% versus 33.2% (P = NS); dust mite allergy 21.8% versus 46.7% (P = 0.016) and fungal allergy 21.8% versus 40.0% (P = 0.079). The higher prevalence of dust mite and fungal allergy in the author's series relative to the series of Asero and Bottazi [2], can be explained by the fact that the latter study did not include intradermal testing.

Does Allergic Status Have an Impact on Postoperative Outcomes Following Sinus Surgery?

Allergy could play a different or perhaps more direct role in sinus mucosal inflammation following sinus surgery by virtue of the fact that allergens now directly impact on the sinus mucosa. One way to examine this would be to assess the impact of allergy on outcomes of endoscopic sinus surgery. This has been done in several studies.

In one of the largest and most comprehensive studies, Kennedy [29] summarized the outcomes of 120 adult patients. Although the method of assessing allergic status was not stated, allergic status was not associated with a difference in surgical outcomes.

The presence of diffuse polyposis preoperatively was the factor most strongly associated with more severe mucosal disease postoperatively.

Emanuel and Shah [30] studied 200 adult patients with refractory CRS all of whom underwent an allergy assessment by skin test or RAST tests to seasonal and perennial allergies and a sinus CT scan prior to undergoing sinus surgery. In all, 84% of the patients had allergies. There was a preponderance of perennial over seasonal allergies in this group, with dust mite allergy being the most common allergy. Sinus CT scans were graded on a scale of 0–4 by the Glicklich grading system [31]. Sinus CT scan severity did not correlate with allergic status. In fact, the subjects with grade 4 disease on CT had the lowest prevalence of allergy (69%). This is consistent with the author's experience that patients with the highest CT scores often have nasal polyps, and 50% of the nasal polyp patients are nonallergic. Finally, neither the type nor the severity of allergen sensitivity correlated with the severity of sinus CT scan mucosal disease.

Robinson et al. [12] examined the need for revision sinus surgery in a group of 193 patients with CRS. Their study population included 127 with CRSsNP and 66 with CRScNP. The prevalence of atopy (positive immunoCAP Rast test to either dust mites, mixed molds, grass pollen, cat or dog dander) was 30% overall and slightly higher in the CRS group. The most important predictor of the need for revision surgery was the presence of nasal polyps. In contrast, allergic status was unassociated with the need for revision surgery. Similarly, Ramadan et al. [32] found no association between allergic status and outcomes 1 year following endoscopic sinus surgery in a group of 141 children, age 3–13 years (mean of 7 years). Outcomes were determined using a nonvalidated questionnaire. The overall prevalence of allergy in this study was 55%.

In summary, a relationship between allergic status and outcomes following sinus surgery has been found in some but not all studies. In contrast, a stronger relationship has been found between the presence of nasal polyps and poorer outcomes following sinus surgery.

Is There a Special Role for Fungal Allergy or Modified Fungal Allergy in CRSsNP, CRSwNP, and AFRS?

Immune hyperresponsiveness to colonizing fungi has also been proposed as a mechanism of disease applicable to all categories of CRS, including CRSsNP, CRSwNP, and AFRS. This can be viewed as a type of "modified allergic" response.

Since the initial publication by Ponikau et al., in 1999, suggesting a role for ubiquitous fungi in CRS pathogenesis [33], there has been an ongoing debate about the significance of colonizing fungi in sinus mucus and their role in causing chronic rhinosinusitis. A major point of contention is whether the low levels of fungal colonization that go undetected by conventional fungal stains or culture but are detected by a highly sensitive immunofluorescent stain [34] are pathologically relevant. Few investigators have actually examined sinus mucus for the presence of fungal specific IgE levels.

In one such study, done by Collins et al. [35], 86 patients were classified into AFS, AFS-like, nonallergic fungal eosinophilic rhinosinusitis (NAEFS) and nonallergic, nonfungal eosinophilic sinusitis (NANFES). As expected, all patients with AFS and NAEFS had positive fungal cultures whereas the AFS-like and NANFES patients had negative cultures. Furthermore, as defined, allergy skin tests were positive in all AFS and AFS-like patients whereas they were negative in the NAEFS patients. In all, 71% of the allergic mucin samples from AFS patients were positive for fungal IgE to *Alternaria alternata* or *Aspergillus fumigatus*. In contrast, only 16% of the allergic mucin samples from AFS-like sinusitis and only 19% of the allergic mucin samples from NAEFS were positive for fungal IgE. In my opinion, the results of this study point to a difference between allergic and nonallergic patients with eosinophilic mucin. The simultaneous presence of fungal-laden allergic mucin, systemic fungal allergy and local fungal IgE truly distinguish AFRS from AFS-like and NAEFS. Out of 51 patients with negative serum fungal specific IgE measurements, only 6 were found to have detectable fungal IgE in the allergic mucin. This suggests that the nearly 90% of cases with negative serum fungal IgE measurements do not have localized fungal IgE-mediated allergy. It is noteworthy that 65% of the patients in this study had fungi identified by culture or fungal staining of the allergic mucin. Therefore, the presence of fungi at some level in allergic mucin is also clearly higher than the prevalence of fungal specific IgE in the allergic mucin.

Wormald and colleagues called into question the role of fungal specific IgE in the pathogenesis of allergic fungal rhinosinusitis (AFRS). Unlike the related condition of classic allergic bronchopulmonary aspergillosis (ABPA), patients with AFRS are indistinguishable from patients with allergic rhinitis and fungal allergy in terms of total serum IgE, levels of *Alternaria alternata* or *Aspergillus fumigatus* specific fungal IgE, IgG or IgA levels or in terms of the percent of fungal specific serum IgE relative to total serum IgE measurements [36]. Furthermore, the prevalence of fungal allergy to *Alternaria alternata* or *Aspergillus fumigatus* in AFRS and AFRS-like patients was no different from that observed in allergic rhinitis with fungal allergy [37]. This study therefore implies that mechanisms other than classic IgE mediated inflammation may account for eosinophilic mucin in CRS. A "modified allergic" systemic T-cell hypersensitivity to certain fungal species, as has been demonstrated in patients with CRS [22], is a plausible means of accounting for the local eosinophil accumulation and subsequent eosinophil-mediated attack of fungal hyphae in mucus.

Unifying Hypothesis of the "Modified Allergic" Response Relevant to CRS

Pathways to Immune Sensitization and Hyperresponsiveness to Fungal Allergens in CRS

A unifying hypothesis of the potential pathway leading to immune sensitization and immune hyperresponsiveness to fungal antigens in CRS is presented in

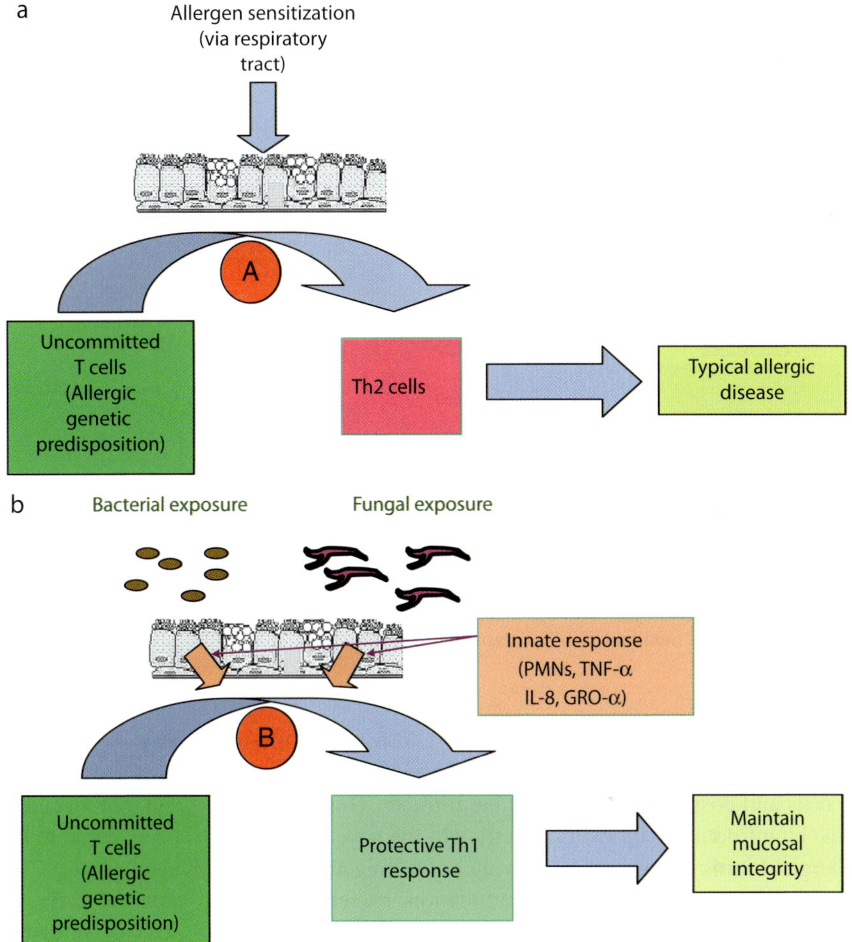

Fig. 2 Pathways leading to allergen sensitization relevant to CRS pathogenesis. (a) Sensitization of normal mucosa gives rise to typical Th2 responses. (b) In the absence of allergic inflammation, bacterial or fungal exposure activates innate responses that protect against infection. Infection activates adaptive Th1 immune responses that eradicate infection. Both innate and adaptive responses help maintain mucosal integrity.

Fig. 2. Fungal spores are widely distributed in nature, although certain fungi, such as *Bipolaris spicifera*, show distinct geographic distributions that likely account for their prevalence in the southern but not northern United States. When present in ambient air, fungal spores are easily trapped in nasal mucus, which may serve as a portal of entry for fungal sensitization.

In seasonal and perennial allergic rhinitis, immune sensitization to fungi presumably occurs in the absence of infection or other perturbation of the nasal mucosa (Fig. 2A). The profile of T cell cytokines elicited in nasal tissue fits the classic Th2 profile, with production of the cytokines IL-4, IL-5, IL-13, and granulocyte-macrophage

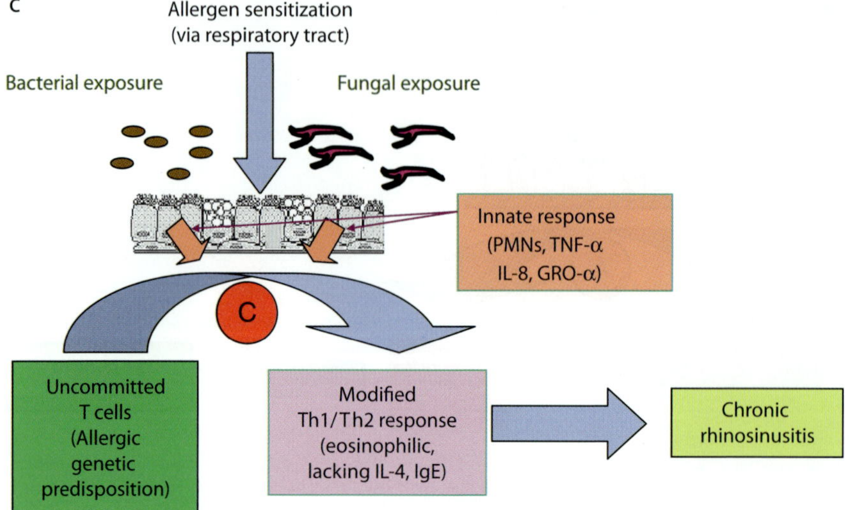

Fig. 2 (continued) (c) In the presence of chronic allergic inflammation, bacterial infection and fungal colonization are promoted and mucosal integrity compromised. Allergic Th2 immune responses are modified by the simultaneous local adaptive Th1 response. Fungal sensitization at this point gives rise to a modified Th1/Th2 response

colony-stimulating factor (GM-CSF) [38]. These cytokines give rise to IgE production with local mast cell degranulation and accumulation of allergen-specific Th2 T cells and eosinophils in allergic nasal tissue. These features can be reproduced *in vivo* by introducing allergens directly into the nose. IL-4 is felt to be essential to the allergic rhinitis disease process owing to its obligatory role in IgE synthesis.

In the absence of allergic inflammation, bacterial or fungal exposure activates innate epithelial responses that protect against infection (Fig. 2B). If infection occurs, adaptive Th1 immune responses are activated that lead to eradication of the infection. Both innate and adaptive responses help maintain mucosal integrity.

A subset of patients with PAR develops other perturbations of the nasal mucosa possibly caused by viral or bacterial infection or inflammatory stimuli, such as cigarette smoke. In the simultaneous presence of chronic allergic inflammation (Fig. 2C), bacterial infection and fungal colonization are promoted and mucosal integrity is compromised. Allergic Th2 immune responses are then modified by the simultaneous local milieu of the adaptive Th1 response. This may alter the nature of the T lymphocyte response to fungal antigens such that fungal sensitization at this point gives rise to a modified Th1/Th2 response (defined previously). Concomitant use of antibiotics and perhaps unknown genetic polymorphisms may also impact on these responses. The result is a modified Th1/Th2 response to fungal allergens and perhaps bacterial proteins in the sinus mucosa leading to chronic eosinophilic inflammation.

In a mouse model, Van de Rijn et al. showed that eosinophilic inflammation could be elicited in the nose of IgE-deficient mice after being sensitized to Aspergillus [39].

This supports the view that eosinophilic nasal inflammation can be driven by cytokines such as IL-5 even in the complete absence of local IgE production. T-lymphocyte sensitization to the fungal antigen, however, is critical to these responses. Of all the cytokines that have been described in CRSsNP and CRScNP, IL-5 is the most consistently found. In addition, we [40] and others [16] found elevated IL-13 levels in both allergic and nonallergic subjects with CRScNP and CRSsNP, respectively.

In nonallergic patients with chronic rhinosinusitis, there is also evidence of Th1 cytokine production. The pattern of T-lymphocyte activation indicates the nature of the immune-specific activation, responding in different ways to different antigenic stimuli. A Th1 profile primarily involves interferon-γ, IL-2, and tumor necrosis factor (TNF)-α. Patients with CRS do not fall strictly into either a Th2 or Th1 category, but rather have a mixture of both Th2 and Th1 cytokines. However, it appears critical that IL-5, and possibly IL-13, are involved. This point is strengthened by studies analyzing infiltrating T-cells in nasal polyps from patients with chronic hyperplastic sinusitis or nasal polyposis [18, 41, 42]. It is also strengthened by the observations of Shin and Kita that peripheral blood lymphocytes from allergic and nonallergic CRS patients stimulated with certain fungal antigens elicit IL-5, IL-13 and IFN-γ *in vitro*, with little production of IL-4 [22]. By comparison, normal control subjects produce very little cytokine response.

The ability of viable fungal spores to become trapped in nasal or sinus mucus and germinate into viable hyphae has been well demonstrated by Ponikau et al. [33] in both CRS patients and normal controls. No difference was seen in the number of different fungal species present in normal versus CRS subjects. Although the amount of fungal antigen present in these two subject populations has not been compared, it is assumed that the amount would be much greater in the CRS subjects owing to local germination and perhaps mucus hypersecretion and local stagnation. The increased burden of fungal antigen may play a role in fungal sensitization and the intense localized inflammatory response.

Once the modified allergic response is initiated, eosinophil infiltration ensues with local eosinophil attack of colonizing fungi and buildup of high levels of eosinophil granular proteins in the mucus [43]. Mucus stagnation and perhaps epithelial damage by eosinophil basic proteins then contribute to bacterial colonization and/or infection. A viscous cycle of colonization and inflammation is therefore set into motion.

In a recent paper, Ponikau et al. have demonstrated that eosinophils in AFRS mucus tend to "line up" next to fungal hyphae [46]. It is presumed that the eosinophils "attack" the fungal hyphae much as they are known to attack parasitic organisms resulting in their degranulation [44].

Summary

By a variety of lines of evidence, a relationship between allergy and chronic rhinosinusitis pathogenesis is suggested. Nasal allergen exposure affects sinus mucosal thickening in a manner and time course consistent with late phase allergic inflammation. Although no studies directly prove the nasal allergen exposure leads to inflammation in the paranasal sinuses, mucosal studies in both CRSsNP and CRScNP confirm that patients with systemic allergy have the classic allergic cytokine profile in their sinus tissues. These studies suggest that sinus allergic mucosal responses are largely concordant with systemic allergic responses. Nonetheless, at most concordant systemic and local classic allergic responses could accounts for only 60% of patients with CRSsNP and 50% of those with CRScNP.

Roughly 40% of CRSsNP and 50% of CRScNP patients are nonallergic by comprehensive allergy evaluations. Yet the majority of these patients have an eosinophil-predominant type of sinus mucosal inflammation suggesting a local allergic mechanism is at play. To account for this phenotype, it has been proposed that "nonallergic" CRS patients exhibit a discordance between local and systemic allergic phenotype (i.e. "local allergy"). Such discordance has been demonstrated between local and systemic IgE responses to certain proteins, such as Staphylococcal superantigens. However, an alternative view is that the predominant allergic mechanism in "nonallergic" CRS patients is actually a "modified allergic" response manifested as a mixed or Th1/Th2 cytokine profile. Although studies of the T lymphocytes within CRS tissue are limited, studies of peripheral blood lymphocytes from CRS patients have found a similar mixed Th1/Th2 cytokine profile in response to certain fungal antigens, lending further support to the concept that fungal allergens play a key role in CRS pathogenesis even if they failed to elicit classic IgE responses. According to this view, local tissue IgE production may be much less important than the local elaboration of Th2 cytokines (IL-5 and IL-13) in terms of accounting for tissue eosinophilia and inflammation. Further investigations of these responses in sinus tissues are needed to confirm the role of colonizing fungi in CRS pathogenesis and to better understand the genesis and regulation of "modified allergic" Th1/Th2 lymphocytes.

Regardless of whether the allergic responses in CRS patients are concordant or discordant with the systemic allergic phenotype, it is clear that several pathologic features of CRS, including the extent of eosinophil infiltration, local production of IL-13, local anti-staphylococcal superantigen-specific IgE levels, epithelial RANTES and eotaxin expression and endothelial VCAM-1 staining, are independent of the systemic IgE-mediated allergic phenotype in CRSsNP and CRScNP. Furthermore, data on eosinophil-mediated local immune attack of fungal hyphae further call into question the importance of local IgE production in CRS tissue pathogenesis and leave open the possibility that the modified Th1/Th2 lymphocyte response may actually be more important pathologically, even in those CRS patients who also have systemic allergies.

References

1. Emanuel IA, Shah SB. Chronic rhinosinusitis: Allergy and sinus computed tomography relationships. Otolaryngol Head Neck Surg. 2000 Dec;123(6):687–91.
2. Asero R, Bottazzi G. Nasal polyposis: A study of its association with airborne allergen hypersensitivity. Ann Allergy Asthma Immunol. 2001 Mar;86(3):283–5.

3. Hamilos DL. Chronic rhinosinusitis patterns of illness. Clin Allergy Immunol. 2007;20:1–13.

4. Asero R, Bottazzi G. Hypersensitivity to molds in patients with nasal polyposis: A clinical study. J Allergy Clin Immunol. 2000 Jan;105(1 Pt 1):186–8.

5. Berrettini S, Carabelli A, Sellari-Franceschini S, Bruschini L, Abruzzese A, Quartieri F, et al. Perennial allergic rhinitis and chronic sinusitis: Correlation with rhinologic risk factors. Allergy. 1999 Mar;54(3):242–8.

6. Blair C, Nelson M, Thompson K, Boonlayangoor S, Haney L, Gabr U, et al. Allergic inflammation enhances bacterial sinusitis in mice. J Allergy Clin Immunol. 2001 Sept;108(3):424–9.

7. Yu X, Sperling A, Blair C, Thompson K, Naclerio R. Antigen stimulation of TH2 cells augments acute bacterial sinusitis in mice. J Allergy Clin Immunol. 2004 Aug;114(2):328–34.

8. Newman LJ, Platts-Mills TA, Phillips CD, Hazen KC, Gross CW. Chronic sinusitis: Relationship of computed tomographic findings to allergy, asthma, and eosinophilia. JAMA. 1994 Feb 2;271(5):363–7.

9. Baroody FM, Suh SH, Naclerio RM. Total IgE serum levels correlate with sinus mucosal thickness on computerized tomography scans. J Allergy Clin Immunol. 1997 Oct;100(4):563–8.

10. Ramadan HH, Fornelli R, Ortiz AO, Rodman S. Correlation of allergy and severity of sinus disease. Am J Rhinol. 1999 Sept–Oct;13(5):345–7.

11. Lund VJ, Mackay IS. Staging in rhinosinusitus. Rhinology. 1993 Dec;31(4):183–4.

12. Robinson S, Douglas R, Wormald PJ. The relationship between atopy and chronic rhinosinusitis. Am J Rhinol. 2006 Nov–Dec;20(6):625–8.

13. Banerji A, Piccirillo JF, Thawley SE, Levitt RG, Schechtman KB, Kramper MA, et al. Chronic rhinosinusitis patients with polyps or polypoid mucosa have a greater burden of illness. Am J Rhinol. 2007 Jan–Feb;21(1):19–26.

14. Suzuki M, Watanabe T, Suko T, Mogi G. Comparison of sinusitis with and without allergic rhinitis: Characteristics of paranasal sinus effusion and mucosa. Am J Otolaryngol. 1999 May–June;20(3):143–50.

15. Demoly P, Crampette L, Mondain M, Campbell AM, Lequeux N, Enander I, et al. Assessment of inflammation in noninfectious chronic maxillary sinusitis. J Allergy Clin Immunol. 1994 July;94(1):95–108.

16. al Ghamdi K, Ghaffar O, Small P, Frenkiel S, Hamid Q. IL-4 and IL-13 expression in chronic sinusitis: Relationship with cellular infiltrate and effect of topical corticosteroid treatment. J Otolaryngol. 1997 June;26(3):160–6.

17. Hamilos DL, Leung DY, Wood R, Meyers A, Stephens JK, Barkans J, et al. Chronic hyperplastic sinusitis: Association of tissue eosinophilia with mRNA expression of granulocyte-macrophage colony-stimulating factor and interleukin-3. J Allergy Clin Immunol. 1993 July;92(1 Pt 1):39–48.

18. Hamilos DL, Leung DY, Wood R, Cunningham L, Bean DK, Yasruel Z, et al. Evidence for distinct cytokine expression in allergic versus nonallergic chronic sinusitis. J Allergy Clin Immunol. 1995 Oct;96(4):537–44.

19. Pelikan Z, Pelikan-Filipek M. Role of nasal allergy in chronic maxillary sinusitis – diagnostic value of nasal challenge with allergen. J Allergy Clin Immunol. 1990 Oct;86(4 Pt 1):484–91.

20. Van Zele T, Gevaert P, Watelet JB, Claeys G, Holtappels G, Claeys C, et al. Staphylococcus aureus colonization and IgE antibody formation to enterotoxins is increased in nasal polyposis. J Allergy Clin Immunol. 2004 Oct;114(4):981–3.

21. Humbert M, Durham SR, Ying S, Kimmitt P, Barkans J, Assoufi B, et al. IL-4 and IL-5 mRNA and protein in bronchial biopsies from patients with atopic and nonatopic asthma: Evidence against "intrinsic" asthma being a distinct immunopathologic entity. Am J Respir Crit Care Med. 1996 Nov;154(5):1497–504.

22. Shin SH, Ponikau JU, Sherris DA, Congdon D, Frigas E, Homburger HA, et al. Chronic rhinosinusitis: An enhanced immune response to ubiquitous airborne fungi. J Allergy Clin Immunol. 2004 Dec;114(6):1369–75.

23. Harlin SL, Ansel DG, Lane SR, Myers J, Kephart GM, Gleich GJ. A clinical and pathologic study of chronic sinusitis: The role of the eosinophil. J Allergy Clin Immunol. 1988 May; 81(5 Pt 1):867–75.

24. Bhattacharyya N, Vyas DK, Fechner FP, Gliklich RE, Metson R. Tissue eosinophilia in chronic sinusitis: Quantification techniques. Arch Otolaryngol Head Neck Surg. 2001 Sept;127(9):1102–5.
25. Yamashita T, Tsuji H, Maeda N, Tomoda K, Kumazawa T. Etiology of nasal polyps associated with aspirin-sensitive asthma. Rhinology Suppl. 1989;8:15–24.
26. Hamilos DL, Leung DY, Huston DP, Kamil A, Wood R, Hamid Q. GM-CSF, IL-5 and RANTES immunoreactivity and mRNA expression in chronic hyperplastic sinusitis with nasal polyposis (NP). Clin Exp Allergy. 1998 Sept;28(9):1145–52.
27. Leung DY. Atopic dermatitis: The skin as a window into the pathogenesis of chronic allergic diseases. J Allergy Clin Immunol. 1995 quiz 319; Sept;96(3):302–18.
28. Straumann A, Bauer M, Fischer B, Blaser K, Simon HU. Idiopathic eosinophilic esophagitis is associated with a T(H)2-type allergic inflammatory response. J Allergy Clin Immunol. 2001 Dec;108(6):954–61.
29. Kennedy DW. Prognostic factors, outcomes and staging in ethmoid sinus surgery. Laryngoscope. 1992 Dec;102(12 Pt 2 Suppl 57):1–18.
30. Emanuel IA, Shah SB. Chronic rhinosinusitis: Allergy and sinus computed tomography relationships. Otolaryngol Head Neck Surg. 2000 Dec;123(6):687–91.
31. Gliklich RE, Metson R. Techniques for outcomes research in chronic sinusitis. Laryngoscope. 1995 Apr;105(4 Pt 1):387–90.
32. Ramadan HH, Hinerman RA. Outcome of endoscopic sinus surgery in children with allergic rhinitis. Am J Rhinol. 2006 July–Aug;20(4):438–40.
33. Ponikau JU, Sherris DA, Kern EB, Homburger HA, Frigas E, Gaffey TA, et al. The diagnosis and incidence of allergic fungal sinusitis. Mayo Clin Proc. 1999 Sept;74(9):877–84.
34. Taylor MJ, Ponikau JU, Sherris DA, Kern EB, Gaffey TA, Kephart G, et al. Detection of fungal organisms in eosinophilic mucin using a fluorescein-labeled chitin-specific binding protein. Otolaryngol Head Neck Surg. 2002 Nov;127(5):377–83.
35. Collins M, Nair S, Smith W, Kette F, Gillis D, Wormald PJ. Role of local immunoglobulin E production in the pathophysiology of noninvasive fungal sinusitis. Laryngoscope. 2004 July;114(7):1242–6.
36. Pant H, Kette FE, Smith WB, Wormald PJ, Macardle PJ. Fungal-specific humoral response in eosinophilic mucus chronic rhinosinusitis. Laryngoscope. 2005 Apr;115(4):601–6.
37. Pant H, Kette FE, Smith WB, Macardle PJ, Wormald PJ. Eosinophilic mucus chronic rhinosinusitis: Clinical subgroups or a homogeneous pathogenic entity?. Laryngoscope. 2006 July;116(7):1241–7.
38. Durham SR, Ying S, Varney VA, Jacobson MR, Sudderick RM, Mackay IS, et al. Cytokine messenger RNA expression for IL-3, IL-4, IL-5, and granulocyte/macrophage-colony-stimulating factor in the nasal mucosa after local allergen provocation: Relationship to tissue eosinophilia. J Immunol. 1992 Apr 15;148(8):2390–4.
39. van de Rijn M, Mehlhop PD, Judkins A, Rothenberg ME, Luster AD, Oettgen HC. A murine model of allergic rhinitis: Studies on the role of IgE in pathogenesis and analysis of the eosinophil influx elicited by allergen and eotaxin. J Allergy Clin Immunol. 1998 July;102(1):65–74.
40. Hamilos DL, Leung DY, Wood R, Bean DK, Song YL, Schotman E, et al. Eosinophil infiltration in nonallergic chronic hyperplastic sinusitis with nasal polyposis (CHS/NP) is associated with endothelial VCAM-1 upregulation and expression of TNF-alpha. Am J Respir Cell Mol Biol. 1996 Oct;15(4):443–50.
41. Miller CH, Pudiak DR, Hatem F, Looney RJ. Accumulation of interferon gamma-producing TH1 helper T cells in nasal polyps. Otolaryngol Head Neck Surg. 1994 July;111(1):51–8.
42. Sanchez-Segura A, Brieva JA, Rodriguez C. T lymphocytes that infiltrate nasal polyps have a specialized phenotype and produce a mixed TH1/TH2 pattern of cytokines. J Allergy Clin Immunol. 1998 Dec;102(6 Pt 1):953–60.

43. Ponikau JU, Sherris DA, Kephart GM, Kern EB, Congdon DJ, Adolphson CR, et al. Striking deposition of toxic eosinophil major basic protein in mucus: Implications for chronic rhinosinusitis. J Allergy Clin Immunol. 2005 Aug;116(2):362–9.
44. Butterworth AE, David JR, Franks D, Mahmoud AA, David PH, Sturrock RF, et al. Antibody-dependent eosinophil-mediated damage to 51Cr-labeled schistosomula of schistosoma mansoni: Damage by purified eosinophils. J Exp Med. 1977 Jan 1;145(1):136–50.

Otitis Media and Sinusitis

Deborah A. Gentile, Timothy J. Schaffner, Christine A. Schad,
and David P. Skoner

Introduction

Otitis media (OM) and sinusitis are common diseases for which both children and
adults receive medical care each year [1]. Life-threatening complications of these
diseases have been minimal following the introduction of antibiotics, but sequelae
occasionally occur and may include bony erosion and facial nerve paralysis [2].
The cost of treating these disorders is between $4 and $6 billion per year. In
addition, the patient or caregiver is absent from work on an average of 2 days per
illness episode, with an estimated cost of $1 billion [3]. The increase in the preva-
lence of these diseases over the last 15–20 years has led to a similar increase in the
use of antibiotics to treat the disease, despite the demonstration of their marginal
efficacy in placebo-controlled trials. This is a credible explanation for the selection
of antibiotic-resistant bacteria, a phenomenon that is generating increasing concern
as inexpensive, first-line antibiotics used to treat common diseases such as OM and
sinusitis are becoming ineffective [4].

vURIs are extremely common in children and adults. For most segments of the
population, this condition is self-limited and associated with relatively short periods of morbidity. However, in infants, the elderly, and the immunocompromised,
infection with some of the causal viruses is associated with significant excess morbidity and, in some cases, even mortality. Also, vURIs are well established as predisposing to other diseases involving the paranasal sinuses, middle ears, and lungs
[5–7]. These complications are characterized by a more prolonged time course
than that of the precipitating vURI and are often refractory to conventional medical
treatment. For example, respiratory synctial virus (RSV) infection, which has been
long recognized as a cause of severe lower respiratory illness and complications in
infants and young children, was recently shown to signficantly increase morbidity
and mortality in the elderly [8]. Medications of questionable efficacy sold for the

D.A. Gentile (✉), T.J. Schaffner, C.A. Schad, and D.P. Skoner
Allegheny General Hospital, Division of Allergy, Asthma and Immunology, Pittsburgh,
PA, USA
e-mail: DGentile@wpahs.org

R. Pawankar et al. (eds.), *Allergy Frontiers: Clinical Manifestations*,
DOI: 10.1007/978-4-431-88317-3_7, © Springer 2009

relief of symptoms and signs of vURIs represent a major component of the over-the-counter drug market, and prescription medications for treating associated complications including sinusitis, OM, and pneumonia represent a significant financial burden to society. These costs are compounded by the decreased economic productivity resulting from the large number of days lost to industry and education.

Pathogenesis of Viral Rhinitis

Viruses that cause URIs include rhinovirus (RV), adenovirus, influenza virus (FLU), parainfluenza virus, coxsackie virus, and RSV. Comparative studies of experimental infection of adult humans with RSV, FLU, RV, and coxsackie A virus show that all of these viruses provoke a similar local symptom-sign presentation (with varying degrees of systemic involvement), nasal secretory response, pattern of complications (with varying frequencies), and a panel of elaborated inflammatory mediators (IMs), leukotrienes, and cytokines [9, 10]. Differences that exist among viruses primarily reflect the types of cells that are infected (tissue tropism) and thus the degree to which the infection is localized. For example, although RVs are generally confined to the upper airways by their sensitivity to temperature, RSV can be disseminated to the lung and middle ear by way of the contiguous mucosa and FLU can infect leukocytes via viremic dissemination. These observations suggest that the pathogenesis of the local, cold-like signs, symptoms, and complications is common to the different etiologic agents and most likely represents the consequences of a generalized host response to viral infection of the nasal mucosa.

The most prominent signs and symptoms of vURIs include rhinorrhea, sneezing, nasal obstruction, sore throat, cough, malaise, fever, and sweats [11]. In some studies, the development of airway hyperreactivity has been reported [7], and complications involving the paranasal sinuses are common [5]. Also reported are otologic complications, including Eustachian tube obstruction, middle ear underpressures, and otitis media [12], although cold-like illness or symptoms are not always associated with viral detection by PCR during OM [13]. Most studies have failed to culture virus from the site of the complication (sinus, lung, or middle ear), and the development of complications has been associated with the extension of the inflammatory response as opposed to *in situ* viral infection.

The pathogenesis of symptoms and signs of illness and the pathophysiologies and complications of vURIs have been studied using epidemiological surveys, animal models, and adults experimentally infected with different respiratory viruses. Importantly, similar patterns and magnitudes of pathophysiologic and symptomatic responses to infection were documented for experimental and natural vURIs [11]. A distinct advantage offered by the experimental model over natural infection is its high degree of control over several factors: the health of the subjects; the dose and nature of the infecting agent; and the precise temporal sequence of infection, signs and symptoms, and elaboration of IMs and cytokines.

Early studies of the host response to vURIs focused on the humoral system. High homotypic serum neutralizing IgG antibody titers have been associated with

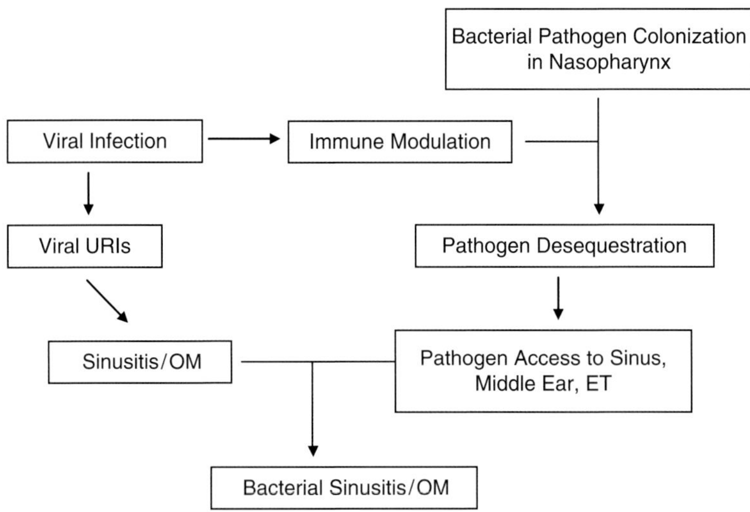

Fig. 1 Immune interaction and sequelae of viral infections

protection from infection and lessened signs and symptoms [14]. Similarly, high nasal IgA antibody titers have been significantly correlated with a decreased duration of viral shedding. There is also evidence that the cellular immune response may play a role in the pathogenesis of vURIs. Phenotypic and functional changes in the circulating immune/inflammatory parameters have been documented during experimental vURIs [15] (Fig. 1).

Role of Inflammatory Mediators

The role of IMs has been the focus of recent studies on vURI pathogenesis. The similarity between the clinical manifestations of allergic rhinitis and the common cold has prompted repeated attempts to establish a role for histamine and other IMs in the pathogenesis of vURIs. Three generalized methods have been used to provide evidence for a role of IMs and cytokines in the pathogenesis of vURIs: (1) documentation of a time-dependent increase in the concentration of the IM/cytokine (in nasal secretion, blood, or urine) during the period of infection that parallels the symptoms; (2) provocation of signs, symptoms, and mucosal inflammation by topical application of the IM/cytokine; and (3) moderation of the inflammatory process or symptom expression by inhibitors of these IMs/cytokines.

Histamine, a classic mediator of allergic rhinitis, is stored in the granules of tissue mast cells and circulating basophils and is released immediately upon cellular contact with a variety of stimuli. Local histamine in nasal secretions [9] and urinary histamine metabolites can be detected during vURIs [16]. Mucosally applied histamine triggers a full spectrum of rhinitis symptoms and is the only mediator studied that provokes sneezing [17]. Of interest, antihistamine treatment during vURIs consistently depresses symptoms and signs of sneezing and rhinorrhea, but has little effect on the other aspects of disease expression [18].

Bradykinin is a potent mediator of inflammation and is synthesized locally from precursors delivered with other serum proteins, by transudation. Application of bradykinin to the nasal mucosa provokes rhinorrhea, congestion, facial pain, and sore throat [17]. Kinins were found in the nasal secretions recovered from subjects with experimental and natural vURIs [19]. The concentration and time course of the production of kinins are correlated with symptom severity. However, steroid therapy significantly reduces kinins in nasal lavage fluids, but has no effect on the symptoms, and bradykinin antagonists have not affected the signs and symptoms in a number of experimental RV studies [20].

LTs are potent mediators generated by different cell types that participate in inflammatory reactions. The sulfidopeptide LTs increase the permeability of post-capillary venules and facilitate plasma leakage, edema formation, and cellular diapedesis [21]. LTB_4 is one of the most potent chemoattractants for neutrophils and, to a lesser degree, eosinophils. Both the sulfidopeptide LTs and LTB_4 are potent enhancers of mucus secretion. According to data on a 5-lipoxygenase knockout mouse model, LTs are critically involved in many, but not all, causes of inflammation. Combined with the results reported for mast cell-deficient mice, chemotactic LTs released by mast cells can be shown to be important in neutrophil recruitment during the early acute inflammatory response to insult. Elevated levels of LTs were observed in nasal secretions of children infected with RSV, parainfluenza virus, and FLU and in experimentally infected adults [22]. Moreover, LTs applied directly to the nasal mucosa in noninfected individuals reproduced symptoms of nasal congestion and rhinorrhea [23]. Both 5-lipoxygenase enzyme inhibitors and LTD_4 antagonists have efficacy in treating nasal congestion in allergic rhinitis. Montelukast, an LT receptor antagonist, has been shown to be effective in reducing cough, wheezing, dyspnea, and limitation of activity in infants during RSV infection, however, its ability to prevent vURIs, otitis media, or sinusitis has not been demonstrated [24].

Recent evidence also implicates a role for nitric oxide (NO) in the pathogenesis of vURIs. NO has been shown to decrease and/or inhibit proliferation of several viral systems (through various pathways) in vitro, including FLU, coronavirus (MHV), poliovirus, and HSV-1 (herpesvirus) [25]. Increased concentrations of nasal NO have been reported during vURIs in vivo. Moreover, NO inhibited RV-induced cytokine production and viral replication in a human respiratory epithelial cell line. Recent studies, however, have failed to find an association between NO and signs, symptoms, and complications during experimental vURIs [26].

Role of Neurogenic Inflammation

Mediators of neurogenic inflammation may also play a role in the pathogenesis of vURIs and complications. It is hypothesized that virus infection provokes the release from epithelial cells of IL-11 and endothelins (ETs), which conjointly and synergistically activate nociceptive nerves, leading to local mucosal axon responses and the subsequent release of inflammatory neuropeptides. These peptides, in turn, cause neurogenic inflammation, which is expressed as nasal irritation, sneezing (nociceptive nerve activation), engorgement of venous sinusoids (mucosal swelling with decreased nasal patency), increased vascular permeability (major source of rhinorrhea fluid), glandular exocytosis, low-grade inflammatory cell infiltration, and reflex obstruction of the eustachian tube and sinus ostia. Evidence also indicates that neurogenic inflammation may be upregulated during allergic inflammation. Nasal secretions obtained from patients with perennial allergic rhinitis (PAR) and healthy controls were compared following whole-nose capsaicin provocation. Subjects from the PAR group exhibited plasma extravasation while the control group did not, likely resulting from neuropeptide release by capsaicin-sensitve fibers [27, 28].

Several lines of evidence support a role for neurogenic inflammation in the pathogenesis and expression of vURIs. These include the following observations: (1) parasympathetic reflexes mediate the glandular exocytosis and mucous hypersecretion; (2) hyperresponsiveness of the nasal mucosa to histamine and cold dry air was reported during RV and FLU infections; (3) viral infection in humans causes release of IL-11, a "neurokine" that increases the sensitivity of nociceptive neurons to activation, increases neural responses to painful stimuli, and provokes bronchial hyperresponsiveness; and (4) ETs are synthesized and secreted by nasal epithelial and glandular cells in response to virus infection [29–31]. In other inflammatory diseases such as asthma and allergic rhinitis, ETs and IL-11 are released, stimulate nociceptive neurons, and recruit parasympathetic reflexes. Also, in allergen challenge studies, the release of substance P, calcitonin gene-related peptide, and vasoactive intestinal peptide is associated with itch, nasal blockage, and rhinorrhea, showing that these nociceptive neuropeptides can be measured in nasal secretions and that their concentrations are related to specific symptoms [32]. Moreover, one study reported that the nasal mucosa of patients with allergic rhinitis contains three times the concentration of substance P as compared with healthy controls [33].

Role of Cytokines

Recent studies have focused on elucidating the role of cytokines in the pathogenesis of vURIs and its complications. The cytokine network provides a complex and highly interactive mechanism for regulation and amplification of the immune system and inflammatory response. During an inflammatory event, proinflammatory cytokines are typically upregulated in a cascading fashion. On the continuum of proinflammatory and immune system-stimulating chemicals, tumor necrosis factor-alpha (TNF-α) and interleukin-1 (IL-1) hold central roles. TNF-α is the first cytokine to be upregulated in response to an inflammatory stimulus, with levels peaking within several hours. IL-1 is the second cytokine to be upregulated, with levels peaking within 24–48 h. TNF-α and IL-1 then trigger the sequential upregulation of other cytokines, including IL-6, IL-8, and IL-10. Interestingly, results from recent studies suggest that the severity of vURI-induced illness and the development of complications are orchestrated by the sequential elaboration of these various proinflammatory cytokines [34–36].

TNF-α and IL-1 also play roles in regulating T-helper type 1 (T_H1) and type 2 (T_H2) immune responses. T-helper lymphocytes can be divided into several subsets including T_H1 and T_H2 cells, which are involved in cellular and humoral immunity, respectively. T_H2 lymphocytes and their cytokines, including IL-4, have been implicated in the pathogenesis of vURI-induced illness and its complications. Increases in local and systemic IL-4 mRNA and protein levels were observed during viral URIs. Several studies reported associations between IL-4 elevations, severity of viral rhinitis, and incidence of virally induced complications [37]. In animal models, overexpression of IL-4 was shown to delay RSV clearance, and treatment with anti–IL-4 was shown to decrease the severity of RSV-induced illness [38].

TNF-α is produced primarily by activated macrophages, induces synthesis of acute phase reactants by the liver, induces fever, and causes the relaxation of the vascular smooth muscle. TNF-α can also activate endothelial cells to upregulate other cytokines and adhesion molecule expression, thus enhancing vascular permeability, cellular adhesion, and procoagulant activity [39]. TNF-α is a proinflammatory cytokine with pleiotropic expression consistent with a primary role in the pathogenesis of virally induced rhinitis. In several studies, release of TNF-α was increased from epithelial cells and monocytes following in vitro infection with respiratory viruses [40]. Elevated levels of TNF-α protein in nasal lavage samples recovered from otherwise healthy infants during primary RSV infection, and from adults following experimental infection with a variety of respiratory viruses have also been reported [41]. Several studies reported that TNF-α production was biphasic with peaks occurring between 6h and 2–3 days following infection with respiratory viruses. Another reported a positive association between local elevations of TNF-α protein and severity of vURIs, particularly RSV infection [42], and a study conducted in our laboratory related elevated TNF-α to the expression of otological complications during FLU infection [39]. These data are consistent with the hypothesis that TNF-α contributes to the pathogenesis of vURIs and complications.

IL-1 is produced by epithelial cells, mononuclear phagocytes, and fibroblasts and shares many of the same activities as TNF-α. The IL-1 family has three members: IL-1α, IL-1β, and an endogenous IL-1 receptor antagonist (IL-1ra). IL-1 has been implicated in the activation of T lymphocytes. Blocking the action of IL-1 has many diverse effects that include inhibiting neutrophil accumulation in the lung tissue of animal models. As with TNF-α, release of IL-1 was increased from nasal epithelial cells following in vitro virus infection [43]. One recent study reported a small increase in IL-1α, a modest increase in IL-1β, and an impressive increase in IL-1ra, in nasal lavages obtained from adults with experimental RV infection [44]. Maximal induction of IL-1α and IL-1β was noted at 48h, whereas, maximal induction of IL-1ra occurred between 48 and 72h. These times corresponded with the peak periods for symptomatology and symptom resolution, respectively. These data support the hypotheses that IL-1 contributes to the pathogenesis of vURIs, and that IL-1ra plays an important role in disease resolution.

IL-1 and TNF-α interact with other cytokines to modulate inflammation. IL-6 is produced by a wide spectrum of cells in response to a number of stimuli, including IL-1–induced activation of transcription factors. IL-6 mediates many biologic functions that are relevant to virus infection. These include its abilities to act as an endogenous pyrogen, stimulate the acute phase response, stimulate T lymphocytes, induce the terminal differentiation of B lymphocytes, and stimulate immunoglobulin production. IL-6 is a potent regulator of pulmonary inflammation and an important component of biologic homeostasis. Dysregulation is implicated in a wide array of inflammatory and viral disorders. Increases in local IL-6 production were reported during vURIs caused by RV, FLU, and RSV, and coincide with peaks in symptomatology and pathophysiology [35, 36, 45]. Moreover, IL-6 causes significant increases in nasal secretions after topical application [46].

Interleukin-8 is a neutrophil-chemotactic cytokine whose production by monocytes, fibroblasts, endothelial cells, epithelial cells, and neutrophils is induced by IL-1 and TNF-α. In addition to its activity as a potent neutrophil chemoattractant, IL-8 activates neutrophil degranulation and respiratory burst, T lymphocyte chemotaxis, and release of histamine and LTs from basophils. IL-8 has been identified in a number of inflammatory conditions (including nasal allergic responses) at plasma concentrations of up to 1.2 mg/ml, which fall within the range at which neutrophils are stimulated in vitro. IL-8 has been detected in nasal secretions of volunteers infected with RV, FLU, and RSV [35, 36, 47]. Moreover, IL-8 causes marked increases in nasal airway resistance and tissue neutrophilia after topical application, and has been associated with disease severity during experimental RV infection [47, 48].

Interleukin-10 is produced by T lymphocytes, blood monocytes, and tissue macrophages and is considered to be an intrinsic anti-inflammatory and immunosuppressive cytokine. IL-10 inhibits cytokine production by T lymphocytes, mononuclear phagocytes, and natural killer cells. Expression of IL-10 by antigen-presenting cells may have a role in lessening inflammation by inhibiting the synthesis of proinflammatory cytokines such as IL-1, IL-6, IL-8, and TNF-α. This role of IL-10 is supported by its ability to induce T-cell tolerance to the antigen. Indeed, lack of macrophage IL-10 production has been purported to underlie the chronic airway inflammation characteristic of asthma [49]. Increases in local IL-10 production were reported during experimental vURIs, and maximal IL-10 levels typically coincide with the onset of resolution of vURI-induced symptomatology and pathophysiology [50].

Genetic factors likely also play a role in the predisposition of certain individuals to vURIs and their complications, most notably OM and chronic sinusitis. Single nucleotide polymorphisms (SNPs) of cytokine-related genes, which result in high cytokine production, may have a role in promoting inflammation during infection [51]. Severity of RSV infection in infants and adults has been shown to be associated with polymorphism in certain alleles of Interferon-gamma (IFN-γ) and TNF-β genotypes, respectively [52, 53]. Polymorphism of the TNF-β gene has also been shown to form a component of genetic predisposition to chronic sinusitis [54]. Likewise, OM susceptibility is linked to specific polymorphisms of TNF-α and IL-6 alleles [51].

Several recently developed tools are available for dissecting the role of various proinflammatory cytokines in the pathogenesis of vURIs and its complications. One such tool is the use of animal models of cytokine knockout and blockade. In mice deficient for IL-6 or in those treated with IL-1ra, symptoms of FLU-induced illness were partially reduced [55]. Moreover, mortality was reduced in those animals treated with IL-1ra. Another recently developed tool is cytokine genotyping. Recent studies demonstrated associations between specific cytokine genotypes associated with high production of TNF-α or IL-1β and increased susceptibility to several infectious diseases [56]. These results suggest that certain cytokines are necessary for the development of symptomatology during vURIs and that specific cytokine polymorphisms may be associated with increased susceptibility to viral rhinitis and its complications.

In summary, cytokines promote the initiation, amplification, and persistence of inflammation by their direct cellular effects and by their role in inducing synthesis or release of other inflammatory chemicals in a cascading fashion. A common pathway in vURIs may be the early release of nonspecific, host-alert cytokines, including TNF-α and IL-1. These have both local effects (e.g., depress protein synthesis and upregulate major histocompatibility complex presentation) and systemic effects (e.g., pyrogenic and stem cell maturation) that are expressed as the more general symptoms and signs of illness (e.g., fever and malaise). They also upregulate integrin and selectin expression and thereby mediate the local recruitment of inflammatory cells, which in turn promotes the release or synthesis of IMs (e.g., histamine, bradykinin, eicosanoids, and other cytokines). Some of those IMs initiate neurogenic inflammation and increased vascular permeability (rhinorrhea) and cause sneezing, cough, and nasal congestion. In a cascading and networking fashion, TNF-a and IL-1 also regulate the production of other pro- or anti-inflammatory cytokines via transcription factor activation in an autocrine or paracrine manner. Additionally, there is strong evidence for cross talk between IMs, especially those products of the lipoxygenase pathway and the cytokines. In spite of the data demonstrating an association between cytokines and symptoms of vURIs, the role of these mediators in pathogenesis will not be clear until specific inhibitors are available for use in clinical trials.

Prevention and Treatment

There are a variety of pharmacologic agents currently available for the treatment and/or prevention of vURIs. For certain pathogens, viral rhinitis and its complications can be prevented by effective immunization against the precipitating virus or by effective antiviral prophylaxis or treatment. For example, populations at risk for severe FLU- or RSV-induced lower respiratory illness can be actively immunized with a FLU vaccine or passively immunized with an anti-RSV monoclonal antibody [57, 58]. Moreover, several antiviral agents are available for prophylaxis or treatment [59]. These include ribavirin for RSV and amantadine, rimantadine, zanamivir, and oseltamivir for FLU. Antiviral agents for RV, such as pleconaril, are currently under development and testing. However, at present, the use of immunization or antiviral agents is not applicable to the majority of episodes of vURIs for several reasons: (1) the large number of causative viruses; (2) the high degree of antigenic variability exhibited by most of these viruses; (3) the limited arsenal, high specificity, and significant side-effects of available antivirals; and (4) concerns regarding selection of resistant virus strains during extended antiviral prophylaxis [60].

Symptomatic therapy, including the use of antihistamine, decongestants, and antichoinergics remains the mainstay of treatment for vURIs [61, 62]. Although several large studies of experimental vURIs have confirmed that these agents have some efficacy in treating the symptoms of vURIs, other studies have shown very minimal or no efficacy in the treatment and/or prevention of complications, including OM and sinusitis.

Numerous studies have examined the efficacy of zinc for the treatment of vURIs. Despite the in vitro effect of zinc on viral replication, there has been no detectable effect of zinc on virus replication in vivo. The effect of zinc on symptoms of viral rhinitis has been inconsistent. Some studies reported dramatic decreases in the duration and severity of symptoms, while other studies have shown no effect [63]. Echinacea has also been widely used for treatment of vURIs, and similar to zinc, efficacy studies have been inconsistent. A recent study by Turner et al. [64] shows that the extract of *Echinacea angustifolia* root had no demonstrable effect on the rates of viral infection or symptom scores following viral challenge.

Conclusions

The majority of current treatments for vURIs and its complications were "borrowed" from other nasal inflammatory diseases (e.g., allergy). The rational development of specific therapies for vURIs and its complications is complicated by our incomplete understanding of the disease pathogenesis, the similar expression of illness for different viruses, and the relatively late presentation of identifiable symptoms and signs. Future studies should contribute to a better understanding of the inflammatory responses to vURIs and clarify the roles of the targeted proinflammatory cytokines and neurogenic inflammation in disease expression. This knowledge will lay the foundation for rationally targeted therapies directed at host inflammatory or immune responses that have the potential to alter the course of a vURI, suppress disease expression, and limit complications, including otitis media and sinusitis.

References

1. Cayce KA, Krowchuk DP, Feldman SR, et al. Healthcare ultilization for acute and chronic disease of young, school-age children in the rural and non-rural setting. *Clin Pediatr* 2005, 44:491–498.
2. Agrawal S, Husein M, MacRae D. Complications of otitis media: an evolving state. *J Otolaryngol* 2005, 34S1:S33–S39.
3. Paramore LC, Ciuryla V, Ciesla G, Liu L. Economic impact of RSV-related illness in the US: an analysis of national databases. *Pharmacoeconomics* 2004, 22:275–284.
4. Glasziou PP, Del Mar CB, Sanders SL, Hayem M. Antibiotics for acute otitis media in children. *Cochrane Database Syst Rev* 2004, CD000219.
5. Gwaltney JM Jr, Phillips CD, Miller RD, Riker DK. Computed tomographic study of the common cold. *N Engl J Med* 1994, 330:25–30.
6. Revai K, Dobbs LA, Nair S, Patel JA, Grady JJ, Chonmaitree T. Incidence of acute otitis media and sinusitis complicated by upper respiratory tract infection: the effect of age. *Pediatrics* 2007 June, 119(6):e1408–e1412.
7. Lemanske RF Jr, Dick EC, Swenson CA, et al. Rhinovirus upper respiratory infection increases airway hyperreactivity and late asthmatic reactions. *J Clin Invest* 1989, 83:1–10.
8. Falsey AR. Respiratory syncytial virus infection in older persons. *Vaccine* 1998 Nov, 16(18):1775–1778.
9. Igarashi Y, Skoner DP, Doyle WJ, et al. Analysis of nasal secretions during phases of experimental rhinovirus upper respiratory tract infection. *J Allergy Clin Immunol* 1993, 92:722–731.
10. Doyle WJ, Skoner DP, White MV, et al. Pattern of nasal secretions during experimental influenza virus infection. *Rhinology* 1996, 34:2–8.
11. Turner RB, Witek TJ, Riker DK. Comparison of symptom severity in natural and experimentally induced colds. *Am J Rhinol* 1996, 10(3):167–172.
12. Doyle WJ, Skoner DP, Hayden F, et al. Nasal and otologic effects of experimental influenza A virus infection. *Ann Otol Rhinol Laryngol* 1994, 103:59–69.
13. Winther B, Alper CM, Mandel EM, Doyle WJ, Hendley JO. Temporal relationships between colds, upper respiratory viruses detected by polymerase chain reaction and otitis media in young children followed through a typical cold season. *Pediatrics* 2007 June, 119(6):1069–1075.
14. Alper C, Doyle W, Skoner D, et al. Prechallenge antibodies moderate disease expression in adults experimentally exposed to rhinovirus strain Hanks. *Clin Infect Dis* 1998, 27:119–128.
15. Skoner DP, Whiteside TL, Wilson JW, et al. Effect of rhinovirus 39 (RV-39) infection on immune parameters in allergic and non-allergic subjects. *J Allergy Clin Immunol* 1993, 92:732–743.
16. Skoner DP, Fireman PF, Doyle WJ. Urine histamine metabolite elevations during experimental colds. *J Allergy Clin Immunology* 1997, 99:S419.
17. Doyle WJ, Boehm S, Skoner DP. Physiologic responses to intranasal dose-response challenges with histamine, methacholine, bradykinin and prostaglandin in adult volunteers with and without nasal allergy. *J Allergy Clin Immunol* 1990, 86:924–935.
18. Doyle WJ, McBride TP, Skoner DP, et al. A double-blind placebo-controlled clinical trial of the effect of chlorpheniramine on the response of the nasal airway, ME and eustachian tube to provocative rhinovirus challenge. *J Pediatr Inf Dis* 1988, 7:229–238.
19. Naclerio RM, Proud D, Lichtenstein LM, et al. Kinins are generated during experimental rhinovirus colds. *J Infect Dis* 1988, 157:133–142.
20. Higgins PG, Barrow GI, Tyrrell DA. A study of the efficacy of the bradykinin antagonist, NPC 567, in rhinovirus infections in human volunteers. *Antiviral Res* 1990, 14(6):339–344.
21. Gentile DA. Evolving role of leukotrienes in pathogenesis of viral infections, including otitis media. *Curr Allergy Asthma Resp* 2006 July, 6(4):316–320.
22. Gentile DA, Patel A, Doyle WJ, et al. Elevations of local leukotriene C4 levels during experimental viral upper respiratory infections. *Am J Respir Crit Car Med* 2000, 161:A179.

23. Bisgaard H, Olsson P, Bende M. Effect of leukotriene D4 on nasal mucosal blood flow, nasal airway resistance and nasal secretion in humans. *Clin Allergy* 1986, 16:289–297.

24. Bisgaard, H. Study Group on Montelukast and Respiratory Syncytial Virus. A randomized trial of montelukast in respiratory syncytial virus postbronchiolitis. *Am J Crit Care Med* 2003, Feb 1, 167(3):379–383.

25. Shoshkes Reiss C, Komatsu, T. Does nitric oxide play a critical role in viral infections? *J Virol* 1998:4546–4551.

26. Kaul P, Singh I, Turner R. Effect of nitric oxide on rhinovirus replication and virus-induced IL-8 elaboration. *Am J Respir Crit Care Med* 1999, 159:1193–1198.

27. Sanico A, Atsuta S, Proud D, Togias A. Plasma extravasation through neural stimulation in human nasal mucosa. *J Appl Physiol* 1998, 84:537–543.

28. Sanico A, Philip G, Proud D, et al. Comparison of nasal mucosal responsiveness to neuronal stimulation in nonallergic and allergic rhinitis: effects of capsaicin nasal challenge. *Clin Exp Allergy* 1998, 28: 92–100.

29. Yuta A, Doyle WJ, Gaumond E, et al. Rhinovirus infection induces mucus hypersecretion. *Am J Physiol* 1998, 274:L1017–L1023.

30. Einarsson O, Geba GP, Zhu Z, et al. Interleukin-11: stimulation in vivo and in vitro by respiratory viruses and induction of airway hyperresponsiveness. *J Clin Invest* 1996, 97:915–924.

31. Mullol J, Chowdoury BA, White MV, et al. Endothelin in human nasal mucosa. *Am J Respir Cell Mol Biol* 1993, 8:393–402.

32. Mosimann BL, White MV, Hohman RJ, et al. Substance P, calcitonin-gene related peptide, and vasoactive intestinal peptide increase in nasal secretions after allergen challenge in atopic patients. *J Allergy Clin Immunol* 1993, 92:95–104.

33. Fang SY, Shen CL, Ohyama M. Distribution and quantity of neuroendocrine markers in allergic rhinitis. *Acta Otolaryngol* (Stockh) 1998; 118:398–403.

34. Gentile D, Doyle W, Whiteside T, et al. Increased IL-6 levels in nasal lavage samples following experimental influenza A virus infection. *Clin Diagn Lab Immunol* 1998, 5:604–608.

35. Skoner DP, Gentile DA, Patel A, Doyle WJ. Evidence for cytokine mediation of symptoms in adults experimentally infected with influenza A virus. *J Infect Dis* 1999, 180:10–14.

36. Hayden FG, Fritz R, Lobo MC, et al. Local and systemic cytokine responses during experimental human influenza A virus infection: relation to symptom formation and host defense. *J Clin Invest* 1998, 101:643–649.

37. Pitkaranta A, Nokso-Koivisto J, Jantti V, et al. Lowered yields of virus-induced interferon production in leukocyte cultures and risk of recurrent respiratory infections in children. *J Clin Virol* 1999, 14:199–205.

38. Tang YW, Graham BS. Anti-IL-4 treatment at immunization modulates cytokine expression, reduces illness, and increases cytotoxic T lymphocyte activity in mice challenged with respiratory syncytial virus. *J Clin Invest* 1994, 94:1953–1958.

39. Doyle WJ, Skoner DP, Gentile D. Nasal cytokines as mediators of illness during the common cold. *Curr Allergy Asthma Rep* 2005 May, 5(3):173–181.

40. Raza M, Essery S, Weir D, et al. Infection with respiratory syncytial virus and water-soluble components of cigarette smoke alter production of TNF-a and nitric oxide by human blood monocytes. *FEMS Immunol Med Microbiol* 1999, 24:387–394.

41. Matsuda K, Tsutsumi H, Okamoto Y, Chiba C. Development of IL-6 and TNF-a activity in nasopharyngeal secretions of infants and children during infection with respiratory syncytial virus. *Clin Diag Lab Immunol* 1995, 2:322–324.

42. Hornsleth A, Klug B, Nir M, et al. Severity of respiratory syncytial virus disease related to type and genotype of virus and to cytokine values in nasopharyngeal secretions. *Pediatr Infect Dis J* 1998, 17:1114–1121.

43. Subauste MC, Jacoby DB, Richards SM, Proud D. Infection of a human respiratory epithelial line with rhinovirus: induction of cytokine release and modulation of susceptibility to infection by cytokine exposure. *J Clin Invest* 1995, 96:549–557.

44. Yoon HJ, Zhu Z, Gwaltney JM, Elias JA. Rhinovirus regulation of IL-1 receptor antagonist in vivo and in vitro: a potential mechanism of symptom resolution. *J Immunol* 1999, 162:7461–7469.

45. Matsuda K, Tsutsumi H, Okamoto Y, Chiba C. Development of IL-6 and TNF-a activity in nasopharyngeal secretions of infants and children during infection with respiratory syncytial virus. *Clin Diag Lab Immunol* 1995, 2:322–324.

46. Gentile DA, Yokitis J, Angelini BL, et al. Effect of intranasal challenge with IL-6 on airway symptomatology and physiology in allergic and non-allergic subjects. *Ann Allergy Asthma Immunol* 2000, 84:130.

47. Turner RB, Weingand KWQ, Yeh CH, Leedy DW. Association between interleukin-8 concentration in nasal secretions and severity of symptoms of experimental rhinovirus colds. *Clin Exp Allergy* 1995, 25:46–49.

48. Douglass JA, Dhami D, Gurr CE, et al. Influence of interleukin-8 challenge in the nasal mucosa in atopic and nonatopic subjects. *Am J Respir Crit Care Med* 1994, 150:1108–1113.

49. Borish L, Aarons A, Rumbyrt J, et al. Interleukin-10 regulation in normal subjects and patients with asthma. *J Allergy Clin Immunol* 1996, 97:1288–1296.

50. Gentile DA, Patel A, Ollila C, et al. Diminished IL-10 production in subjects with allergy after infection with influenza A virus. *J Allergy Clin Immunol* 1999, 103:1045–1048.

51. Patel JA, Nair S, Revai K, Grady J, Saeed K, Matalon R, Block S, Chonmaitree T. Association of proinflammatory cytokine gene polymorphisms with susceptibility to otitis media. *Pediatrics* 2006 Dec, 118(6):2273–2279. Erratum in: *Pediatrics* 2007 June, 119(6):1270.

52. Gentile DA, Doyle WJ, Zeevi, A, Piltcher O, Skoner DP. Cytokine gene polymorphisms moderate responses to respiratory syncytial virus in adults. *Hum Immunol* 2003 Jan, 64(1):93–98.

53. Gentile DA, Doyle WJ, Zeevi A, Howe-Adams J, Kapadia S, Tecki J, Skoner DP. Cytokine gene polymorphisms moderate illness severity in infants with respiratory syncytial virus infection. *Hum Immunol* 2003 Mar, 64(3):338–344.

54. Takeuchi K, Majima Y, Sakakura Y. Tumor necrosis factor gene polymorphism in chronic sinusitis. *Laryngoscope* 2000 Oct, 110(10 Pt 1):1711–1714.

55. Swiergiel AH, Smagin GN, Johnson LJ, Dunn AJ. The role of cytokines in the behavioral responses to endotoxin and influenza virus infection in mice: effects of acute and chronic administration of the interleukin-1 receptor antagonist (IL-1ra). *Brain Res* 1997, 776:96–104.

56. Mira J, Cariou A, Grall F, Delclaux C. Association of TNF2, a TNF-a promoter polymorphism, with septic shock and susceptibility to mortality. *JAMA* 1999, 282:561–568.

57. Sawyer LA. Antibodies for the prevention and treatment of viral diseases. *Antiviral Res* 2000, 47(2):57–77.

58. Deguchi Y, Takusugi Y. Efficacy of influenza vaccine in the elderly: reduction in risks of mortality and morbidity during an influenza A (H3N2) epidemic for the elderly in nursing homes. *Int J Clin Lab Res* 2000, 30(1):1–4.

59. Doyle WJ, Skoner DP, Alper CM, et al. Effect of rimantadine treatment on clinical manifestations and otologic complications in adults experimentally infected with influenza A (H1N1) virus. *J Infect Dis* 1998, 177:1260–1265.

60. Hayden FG, Hay AJ. Emergence and transmission of influenza A viruses resistant to amantadine and rimantadine. *Curr Top Microbiol Immunol* 1992, 176:119–1130.

61. Gentile DA, Friday G, Skoner DP. Management of rhinitis: antihistamines and decongestants. *Immunology and Allergy Clinics of North America*. Edited by Vassallo J. Philadelphia, PA: W.B. Saunders; 2000, pp.355–368.

62. Dykewicz MS, Fineman S, Skoner DP, et al. Diagnosis and management of rhinitis: parameter documents of the joint task force on practice parameters for allergy, asthma and immunology. *Ann Allergy Asthma Immunol* 1998, 36:2992–3000.

63. Prasad AS, Fitzgerald JT, Bao B, et al. Duration of symptoms and plasma cytokine levels in patients with the common cold treated with zinc acetate: a randomized, double-blind, placebo-controlled trial. *Ann Intern Med* 2000, 133:245–252.

64. Turner RB, Bauer R, Woelkart K, Hulsey TC, Gangemi JD. An evaluation of Echinacea angustifolia in experimental rhinovirus infections. *N Engl J Med* 2005 July 28, 353(4):341–348.

Allergic Rhinitis, Asthma, and Obstructive Sleep Apnea: The Link

Jeffrey R. Stokes and Thomas B. Casale

Background

Atopic diseases, including allergic rhinitis and allergic asthma have increased worldwide over the last 3 decades. Rhinitis is extremely common globally affecting 10–25% of the population including 1.4–39.7% children [1, 2]. Allergic rhinitis is an inflammatory disorder induced by an IgE-mediated type 1 hypersensitivity reaction. Typical symptoms associated with allergic rhinitis include sneezing, nasal pruritis, rhinorrhea, and nasal congestion with associated eye symptoms. Allergic rhinitis typically had been categorized based on the timing of the rhinitis symptoms as either seasonal or perennial. However, the recent ARIA (Allergic Rhinitis and its Impact on Asthma) guidelines reclassified allergic rhinitis based on a patient's symptom frequency (intermittent and persistent) and severity (mild and moderate/severe) [1]. Allergic rhinitis has a significant effect on daily living including time missed from work/school. Both direct and indirect costs for allergic rhinitis make it a significant disease worldwide.

Asthma is also a chronic inflammatory disease associated with lower airway dysfunction. The airways demonstrate hyperresponsiveness with variable airflow obstruction that is often reversible. Triggers for asthma include allergens, infection, exercise, and cold weather. Asthma symptoms include recurrent episodes of wheezing, breathlessness, chest tightness, and coughing often worse at night or in the early morning [3]. It is estimated that 300 million people in the world have asthma, with an additional 100 million predicted by 2025. Globally, asthma accounts for 1 in every 250 deaths with many of these deaths being preventable [4]. The airway inflammation in asthma is characterized by activated mast cells, increased numbers

J.R. Stokes
Associate Professor Department of Medicine, Program Director Allergy/Immunology, Creighton University, Division of Allergy/Immunology, Suite 5850, Omaha, NE 68131, USA
e-mail: jstokes@creighton.edu

T.B. Casale
Professor, Department of Medicine, Chief, Allergy/Immunology, Creighton University, Division of Allergy/Immunology Suite 5850, Omaha, NE 68131, USA
e-mail: tbcasale@creighton.edu

R. Pawankar et al. (eds.), *Allergy Frontiers: Clinical Manifestations,*
DOI: 10.1007/978-4-431-88317-3_8, © Springer 2009

of activated eosinophils, and increased numbers of T helper type 2 lymphocytes. In addition to the inflammatory response in the airways, structural changes often described as remodeling are present. This inflammatory response in combination with the airway remodeling predispose the airways to narrowing in response to triggers leading to smooth muscle contraction, airway edema, airway thickening, and mucus hypersecretion [3, 4].

Obstructive sleep apnea (OSA) has been a clinically recognized entity for over 30 years [5]. Obstructive sleep apnea syndrome (OSAS) is characterized by recurrent episodes of upper airway collapse and obstruction during sleep leading to multiple arousals from sleep associated with symptoms of OSA. Classic symptoms associated with OSA include, snoring, daytime sleepiness, restless sleep, and awakening with sensation of choking, gasping, or smothering. The definitive diagnosis requires polysomnography to determine the level of sleep disturbance. Two commonly used measures are the apnea-hypopnea index (AHI), which is the number of apnea plus hypopnea episodes per hour of sleep and the respiratory disturbance index (RDI), which includes apneas, hypopneas and all airflow limitations with and without oxygen desaturation [6]. In Western countries, it has been estimated that 5% of adults have OSAS while 20% or more may have minimally symptomatic or asymptomatic OSA [5]. A survey of adults in primary care settings from the United States, Germany, and Spain reports symptoms of OSA with a high frequency. Symptoms consistent with OSA were noted in 26% of the European patients and 35% of the American patients [7]. The cause of OSA is multifactorial with several factors contributing to the upper airway obstruction. These factors include anatomical narrowing of the upper airway, increased collapsibility of upper airway tissues, and reflexes affecting upper airway caliber and pharyngeal inspiratory muscle function [8]. As a result of the poor sleep quality, OSAS patients have a decreased quality of life and are at increased risk for automobile accidents which may account for 1,400 fatalities annually in the United States alone [9]. OSAS is associated with cardiac diseases including atrial hypertension, ischemic heart disease, stroke, heart failure, atrial fibrillation, and sudden cardiac death [10].

Asthma has been associated with poor sleep quality and increased daytime sleepiness, symptoms of OSAS. Allergic rhinitis has been show to be independently related to difficulties inducing sleep and daytime sleepiness [11]. There are a number of factors that may explain these associations.

Allergic Rhinitis and Asthma

The association between rhinitis and asthma has been noted since the 1800s [12]. The estimates of concomitant allergic rhinitis (AR) in patients with asthma in the United States and in Europe is in excess of 50%, with up to 100% prevalence reported in patients with allergic asthma [13]. In addition, more than 22% of patients with AR have been reported to have asthma [14]. In asthmatic patients with concomitant AR, asthma-related medical resource use, including emergency room visits, physician visits, and prescription medication use, is higher than in asthmatics without AR. These patients also experience more frequent absence from work and decreased productivity [13].

Genetics may play a significant role in this association as children are more likely to develop asthma or AR if one of their parents has asthma compared to children with no family history of allergy [15]. AR is also a risk factor for asthma as rhinitis patients have a threefold greater risk of developing asthma then healthy people [16, 17]. The ARIA report in 2001 described the association between asthma and AR and the detrimental impact of AR on asthma. This concept has been termed "one airway, one disease" or the unified airway.

Several possible mechanisms have been suggested to explain the connection between the upper and lower airway in allergic rhinitis and asthma [18, 19] (Table 1). The first involves a shift from nasal to mouth breathing due to nasal congestion. This bypasses warming and humidifying the air thus increasing the likelihood of cold; dry air inspired directly into the lungs leading to bronchoconstriction. A second proposed mechanism involves the activation of the nasobronchial reflex. Reflexes arising from receptor sites in the nose and nasopharynx, mediated by sensory and vagal nerve fibers, mediate lower airway changes. For example, nasal provocation to substances such as capsaicin and silica particles causes a reflex-mediated decline in pulmonary function, which is inhibited by atropine. A third possibility involves aspiration of postnasal drainage of inflammatory material from the upper airway into the lower airway. Another putative mechanism is the absorption of inflammatory mediators systemically from the upper airway which then act on the lower airway. Most data suggest the first two mechanisms as the most likely interactions between upper and lower airway events.

Similarities observed between the two diseases may in part result from common structural and inflammatory components (Table 2). Embryologically the upper and lower airways share respiratory epithelium This ciliated pseudostratified columnar

Table 1 Allergic rhinitis contributing factors to asthma

Shift from nasal to mouth breathing
Activation of nasobronchial reflex
Aspiration of postnasal inflammatory secretions
Systemic absorption of inflammatory mediators from the upper airway

Table 2 Allergic rhinitis and asthma: similarities and differences

In common	Differences
Share respiratory epithelium	Different embryonic source
Similar inflammatory cells	Remodeling more prevalent in asthma
Both diseases respond to same treatments	Different cause of obstruction
• Antihistamines	
• Leukotriene modifying agents	
• Topical corticosteroids	
• Anti-IgE antibody	
• Allergen-specific immunotherapy	

epithelium with goblet cells gradually looses height, cilia and goblet cells as it progresses distally toward the alveoli [20]. Despite this similarity embryologically, the nose arises from ectodermal cells while the bronchi has an endodermal origin.

Both AR and asthma are inflammatory airway diseases and share similar inflammatory mechanisms. Key inflammatory cells include CD4 + T-lymphocytes (TH2 phenotype), eosinophils, basophils, and mast cells. Mediators such as histamine, cysteinyl leukotrienes, prostaglandins, platelet activating factor, and cytokines (e.g. IL-4, IL-13, IL-5, GM-CSF, RANTES, and IL-3), and adhesion molecules are numerous and important in both diseases [21]. In fact, eosinophils are present in the nasal mucosa in non-atopic asthmatics even in the absence of rhinitis symptoms. Furthermore there is a correlation between the eosinophil cell counts in the nose and lower airway [22]. Nonasthmatic patients with AR may still develop lower airway hyperresponsiveness to nonspecific stimuli, especially during their relevant pollen season [23]. When AR patients without associated asthma undergo nasal allergen provocation, the lower airway inflammatory responses mimic the upper airway response with increases in mucosal eosinophils and upregulation of adhesion molecules [24]. Furthermore, when nonasthmatic patients with AR undergo segmental bronchial allergen challenges, AR symptoms worsen and inflammatory cells in the nasal mucosa as well as total blood eosinophil counts increase [25]. Moreover, both AR and asthma have an early phase response to allergen and a late phase inflammatory reaction [1]. One of the key features of asthma is airway remodeling due to chronic inflammation, but this is not present to the same degree in AR despite a similar inflammatory pattern. Patients with asthma have substantial epithelial shedding and smooth muscle hypertrophy/hyperplasia in the lower airway [26]. The nasal obstruction in AR is due to nasal vasculature dilatation, especially of the venous cavernous sinusoids, whereas in asthma, smooth muscle contraction is an important source of airway obstruction.

In patients with asthma, treatment of concomitant AR with either nasal corticosteroids or second-generation antihistamines reduces asthma related emergency room visits and hospitalizations [27]. The use of second-generation antihistamines in patients with both AR and asthma improves both upper and lower airway symptoms [28]. Combination therapy with a second-generation antihistamine and decongestant not only improved asthma and rhinitis symptoms and quality of life, but also increased pulmonary function [29]. Systemic agents used to treat AR have been shown to improve concomitant allergic asthma. The reverse is also true, as leukotriene modifying agents improve AR symptoms and quality of life in the presence or absence of asthma [30, 31]. Leukotriene modifiers have demonstrated efficacy for AR symptom relief equal to that of second-generation antihistamines [32].

Topical agents used to treat AR also affect asthma in patients with both diseases. Nasal corticosteroid therapy can prevent lower airway hyperresponsiveness associated with seasonal pollen exposure in patients with both AR and asthma [33]. An early study demonstrated that topical agents such as intranasal corticosteroids and intranasal cromolyn sodium were effective in reducing asthma symptoms during ragweed season, in patients with AR, but the nasal corticosteroid preparations were more effective than cromolyn [34]. For patients with perennial AR and asthma, treatment with intranasal corticosteroids did not significantly improve either global asthma symptoms or peak flow measurements. Nasal corticosteroids did reduce evening asthma symptoms and significantly decreased lower airway hyperresponsiveness. These effects did not appear to be due to the corticosteroid reaching the lung as less than 2% of the drug was deposited in the lower airways [35]. However, a recent Cochrane meta-analysis evaluated 14 trials of intranasal corticosteroid use in patients with coexisting asthma and rhinitis. While individual studies found nasal corticosteroids improved asthma symptoms and measurements, only a non-significant beneficial trend for asthma symptom scores and forced expiratory volume in 1 s (FEV_1) was noted in the meta-analysis [36].

Since allergic asthma and AR both have elevated total IgE, therapy aimed at decreasing IgE may benefit both diseases. Omalizumab is a humanized anti-IgE monoclonal antibody that decreases total serum IgE levels. Over 400 patients with concomitant moderate-to-severe asthma and persistent AR were treated with either omalizumab or placebo for 28 weeks [37]. Similar to previous studies, omalizumab decreased asthma exacerbations and improved asthma quality of life. Patients treated with omalizumab also had less rhinitis symptoms and improved rhinitis quality of life [37].

Allergic Rhinitis and Obstructive Sleep Apnea

The relationship between AR and OSA is likely related to nasal congestion. Several mechanisms may play a role in this association. Nasal resistance accounts for two thirds of the total airway resistance and nasal patency is primarily controlled by the capacitance vessels of the nasal turbinates. AR causes the capacitance vessels to dilate leading to mucosal edema and increased secretions. Any anatomical reasons for narrowing of the upper airway such as hypertrophy of nasal turbinates or adenoid or tonsillar enlargement can also affect airway resistance [38]. Nasal congestion causes increased pressure differences between ambient air and the intrathoracic space. This leads to an increase in negative luminal upper airway pressure predisposing to upper airway collapse [39, 40]. Nasal congestion has been shown to be an independent risk factor for both OSA and habitual snoring. Patients with chronic nasal congestion are at an increased risk of having habitual snoring as well as developing snoring later in life if congestion persists [40–42]. Treating nasal congestion has been shown to reduce mouth breathing and OSA severity but does not alleviate OSA in adults [43]. Adults who reported nasal congestion due to allergy were more likely to have moderate to severe sleep-disordered breathing than were individuals without nasal congestion due to allergy [44].

In a small group of ragweed allergic adults nasal resistance and apnea episodes were worse during ragweed season. Despite this, the episodes of apnea were rarely associated with significant oxygen desaturation and were fewer in number than typically seen in a clinically significant sleep apnea syndrome [45]. In 11% of adult patients with nasal symptoms and sleep disturbances, perennial AR was thought to be a contributing factor [46]. Other investigators found that nearly 12% of patients presenting with symptoms of OSAS had AR but only 50% of those allergic patients had OSAS while 60% of the nonallergic patients had OSAS by polysomography [47]. Patients in whom AR affects sleep quality, but not necessarily leading to apnea, have been found to have sleep quality improvement with nasal corticosteroids or leukotriene receptor antagonists [48]. Overall, the connection between AR and OSA in adults is still somewhat controversial, despite several studies implicating a link.

Snoring occurs in 3–12% of children, but only about 2% of children develop OSAS [38, 49]. Atopic disease in children has been strongly associated with snoring [50, 51]. This was most significant with AR (odds ratio (OR) 2.90), but if a child had three atopic diseases (asthma, AR and atopic dermatitis), the effect appears cumulative with an OR of 7.45 for habitual snoring [51]. In one study the incidence of allergic sensitization in children who snored was estimated to be three times that reported in the general pediatric population [52]. In a study of children with habitual snoring referred for polysomnography, the overall frequency of OSAS was increased in allergic subjects, 57% compared to the nonatopic group that snored, 40% [52]. Other investigators have found that up to 80% of children with OSAS were atopic and these children tended to have higher BMIs than nonatopic children with OSAS [53].

Another reason why children appear to demonstrate a closer association between AR and OSA is the relationship between tonsillar and adenoidal hypertrophy and AR. Surgery to remove the tonsils and adenoids has been shown to resolve the OSA. In a study of sixth grade children, only 8% of the children without tonsillar hypertrophy had AR while nearly 30% of those with tonsillar hypertrophy had AR [54]. Intranasal corticosteroids are the most effective medication for treating nasal congestion due to AR. Children with sleep disordered breathing due to AR treated with nasal corticosteroids have less nasal congestion and improved sleep quality [55]. When used for children with OSA, polysomnography values and clinical symptoms improved [56, 57]. It is unclear if the beneficial effects of corticosteroids on OSA are due to improving tonsillar or adenoidal hypertrophy as oral corticosteroids have been ineffective in treating children with OSAS due to adenotonsillar hypertrophy [58]. In one study using nasal corticosteroids, it was observed that corticosteroids while decreasing the frequency of apnea and hypopnea in children with AR did not change tonsillar or adenoidal size [56]. A recent study evaluated the effect of regular nasal corticosteroids in non-atopic children with adenoidal hypertrophy. The severity of symptoms and adenoid size decreased in those children treated with nasal corticosteroids compared to the placebo group [59]. Although the evidence for a relationship between OSA and AR is somewhat debatable in adults, the association in children appears more straightforward (Table 3).

Table 3 Allergic rhinitis and obstructive sleep apnea (OSA)

Relationship based upon nasal congestion
An association between allergic rhinitis and snoring
Adults: allergic rhinitis and OSA relationship unclear
Pediatrics: allergic rhinitis and OSA relationship apparent (e.g. treatment of nasal symptoms with nasal corticosteroids improves OSA symptoms)

Asthma and Obstructive Sleep Apnea

In children, snoring and apnea related events are more prevalent in those with asthma-related symptoms than those without [60]. Asthma is a frequent comorbidity in adult patients with OSAS, and there is a higher prevalence of OSAS in patients with asthma [61, 62]. In difficult-to-control asthmatics, those with more than three severe exacerbations per year were more likely to suffer from OSA than those with only one severe exacerbation per year [63]. In patients with difficult-to-control asthma requiring oral corticosteroids, OSA is extremely prevalent. In a small population of 22 such patients, 95% had significant sleep disturbance consistent with OSAS [64]. The mechanism underlying this relationship is unclear, but several hypotheses have been put forth. OSA and asthma have several common risk factors such as obesity, nasal congestion, and nasal polyps [65]. Possible mechanisms for asthma promoting OSA include chronic disruption of sleep architecture, or anatomical abnormalities that decrease pharyngeal area (chronic inflammation and pharyngeal wall fat deposition). The worsening of asthma symptoms in patients with OSAS may be due to obesity, activation of inflammatory pathways, Gastroesophageal reflux disease (GERD), and cardiac pathology [65]. The inflammation due to OSA may not be localized in just the upper airway. When sputum samples were examined increased IL-8 levels and neutrophils were noted. The IL-8 levels correlated to the API and oxygen desaturation. This lower airway inflammatory pattern is unaffected by nasal Continuous positive airway pressure (CPAP) [66]. In patients without a history of asthma, the use of CPAP increased airway hyperresponsiveness unrelated to atopic status [66]. The reason for this association in non-asthmatics is unknown.

The recommended initial treatment for OSAS is nasal CPAP [67]. Several studies have demonstrated the benefit of nasal CPAP in patients with OSAS and nocturnal asthma. It is thought that a subgroup of asthmatic patients with small pharynxes may have increased vagal stimulation during sleep that could precipitate nocturnal asthma attacks which are alleviated by CPAP [68].

In a small group of nocturnal asthma patients with frequent asthma exacerbations (leading to respiratory arrest in three of the nine patients), treatment with nasal CPAP improved peak flow measurements and asthma control after only a week of therapy [69]. In a larger group of symptomatic nocturnal asthmatic adults with an AHI 15 or greater (moderate–severe OSA), treatment with CPAP for 2 months did not improve pulmonary functions despite improvement in asthma symptoms [70]. In 20 patients with OSA and mild–moderate nocturnal asthma, CPAP improved quality of life but did not affect airway hyperresponsiveness or FEV_1 [71]. In a small group of patients with nocturnal asthma but without OSA, CPAP worsened sleep architecture, increased awake time and decreased REM sleep. Only two patients demonstrated improvements in FEV_1 with CPAP, but a similar improvement was also noted in the same two patients with only supplemental oxygen. This study suggested that nocturnal oxygen desaturation may play a role in nocturnal asthma even in the absence of OSA [72]. Thus, the true association between nocturnal asthma and OSAS may be related to oxygenation, and not actual obstruction. Overall, the relationship between OSAS and nocturnal asthma appears to be multifactorial (Table 4).

Table 4 Asthma and obstructive sleep apnea (OSA)

Share several common risk factors
  • Obesity
  • Nasal congestion
  • Nasal polyps
Possible contributing factors to both diseases
  • Chronic disruption of sleep architecture
  • Anatomical issues decreasing pharyngeal area
Both diseases involve airway inflammation
Association between OSA and nocturnal asthma
CPAP effective in reducing asthma symptoms in patients with both disease states
CPAP in patients without asthma but OSA may increase airway hyperresponsiveness
CPAP in patients with nocturnal asthma but not OSA worsens sleep quality

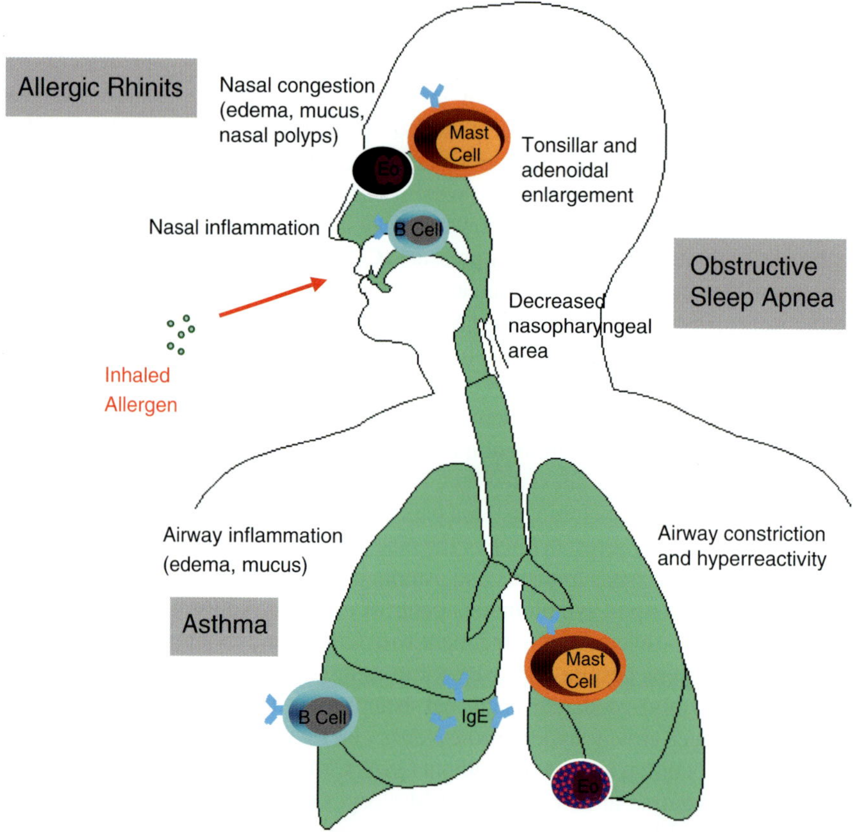

Fig. 1 "One Airway": Implications of the association of the upper and lower airways. The relationships of allergic rhinitis (nasal congestion and inflammation), obstructive sleep apnea (decreased nasopharyngeal area with increased adenoidal enlargement), and asthma (airway inflammation, airway obstruction and hyperreactivity). Inflammatory pattern similar in upper and lower airways with mast cells, eosinophils, and IgE producing B-cells

Conclusion and Summary

The studies reported herein support the united airway theory (Fig. 1). Epidemiologic, pathologic and physiologic links have clearly been found between AR, asthma, and OSA. Furthermore, treatment of one condition can lead to improvements in another. The exact mechanisms underlying these associations are unknown, but appear to involve common inflammatory and neurogenic pathways. It is likely that better understanding of the disease processes and common underlying mechanisms will provide better therapeutic options for all three disorders, and more importantly, perhaps the ability to halt the progression of one to another. In this regard, systemic treatments that attack common inflammatory mechanisms could be important. This is illustrated by the data from the Prevention of Asthma Trial, in which children with AR and high risk for developing asthma receiving allergen-specific immunotherapy had a substantially lower rate of asthma development than did their peers treated with conventional therapy alone [73]. Whether this or other treatments might also prevent OSA from occurring is unknown. Nonetheless, because AR, asthma, and OSA often occur together, it behooves physicians to closely assess their patients for all three conditions when they present with one or two.

References

1. Bousquet J, van Cauwenberge P, Khaltaev N, World Health Organization. Allergic rhinitis and its impact on asthma. J Allergy Clin Immunol 2001;108:S147–S336.
2. The International Study of Asthma and Allergies in Childhood (ISAAC) Steering Committee, Worldwide variation in prevalence of symptoms of asthma, allergic rhinoconjunctivitis, and atopic eczema: ISAAC. Lancet 1998;351:1225–1232.
3. Global strategy for asthma management and prevention, Global Initiative for Asthma (GINA) 2006. Available from: http://www.ginasthma.org
4. Masoli M, Fabian D, Holt S, Beasley R, Global Initiative for Asthma (GINA) Program. The global burden of asthma: executive summary of the GINA dissemination committee report. Allergy 2004;59:469–478.
5. Young T, Peppard PE, Gottlieb DJ. Epidemiology of obstructive sleep apnea: a population health perspective. Am J Respir Crit Care Med 2002;165:1217–1239.
6. Hosselet JJ, Ayuappa I, Norman RG, Krieger AC, Rapoport DM. Classification of Sleep-disordered Breathing. Am J Respir Crit Care Med, 2001;163:398–405.
7. Netzer NC, Hoegel JJ, Loube D, Netzer CM, Hay B, Alvarex-Sala R, Strohl KP. Sleep in primary care international study group. Prevalence of symptoms and risk of sleep apnea in primary care. Chest 2003;124:1406–1414.
8. Hudgel DW. Mechanisms of obstructive sleep apnea. Chest 1992;101:541–549.
9. Sassani A, Findley LJ, Kryger M, Goldlust E, George C, Davidson TM. Reducing motor-vehicle collisions, costs, and fatalities by treating obstructive sleep apnea syndrome. Sleep 2004;27:453–458.
10. McNicholas WT, Bonsignore MR. Management Committee of EU COST ACTION B26. Sleep apnoea as an independent risk factor for cardiovascular disease: current evidence, basic mechanisms and research priorities. Eur Respir J 2007;29:156–178.
11. Janson C, De Backer W, Gislason T, Plaschke P, Björnsson E, Hetta J, Kristbjarnarson H, Vermeire P, Boman G. Increased prevalence of sleep disturbances and daytime sleepiness

in subjects with bronchial asthma: a population study of young adults in three European countries. Eur Respir J 1996;9:2132–2138.

12. Demoly P, Bousquet. The relationship between asthma and allergic rhinitis. Lancet 2006;368: 711–713.

13. Gaugris S, Sazonov-Kocevar V, Thomas M. Burden of concomitant allergic rhinitis in adults with asthma. J Asthma 2006;43:1–7.

14. Greiner AN. Allergic rhinitis: Impact of the disease and considerations for management. Med Clin North Am 2006;90:17–38.

15. Dold S, Wjst M, von Mutius E, Reitmeir P, Stiepel E. Genetic risk for asthma, allergic rhinitis, and atopic dermatitis. Arch Dis Child 1992;67:1018–1022.

16. Settipane RJ, Hagy G, Settipane GA. Long-term risk factors for developing asthma and allergic rhinitis: A 23-year follow-up study of college students. Allergy Proc 1994;15:21–25.

17. Guerra S, Sherrill DL, Martinez FD, Barbee RA. Rhinitis as an independent risk factor for adult-onset asthma. J Allergy Clin Immunol 2002;109:419–425.

18. Togias A. Mechanisms of nose-lung interaction. Allergy 1999;54:S94–S105.

19. Braunstahl GJ. The unified immune system: respiratory tract-nasaobronchial interaction mechanisms in allergic airway disease. J Allergy Clin Immunol 2005;115:142–148.

20. Simons FER. Allergic rhinobronchitis: the asthma-allergic rhinitis link. J Allergy Clin Immunol 1999;104:534–540.

21. Kay AB. Allergy and allergic diseases. N Engl J Med 2001;344:30–37.

22. Gaga M, Lambrou P, Papageorgiou N, Koulouris NG, Kosmas E, Fragakis S, Sofios C, Rasidakis A, Jordanoglou J. Eosinophils are a feature of upper and lower airway pathology in non-atopic asthma, irrespective of the presence of rhinitis. Clin Exp Allergy 1998;30:663–669.

23. Madonini E, Briatico-Vangosa G, Pappacoda A, Maccagni G, Cardani A, Saporiti F. Seasonal increase of bronchial reactivity in allergic rhinitis. J Allergy Clin Immunol 1987;79:358–363.

24. Braunstahl GJ, Overbeek SE, KleinJan A, Prins JB, Hoogsteden HC, Fokkens WJ. Nasal allergen provocation induces adhesion molecule expression and tissue eosinophilia in upper and lower airways. J Allergy Clin Immunol 2001;107:469–476.

25. Braunstahl G-J, Kleinjan A, Overbeek SE, et al. Segmental bronchial provocation induces nasal inflammation in allergic rhinitis patients. Am J Respir Crit Care Med 2000;161(6):2051–2057.

26. Demoly P, Bousquet J. The relationship between asthma and allergic rhinitis. Lancet 2006;368:711–713.

27. Corren J, Manning BE, Thompson SF, Hennessy S, Strom BL. Rhinitis therapy and prevention of hospital care for asthma: a case-control study. J Allergy Clin Immunol 2004;113:415–419.

28. Grant JA, Nicodemus CF, Findlay SR, Glovsky M, Grossman J, Kaiser H, Meltzer EO, Mitchell DQ, Pearlman D, Selner J, Settipane G, Silvers W. Cetirizine in patients with seasonal rhinitis and concomitant asthma: prospective, randomized, placebo-controlled trial. J Allergy Clin Immunol 1995;95:923–932.

29. Corren J, Harris AG, Aaronson D, Beaucher W, Berkowitz R, Bronsky E, Chen R, Chervinsky P, Cohen R, Fourre J, Grossman J, Meltzer E, Pedinoff A, Stricker W, Wanderer A. Efficacy and safety of loratadine plus pseudoephedrine in patients with seasonal allergic rhinitis and mild asthma. J Allergy Clin Immunol 1997;100:781–788.

30. Philip G, Malmstrom K, Hampel Jr FC, Weinstein SF, LaForces CF, Ratner PH, Malice MP, Reiss TF. Montelukast Spring Rhinitis Study Group. Montelukast for treating seasonal allergic rhinitis: a randomized, double-blind, placebo-controlled trial performed in the spring. Clin Exp Allergy 2002;32:1020–1028.

31. Donnelly AL, Glass M, Minkwitz MC, Casale TB. The leukotriene D4-receptor antagonist, ICI 204,219, relieves symptoms of acute seasonal allergic rhinitis. Am J Resp Crit Care Med 1995;151:1734–1739.

32. Meltzer EO, Malmstrom K, Lu S, Prenner BM, Wei LX, Weinstein SF, Wolfe JD, Reiss TF. Concomitant montelukast and loratadine as treatment for seasonal allergic rhinitis: a randomized, placebo-controlled clinical trial. J Allergy Clin Immunol 2000;105:917–922.

33. Corren J, Adinoff AD, Buchmeier AD, Irvin CG. Nasal beclomethasone prevents the seasonal increase in bronchial responsiveness in patients with allergic rhinitis and asthma. J Allergy Clin Immunol 1992;90:250–256.

34. Welsh PW, Striker WE, Chu CP, Naessens JM, Reese ME, Reed CE, Marcoux JP. Efficacy of beclomethasone nasal solution, flunisolide, and cromolyn in relieving symptoms of ragweed allergy. Mayo Clin Proc 1987;62:125–134.

35. Watson WT, Becker AB, Simons FE. Treatment of allergic rhinitis with intranasal corticosteroids in patients with mild asthma: effect on lower airway responsiveness. J Allergy Clin Immunol 1993;91:97–101.

36. Taramarcaz P, Gibson PG. Intranasal corticosteroids for asthma control in people with coexisting asthma and rhinitis. Cochrane Database of Systemic Reviews 2003, Issue 3. Art. No.: CD003570. DOI:10.1002/14651858.CD003570.

37. Vignola AM, Humbert M, Bousquet J, Boulet L-P, Hedgecock S, Blogg M, Fox H, Surrey K. Efficacy and tolerability of anti-immunoglobulin E therapy with omalizumab in patients with concomitant allergic asthma and persistent allergic rhinitis: SOLAR. Allergy 2004;59:709–717.

38. Ng DK, Chan CH, Wang GY, Chow P, Kwok K. A review of the roles of allergic rhinitis in childhood obstructive sleep apnea syndrome. Allergy Asthma Proc 2006;27:240–242.

39. Shepard JW Jr, Burger CD. Nasal and oral flow–volume loops in normal subjects and patients with obstructive sleep apnea. Am Rev Respir Dis 1990;142:1288–1293.

40. Scharf MB, Cohen AP. Diagnostic and treatment implications of nasal obstruction in snoring and obstructive sleep apnea. Ann Allergy Asthma Immunol 1998;81:279–290.

41. Young T, Finn L, Palta M. Chronic nasal congestion at night is a risk factor for snoring in a population-based cohort study. Arch Intern Med 2001;161:1519.

42. Staevska MT, Mandajieva MA, Dimitrov VD. Rhinitis and sleep apnea. Curr Allergy Asthma Rep 2004;4:193–199.

43. McLean HA, Urton AM, Driver HS, Tan AKW, Day AG, Munt PW, Fitzpatrick. Effect of treating severe nasal obstruction on the severity of obstructive sleep apnoea. Eur Respir J 2005;25:521–527.

44. Young T, Finn L, Kim H. Nasal Obstruction as a risk factor for sleep-disordered breathing. The University of Wisconsin Sleep and Respiratory Research Group. J Allergy Clin Immunol 1997;99:S757–S762.

45. McNicholas WT, Tarlo S, Cole P, Zamel N, Rutherford R, Griffin D, Phillipson EA. Obstructive apneas during sleep in patients with seasonal allergic rhinitis. Am Rev Respir Dis 1982;126:625–628.

46. Canova CR, Downs SH, Knoblauch A, Andersson M, Tamm M, Leuppi JD. Increased prevalence of perennial allergic rhinitis in patients with obstructive sleep apnea. Resp 2004;71:138–143.

47. Kramer MF, De La Chaux R, Dreher A, Pfrongner E, Rasp G. Allergic rhinitis does not constitute a risk factor for obstructive sleep apnea syndrome. Acta Otolaryngol 2001;121:494–499.

48. Craig TJ, McCann JL, Gurevich F, Davies MJ. The correlation between allergic rhinitis and sleep disturbance. J Allergy Clin Immunol 2004;114:S139–S145.

49. Chau K, Ng K, Kwok K, Cheung M. Survey of children with obstructive sleep apnea syndrome in Hong Kong of China. Chin Med J 2004;117:657–660.

50. Anuntaseree W, Rookkapan K, Kuasirikul S, Thongsuksai P. Snoring and obstructive sleep apnea in Thai school-age children: prevalence and predisposing factors. Pediatr Pulmonol 2001;32:222–227.

51. Chng SY, Goh DYT, Wang XS, Tan TN, Ong NBH. Snoring and atopic disease: a strong association. Pediatr Pulmonol 2004;38:210–216.

52. McColley SA, Carroll JL, Curtis S, Loughlin GM, Sampson HA. High prevalence of allergic sensitization in children with habitual snoring and obstructive sleep apnea. Chest 1997;111:170–173.

53. Ramirez PL, Umre U, Schneider A. Association between obstructive sleep apnea syndrome and atopy in children. J Allergy Clin Immunol 2006;117:s297 (abstract).

54. Yumoto E, Kozawa T, Yanagihara N. Influence of tonsillar hypertrophy to physical growth and diseases of the nose and ear in school-age children. Nippon Jibiinkoka Gakkai Kaiho 1991;94:534–540.
55. Mansfield LE, Diaz G, Posey CR, Flores-Neder J. Sleep disordered breathing and daytime quality of life in children with allergic rhinitis during treatment with intranasal budesonide. Ann Allergy Asthma Immunol 2004;92:240–244.
56. Brouillette RT, Manouklan JJ, Ducharme FM, et al. Efficacy of fluticasone nasal spray for pediatric obstructive sleep apnea. J Pediatr 2001;138:838–844.
57. Chau KW, Ng KK, Kwok KL, et al. Survey of children with obstructive sleep apnea syndrome in Hong Kong of China. Chin Med J (Engl) 2004;117:657– 660.
58. Al-Ghamdi SA, Manoukian JJ, Morielli A, et al. Do systemic corticosteroids effectively treat obstructive sleep apnea secondary to adenotonsillar hypertrophy? Laryngoscope 1997;107:1382–1387.
59. Berlucchi M, Salsi D, Valetti L, Parrinello G, Nicolai P. The role of mometasone furoate aqueous nasal spray in the treatment of adenoidal hypertrophy in the pediatric age group: preliminary results of a prospective randomized study. Pediatrics 2007;119:e1392–e1397.
60. Ekici A, Ekici M, Kurtipek E, Keles H, Kara T, Tunckol M, Kocyigit P. Association of asthma-related symptoms with snoring and apnea and effect on health-related quality of life. Chest 2005;128:3358–3363.
61. Larsson LG, Lindberg A, Franklin KA, Lundback B. Symptoms related to obstructive sleep apnoea are common in subjects with asthma, chronic bronchitis and rhinitis in a general population. Respir Med 2001;95:423–429.
62. Kalra M, Biagini J, Bernstein D, Stanforth S, Burkle J, Cohen A, LeMasters G. Effect of asthma on the risk of obstructive sleep apnea syndrome in atopic women. Ann Allergy Asthma Immunol 2006;97:231–235.
63. ten Brinke A, Sterk PJ, Masclee AAM, Spinhoven P, Schmidt JT, Zwinderman AH, Rabe KF, Bel EH. Risk factors of frequent exacerbations in difficult-to treat asthma. Eur Respir J 2005;26:812–818.
64. Yigla M, Tov N, Solomonov A, Rubin AH, Harley D. Difficult-to-control asthma and obstructive sleep apnea. J Asthma 2003;40:865–871.
65. Kasasbeh A, Kasasbeh E, Krishnaswamy G. Potential mechanisms connecting asthma, esophageal reflux, and obesity/sleep apnea complex: a hypothetical review. Sleep Med Rev 2007;11:47–58.
66. Devouassoux G, Lévy P, Rossini E, Pin I, Fior-Gozlan M, Henry M, Seigneurin D, Pépin JL. Sleep apnea is associated with bronchial inflammation and continuous positive airway pressure-induced airway hyperresponsiveness. J Allergy Clin Immunol 2007;119:597–603.
67. Basner RC. Continuous positive pressure for obstructive sleep apnea. N Engl J Med 2007;356:1751–1758.
68. Guilleminault C, Quera-Salva MA, Powell N, Riley R, Romaker A, Partinen M, Baldwin R, Nino-Murcia G. Nocturnal asthma: snoring, small pharynx and nasal CPAP. Eur Respir J 1988;10:902–907.
69. Chan CS, Woolcock AJ, Sullivan CE. Nocturnal asthma: role of snoring and obstructive sleep apnea. Am Rev Respir Dis 1988;137:1502–1504.
70. Ciftci TU, Ciftci B, Guven SF, Kokturk O, Turktas H. Effect of nasal continuous positive airway pressure in uncontrolled nocturnal asthmatic patients with obstructive sleep apnea syndrome. Resp Med 2005;99:529–534.
71. Lafond C, Series F, Lemiere C. Impact of CPAP on asthmatic patients with obstructive sleep apnoea. Eur Respir J 2007;29:307–311.
72. Martin RJ, Pak J. Nasal CPAP in non-apneic nocturnal asthma. Chest 1991;100:1024–1027.
73. Moller C, Dreborg S, Ferdousi HA, Halken S, Host A, Jacobsen L, Koivikko A, Koller DY, Niggemann B, Norberg LA, Urbanek R, Valovirta E, Wahn U. Pollen immunotherapy reduces the development of asthma in children with seasonal rhinoconjunctivitis (the PAT-study). J Allergy Clin Immunol 2002 Feb;109(2):251–256.

Common Colds and Respiratory Viruses:
Impact on Allergy and Asthma

Ioanna M. Velissariou, Paraskevi Xepapadaki,
and Nikolaos G. Papadopoulos

Introduction

The association between common colds and acute wheezing episodes has been recognized for decades [1]. Indeed, wheezing associated with colds is the most common form of wheezing at all ages [2]. Although the nature of the debate has evolved over the years, many of the contradictory issues are still relevant, including whether episodic virus-induced wheezing in young children should be considered asthma. Furthermore, the debate continues over whether severe early viral infections have a causative role in the development of asthma, by immune modulation, airway damage, or both, or whether children who present with virus-induced wheezing have a pre-existing predisposition.

The clinical correlation of the common cold with asthma episodes is not recent. However, it is only in the last 10–15 years, with using sensitive methodologies for the detection of the most prevalent respiratory viruses, such as rhinoviruses and coronaviruses, we have been able to appreciate their importance [3, 4]. Furthermore, some of the most obvious changes in affluent societies, such as family structure, congregation, and hygiene, have implications for the epidemiology of infections, leading to speculation that infection-associated factors may be related to the asthma epidemic [5].

Using the polymerase chain reaction (PCR) and detailed analysis of epidemiological data, our understanding of the relationship between viral infections and asthma exacerbations has improved [6]. Nevertheless, there still are some apparently contradictory effects and many unexplored aspects to be addressed. The mechanisms by which respiratory viruses exacerbate asthma are under scrutiny. In addition, the possibility that some viral or intracellular bacterial infections may initiate asthma is still disputed. The subject has become more complicated since it was recognized that early exposure to microorganisms and/or different infections may actually protect against asthma, the so-called "hygiene hypothesis" [7].

I.M. Velissariou, P. Xepapadaki and N.G. Papadopoulos
Allergy Research Center, 2nd Pediatric Clinic, University of Athens, 41, Fidippidou Street, 11527, Goudi, Greece

R. Pawankar et al. (eds.), *Allergy Frontiers: Clinical Manifestations,*   141
DOI: 10.1007/978-4-431-88317-3_9, © Springer 2009

Understanding the role of viral infections in the development of allergy and asthma may have implications on designing and selecting optimal therapeutic strategies, while indirectly affecting immunization programs, antibiotic use, and marketing of antiviral drugs, as well as the development of new approaches to therapy. This chapter addresses the interplay between viral infections, the immune system, and lung development, focusing on the possible role of respiratory viruses in the origin and exacerbations of asthma and allergy. Also presented are antiviral strategies for the prevention and treatment of virus-induced asthma exacerbations that have been investigated recently.

Viral Infections and the Development of Allergy and Asthma

To understand the potential implications of viral infections in the development of asthma, it has to be kept in mind that asthma has a complex natural history that includes different phenotypes, which may differ in their pathogenesis. It is well established that a majority of asthma cases start early in life. However, a significant proportion of children who wheeze at a young age, mostly after upper respiratory tract infections (URTIs), overcome their problem before school age. These subjects, characterized as 'transient early wheezers', have reduced airway function at birth; thus it is likely that their disease is at least partly mechanical rather than immunological in nature [8]. Other children commence wheezing early and continue to do so at least until adolescence. These persistent wheezers have an altered immune response with a rise in IgE levels during their first reported URTI, and no reduction in eosinophil numbers during the acute phase of the URTI, in contrast to transient wheezers [9].

The virus, most frequently associated with severe bronchiolitis in the first years of life, is the respiratory syncytial virus (RSV). RSV infection occurs in almost all children before their second birthday, and clinical presentations vary from subclinical to severe, life-threatening bronchiolitis [10]. Early studies have pointed out that children suffering from severe bronchiolitis have an increased risk of developing asthma in subsequent years [11]. Whether RSV bronchiolitis represents a marker of susceptibility to wheezing or it can per se divert the immune system or affect the lung and initiate asthma is not yet concluded. It is also possible that these pathways are not mutually exclusive: a pre-existing susceptibility may become clinically relevant once an exceptionally severe infection occurs (Fig. 1).

In 1971, Rooney and Williams [11] found that 56% of children hospitalized for bronchiolitis would continue to wheeze 2–7 years later, and this has been confirmed in several subsequent studies. However, it has been difficult to ascertain whether this is solely an association or whether causation is also involved, resulting from either direct lung damage or an RSV-mediated immunological deviation toward type-2 cytokine production [12]. Although pulmonary function is reduced many years later in children with a history of lower respiratory tract infection, it seems that this is a pre-existing feature of these children [8, 13].

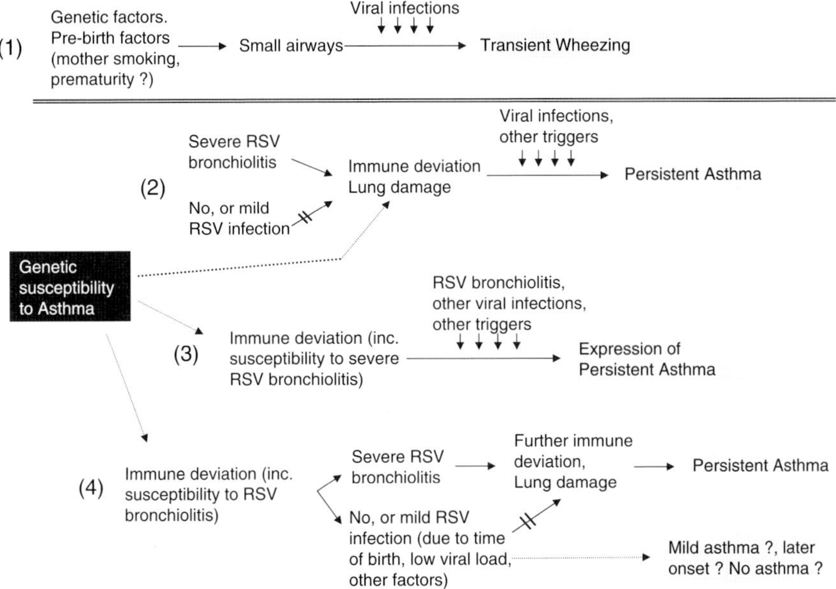

Fig. 1 Transient wheezing may be associated mostly with airway size at birth, resoling before school-age (1) severe RSV bronchiolitis in early life may be either the cause (2) or a marker of susceptibility (3) of asthma. These possibilities are not mutually exclusive, as it is possible that a viral attack may further affect immune programming in a susceptible host (4)

When bronchial responsiveness was assessed, the results were conflicting; either no difference or an increase in bronchial reactivity several years after bronchiolitis has been reported [14]. Equally conflicting are the results relating to the potential effects of RSV in allergic sensitization. One group has shown that RSV bron-chiolitis is an independent risk factor for the development of asthma and allergic sensitization at age 7 years, in fact a stronger risk factor than a family history of asthma [15]. In contrast, other studies have failed to establish such an effect [16, 17]. Differences in disease severity and age of evaluation may partly account for this discrepancy. It is conceivable that severe RSV disease may be required for the establishment of long-lasting effects. In another study, the correlation of RSV bronchiolitis with sensitization that was observed at the age of 6 was not present at age 9–10 years [18]. Importantly, RSV-related effects on wheezing and asthma decline with age, becoming nonsignificant by adolescence [17–19]. These findings should also be interpreted with caution: asthma symptoms may be undervalued in adolescence or may relapse later in life [20]; thus, prospective evaluation of the current cohorts is required to evaluate these possibilities. Most data relating to acute severe infections early in life and the increased risk of asthma implicate RSV, but most of the studies on which these conclusions are based have not adequately looked for other respiratory viruses, in particular rhinovirus (RV). Stein et al. [17] reported a fourfold increased risk of asthma later in life in children with RSV infections that were severe enough to lead to a pediatric consultation early in life. However, increased risks, —twofold to threefold, were observed with other respiratory viruses, suggesting that any single acute infection severe enough to lead to a pediatric consultation early in life is also a risk factor for asthma later in life. Although important as an observation, this lasting effect, possibly associated with human RV infections that were not virologically confirmed at the time, has not gained enough attention [17]. Nevertheless, it is supported by more recent findings showing that infection with human RV is more frequent during infancy than previously thought [21], can induce severe bronchiolitis [22], is associated with increased airway resistance [23], and is also more strongly associated with persistence of wheezing in the first 3 years of life [24].

A type-2/type-1 cytokine imbalance in favor of type-2 responses or with impaired type-1 responses in acute RSV bronchiolitis has been reported in several instances [25, 26]. These findings could be explained as either an inherent defect or a direct result of the RSV infection itself. A profound imbalance in infants with acute RSV bronchiolitis has been observed, with significantly reduced production of the type-1 cytokines interferon (IFN)-γ, interleukin (IL)-12, and IL-18 and increased production of IL-4 [27]. This imbalance was associated with impaired virus clearance, suggesting that it may be an important determinant of disease severity. In addition, because the imbalance was observed as early as the 1st or 2nd day after initiation of disease, the immune deviation was most probably already present in these infants before RSV infection; deviation of the immune response by the virus itself was unlikely to have occurred so early in the course of the illness, when virus-specific immunity was only beginning to develop [27].

From the above, it is obvious that no safe conclusion about whether RSV bronchiolitis may cause or is only associated with asthma in later life (through common causality) can be currently reached. Nevertheless, these two possibilities are not mutually exclusive. Children with a predisposition to asthma may be prone to develop severe RSV bronchiolitis; however, this infection may also further affect their immune responses and/or lung structure, leading to the development of asthma symptoms (Fig. 1) [28]. With the advent of effective RSV prevention modalities it is now possible to design randomized intervention studies. In these studies, confounding factors should be ruled out by randomization; thus they may offer more conclusive evidence. In one such study, modest differences in pulmonary function were observed between infants treated with ribavirin versus placebo-treated control infants, but the number of subjects was small [29]. Later intervention studies are awaited.

The Protective Effect of Respiratory Viruses on the Development of Allergy and Asthma

As respiratory viral infections are frequently the most apparent event in the presentation of asthma, either as a cause or as a marker, it seems contradictory that similar infections may protect against development of the disease. Nevertheless, the "hygiene hypothesis", first suggested by Strachan [5], is a dominant theory used to explain the increasing prevalence of allergies and asthma, based on our understanding of these diseases as dysregulations of the immune system. This subject has aroused much interest because of the findings of an effect of birth order and family size, as surrogate markers of infectious load, on the development of allergy [7, 29]. A protective role of infections also has been seen in developing countries, where an inverse relationship between evidence of respiratory infections and later development of atopy has been observed [30]. One possibility is that these findings could have resulted from a genetic bias in confined communities. However, this is unlikely, as there was a similarly reduced prevalence of atopic disease in East Germany compared with the genetically similar population of West Germany [31]. The East German children were assumed to have been exposed to more infections because of the much greater use of early childhood daycare facilities, which has been associated with less subsequent asthma [31].

There is a paradox, however, as several studies show that parental reports of lower respiratory illnesses are associated positively with later asthma [7]. A possible explanation is that daycare use and large family size are associated with an increased microbial load, which includes gastrointestinal viruses and other potentially protective microbes and is independent of the host response [7]. In contrast, parental reporting of symptoms reflects the host response. Children destined to have asthma have an impaired type-1 response to virus infections and are therefore at a risk of more frequent and severe symptoms, which are more likely to be reported.

In a prospective birth cohort study, children who had more than one respiratory illness confined to the upper respiratory tract during the first 3 years of life were at lower risk of having asthma symptoms at age 7 [31]. In contrast, when the infections were located in the lower airways, the risk for asthma increased significantly in a dose-dependent manner. Although the authors concluded that upper respiratory infections early in life may protect infants against the development of asthma, it is also possible that the development of upper or lower respiratory infectious disease is influenced to a considerable extent by the susceptibility of the host.

Another large birth cohort study found that personal and sibling viral infections (e.g., measles, mumps, rubella, hepatitis, chickenpox, herpes, mononucleosis) during the first year of life resulted in a small protective effect against the development of asthma (but not hay fever or eczema) later in childhood [32]. However, a strong protective birth order effect against all atopic diseases was present in that cohort. When respiratory tract infections as a whole were analyzed, a dose-dependent increased risk for asthma and hay fever was noted. Further, exposure to antibiotics was associated with an increased risk of developing allergic disease.

In another study, the detrimental effect of lower respiratory episodes during the first year of life in the expression of asthma at age 4 was confirmed, while no significant protective effect of upper respiratory infection was found in that setting [33]. An increased number of respiratory infections (e.g., measles, mumps, rubella, varicella) conferred increased risk for atopy in a Danish cohort, irrespective of the age of exposure: the presence of asthma was not assessed in that study [34].

It is probably too early to confirm a possible protective effect of respiratory viruses on the development of allergy and asthma. Prospective studies evaluating exposure to microorganisms, pathogenic or not, as well as symptomatic infection, will be required to differentiate between the effect of these two factors, also taking into account possible confounders such as birth order and antibiotic use.

We recently proposed an alternative explanation for this apparent contradiction, using the term "incoordination" hypothesis [35]: the physiological rate of development and response of the human immune system may not match the rate of exposure to various stimuli as they currently appear in modern (especially "Westernized") environments. Infectious agents, including viruses, are prominent, but not unique among these stimuli, as they are major determinants of immune maturation and their ecology is affected considerably by environmental changes, including, but not uniquely depending on, hygiene.

Epidemiology of Viruses in Asthma Exacerbations

Although the role of viruses in the induction of, or protection from allergy and asthma is still inconclusive, the evidence for the participation of these pathogens in asthma exacerbations is much stronger. The observation that asthma exacerbations often follow common colds is old and a daily experience of practicing physicians, especially pediatricians. Early reports documented that viral shedding decreased soon after the cold, before the patient referred to their physician or the hospital, indicating that early sampling was necessary for viral detection [36]. Furthermore, virus detection rates in these studies fluctuated considerably; this was attributed to difficulties in RV and corona virus identification. With the use of PCR-based detection for RV and prospective designs, the magnitude of the problem was revealed.

In a prospective study in the community, asthmatic children aged 9–11 years were followed up for 1 year and sampled as soon as they reported cold symptoms [37]. The percentage of asthma exacerbations following virologically confirmed colds was 80–85%. In children hospitalized with severe asthma exacerbations, the viral detection rate was 82% [38]. In adults, the proportion of virus-attributed asthma exacerbations was generally lower. However, it was possible that viral shedding was less or of a shorter duration in adults than in children. In one of the first community-based prospective studies using polymerase chain reaction (PCR) detection for rhinoviruses, virus detection rates were 44%, although cold symptoms preceded 70% of the episodes [39]. In another study (with a combined longitudinal and cross-sectional design) of inner-city asthmatic adults [40], virus detection was once again 44% in followed-up subjects and 50–55% in subjects presenting to the Emergency Department. In another study, virological confirmation was achieved in 60% of asthma exacerbations in adults [40]. Additional studies of similar designs have confirmed the high prevalence of viral infections in association with asthma exacerbations, with RV being the dominant pathogen [41–43].

The conclusion from the above is that respiratory viruses are the most common triggers of asthma attacks, and it is shown that such attacks can be severe, leading to hospital admissions [44]. Peak in hospital admissions for asthma and virus isolation occurs, in most instances, immediately after school vacations. This pattern of a segregation-dependent disease is a characteristic of rhinovirus colds [45]. Similar seasonal variation has been partly observed in asthma mortality, especially among young children and the elderly, who are most susceptible to viral infections [46].

Another important point, on which all of these studies agree, is that RVs are the most prevalent agents, accounting for 50–60% of all detected viruses. This is thought to reflect the prevalence of these viruses in common colds, rather than any specific asthmagenic properties, because there are minor or no differences in symptoms produced by different viruses [37] or in the proportion of asthma episodes resulting from colds by any specific virus [36]. However, recent evidence from our laboratory suggests that RVs may have increased propensity toward inducing asthma in comparison to influenza viruses (NG Papadopoulos, unpublished data).

Virus-Induced Changes in Airway Reactivity

The above epidemiological data have raised considerable interest regarding the mechanisms of virus-induced asthma exacerbations, the understanding of which may suggest potential therapeutic targets. Airway hyperresponsiveness is one of the most prominent functional abnormalities in asthma that can be objectively assessed in human and animal models. An increase in airway responsiveness to histamine in normal subjects after URTIs, lasting as long as 7 weeks, was observed more than 20 years ago [47]. Although results have varied, probably because of differences in methodology, models, viral strains, and so on; increased airway reactivity has since been documented after RSV, influenza, parainfluenza, and adenovirus infections, mostly in animal models [48].

Because of the lack of appropriate animal models, human experimental infections have been used as a model for RV infection. Using this model, the increased airway responsiveness to histamine after RV infection in atopic asthmatic subjects was correlated with the severity of the experimental cold, which was paralleled by an increase in IL-8 in nasal lavage fluid [49]. In addition, when daily forced expiratory volume in 1 s (FEV_1) was monitored, a variable airway obstruction was observed [50]. When normal and atopic rhinitic subjects were compared, lower airway responsiveness was more affected in the allergic group [51]. However, in another study, experimental RV infection induced small changes in either upper or lower airway symptoms in normal and asthmatic subjects, with no effect on bronchial reactivity, leading the authors to suggest that RV infection by itself may not be sufficient to provoke clinical worsening of asthma [52]. Exposure to allergens during respiratory viral infection is the most obvious cofactor, because it is well known that rhinovirus experimental infection enhances the responses to inhaled allergens [53] and potentiates inflammation after segmental allergen bronchoprovocation [54]. Most surprisingly, Avila et al. [55], using the same human model in allergic rhinitis subjects, showed that pre-exposure of the nose to an allergen significantly delayed the onset of cold symptoms, reduced the duration of the illness, and delayed the appearance of proinflammatory cytokines locally. An inverse correlation between nasal eosinophils at the time of inoculation and eventual cold symptoms was also observed, suggesting that an allergic response might protect from RV colds. Although this evidence seemed contradictory to most previous findings, it could prove helpful in several ways. First, it suggested that eosinophils could be involved in RV immunity [56]. Furthermore, it indicated that allergen exposure and viral infection did not have a simple additive effect, and timing or dosage may be important.

Mechanisms of Virus-Induced Inflammation

Several characteristics of virus-mediated pathology can also be seen in asthma. Among these, direct virus-mediated damage to lower airway epithelium is a characteristic of several viruses including influenza and RSV. Dead epithelial cells drop into the airway lumen, inducing or increasing airway obstruction. Although to a lesser extent, this is also the case for RV, which can infect the lower airways and induce cytotoxicity [57–59] (Fig. 2). Furthermore, RV infection induces the production of several cytokines and chemokines, including IL-6 and IL-8, regulated upon activation normal T cell expressed and secreted (RANTES), granulocyte-macrophage colony-stimulating factor (GM-CSF), and IL-16 [58, 59]. These studies strongly suggest that lower airway infection and local inflammation may represent the first step in the pathogenesis of an asthma episode, adding to and clarifying previous attempts to prove this notion [60, 61]. It is possible that the degree of inflammation, which is similar to other respiratory viruses [62], and not the degree of cytotoxicity, is more relevant in the induction of an exacerbation.

Epithelial damage and mediator production after viral infection are only some of the mechanisms that could initiate or sustain an asthma exacerbation. A dysfunction of the inhibitory M2 muscarinic receptor has been documented after viral infection, which could lead to increased reflex bronchoconstriction [63]. The role of tachykinins has also been suggested, partly explained by the reduction of neutral endopeptidase activity, which is the major metabolizing enzyme for substance P and neurokinin A

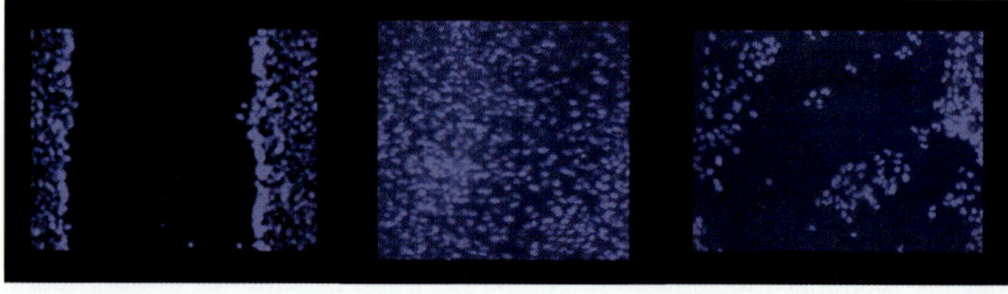

Fig. 2 In a simple model of epithelial wound healing, damaged epithelium ($t = 0$) is suboptimally repopulated after RV-infection in comparison to sham-infected control. DAPI stained cells (Published in *Respiratory Research* [57])

[64]. Most of the above studies have been performed in animal models with cytotoxic viruses such as influenza, parainfluenza, and RSV. A neurally mediated effect does not seem to be a prominent feature of human experimental RV infections [65].

Most puzzling is the potential involvement of the immune response to respiratory viruses in asthma exacerbations. Although the asthmatic phenotype is paradigmatically related to type-2 lymphocyte responses, predominantly IL-4 and IL-5, viral infections induce strong type-1 responses with high levels of IFN-γ that would be expected to downregulate, rather than augment, "allergic" immune responses. Among respiratory viruses, RSV, influenza, and parainfluenza are more extensively studied in animal models. Sensitization of BALB/c mice to the virus attachment protein G of RSV, followed by live virus infection, leads to pulmonary eosinopihlia and type-2 cytokine production. Although IFN-γ is still the dominant T-cell cytokine, a localized relative reduction of IFN-γ mRNA expression with a concomitant increase in IL-4 and IL-5 transcripts has been reported [66]. When *Dermatophagoides farinae*-sensitized mice were repeatedly infected with RSV, an increased production of type-2 cytokines was observed [67]. In the presence of IL-4, virus-specific CD8 T cells can switch to IL-5 production and induce airway eosinophilia [68]. Interestingly, IL-4 can also inhibit antiviral immunity, delaying both influenza [69] and RSV clearance.

RV-infected peripheral blood mononuclear cells from atopic asthmatic subjects produce significantly lower IFN-γ and IL-12 and significantly higher IL-10 and IL-4 than do cells from normal individuals [70]. Although IFN-γ remained the dominant T cell cytokine in this model, a shift toward a type-2 response may be involved in the induction of an asthma exacerbation, by mechanisms similar to the ones described above, for RSV in the mouse.

The recent discovery that airway epithelial cells are deficient in their capacity to generate INF-β when infected with RV raises the possibility that a defect in innate immunity might underlie exacerbations of asthma [71]. The normal response of the airway epithelium to virus infection is the induction of primary IFNs, such as IFN-β, through activation of the Toll-like receptor 3, which recognizes viral double-stranded RNA, leading to apoptosis that is able to effectively eliminate the infected cell and therefore limit viral replication and release. However, in asthmatic epithelial cells a major defect in this pathway leads to enhanced viral replication and virus-induced cell cytotoxicity [72]. Evidence that this pathway might be relevant to the persistence of asthma, as well as exacerbation, comes from the demonstration that in asthmatic patients RV can persist up to 6 weeks after infection [73] and in patients with severe asthma, RV is detectable in airway biopsy specimens between exacerbations [74].

Can Virus-Induced Wheeze Predict Later Asthma?

Most young children who wheeze initially present with episodes related to viral infections. Only a proportion of these children will continue to wheeze in later childhood and adulthood. For the first few years of life, these latter children remain clinically indistinguishable from those with a transient wheeze. Therefore, it has been a long-standing aim of pediatricians to predict those who will have asthma later in life. In theory, anti-inflammatory remedies given early might modify the outcome [75], although recently it has been shown that early use of inhaled steroids for wheezing in preschool children had no effect on the natural history of asthma or wheeze later in childhood and did not prevent lung function decline or reduce airway reactivity [76]. From population studies, risk factors such as personal atopy or a family history of asthma could predict the relative risk of developing asthma with considerable accuracy, but for use in an individual, this approach is not sufficiently sensitive [77].

Because increased IgE levels and relative eosinophilia can be seen in infants that continue to have persistent wheeze, information obtained from a blood test during the initial episode could have some predictive potential [9]. However, this information has relatively low specificity and may not be ideal for day-to-day practice. It seems, therefore, that currently, a precise prediction of asthma persistence cannot be attempted from the initial virus-induced wheezing episodes.

Antiviral Strategies

Although possible, it is not certain whether a window of opportunity exists from the occurrence of a viral upper respiratory infection to the development of an acute asthma exacerbation, during which an antiviral strategy may be effective. In addition, we cannot predict whether immunization against one or more of the viruses involved will reduce virus-induced asthma exacerbations or it may simply shift the problem to different strains. To answer the above questions, reliable antiviral tools are required.

RVs represent the major causes of virus-induced asthma exacerbations; however, immunization options remain unsatisfactory, mainly due to the large number of

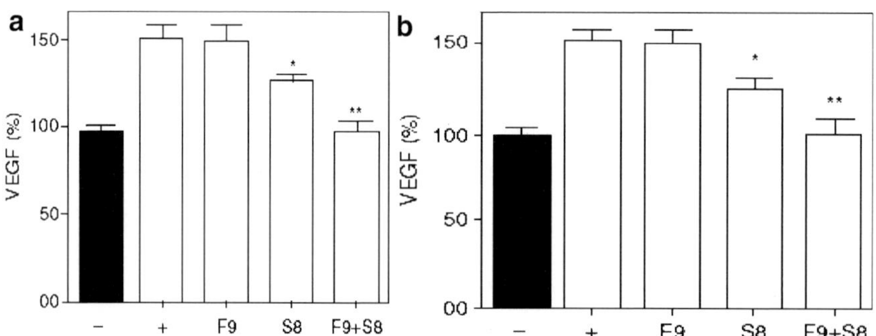

Fig. 3 Addition of salmeterol (S) either at 10^{-8}(A) or 10^{-9}(B) M to fluticasone propionate (F) at 10^{-9} M resulted in a significant reduction of RV-mediated VEGF production by epithelial cells, in a synergistic manner. $n = 4$–6, $^{*}p < 0.05$, $^{**}p < 0.001$ (Adapted from Volonaki et al. [84])

different serotypes [29, 78]. A variety of antiviral agents against RV have been studied. Additional antiviral and anti-inflammatory strategies against common cold have been suggested with varying, but usually little, success [79]. Such strategies include the regularly used ascorbic acid, zinc, and Echinacea, which have little therapeutic value [78]. Macrolide antibiotics, batilomycin A1, erythromycin, and telithromycin have been shown to be effective as potential anti-inflammatory agents in vitro, but clinical proof is still insufficient [80, 81]. During the past few years antirhinoviral compounds such as pleconaril, acting by preventing the uncoating of picornaviruses [82], and the RV protease inhibitor ruprintrivir [83], have shown promising results, but only in early-stage clinical trials.

Based on the above, strategies against virus-induced asthma and related exacerbations are, in principle, anti-inflammatory, following strategies against persistent asthma. Steroids combined with long-acting beta agonists may be effective in this setting: recent studies have shown that such combinations are synergistically effective in reducing RV-induced inflammation in vitro [84] (Fig. 3). Nevertheless, the extent to which these findings translate in clinical practice is still unspecified [85].

References

1. McIntosh K, Ellis EF, Hoffman LS, Lybass TG, Eller JJ, Fulqiniti VA (1973) The association of viral and bacterial respiratory infections with exacerbations of wheezing in young asthmatic children. J Pediatr 82(4): 578–590
2. Dodge RR, Burrows B (1980) The prevalence and incidence of asthma and asthma-like symptoms in a general population sample. Am Rev Respir Dis 122(4): 567–575
3. Papadopoulos NG, Hunter J, Sanderson G, Meyer J, Johnston SL (1999) Rhinovirus identification by BgI I digestion of picornavirus RT-PCR amplicons. J Virol Methods 80: 179–185
4. Xepapadaki P, Psarras S, Bossios A, Tsolia M, Gourgiotis D, Liapi-Adamidou G, Constantopoulos AG, Kafetzis D, Papadopoulos NG (2004) Human Metapneumovirus as a causative agent of acute bronchiolitis in infants. J Clin Virol 30: 267–270
5. Strachan DP (1989) Hay fever, hygiene, and household size. BMJ 299: 1259–1260
6. Johnston SL, Sanderson G, Pattemore PK, Smith S, Bardin PG, Bruce CB, Lambden PR, Tyrrell DA, Holgate ST (1993) Use of polymerase chain reaction for diagnosis of picornavirus infection in subjects with and without respiratory symptoms. J Clin Microbiol 31: 111–117
7. Mallia P, Johnston SL (2002) Respiratory viruses: do they protect from or induce asthma? Allergy 57: 1118–1129
8. Martinez FD, Morgan WJ, Wright AL, Holberg CJ, Taussig LM (1988) Diminished lung function as a predisposing factor for wheezing respiratory illness in infants. New Engl J Med 319: 1112–1117
9. Martinez FD, Stern DA, Wright AL, Taussig LM, Halonen M (1998) Differential immune responses to acute lower respiratory illness in early life and subsequent development of persistent wheezing and asthma. J Allergy Clin Immunol 102: 915–920
10. Glezen WP, Taber LH, Frank AL, Kasel JA (1986) Risk of primary infection and reinfection with respiratory syncytial virus. Am J Dis Child 140: 543–546
11. Rooney JC, Williams HE (1971) The relationship between proved viral bronchiolitis and subsequent wheezing. J Pediatr 79: 744–747
12. Smyth RL, Fletcher JN, Thomas HM, Hart CA, Openshaw PJM (1999) Respiratory syncytial virus and wheeze [letter]. Lancet 354: 1997–1998

13. Tager IB, Hanrahan JP, Tosteson TD, Castile RG, Brown RB, Weiss ST (1993) Lung function, pre- and post-natal smoke exposure, and wheezing in the first year of life. Am Rev Respir Dis 47: 811–817
14. Kattan M (1999) Epidemiologic evidence of increased airway reactivity in children with a history of bronchiolitis. J Pediatr 135: 8–13
15. Sigurs N, Bjarnason R, Sigurbergsson F, Kjellman B (2000) Respiratory syncytial virus bronchiolitis in infancy is an important risk factor for asthma and allergy at age 7. Am J Respir Crit Care Med 161: 1501–1507
16. Toms GL, Quinn R, Robinson JW (1996) Undetectable IgE responses after respiratory syncytial virus infection. Arch Dis Child 74: 126–130
17. Stein RT, Sherrill D, Morgan WJ, Holberg CJ, Halonen M, Taussig LM, Wright AL, Martinez FD (1999) Respiratory syncytial virus in early life and risk of wheeze and allergy by age 13 years. Lancet 354: 541–545
18. Noble V, Murray M, Webb MS, Alexander J, Swarbrick AS, Milner AD (1997) Respiratory status and allergy nine to 10 years after acute bronchiolitis. Arch Dis Child 76: 315–319
19. McConnockie KM, Roghmann KJ (1989) Wheezing at 8 and 13 years: changing importance of bronchiolitis and passive smoking. Pediatr Pulmonol 6: 138–146
20. Roorda RJ (1996) Prognostic factors for the outcome of childhood asthma in adolescence. Thorax 51(Suppl 1): S7–S12
21. van Benten I, Koopman L, Niesters B, Hop W, van Middelkoop B, de Waal L, van Drunen K, Osterhaus A, Neijens H, Fokkens W (2003) Predominence of rhinovirus in the nose of symptomatic and asymptomatic infants. Pediatr Allergy Immunol 14(5): 363–370
22. Papadopoulos NG, Moustaki M, Tsolia M, Bossios A, Astra E, Prezerakou A, Gourgiotis D, Kafetzis D (2002) Association of rhinovirus infection with increased disease severity in acute bronchiolitis. Am J Respir Crit Care Med 165(9): 1285–1289
23. Malmstrom K, Pitkaranta A, Carpen O, Pelkonen A, Malmberg LP, Turpeinen M, Kajosaari M, Sarna S, Lindahl H, Haahtela T, Makela MJ (2006) Human rhinovirus in bronchial epithelium of infants with recurrent respiratory symptoms. J Allergy Clin Immunol 118(3): 591–596
24. Lemanske RF Jr, Jackson DJ, Gangnon RE, Evans MD, Li Z, Shult PA, Kirk CJ, Reisdorf E, Roberg KA, Anderson EL, Carlson-Dakes KT, Adler KJ, Gilbertson-White S, Pappas TE, Dasilva DF, Tisler CJ, Gern JE (2005) Rhinovirus illnesses during infancy predict subsequent childhood wheezing. J Allergy Clin Immunol 116(3): 571–577
25. Aberle JH, Aberle SW, Dworzak MN, Mandl CW, Rebhandl W, Vollnhofer G, Kundi M, Popow-Kraupp T (1999) Reduced interferon-gamma expression in peripheral blood mononuclear cells of infants with severe respiratory syncytial virus disease. Am J Respir Crit Care Med 160: 1263–1268
26. Openshaw PJ, Lemanske RF (1998) Respiratory viruses and asthma: can the effects be prevented? Eur Respir J (Suppl 27): 35–39
27. Legg JP, Hussain IR, Warner JA, Johnston SL, Warner JO (2003) Type 1 and type 2 cytokine imbalance in acute respiratory syncytial virus bronchiolitis. Am J Respir Crit Care Med 168(6): 633–639
28. Rodriguez WJ, Arrobio J, Fink R, Kim HW, Milburn C (1999) Prospective follow-up and pulmonary functions from a placebo-controlled randomized trial of ribavirin therapy in respiratory syncytial virus bronchiolitis : Ribavirin Study Group. Arch Pediatr Adolesc Med 153: 469–474
29. Papadopoulos NG, Psarras S (2003) Rhinoviruses in the pathogenesis of asthma. Curr Allergy Asthma Rep 3: 137–145
30. Openshaw PJ, Hewitt C (2000) Protective and harmful effects of viral infections in childhood on wheezing disorders and asthma. Am J Respir Crit Care Med 162: 540–543
31. Illi S, von Mutius E, Lau S, Bergmann R, Niggemann B, Sommerfeld C Wahn U:MAS Group (2001) Early childhood infectious diseases and the development of asthma up to school age: a birth cohort study. BMJ 322: 390–395
32. McKeever TM, Lewis SA, Smith C, Collins J, Heatlie H, Frischer M, Hubbard R (2002) Early exposure to infections and antibiotics and the incidence of allergic disease: a birth cohort

study with the West Midlands General Practice Research Database. J Allergy Clin Immunol 109: 43–50

33. Celedon JC, Litonjua AA, Ryan L, Weiss ST, Gold DR (2002) Day care attendance, respiratory tract illnesses, wheezing, asthma, and total serum IgE level in early childhood. Arch Pediatr Adolesc Med 156: 241–245

34. Bager P, Westergaard T, Rostgaard K, Hjalgrim H, Melbye M (2002) Age at childhood infections and risk of atopy. Thorax 57: 379–382

35. Papadopoulos NG, Foteinos G (2007) Is allergy a result or a modifier of viral infections? An incoordination hypothesis. Allergy Clin Immunol Int (in press)

36. Pattemore PK, Johnston SL, Bardin PG (1992) Viruses as precipitants of asthma symptoms: I. Epidemiology. Clin Exp Allergy 22: 325–336

37. Johnston SL, Pattemore PK, Sanderson G, Smith S, Lampe F, Josephs L, Symington P, O'Toole S, Myint SH, Tyrrell DA (1995) Community study of role of viral infections in exacerbations of asthma in 9–11 year old children. BMJ 310: 1225–1228

38. Freymuth F, Vabret A, Brouard J, Toutain F, Verdon R, Petitjean J, Gouarin S, Duhamel JF, Guillois B (1999) Detection of viral, *Chlamydia pneumoniae* and *Mycoplasma pneumoniae* infections in exacerbations of asthma in children. J Clin Virol 13: 131–139

39. Nicholson KG, Kent J, Ireland DC (1993) Respiratory viruses and exacerbations of asthma in adults. BMJ 307: 982–986

40. Atmar RL, Guy E, Guntupalli KK, Zimmerman JL, Bandi VD, Baxter BD, Greenberg SB (1998) Respiratory tract viral infections in inner-city asthmatic adults. Arch Intern Med 158: 2453–2459

41. Ong BH, Gao Q, Phoon MC, Chow VT, Tan WC, Van Bever HP (2007) Identification of human metapneumovirus and Chlamydophila pneumoniae in children with asthma and wheeze in Singapore. Singapore Med J 48(4): 291–293

42. Joao SM, Ferraz C, Pissarra S, Cardoso MJ (2007) Role of viruses and atypical bacteria in asthma exacerbations among children in Oporto (Portugal). Allergol Immunopathol (Madr) 35(1): 4–9

43. Jartti T, Lehtinen P, Vuorinen T, Osterback R, van der Hoogen B, Osterhaus AD, Ruuskanen O (2004) Respiratory picornaviruses and respiratory syncytial virus as causative agents of acute expiratory wheezing in children. Emerg Infect Dis 10(6): 1095–1101

44. Johnston SL, Pattemore PK, Sanderson G, Smith S, Campbell MJ, Josephs LK, Cunningham A, Robinson BS, Myint SH, Ward ME, Tyrrell DA, Holgate ST (1996) The relationship between upper respiratory infections and hospital admissions for asthma: a time-trend analysis. Am J Respir Crit Care Med 154: 654–660

45. Johnston NW, Johnston SL, Norman GR, Dai J, Sears MR (2006) The September epidemic of asthma hospitalization: school children as disease vectors. J Allergy Clin Immunol 117(3): 557–562

46. Campbell MJ, Holgate ST, Johnston SL (1997) Trends in asthma mortality: data on seasonality of deaths due to asthma were omitted from paper but editorial's author did not know [letter]. BMJ 315: 1012

47. Empey DW, Laitinen LA, Jacobs L, Gold WM, Nadel JA (1976) Mechanisms of bronchial hyperreactivity in normal subjects after upper respiratory tract infection. Am Rev Respir Dis 113: 131–139

48. Folkerts G, Busse WW, Nijkamp FP, Sorkness R, Gern JE (1998) Virus-induced airway hyperresponsiveness and asthma. Am J Respir Crit Care Med 157: 1708–1720

49. Grunberg K, Timmers M, Smits H, de Klerk EP, Dick EC, Spaan WJ, Hiemstra PS, Sterk PJ (1997) Effect of experimental rhinovirus 16 colds on airway hyperresponsiveness to histamine and interleukin-8 in nasal lavage in asthmatic subjects in vivo. Clin Exp Allergy 27: 36–45

50. Grunberg K, Timmers MC, de Klerk EP, Dick EC, Sterk PJ (1999) Experimental rhinovirus 16 infection causes variable airway obstruction in subjects with atopic asthma. Am J Respir Crit Care Med 160: 1375–1380

51. Gern J, Calhoun W, Swenson C, Shen G, Busse WW (1997) Rhinovirus infection preferentially increases lower airway responsiveness in allergic subjects. Am J Respir Crit Care Med 155: 1872–1876

52. Fleming HE, Little FF, Schnurr D, Avila PC, Wong H, Liu J, Yagi S, Boushey HA (1999) Rhinovirus-16 colds in healthy and in asthmatic subjects: similar changes in upper and lower airways. Am J Respir Crit Care Med 160: 100–108

53. Lemanske RF Jr, Dick EC, Swenson CA, Vrtis RF, Busse WW (1989) Rhinovirus upper respiratory infection increases airway hyperreactivity and late asthmatic reactions. J Clin Invest 83: 1–10

54. Calhoun W, Dick E, Schwartz L, Busse W (1994) A common cold virus, rhinovirus 16, potentiates airway inflammation after segmental antigen bronchoprovocation in allergic subjects. J Clin Invest 94: 2200–2208

55. Avila PC, Abisheganaden JA, Wong H, Liu J, Yagi S, Schnurr D, Kishiyama JL, Boushey HA (2000) Effects of allergic inflammation of the nasal mucosa on the severity of rhinovirus 16 cold. J Allergy Clin Immunol 105: 923–932

56. Busse WW, Gern JE (2000) Do allergies protect against the effects of a rhinovirus cold? [editorial]. J Allergy Clin Immunol 105: 889–891

57. Bossios A, Psarras S, Gourgiotis D, Skevaki CL, Constantopoulos AG, Saxoni-Papageorgiou P, Papadopoulos NG (2005) Rhinovirus infection induces cytotoxicity and delays wound healing in bronchial epithelial cells. Respir Res 6: 114

58. Schroth MK, Grimm E, Frindt P, Galagan DM, Konno SI, Love R, Gern JE (1999) Rhinovirus replication causes RANTES production in primary bronchial epithelial cells. Am J Respir Cell Mol Biol 20: 1220–1228

59. Papadopoulos NG, Bates PJ, Bardin PG, Papi A, Leir SH, Fraenkel DJ, Meyer J, Lackie PM, Sanderson G, Holgate ST, Johnston SL (2000) Rhinoviruses infect the lower airways. J Infect Dis 181 : 1875–1884

60. Gern JE, Galagan DM, Jarjour NN, Dick EC, Busse WW (1997) Detection of rhinovirus RNA in lower airway cells during experimentally induced infection. Am J Respir Crit Care Med 155: 1159–1161

61. Subauste MC, Jacoby DB, Richards SM, Proud D (1995) Infection of a human respiratory epithelial cell line with rhinovirus: induction of cytokine release and modulation of susceptibility to infection by cytokine exposure. J Clin Invest 96: 549–557

62. Olszewska-Pazdrak B, Casola A, Saito T, Alam R, Crowe SE, Mei F, Oqra PL, Garofalo RP (1998) Cell-specific expression of RANTES, MCP-1, and MIP-1alpha by lower airway epithelial cells and eosinophils infected with respiratory syncytial virus. J Virol 72: 4756–4764

63. Jacoby DB, Fryer AD (1999) Interaction of viral infections with muscarinic receptors. Clin Exp Allergy 29(Suppl 2): 59–64

64. Jacoby DB, Tamaoki J, Borson DB, Nadel JA (1988) Influenza infection causes airway hyperresponsiveness by decreasing enkephalinase. J Appl Physiol 64: 2653–2658

65. Grunberg K, Kuijpers E, de Klerk E, de Gouw HW, Kroes AC, Dick EC, Sterk PJ (1997) Effects of experimental rhinovirus 16 infection on airway hyperresponsiveness to bradykinin in asthmatic subjects in vivo. Am J Respir Crit Care Med 155: 833–838

66. Spender LC, Hussell T, Openshaw PJ (1998) Abundant IFN-gamma production by local T cells in respiratory syncytial virus-induced eosinophilic lung disease. J Gen Virol 79: 1751–1758

67. Matsuse H, Behera AK, Kumar M, Rabb H, Lockey RF, Mohapatra SS (2000) Recurrent respiratory syncytial virus infections in allergen-sensitized mice lead to persistent airway inflammation and hyperresponsiveness. J Immunol 164: 6583–6592

68. Coyle AJ, Erard F, Bertrand C, Walti S, Pircher H, Le Gros G (1995) Virus-specific CD8 cells can switch to interleukin 5 production and induce airway eosinophilia. J Exp Med 181: 1229–1233

69. Moran TM, Isobe H, Fernandez-Sesma A, Schulman JL (1996) Interleukin-4 causes delayed virus clearance in influenza virus-infected mice. J Virol 70: 5230–5235

70. Papadopoulos NG, Stanciu LA, Papi A, Holgate ST, Johnston SL (2002) A defective type 1 response to rhinovirus in atopic asthma. Thorax 57(4):328–332.

71. Wark PA, Johnston SL, Bucchieri F, Powell R, Puddicombe S, Laza-Stanca V, Holgate ST, Davies DE (2005) Asthmatic bronchial epithelial cells have a deficient innate immune response to infection with rhinovirus. J Exp Med 201: 937–947

72. Holgate ST (2006) Rhinoviruses in the pathogenesis of asthma: the bronchial epithelium as a major disease target. J Allergy Clin Immunol 118: 587–590
73. Kling S, Donninger H, Williams Z, Vermeulen J, Weinberg E, Latiff K, Ghildyal R, Bardin P (2005) Persistence of rhinovirus RNA after asthma exacerbation in children. Clin Exp Allergy 35: 672–678
74. Crisafi GM, Billmeyer EE, Sorkness RL (2006) The detection of rhinovirus RNA in severe asthma. Proc Am Thorac Soc 3: A15
75. Wilson NM (2003) Virus infections, wheeze and asthma. Paediatr Respir Rev 4(3): 184–192
76. Murray CS, Woodcock A, Langley SJ, Morris J, Custovic A, IFWIN study team (2006) Secondary prevention of asthma by the use of Inhaled Fluticasone Propionate in Wheezy Infants (IFWIN): double-blind, randomised, controlled study. Lancet 368(9537): 754–762
77. Castro-Rodriguez JA, Holberg CJ, Wright AL, Martinez FD (2000) A clinical index to define risk of asthma in young children with recurrent wheeze. Am J Respir Crit Care Med 162(4 Pt1): 1403–1406
78. Papadopoulos NG, Papi A, Psarras S, Johnston SL (2004) Mechanisms of rhinovirus-induced asthma. Paediatr Respir Rev 5(3): 255–260
79. Yamaya M, Sasaki H (2003) Rhinovirus and asthma. Viral Immunol 16(2): 99–109
80. Suzuki T, Yamaya M, Sekizawa K, Hosoda M, Yamada N, Ishizuka S, Yoshino A, Yasuda H, Takahashi H, Nishimura H, Sasaki H (2002) Erythromycin inhibits rhinovirus infection in cultured human tracheal epithelial cells. Am J Respir Crit Care Med 165(8): 1113–1118
81. Johnston SL, Blasi F, Black PN, Martin RJ, Farrell DJ, Nieman RB, TELICAST Investigators (2006) The effect of telithromycin in acute exacerbations of asthma. N Engl J Med 354(15): 1589–1600
82. Ledford RM, Patel NR, Demenczuk TM, Watanyar A, Herbertz T, Collett MS, Pevear DC (2004) VP1 sequencing of all human rhinovirus serotypes: insights into genus phylogeny and susceptibility to antiviral capsid-binding compounds. J Virol 78(7): 3663–3674
83. Hayden FG, Turner RB, Gwaltney JM, Chi-Burris K, Gersten M, Hsyn P, Patick AK, Smith GJ 3rd, Zalman LS (2003) Phase II, randomized, double-blind, placebo-controlled studies of ruprintrivir nasal spray 2-percent suspension for prevention and treatment of experimentally induced rhinovirus colds in healthy volunteers. Antimicrob Agents Chemother 47(12): 3907–3916
84. Volonaki E, Psarras S, Xepapadaki P, Psomali D, Gourgiotis D, Papadopoulos NG (2006) Synergistic effects of fluticasone propionate and salmeterol on inhibiting rhinovirus-induced epithelial production of remodelling-associated growth factors. Clin Exp Allergy 36(10): 1268–1273
85. O'Byrne PM, Bisgaard H, Godard PP, Pistolesi M, Palmqvist M, Zhu Y, Ekstrom T, Bateman ED (2005) Budesonide/formoterol combination therapy as both maintenance and reliever medication in asthma. Am J Respir Crit Care Med 17(2): 129–136

Cold, Dry Air, and Hyperosmolar Challenges in Rhinitis

Paraya Assanasen and Robert M. Naclerio

Introduction

Rhinitis implies inflammation of the nasal mucosa. Inflammation is caused by many stimuli, including ambient conditions. The environmental conditions can also act as a trigger of symptoms. The interaction of environmental temperatures and humidity, especially dry conditions, and nasal inflammation are reviewed in this chapter. Also reviewed is the hyperosmolar challenge, which can serve as a surrogate for cold, dry air (CDA) challenge.

Many individuals experience symptoms of rhinitis, primarily rhinorrhea and nasal congestion, on exposure to cold, windy environments [1]. Some individuals are exquisitely sensitive to CDA; for example, patients with nonallergic rhinitis react to CDA more vigorously than do healthy individuals [2]. There has also been an interest in the nasal reaction to CDA, to understand the physiology of the nose.

The prevalence of cold-air-induced rhinitis is not clear, but in a 1980/81 survey of 912 police officers in Paris, France, 5.4% reported this problem [3]. A database of 206 individuals with objectively confirmed perennial allergic rhinitis and 150 with seasonal allergic rhinitis indicated that cold air is considered a stimulus for nasal symptoms in 55% and 28% of the individuals, respectively [4]. Additionally, individuals who go skiing almost uniformly have rhinitis, and hence the placement of tissues on the lift lines is commonly seen.

Nasal inhalation of CDA causes drying of the nasal mucosa, resulting in increased tonicity and osmolarity of nasal secretions [5]. Hyperosmolar stimuli can trigger nerves, leading to reflex stimulation of the parasympathetic system. In support of this concept, unilateral challenge with CDA leads to bilateral choliner-

P. Assanasen
The Department of Otorhinolaryngology, Faculty of Medicine, Siriraj Hospital,
Mahidol University, Bangkok, Thailand

R.M. Naclerio (✉)
Professor and Chief, Section of Otolaryngology-Head and Neck Surgery,
The University of Chicago, 5841 S. Maryland Ave., MC 1035, Chicago, IL 60637, USA
e-mail: rnacleri@surgery.bsd.uchicago.edu

R. Pawankar et al. (eds.), *Allergy Frontiers: Clinical Manifestations,*
DOI: 10.1007/978-4-431-88317-3_10, © Springer 2009

gic secretory response via a nasonasal reflex, and this secretory response can be reduced by topical treatment with atropine [6, 7]. The complex structure of the nasal vasculature performs air conditioning by dilatation of the resistance vessels and increasing blood flow [8]. Passive vasodilatation of the nasal vascular bed in response to CDA is mediated by the parasympathetic system [9–11]. These effects lead to increased speed of airflow, increased evaporation of water from the nasal mucosal surface, and hence increased osmolarity of nasal secretions.

The Conditioning Capacity of the Human Nose

A major function of the nose is to condition the temperature and humidity of inspired air [12]. In the healthy state, the reserve of the nose to perform this function is enormous. Prior investigations of nasal conditioning have led to several observations. First, exhaled air is fully humidified [12]. Second, its temperature is slightly below body temperature because of a mucosal temperature gradient caused by inspiration. This gradient leads to a recovery of heat and water estimated to be 30% of that needed for conditioning of inspired air [13, 14]. Inspiring hot, dry air interferes with the establishment of the gradient and allows for less recovery of heat and water during expiration [14]. Third, there is wide individual variability in the temperature recorded in the nasopharynx [12–14]. Fourth, despite the wide variability in nasopharyngeal temperature, the relative humidity is 100% [12–14]. Finally, ventilation between 10 and 40 litres has no effect on the temperature and humidity of inspired air [13].

The theoretical model of Hanna and Scherer predicts that the blood temperature distribution along the airway wall, and the total cross-sectional area and perimeter of the nasal cavity, are the two most important parameters of the human air-conditioning response [15]. Other factors, such as the thickness of liquid on the airway surface, blood perfusion rates, and the thickness of the mucosal-submucosal layers, are thought to be less important. As discussed below, parts of this model can be supported, but others cannot.

A part of the importance of nasal air conditioning is its impact on the lower airway. Air that is not fully conditioned when it exits the nasal cavity requires further conditioning by the lower airways [16]. This fact has been amply demonstrated and relates to minute ventilation, tidal volume, and the temperature and water content of the inspired air [17]. Transferring this function from the nose to other parts of the airway for prolonged periods may alter the airway physiology. This notion is supported in part by several lines of evidence: epidemiologic studies by Annensi et al. showed that subjects reporting nasal sensitivity to CDA had a more rapid decline in FEV_1 over 5 years, compared to those without such sensitivity [18]; inhalation of the same volume of dry air through the mouth, in contrast to the oronasal route, causes a greater reduction in FEV_1 in asthmatics [19]; temperature changes can affect ciliary activity *in vitro*; and subjects requiring a tracheotomy or endotracheal intubation for protracted periods of time have changes in the tracheal epithelium [12]. Also, studies of the lower airways of elite athletes, who exercise in cold environments for prolonged periods of time, have changes in structure.

Exposure to unconditioned air also has been shown to affect the nose itself. Nasal congestion is a physiologic response to breathing of cold air [20]. Prolonged exposure of rats to cold environments results in nasal mucosal damage, with decreased goblet cells and intraepithelial glands as well as fibrotic changes [21, 22]. Intermittent exposure of guinea pigs to cold air induces upregulation of muscarinic receptors and increased responsiveness to methacholine and antigen provocation, but not to histamine provocation [23]. The use of nasal continuous positive airway pressure (CPAP), which involves high flows of dry air, for treatment of sleep apnea leads to significant rhinitis, which is in part reduced by heated humidification of the inspired air. Additionally, subjects who have had total laryngectomy and hence are no longer passing air through their nose undergo structural changes in their nasal mucosa [14]. These lines of evidence suggest that the mucosa of the upper and lower airway changes in response to the air-conditioning demands dictated by the environment.

When air is inspired through the nose, not only the warming process, but also the humidification process leads to cooling of the mucosal surface [24], because vaporization of water from the epithelial lining fluid into the airstream requires heat. With water leaving the epithelial-lining fluid, transient increases in the osmolarity of this fluid occur. With increasing ventilation rates through the nose or when the ambient air is at a temperature much lower than room air (and, consequently, water content), the nasal heat and water losses are increased and the cooling as well as the drying effects on the nasal mucosa are greater.

The anatomy of the nasal mucosa is of major importance in the ability of the nasal passages to condition air while retaining homeostasis of mucosal heat and water. One of the characteristic mucosal structures is the dense, subepithelial capillary network. These capillaries have fenestrations that are polarized toward the luminal surface [25]. Blood flow through this network provides heat, and the fenestrae probably facilitate water transportation into the interstitium, the epithelial cells, and the epithelial lining fluid. The other important structural elements of the nasal submucosa are the venous sinusoids, which lie below the subepithelial capillary network. These blood vessels have the ability to rapidly pool large volumes of blood because they are supplied by many arteriovenous anastomoses and because their draining veins (cushion veins) can contract and stop the blood outflow [26]. Blood pooling leads to engorgement of the nasal mucosa, and this increases the airstream contact surface.

There is no agreement on which the structural element of nasal mucosa mainly contributes to water transportation and air humidification. The abundance of seromucous submucosal glands, especially in the anterior portions of the nasal cavity, suggests that their secretions could provide most of the water needed for humidification [27]. Cauna contended that the role of humidification belongs to water from the fenestrated subepithelial capillaries, which continuously diffuses through the epithelium [28]. However, Ingelstedt, who injected fluorescein intravenously in normal human subjects, was not subsequently able to detect it in their nasal secretions [29]. Fluorescein is supposed to move freely across capillaries into the adjacent tissues, and its absence in these experiments suggests that transudation does not occur. However, it is not known whether fluorescein can cross the nasal basement membrane and diffuse between epithelial cells. Osmotic drives generated by water loss during the inspiratory phase may move water from the intraepithelial spaces into the airway lumen [30]. Under basal conditions, no osmotic drive for water to reach the lumen is generated by the apical surface of the nasal epithelium, which predominantly absorbs sodium ions [31]. However, hypertonicity of the periciliary fluid, which may occur as a result of water loss into the airstream, may lead to a reduction of sodium absorption, followed by induction of chloride secretion [31].

Agents that induce cAMP also increase chloride secretion. These include α_2- and β-agonists and prostaglandins E_1, E_2, and $F_{2\alpha}$. In addition, bradykinin, adenosine, eosinophil major basic protein, substance P, and mast cell mediators have shown similar effects [32, 33]. From this list, it becomes evident that sympathetic and neuropeptide-containing nerve activation as well as allergic or nonallergic inflammation can increase chloride secretion, leading to osmotic water diffusion into the airway lumen [34, 35].

Evidence for Hyperosmolarity Occurring Because of Water Loss from the Nasal Surface

An experimental model of nasal provocation with CDA was developed in 1985 [36]. Nasal inhalation of CDA led to hypertonicity of the nasal lining fluid [5, 37]. Secretions produced by inhalation of hot (40–45°C) dry air through the nose were more hyperosmolar than those for the respective CDA challenge [38]. These studies suggest that hydration of the nasal mucosa and water loss caused by CDA challenge are important factors for determining the osmolarity of nasal secretions. Individuals who do not develop a symptomatic response to CDA do not have increased post-CDA osmolarity [5], indicating that they have a greater capacity to achieve osmotic homeostasis. No change in the number of epithelial cells in nasal lavage fluids was observed after CDA provocation in nonresponders, whereas, the number of epithelial cells in nasal lavage fluids increased sixfold immediately after CDA provocation in CDA-reactive individuals. It is possible that the epithelial detachment occurred as a result of mucosal desiccation, due to the inability to compensate for dry-air-induced water loss [39].

Human Model for the Study of Dry-Air and Hyperosmolar Challenge

Models of nasal challenge with dry air or with hyperosmolar stimuli (hypertonic saline, mannitol) have helped investigators to understand the pathophysiology of CDA-induced nasal inflammation [40]. The model of nasal CDA challenge developed by Togias is characterized by: (a) breathing of air through a nasal CPAP mask placed over the nose; (b) subfreezing air temperatures (0–10°C); (c) moderately high airflow (around 26 l/min); and (d) a 10–15-min duration of challenge [36]. Subjects were asked to inhale through the nose and exhale through the mouth to maximize the potency of the stimulus. Nasal inhalation of warm, moist air (around 37°C, 100%

relative humidity) was used as a negative control. Braat and colleagues [41] used air at −10°C with a relative humidity of <10% via a porpoise-shaped nose cap. The dosage was increased in steps as follows: 12.5, 25, 50, 100, 200, and 400 liters/min. This involved CDA provocation steps of 1, 1, 2, 4, 8, and 16 min with a flow of 12.5 for the first step and 25 l/min for the following steps. With this model, they could differentiate patients with nonallergic, noninfectious, and perennial rhinitis from control subjects.

Hyperosmolar challenge of the nose involves the instillation of 10 ml of hyperosmolar mannitol solution (around 800 mosmol/kg) into the nose (in the form of a nasal lavage), where it remains for 10 s [37, 42] before being expelled. This can lead to nasal symptoms (burning is the most prominent symptom) and histamine release in returned nasal lavage fluids. One can access the capacity of the nasal mucosa to correct acutely the hypertonic load by measuring the osmolarity of the mannitol solution before instillation and after it is expelled from the nose [37]. Hypertonic saline spray with increasing concentrations (0.9–22% NaCl solutions) have been used in a stepwise protocol for challenge of the nose [43, 44]. Furthermore, localized hyperosmolar nasal provocation can be done by application of a filter paper disk soaked with NaCl solution on the septal or conchal mucosa [45, 46].

For experimental research, quantitative measurements with high reproducibility are essential [47]. The interpretation of the results demands a basic knowledge of the techniques employed as well as of the study design. All provocation studies require careful selection of subjects, and the disease state and the symptomatic status of the subject must be clearly defined by subjective and objective parameters. The selected subjects should be free of other underlying diseases and of the need for medications that may confound the interpretation of results.

Assessment of the Response

Subjective

Symptoms produced after nasal challenge can be recorded by different techniques, such as, symptom scores or a visual analog scale. Congestion and rhinorrhea are easy to assess by the subject and yield valuable information. Counting of sneezes by the investigator provides an objective symptom assessment.

Objective

1. *Nasal airway resistance (NAR)*: Rhinomanometry measures NAR by quantitatively measuring nasal airflow and pressure. Active anterior rhinomanometry is most frequently used because it is well tolerated by the patients. Unfortunately, the correlation between the objective and subjective response is weak.
2. *Nasal peak inspiratory flow*: This is the simplest technique for detecting changes in nasal patency for repeated measurements before and after a nasal challenge.

It can also be used at home to monitor the airflow or the response to treatment over a more prolonged time period.

3. *Nasal volume*: The geometric cross-sectional area and nasal volume can be measured using acoustic rhinometry.

4. *Nasal secretions*: Several methods have been used for collecting and quantifying nasal secretions: suction, blowing, dripping, lavage, and absorption. Blown secretions can be quantified by weighing of handkerchiefs. An amount of nasal secretions can be obtained by placement of disks on the nasal mucosa for a fixed period of time. Disks used for secretion collection are first kept in Eppendorf tubes, and the disk-tube combinations are weighed before the collection of secretions. After collection, the disks are replaced in the Eppendorf tubes and weighed. The precollection weight is then subtracted from the postcollection weight for determining the weight of secretions generated in a fixed period [48]. Nasal lavage samples secretions from a large mucosal area, whereas, disks sample secretions from a localized area. Importantly, the collection of nasal secretions is useful for the assessment of both cellular and biochemical changes in nasal secretions and change in the osmolarity of nasal secretions.

5. *Biological markers*: Biological markers in the collected secretions can be measured for understanding the underlying pathophysiology. These include histamine and other mast-cell-associated mediators, cytokines, plasma protein, and glandular secretory products. It is important to know the stability of each marker after recovery, as well as the validity of each measurement, when interpreting changes in the levels of these markers. The amount of markers obtained reflects their levels on the mucosal surface, which may not be the true amount of the released substances. However, the level of mediators obtained at fixed time intervals best reflects the total amount of the mediator collected.

6. *Cells*: Cells can be obtained from the nasal cavity by multiple techniques. The epithelial layer can be scraped or brushed. Nasal scrapings and brushing allow mucosal sampling from a wide area of the nasal cavity and contain a large number of epithelial cells. Blown secretions are simple and painless to collect, but are dependent on the spontaneous exfoliation of cells. The specimen reflects activity only in the upper level of the nasal mucosa and yields low cellularity. Nasal lavage samples the entire nasal cavity and reflects changes in the upper mucosa only. Nasal biopsy provides information about structural elements and cellular contents of the epithelial layer and the deeper submucosa. A wide range of histochemical or immunohistochemical techniques can be employed for light microscopy.

Comparison Between Dry-Air and Hyperosmolar Challenge

Hyperosmolar provocation in the human nose activates nasal glands [42, 44, 49]. However, plasma extravasation has not been demonstrated [44, 49]. Unilateral stimulation of the nasal mucosa with hyperosmolar stimuli results in bilateral secretory response [46]. Treatment of the ipsilateral site to the hyperosmolar challenge with topical anesthetic (lidocaine) inhibits both the ipsilateral and the contralateral secretory response. Repetitive, unilateral application of capsaicin for several days before hyperosmolar challenge inhibits both the ipsilateral and the contralateral secretory response [45]. This demonstrates that a hypertonic stimulus can activate sensory nerves and induce central reflexes with efferent glandular responses in both nasal cavities.

Hyperosmolar provocation results in the release of histamine and leukotriene C_4 [42], generating the hypothesis that hyperosmolarity leads to mast cell activation. Human lung mast cells release inflammatory mediators upon exposure to a hyperosmolar medium *in vitro* [50, 51]. However, mast cell tryptase cannot be detected after hyperosmolar nasal challenge [49].

The similarities between the nasal response to a hyperosmolar stimulus and to CDA are: (1) Individuals who develop nasal symptoms after CDA challenge are more responsive to challenge with hyperosmolar mannitol [37]; (2) CDA provocation in CDA-sensitive subjects can activate nasal glands [49, 52]; (3) In cold-air-sensitive individuals, CDA activates sensory nerve endings and produces a central secretory reflex [7]; and (4) CDA provocation in the CDA-sensitive subjects leads to mast cell activation [36, 49, 53]. The difference between the nasal response to a hyperosmolar stimulus and that to CDA is that plasma extravasation has been demonstrated after CDA challenge, but not after hyperosmolar challenge [35, 36]. Late-phase responses after nasal provocation with CDA have been shown [54]. Unfortunately, no one has examined the occurrence of a late response after nasal challenge with hyperosmolar stimuli.

Assessment of the Ability of the Nose to Warm and Humidify Air

Nasal Probe: We developed a probe with a thermistor and a humidity sensor that is placed in the nasopharynx [55]. We selected the nasopharynx for these studies because it represented the end result of nasal conditioning. Although the exact location for conditioning of air within the nose will shift, such a shift occurring before the exit of air from the nose would not be expected to influence the lower airway. The technique involved placing a nasal CPAP mask over the probe with head straps. Air from the compressed air tanks was passed through a flow meter into a cold-air machine. CDA at 0% relative humidity was then delivered to the patient's nose via the mask at flow rates of 5, 10, and 20 l/min. The air temperature was approximately 19°C, 10.5°C, and 0.8°C at 5, 10, and 20 l/min, respectively [56]. The subjects were instructed to breathe in and out through the mouth. Nasopharyngeal temperatures at 5, 10, and 20 l/min for subjects during exposure to CDA were $33.4 \pm 0.7°C$, $30.5 \pm 1.1°C$, and $25.9 \pm 1.4°C$, respectively [55]. The difference between the water content of air prior to entry into the nose and that in the nasopharynx was the water gradient (WG) across the nose, which represented the amount of water evaporated by the nose to condition air. After exposure to CDA, the WG at 5, 10, and 20 l/min. was 297.6 ± 12.6 mg, 509.1 ± 32.0 mg, and 794.1 ± 62.1 mg, respectively. Individuals showed wide variability in their ability to condition air. This ability did not correlate with the baseline nasal airway resistance, nasal volume, nasopharyngeal mucosal temperature, or body temperature. Proctor et al. speculated that prior viral infections may have altered the epithelium, thus producing the variability [56]. However, it could reflect an intrinsic capacity of the nasal surface to condition inhaled air. A recent study showed that siblings condition air similarly, suggesting a hereditary component to nasal conditioning [77].

Surface Temperature: Multiple factors can contribute to the amount of water delivered to inspired air. Among these, the geometry of the nasal cavity and the temperature of the nasal mucosa appear to be key factors [15]. Keck and colleagues measured intranasal temperature at different locations in 50 volunteers, after inspiration, and found that the greatest increase in temperature was observed in the nasal valve area [57]. We studied the effects of raising the nasal mucosal surface temperature by immersion of the feet in warm water [58–60]. Increased nasal mucosal temperature improved the ability of the nose to condition inspired air without a significant change in the volume of the nasal cavity [61].

Application of a topical vasoconstrictor drug, oxymetazoline, decreased the nasal mucosal temperature [62] and the temperature of inspired air at the oropharynx [24]. Application of an alpha-adrenoreceptor antagonist, which increased the temperature of the nasal mucosa, had no impact on the ability of the nose to condition air [62]. Furthermore, we reduced the nasal volume without altering the mucosal temperature by placing subjects in the supine position, and we studied this effect on the nasal conditioning capacity. Contrary to the theoretical model, in the supine position, subjects were less able to condition CDA compared to the upright position [63]. Based on these observations, the theoretical model of Hanna and Sherer is only partially supported [15]. It is quite possible that surface temperature and nasal volume are only partially responsible for the water transportation capacity across the nasal mucosa. There are many complex factors (e.g., electrolyte transportation across the nasal mucosa, tight junction transport, or aquaporin function) which have not been assessed.

Nasal Inflammation: We previously showed that subjects with seasonal allergic rhinitis, out of season, had a reduced ability to warm and humidify air compared with normal subjects [55]. We studied the effect of allergic responses induced by either seasonal exposure or nasal challenge with antigen on nasal conditioning of CDA. An allergic response caused by either seasonal exposure or allergen challenge increased the ability of the nose to condition inspired air [64]. The allergen challenge-induced observation was subsequently confirmed in subjects with perennial allergic rhinitis [65, 66]. We also showed that subjects with asthma had a decreased ability to condition air [67]. The more severe the asthma, the worse was the ability of the nose to condition air, indicating that the reduced nasal conditioning capacity of subjects with asthma could adversely affect the lower airway.

Parasympathetic Nervous System: The parasympathetically driven glands in the nose, approximately 45,000 per nasal cavity, are the major contributors to the volume of surface secretions [27, 68]. Local application of atropine sulfate significantly inhibits rhinorrhea in nasal lavage fluids, suggesting that parasympathetic neuronal activity occurs during the nasal response to CDA [35]. We were concerned that, although ipratropium bromide treated the rhinorrhea, it might worsen the ability of the nose to condition air. It had been shown that subcutaneous injection of 1 mg atropine decreased the ability of the nose to humidify air [69]. However, application of homatropine or ipratropium bromide to the nasal surface did not impair its humidification function [70, 71]. We studied the effect of treatment with ipratropium bromide on the ability of the nose to condition CDA. Ipratropium bromide improved the conditioning of inspired air, despite the fact that the secretory response measured after the end of cold-air exposure was decreased [72]. This experiment suggested that glandular secretion was not a major contributor to nasal conditioning, and blocking of secretions did not adversely affect the ability of the nose to warm and humidify air.

Mechanism of CDA-Induced Rhinitis

CDA challenge to the nose led to mast cell and glandular activation [49, 52] and plasma extravasation [35] (Fig. 1). This was observed only in cold-air-sensitive individuals, but not in nonsensitive controls and correlated well with the development of nasal symptoms [48].

Inhalation of CDA stimulates sensory nerves and generates a cholinergic secretory response. The cholinergic secretory response was demonstrated by the reduction of the contralateral secretory response after ipsilateral CDA provocation when the contralateral nostril was pretreated with atropine [7]. Furthermore, atropine was shown to reduce rhinorrhea scores and a biomarker of glandular activation after CDA challenge, without affecting exudation [35].

Although the nasal reaction to cold air has been found to involve both mast cell activation and sensorineural stimulation, the clinical significance of the former pathway is unknown. For example, a topical antihistamine (azatadine base) had been shown, previously, to inhibit allergen-induced symptoms and release mast cell mediators in individuals with allergic rhinitis [73]. However, it had no effect on either symptoms or histamine release after CDA provocation [74]. Furthermore, the use of topical glucocorticosteroid (beclomethasone), for 7 days, significantly reduced histamine release, but not in the TAME-esterase activity, albumin levels, or in symptoms after CDA challenge [34]. These results indicate that histamine may not be essential for the development of the immediate nasal reaction to CDA. The clinical response to CDA seems to be mediated primarily by neural mechanisms, with a sensory element that is located in the nasal mucosa and an effector element that is mostly cholinergic. In support of this concept, objective measures of the nasal reaction (decreased nasal patency and secretion weight) to CDA have been

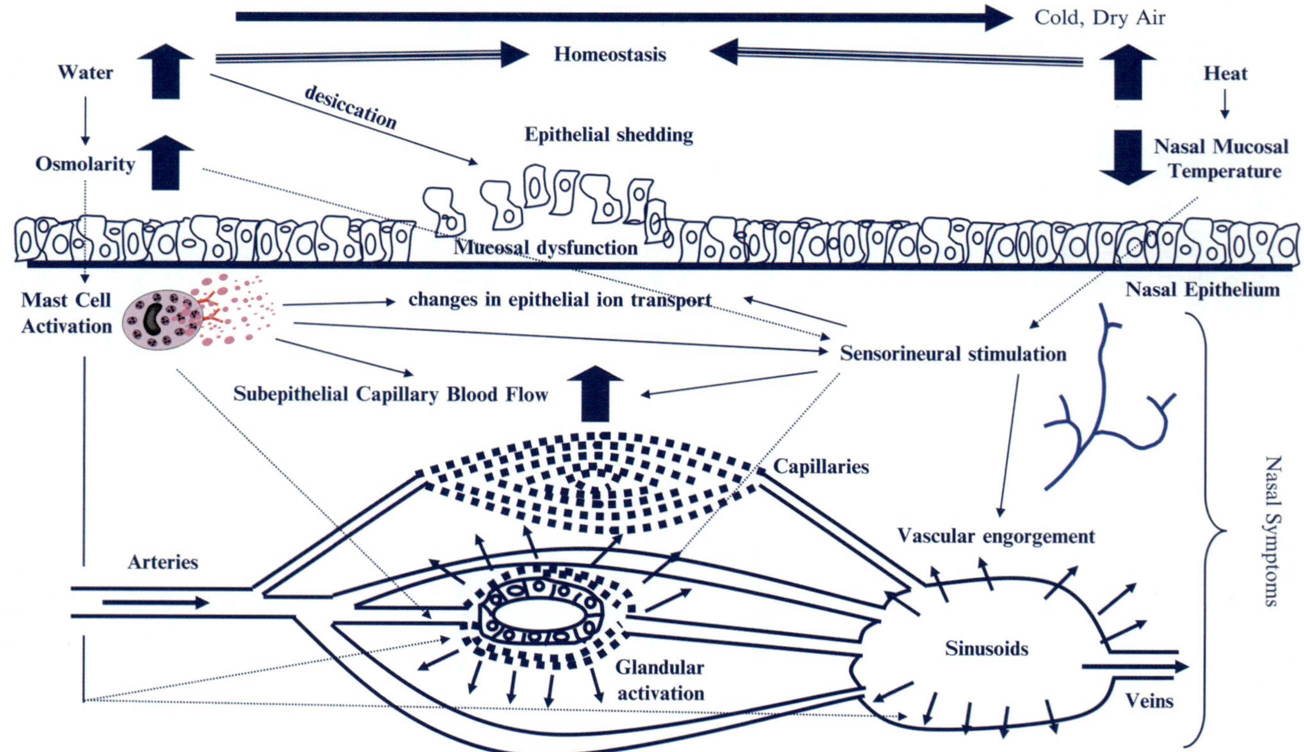

Fig. 1 Pathophysiology of CDA-induced rhinitis

reduced successfully with intranasal capsaicin treatment, which defunctionalizes nociceptor c-fibers [75]. Also, intranasal anticholinergic agents reduce rhinorrhea in skiers [76].

During cold-air breathing, there is loss of heat and water from the mucosal surface, resulting in mucosal cooling and hyperosmolarity of nasal secretions. The effect of cooling of the mucosa is unknown. Evidence has shown that hyperosmolarity is a known trigger for mast cell and sensory nerve activation in the human nose. Water loss leading to hypertonicity is more likely to be the key stimulus rather than heat loss.

One hypothesis for CDA-induced symptoms of rhinitis is that the respiratory mucosa of individuals with CDA sensitivity cannot compensate for the loss of water that occurs on exposure to the stimulus, leading to epithelial damage. Cruz et al. found a sixfold increase in nasal-lavage epithelial cells in the CDA-sensitive group after CDA, but not after exposure to warm, moist air [39]. This finding shows that epithelial cell shedding accompanies clinical responses to CDA in the human nose, supporting the above hypothesis.

Why does cold-air-induced rhinitis affect a subgroup of individuals more than others? Neither the presence of atopy nor nasal responsiveness to histamine has predicted CDA responsiveness [37]. The osmolarity of the epithelial lining fluid was increased after CDA provocation in a CDA-sensitive group, but not in an insensitive group [5]. In addition, when nasal challenge with a hyperosmolar solution was performed in both groups, CDA-sensitive subjects released significantly more histamine in nasal lavage fluids than did CDA-insensitive subjects [37]. The underlying difference between CDA-sensitive and CDA-insensitive individuals probably relates to the ability of the mucosa to cope with conditions that demand an increased water supply to inhaled air or to the epithelial surface, either after the inhalation of dry air or after application of a hyperosmolar stimulus. The airway mucosa of CDA-sensitive individuals cannot compensate for the water loss that occurs under extreme conditions, leading to epithelial damage [39], whereas, CDA-insensitive individuals have an adequate water supply to the epithelial surface under stressful conditions, resulting in no reaction to the stimulus.

Conclusion

Nasal provocation tests with cold air have been used for the study of one of the major functions of the nose, the nasal conditioning capacity, and pathophysiology of cold-air-induced rhinitis and its treatment. Because one of the mechanisms underlying cold-air-induced rhinitis is hyperosmolarity of the epithelial lining fluid, a nasal provocation test using hyperosmolar stimuli has been developed. These tests help us to better understand how the environment interacts with the nasal mucosa, and it may improve treatment strategies for rhinitis in the future.

References

1. Togias A (1998) Non-allergic rhinitis. In: Mygind N, Naclerio R, Durham S (eds) Rhinitis. Marcel Dekker, New York, pp 383–399
2. Braat J, Mulder P, Fokkens W, van Wijk R, Rijntjes E (1998) Intranasal cold dry air is superior to histamine challenge in determining the presence and degree of nasal hyperreactivity in nonallergic noninfectious perennial rhinitis. Am J Respir Crit Care Med 157:1748–1755
3. Kauffmann F, Neukirch F, Annesi I, Korobaeff M, Dore MF, Lellouch J (1988) Relation of perceived nasal and bronchial hyperresponsiveness to FEV_1, basophil counts, and methacholine response. Thorax 43:456–461
4. Diemer F, Sanico A, Horowitz E, Togias A (1999) Non-allergenic inhalant triggers in seasonal and perennial allergic rhinitis. J Allergy Clin Immunol 103:S2
5. Togias AG, Proud D, Lichtenstein LM, Adams GK, Norman PS, Kagey-Sobotka A, Naclerio RM (1988) The osmolality of nasal secretions increases when inflammatory mediators are released in response to inhalation of cold, dry air. Am Rev Respir Dis 137(3):625–629
6. Jankowski R, Philip G, Togias AG, Naclerio RM (1993) Demonstration of bilateral cholinergic secretory response after unilateral nasal cold, dry air challenge. Rhinology 31:97–100
7. Philip G, Jankowski R, Baroody F, Naclerio RM, Togias AG (1993) Reflex activation of nasal secretion by unilateral inhalation of cold, dry air. Am Rev Respir Dis 148:1616–1622
8. Slome D (1956) Physiology of nasal circulation. Sci Basis Med 5:451–468
9. Änggärd A (1974) The effects of parasympathetic nerve stimulation on the microcirculation and secretion in the nasal mucosa of the cat. Acta Otolaryngol 78: 98–105
10. Eccles R, Wilson H (1974) The autonomic innervation of the nasal blood vessels of the cat. J Physiol (Lond) 238:549–560
11. Gadlage R, Behnke EE, Jackson RT (1975) Is the vidian nerve cholinergic? Arch Otolaryngol 101:422–425
12. Ingelstedt S (1956) Studies on the conditioning of air in the respiratory tract. Acta Otolaryngol Suppl:131:1–80
13. Ingelstedt S (1970) Humidifying capacity of the nose. Ann Otol Rhinol Laryngol 79: 475–480
14. Cole P (1953) Some aspects of temperature, moisture and heat relationships in the upper respiratory tract. J Laryngol Otol 67:449–456
15. Hanna LM, Scherer PW (1986) A theoretical model of localized heat and water vapor transport in the human respiratory tract. J Biomech Eng 108:19–27
16. McFadden ER Jr, Pichurko BM, Bowman HF, Ingenito E, Burns S, Dowling N, Solway J (1985) Thermal mapping of the airways in humans. J Appl Physiol 58:564–570
17. Tsai C-L, Saidel GM, McFadden ER Jr, Fouke JM (1990) Radial heat and water transport across the airway wall. J Appl Physiol 69:222–231
18. Annesi I, Neukirch F, Orvoen-Frija E, Oryszczyn MP, Korobaeff M, Dore MF, Kauffmann F (1987) The relevance of hyperresponsiveness but not of atopy to FEV1 decline: preliminary results in a working population. Bull Eur Physiopath Resp 23:397–400
19. Griffin MP, McFadden ER Jr, Ingram RH Jr (1982) Airway cooling in asthmatic and nonasthmatic subjects during nasal and oral breathing. J Allergy Clin Immunol 69:354–359
20. Laine MT, Huggare JAV, Ruoppi P (1994) A modification of the pressure-flow technique for measuring breathing of cold air and its effect on nasal cross-sectional area. Dentofac Orthop 105:265–269
21. Gusi B, Krajina Z, Larie J (1969) Damage of the respiratory mucous membrane of rats exposed to cold. Acta Otolaryngol (Stockh) 57:343
22. Jeffery PK, Godfrey RW, Adelroth E, Nelson F, Rogers A, Johansson SA (1992) Effects of treatment on airway inflammation and thickening of basement membrane reticular collagen in asthma. Am Rev Respir Dis 145:890–899
23. Namimatsu A, Go K, Hata T (1991) Nasal mucosal hypersensitivity in guinea pigs intermittingly exposed to cold. Intl Arch Allergy Appl Immunol 96:107–112

24. Cole P (1954) Respiratory mucosal vascular responses, air conditioning and thermo regulation. J Laryngol Otol 68:613–622
25. Cauna N (1970) The fine structure of the arteriovenous anastomosis and its nerve supply in the human nasal respiratory mucosa. Anat Rec 168:9–21
26. Cauna N, Cauna D (1975) The fine structure and innervation of the cushion veins of the human nasal respiratory mucosa. Anat Rec 181:1–16
27. Tos M (1982) Goblet cells and glands in the nose and paranasal sinuses. In: Proctor DF, Andersen IB (eds) The nose: upper airway physiology and the atmospheric environment. Elsevier Biomedical, Amsterdam, The Netherlands, pp 99–144
28. Cauna N (1982) Blood and nerve supply of the nasal lining. In: Proctor DF, Andersen IB (eds) The nose. Elsevier Biomedical, Oxford, pp 44–169
29. Ingelstedt S, Ivstam B (1949) The source of nasal secretion in infectious, allergic, and experimental conditions. Acta Otolaryngol 37:451–455
30. Yankaskas JR, Gatzy JT, Boucher RC (1987) Effects of raised osmolarity on canine tracheal epithelial ion transport function. J Appl Physiol 62: 2241–2245
31. Knowles, MR, Clark CE, Fischer ND (1983) Nasal secretions: role of epithelial ion transport. In: Mygind N, Pipkorn U (eds) Allergic and vasomotor rhinitis: pathophysiological aspects. Munksgaard, Copenhagen, pp 77–90
32. Welsh MJ (1987) Electrolyte transport by airway epithelia. Physiol Rev 67:1143–1184
33. Boucher RC, Cheng EH, Paradiso AM, Stutts MJ, Knowles MR, Earp HS (1989) Chloride secretory response of cystic fibrosis human airway epithelia. Preservation of calcium but not protein kinase C- and A-dependent mechanisms. J Clin Invest 84:1424–1431
34. Cruz AA, Togias AG, Lichtenstein LM, Kagey-Sobotka A, Proud D, Naclerio RM (1991) Steroid-induced reduction of histamine release does not alter the clinical nasal response to cold, dry air. Am Rev Respir Dis 143:761–765
35. Cruz AA, Togias AG, Lichtenstein LM, Kagey-Sobotka A, Proud D, Naclerio RM (1992) Local application of atropine attenuates the upper airway reaction to cold, dry air. Am Rev Respir Dis 146:340–346
36. Togias AG, Naclerio RM, Proud D, Fish JE, Adkinson NF Jr, Kagey-Sobotka A, Norman P, Lichtenstein LM (1985) Nasal challenge with cold, dry air results in release of inflammatory mediators: possible mast cell involvement. J Clin Invest 76:1375–1381
37. Togias AG, Lykens K, Kagey-Sobotka A, Eggleston PA, Proud D, Lichtenstein LM, Naclerio RM (1990) Studies on the relationships between sensitivity to cold, dry air, hyperosmolal solutions, and histamine in the adult nose. Am Rev Respir Dis 141:1428–1433
38. Togias AG, Proud D, Lichtenstein LM, Naclerio RM (1991) Hot, dry air is more potent stimulus than cold, dry air for causing rhinitis and for increasing the osmolality of nasal secretions. Allergy Clin Immunol News (Suppl. 1):114
39. Cruz AA, Naclerio RM, Proud D, Togias A (2006) Epithelial shedding is associated with nasal reactions to cold, dry air. J Allergy Clin Immunol 117:1351–1358
40. Naclerio RM, Meier HL, Kagey-Sobotka A, Adkinson NF Jr, Meyers DA, Norman PS, Lichtenstein LM (1983) Mediator release after nasal airway challenge with allergen. Am Rev Respir Dis 128:597–602
41. Braat JP, Mulder PG, Fokkens WJ, van Wijk RG, Rijntjes E (1998) Intranasal cold dry air is superior to histamine challenge in determining the presence and degree of nasal hyperreactivity in nonallergic noninfectious perennial rhinitis. Am J Respir Crit Care Med 157: 1748–1755
42. Silber G, Proud D, Warner J, Naclerio RM, Kagey-Sobotka A, Lichtenstein LM, Eggleston P (1988) In vivo release of inflammatory mediators by hyperosmolar solutions. Am Rev Respir Dis 137:606–612
43. Krayenbuhl MC, Hudspith BN, Scadding GK, Brostoff J (1988) Nasal response to allergen and hyperosmolar challenge. Clin Allergy 18:157–164
44. Baraniuk JN, Ali M, Yuta A, Fang SY, Naranch K (1999) Hypertonic saline nasal provocation stimulates nociceptive nerves, substance P release, and glandular mucous exocytosis in normal humans. Am J Respir Crit Care Med 160:655–662

45. Lai G, Philip G, Togias A (1996) The nasal response to hyperosmolar saline is inhibited by capsaicin treatment. J Allergy Clin Immunol 97:A431
46. Sanico AM, Philip G, Lai GK, Togias A (1999) Hyperosmolar saline induces reflex nasal secretions, evincing neural hyperresponsiveness in allergic rhinitis. J Appl Physiol 86:1202–1210
47. Andersson M, Greiff L, Svensson C, Persson C (1995) Various methods for testing nasal responses in vivo: a critical review. Acta Otolaryngol Stockh 115:705–713
48. Naclerio RM, Proud D, Kagey-Sobotka A, Lichtenstein LM, Togias A (1995) Cold dry air-induced rhinitis: effect of inhalation and exhalation through the nose. J Appl Physiol 79: 467–471
49. Proud D, Bailey GS, Naclerio RM, Reynolds CJ, Cruz AA, Eggleston PA, Lichtenstein LM, Togias AG (1992) Tryptase and histamine as markers to evaluate mast cell activation during the responses to nasal challenge with allergen, cold, dry air, and hyperosmolar solutions. J Allergy Clin Immunol 89: 1098–1110
50. Eggleston PA, Kagey-Sobotka A, Schleimer RP, Lichtenstein LM (1984) Interaction between hyperosmolar and IgE-mediated histamine release from basophils and mast cells. Am Rev Respir Dis 130:86–91
51. Eggleston PA, Kagey-Sobotka A, Lichtenstein LM (1987) A comparison of the osmotic activation of basophils and human lung mast cells. Am Rev Respir Dis 135:1043–1048
52. Hanes LS, Issa E, Proud D, Togias A (2006) Stronger nasal responsiveness to cold air in individuals with rhinitis and asthma, compared with rhinitis alone. Clin Exp Allergy 36:26–31
53. Togias AG, Naclerio RM, Peters SP, Nimmagadda I, Proud D, Kagey-Sobotka A, Adkinson NF Jr, Norman PS, Lichtenstein LM (1986) Local generation of sulfidopeptide leukotrienes upon nasal provocation with cold, dry air. Am Rev Respir Dis 133:1133–1137
54. Iliopoulos O, Proud D, Norman PS, Lichtenstein LM, Kagey-Sobotka A, Naclerio RM (1988) Nasal challenge with cold, dry air induces a late-phase reaction. Am Rev Respir Dis 138:400–405
55. Rouadi P, Baroody FM, Abbott D, Naureckas E, Solway J, Naclerio RM (1999) A technique to measure the ability of the human nose to warm and humidify air. J Appl Physiol 87:400–406
56. Proctor D, Andersen IB, Lundqvist GR (1977) Human nasal mucosa function at controlled temperatures. Respir Physiol 30:109–124
57. Keck T, Leiacker R, Riechelmann H, Rettinger G (2000) Temperature profile in the nasal cavity. Laryngoscope 110:651–654
58. Cole P (1954) Recordings of respiratory air temperature. J Laryngol Otol 68:295–307
59. Grayson J (1990) Responses of the microcirculation to hot and cold environments. In: Schonbaum E, Lomax P (eds) Thermoregulation: physiology and biochemistry. Pergamon, New York, pp 221–234
60. Assanasen P, Baroody FM, Haney L, deTineo M, Naureckas E, Solway J, Naclerio RM (2003) Elevation of the nasal mucosal surface temperature after warming of the feet occurs via a neural reflex. Acta Otolaryngol 123:627–636
61. Abbott DJ, Baroody FM, Naureckas E, Naclerio RM (2001) Elevation of nasal mucosal temperature increases the ability of the nose to warm and humidify air. Am J Rhinol 15:41–45
62. Pinto JM, Assanasen P, Baroody FM, Naureckas E, Naclerio RM (2005) Alpha-adrenoreceptor blockade with phenoxybenzamine does not affect the ability of the nose to condition air. J Appl Physiol 99:128–133
63. Assanasen P, Baroody FM, Naureckas E, Solway J, Naclerio RM (2001) Supine position decreases the ability of the nose to warm and humidify air. J Appl Physiol 91:2459–2465
64. Assanasen P, Baroody FM, Abbott DJ, Naureckas E, Solway J, Naclerio RM (2000) Natural and induced allergic responses increase the ability of the nose to warm and humidify air. J Allergy Clin Immunol 106:1045–1052
65. Rozsasi A, Leiacker R, Keck T (2004) Nasal conditioning in perennial allergic rhinitis after nasal allergen challenge. Clin Exp Allergy 34:1099–1104
66. Pinto JM, Assanasen P, Baroody FM, Naureckas E, Solway J, Naclerio RM (2004) Treatment of nasal inflammation decreases the ability of subjects with asthma to condition inspired air. Am J Respir Crit Care Med 170:863–869

67. Assanasen P, Baroody FM, Naureckas E, Solway J, Naclerio RM (2001) The nasal passage of subjects with asthma has a decreased ability to warm and humidify inspired air. Am J Respir Crit Care Med 164:1640–1646
68. Baroody FM, Majchel AM, Roecker MM, Roszko PJ, Zegarelli EC, Wood CC, Naclerio RM (1992) Ipratropium bromide (Atrovent nasal spray) reduces the nasal response to methacholine. J Allergy Clin Immunol 89:1065–1075
69. Ingelstedt S and Ivstam B (1951) Study in the humidifying capacity of the nose. Acta Otolaryngol 39:286–290
70. Drettner B, Falck B, Simon H (1977) Measurements of the air conditioning capacity of the nose during normal and pathological conditions and pharmacological influence. Acta Otolaryngol 84:266–277
71. Kumlien J, Drettner B (1985) The effect of ipratropium bromide (Atrovent) on the air conditioning capacity of the nose. Clin Otolaryngol Allied Sci 10:165–168
72. Assanasen P, Baroody FM, Rouadi P, Naureckas E, Solway J, Naclerio RM (2000) Ipratropium bromide increases the ability of the nose to warm and humidify air. Am J Respir Crit Care Med 162:1031–1037
73. Togias AG, Naclerio RM, Warner J, Proud D, Kagey-Sobotka A, Nimmagadda I, Norman PS, Lichtenstein LM (1986) Demonstration of inhibition of mediator release from human mast cells by azatadine base. In vivo and in vitro evaluation. JAMA 255:225–229
74. Togias AG, Proud D, Kagey-Sobotka A, Norman P, Lichtenstein L, Naclerio RM (1987) The effect of a topical tricyclic antihistamine on the response of the nasal mucosa to challenge with cold, dry air and histamine. J Allergy Clin Immunol 79:599–604
75. Van Rijswijk JB, Boeke EL, Keizer JM, Mulder PG, Blom H M, Fokkens WJ (2003) Intranasal capsaicin reduces nasal hyperreactivity in idiopathic rhinitis: a double-blind randomized application regimen study. Allergy 58:754–761
76. Silvers WS (1991) The skier's nose: model of cold-induced rhinorrhea. Ann Allergy 67:32–36
77. Sahin-Yilmaz A, Pinto JM, deTineo M, Elwany S, Naclerio RM (2007) Familial aggregation of nasal conditioning capacity. J Appl Physiol 103:1078–1081

Mechanisms of Mucus Induction in Asthma

Lauren Cohn

Introduction

In asthma, mucus obstruction is a long recognized cause of morbidity. Sir William Osler described airway obstruction as resulting from mucous secretions [1]. Early in the 20th century, anatomic obstruction by mucus was observed in autopsies in fatal asthma [2]. Mucous secretions in the airways in asthma appeared to be a major cause of airway obstruction, ventilation-perfusion mismatching, and hypoxemia, leading to wheezing and dyspnea [3–5]. Despite this age-old recognition of mucus collection in asthma, the mechanisms regulating mucus hypersecretion were poorly understood. Recently, major strides have been made to define specific molecular pathways that lead to excess mucus production.

Basic Biology of Mucus in the Respiratory Tract

Mucus Composition

In the bronchial airways, surface epithelial cells with secretory features and a classical goblet shape, called goblet cells, produce mucus. Goblet cells produce mucins that are stored in secretory granules and released into the airway lumen. In the large airways mucous glands also produce mucus. Under basal conditions the columnar epithelial surface is comprised of a few percent of goblet cells and a majority of ciliated cells. These structures provide adequate mucus to capture particles and remove them from the air we breathe.

Mucus is composed of a sticky "gel" layer that traps particles in the airway lumen and the "sol" layer, which is predominantly water. The sol layer contacts the surface of the ciliated cells to permit sweeping the gel out of the lower airways

L. Cohn (✉)
Section of Pulmonary and Critical Care Medicine, Yale University School of Medicine,
333 Cedar Street, P.O. Box 208057, New Haven, CT 06520, USA

R. Pawankar et al. (eds.), *Allergy Frontiers: Clinical Manifestations,*
DOI: 10.1007/978-4-431-88317-3_11, © Springer 2009

toward the larynx, like an escalator, to be ultimately cleared by coughing or swallowing. Mucus also contains other macromolecules, including antibacterial agents, to enhance its defense function. Thus, mucus is important in the innate host defense system, as pathogens, proteins, and other inhaled particles are inhibited and eliminated from the respiratory tract.

The functions of mucus rely on its specific viscoelastic properties. The matrix is formed by mucins: high molecular weight, oligomeric glycoproteins. More than 20 mucin genes have been identified and 12 of these have been shown to be expressed in the respiratory tract [6]. The gel-forming mucins are most prominent in respiratory tract secretions in both basal conditions in the healthy lung and in chronic airway diseases. These are huge molecules characterized by multi-domain polypeptide chains with thousands of amino acid residues, large, heavily O-glycosylated apoprotein cores, and cysteine-rich N- and C-terminal domains that permit oligimerization. When secreted, gel-forming mucins form a dense macromolecular matrix [7]. MUC5AC and MUC5B are the most prominent mucins secreted in the lower respiratory tract [6]. MUC5AC is produced exclusively in the airway epithelium, while mucous cells in the submucosal glands typically produce MUC5B. Both MUC5AC and MUC5B are identified in mucus in the lungs of nonasthmatics, mild asthmatics, and those with fatal asthma [8]. While there is an increase in mucin content in sputum from asthmatics compared to sputum from normal controls, the ratio of the major mucins, MUC5AC and MUC5B, is not altered. This suggests that changes in mucus properties, such as increased volume and/or viscosity, observed in asthma, are not a result of a shift to production of different mucins [8–10].

Mucus Secretion

Gel-forming mucins are synthesized and stored in a condensed form as large, covalent disulfide-linked oligomers and multimers in large secretory vesicles that occupy most of the apical surface of the goblet cell (Fig. 1). Numerous inflammatory mediators

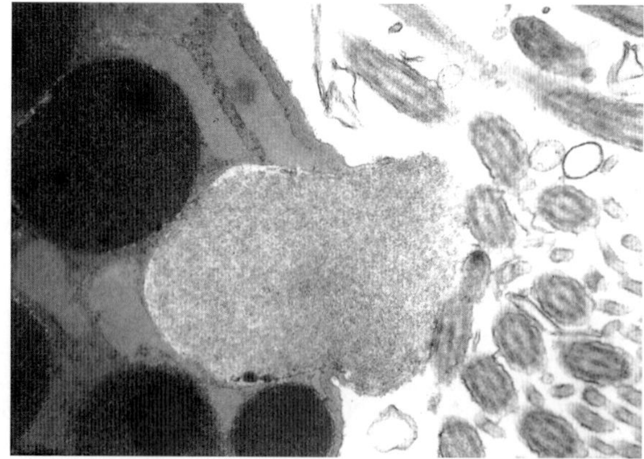

Fig. 1 Apical surface of a goblet cell secreting mucin. Electron micrograph of a murine goblet cell discharging mucin into the airway lumen. Note the electron dense mucin material in the stored vesicles and the flocculent, now hydrated, mucins being discharged. Cross-sections of cilia from adjacent cells are seen in the airway lumen

have been shown to stimulate mucus secretion including cholinergic agonists, lipid mediators, oxidants, cytokines, neuropeptides, Adenosine-5´-triphosphate (ATP), uridine 5´-triphosphate (UTP), and neutrophil elastase [11]. The mechanism of mucin discharge involves interactions of the actin cytoskeleton with the plasma membrane, possibly through their physical association with myristolated, alanine-rich C-kinase substrate (MARCKS). MARCKS is a target of phosphorylation by protein kinase C and is identified in mucin secretory granules [12]. It was shown to be essential for mucin release *in vitro* and *in vivo* in a model of allergic airway inflammation [12, 13]. Mucus secretagogues, many of which have been shown to activate protein kinases, may activate MARCKS and stimulate cytoskeletal changes that allow intracytoplasmic vesicles to move to the cell surface for discharge.

Inflammation and Mucus in Asthma

Pathology of Mucus in Asthma

In lung biopsies of severe asthmatics and in autopsy specimens from patients with fatal asthma, obstructing plugs of mucus and cellular debris have been identified in small- and medium-sized airways (Fig. 2). The pathological lesions that lead to increased mucus production in the respiratory tract, goblet cell metaplasia, and mucous gland hypertrophy, were present in all asthmatics and were not observed in normal control patients [9, 14, 15]. These characteristic pathological findings are believed to contribute to clinical symptoms of wheezing and coughing.

Marked changes in mucus-producing organs are required to accommodate the increased mucus production in asthma. Goblet cells increase in number and percentage of total airway epithelial cells. While less than 5% of airway epithelial cells are goblet cells in healthy individuals, in fatal asthma 20–25% of airway epithelial cells are goblet cells [14]. In autopsies in fatal asthma there was a 20-fold increase

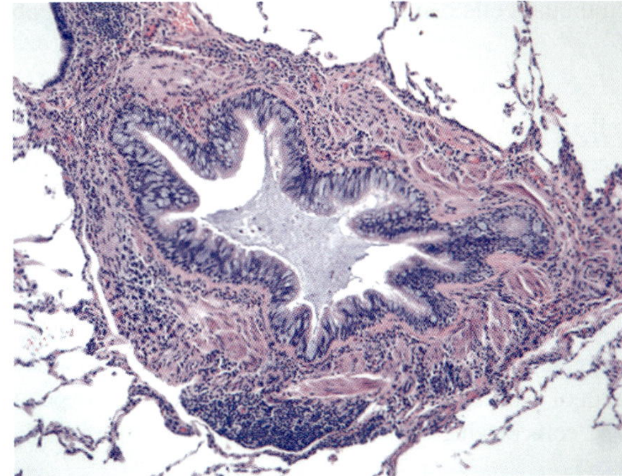

Fig. 2 Lung biopsy of severe asthmatic. Lung biopsy of a 44-year-old woman with asthma and an FEV$_1$ of 35% predicted. Mucus occupies most of the lumen of this large airway. Goblet cells are prominent. Note the intense inflammatory infiltrate around the airways, thickened subepithelial membrane, and smooth muscle hypertrophy

in goblet cells in the peripheral airways compared to nonasthmatic controls [15]. In fatal asthma, intralumenal mucus was also markedly increased in asthmatics compared to control patients without asthma [8, 14, 15]. Asthmatics exhibited mucous glands that were two- to four-times greater in size compared to controls [15, 16].

Increased mucus secretion also appeared to correlate with disease severity. Airway biopsies of mild and moderate asthmatics exhibited a threefold increase in secreted mucin compared to mild asthmatics [9]. In the airways of patients with fatal asthma, compared to asthmatics who died of other causes, there was three times more mucus within the airway lumen [15]. While the number of goblet cells in airway biopsies of mild-to-moderate asthmatics was comparable [9], there was a 30-fold increase in goblet cells in autopsies of fatal asthma compared to those with asthma who died of other causes [15]. This suggested that goblet cell metaplasia was associated with disease severity. The mucous gland size was comparable in autopsies of both fatal and nonfatal asthma [15]. In asthma, it was clear that mucus hyperproduction was reflected in a pathological increase in goblet cells and hypertrophy of mucous glands. In the most severe cases of asthma these effects could be dramatic, and pathological evidence suggested that mucus plugging might be the cause of death in fatal asthma.

Goblet Cell Transition

The process by which goblet cells arise and increase in number and percentage in the airways appears to be a result of epithelial cell transition or transdifferentiation. In murine models of asthma, metaplasia accounts for the majority of increased goblet cells, while proliferation plays a minor role [17]. Animal studies show that when goblet cells increase there is a loss of both ciliated and nonciliated Clara cells [17, 18]. Goblet cells, in some cases, retain the features of Clara cells, indicating their likely origin [19, 20]. In humans and in mice, single cells with features of both ciliated and goblet cells or Clara and goblet cells have been observed. These findings suggest that when provided with an appropriate stimulus various airway epithelial cells can be pushed to differentiate into goblet cells [18–20].

Th2 Inflammation and Mucus

Chronic diseases with airway mucus hyperproduction are typically characterized by airway inflammation. In asthma, the bronchial airways exhibit infiltration of the mucosa and submucosa with inflammatory cells, including lymphocytes, eosinophils, and mast cells [21]. Bronchial biopsies and bronchoalveolar lavage (BAL) indicate that Th2 cells are represented at an increased frequency in the respiratory tract of asthmatics and are activated locally after specific antigen challenge [22, 23]. Th2 cells produce a panel of cytokines including IL-4, IL-5, IL-9, IL-10, and IL-13.

Th2 cells are particularly potent in activating B cells to secrete an antibody, and are essential for IgE production through effects of IL-4 and IL-13. IL-5 influences eosinophil differentiation, maturation, and activation [24]. In asthma, the obvious associations with high IgE levels and airway eosinophilia have implicated the Th2 cell and its cytokines in chronic inflammation and airway remodeling. Furthermore, the presence of cells secreting IL-4 and IL-5 correlate with airway obstruction, and the number of eosinophils in the sputum correlates with its expectorated volume [25, 26]. Thus, it appears that the inflammatory response in asthma is skewed toward Th2, and the airway inflammatory response induced by Th2 cytokines controls mucus production [24].

To understand how inflammation is responsible for mucus induction, investigation of different models of airway inflammation were employed. Mice with airway inflammation induced by Th2 lymphocytes exhibited marked inflammation characterized by eosinophilia [27–29]. These animals showed goblet cell hyperplasia with extensive mucus collections in the proximal airways and increased mucus in the airway lumen. Mice have limited numbers of mucous glands in the lower respiratory tract, so murine studies of mucus hyperproduction have focused on goblet cell metaplasia. Interestingly, airway inflammation with Th1 lymphocytes that produced IFN-gamma (IFN-γ) in the respiratory tract showed airway neutrophilia and low, basal numbers of goblets cells [27]. This suggested that Th2 inflammation had a unique effect on mucus production. Chronic overexpression of individual Th2 cytokines in the murine respiratory tract had been achieved using lung-specific promoters. Overexpresser transgenic mice with the Clara cell 10-kDa (CC10) promoter driving the Th2 cytokines, IL-4, IL-5, IL-9, or IL-13, exhibited characteristic allergic inflammatory features in the airways, including eosinophilia and mucus overproduction [30–33]. These studies showed that mucus metaplasia was induced in a variety of Th2 inflammatory conditions.

A number of studies addressed which specific Th2 inflammatory mediators led to goblet cell metaplasia. While mucus production appeared to correlate with both eosinophilia and IL-4 production in the respiratory tract, mucus was readily inducible by Th2 cells in mice that lacked IL-4 and eosinophils [27, 28, 34, 35]. In mice deficient in the IL-4/IL-13 signaling pathway, either by lack of IL-4 receptor alpha-1 (IL-4Rα1) or Stat6, neither Th2 cells nor IL-13 could induce goblet cell metaplasia or increase mucin gene expression [36–38]. In the absence of IL-13, the Th2 cells that produced IL-4 and IL-5 could no longer stimulate mucus [39–41]. Furthermore, in transgenic mice with lung-specific overexpression of IL-4, IL-5, or IL-9, in which mucus was induced, the effect was IL-13-dependent [39, 42, 43]. For example, mucus metaplasia was blocked in mice overexpressing IL-9 when IL-13 was inhibited, and this effect could be due to IL-9 stimulation of epithelial IL-13 production [44]. These studies show that IL-13 is required for Th2-induced mucus in mice. IL-13 is highly potent and at very low levels can effectively promote mucus metaplasia [39]. IL-13 appears to act via direct effects on airway epithelial cells. Th2 cells could not stimulate mucus in mice with conditional deletion of Stat6 in the airway epithelium [45], and these findings were corroborated by studies using IL-4Rα1-/- bone marrow chimeric mice and airway epithelial Stat6 "knock-in" mice [39, 46]. Taken together, IL-13 is an essential factor for Th2-induced mucus metaplasia through its epithelial specific effects.

In humans, it is not clear if IL-13 has an exclusive role in inducing mucus, as it does in mice. Human airway epithelial cells cultured with IL-13 differentiate into goblet cells over a period of days. Similarly, IL-4 can induce mucus staining and mucin gene induction [47, 48]. The concentrations of IL-4 used in these studies are likely higher than those observed under physiological conditions and may explain the differences observed *in vivo* in murine and *in vitro* in human systems.

In addition to its effects on goblet cell induction, IL-13 appears to be important for maintenance of epithelial mucus production. In epithelial cells cultured with IL-13 there is induction of MUC5AC expression and goblet cell differentiation. On removal of IL-13, the goblet cells reverted to ciliated cells and MUC5AC expression was reduced [49].

Epidermal Growth Factor Receptor

Epidermal growth factor receptor (EGFR) ligands were also shown to be essential for mucus metaplasia. EGRF had critical functions in growth, differentiation, and repair of airway epithelial cells [50, 51]. In cultured human airway epithelial cells, administration of EGFR ligands, TGF-α, and EGF, stimulated MUC5AC expression and goblet cell development [52–54]. Application of these ligands in the airways of animals led to induction of mucus metaplasia. When inhibitors of EGFR signaling were applied *in vitro* and *in vivo*, the effects on the mucus were inhibited [53]. Thus, EGFR was another necessary signal for mucus metaplasia.

EGFR and IL-13 Control Goblet Cell Transition

A two-signal model that controls goblet cell transdifferentiation has been proposed and it explains how mucous cell metaplasia is dependent on both EGFR ligands and IL-13 [18] (Fig. 3). This sequence was defined in mice and it also appears to control goblet cell differentiation in human epithelial cells. To initiate transition of a non-goblet cell into a goblet cell, EGFR activation must occur. EGFR ligands, including TGF-α and reactive oxygen species, have been identified in Th2 inflammatory responses. Activation of EGFR in murine and human bronchial epithelial cultures leads to receptor phosphorylation and results in an increase in markers of epithelial apoptosis, including Akt and activated caspase 3 [18, 55]. Thus, it is hypothesized that EGFR activation inhibits epithelial apoptosis and "primes" the epithelial cell to respond to the second signal, IL-13, which allows for full goblet cell transition. IL-13 leads to the induction of MUC5AC gene expression, which is a defining characteristic of goblet cells. IL-13 activates multiple other genes that support goblet cell secretory functions, such as ClCa1, a calcium activated chloride

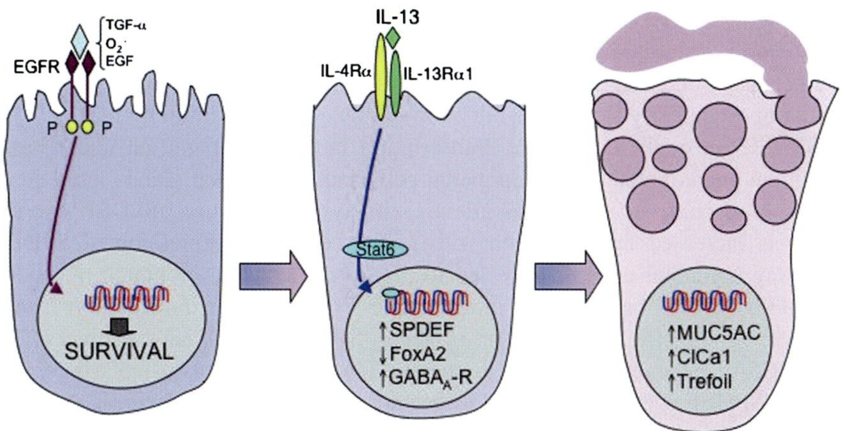

Fig. 3 Goblet cell differentiation requires two signals. The hypothesis: Signal 1 activates the EGFR on the ciliated cells and induces EGFR phosphorylation and activation of PI3 kinase. This pathway leads to inhibition of epithelial cell apoptosis. Epithelial cells that survive have the potential to become goblet cells if provided with Signal 2, IL-13 binding to its receptor. Upon IL-13R activation and Stat6 signaling, epithelial cells show an increase in SPDEF and reduced FoxA2 expression. These effects are IL-13 dependent, yet their blockade inhibits goblet cell induction, placing them early in goblet cell transition. GABA$_A$-R responsiveness is required for goblet cell metaplasia and is induced by IL-13. The precise functions of these early events in goblet cell transdifferentiation are unknown. Following IL-13 activation, cells lose the features of epithelial cells from which they arose, taking on the features of mucus-producing goblet cells and begin to produce mucins and other factors necessary for secretory functions

channel, and trefoil factors that are secreted by goblet cells and maintain the surface integrity of mucosal surfaces [55–58]. Thus, IL-13 has a unique function in promoting goblet cells. Goblet cells were absent when EGFR was blocked, despite the presence of IL-13 [18, 55, 59]. EGFR activation alone cannot induce goblet cell metaplasia unless IL-13 is present. Thus, it appears that EGFR activation is a critical signal that promotes epithelial cell survival, permitting the cell to respond to IL-13 and differentiate into a mucus-producing goblet cell.

A number of transcription factors known to be important in lung development have been identified in the conducting airways. The transcription factors FoxA2 and SAM pointed domain-containing ETS transcription factor (SPDEF) appear to be key elements in goblet cell development. FoxA2 is known to play a critical role in lung morphogenesis and differentiation, and under basal conditions, in the adult lung, is expressed in airway epithelial cells [60, 61]. Th2 inflammation and mucus metaplasia are associated with loss of expression of FoxA2 [60, 62]. This downregulation is limited to proximal airway cells where mucus is produced. Distal airway epithelial cells, which do not produce mucus, respond to IL-13, but FoxA2 expression does not change [62]. Thus, FoxA2 is inversely associated with the development of goblet cells. Mice with conditional deletion of FoxA2 in the respiratory epithelium exhibit spontaneous mucus metaplasia [60]. *In vitro* reporter assays show that FoxA2 inhibits MUC5AC gene expression. Furthermore, FoxA2 expression is inhibited by IL-13. These data suggest that FoxA2 is required for maintenance of normal (non-goblet) epithelial cells. Inhibition of FoxA2 appears to be an important early step in the initiation of goblet cell transition by IL-13.

SPDEF, an epithelial specific transcription factor was identified under basal conditions in proximal airway epithelial cells and submucosal glands in an adult mouse lung [63]. In models of allergic airway inflammation, SPDEF expression was increased in association with goblet cells. Overexpression of SPDEF in airway epithelial cells in mice led to the spontaneous development of mucus metaplasia. SPDEF appeared to interact with TTF1, another transcription factor, for a synergistic effect on a number of genes. SPDEF did not have a direct effect on MUC5AC gene expression, so its specific function in mucus metaplasia remain unclear. SPDEF overexpression led to downregulation of FoxA2 expression, placing it upstream of FoxA2 in the goblet cell transition. The induction of SPDEF was both Stat6 and IL-13 dependent, suggesting it was another key factor that was downstream of IL-13 and controlled goblet cell transition.

γ-Aminobutyric acid (GABA) also appears to transmit a signal via the $GABA_A$-receptor, which is critical for the induction of goblet cell metaplasia. $GABA_A$-receptors (-R) are pentameric chloride channels known to be important for maintenance of normal brain function [64]. $GABA_A$-R are hypothesized to play a role in airway mucus because of their chloride transport function and their presence on the surface of a subpopulation of bronchial epithelial cells [65]. A GABA-R antagonist blocks mucus, despite the presence of Th2 inflammation and high levels of IL-13. Furthermore, IL-13 induces $GABA_A$-receptor expression on airway epithelial cells. Thus, it is likely that $GABA_A$-R promotes goblet cell metaplasia by effects that are downstream of IL-13.

IL-13 does not appear to directly regulate MUC5AC gene expression, since a Stat6 binding site is not identified in the MUC5AC promoter [66]. IL-13 induced signals, such as, TGF-β2/SMAD4, EGFR, and HIF-1 have been proposed as possible activators of mucin production [66]. These studies highlight a complex, organized process by which goblet cell differentiation occurs. Inflammation initiates activation of EGFR, promoting cell survival and permitting proximal airway epithelial cells to respond to IL-13. IL-13 controls the multiple steps in the differentiation and function of goblet cells. Many features of goblet cell induction parallel the events in epithelial repair from injury and suggest that Th2 inflammation is a form of epithelial injury requiring mucus-producing cells for protection of the host and maintenance of epithelial integrity.

Goblet Cell Inhibition

Mucus metaplasia did not occur in all immune responses, particularly those rich in IFN-γ. Th1 cell-induced airway inflammation did not stimulate mucus metaplasia [27]. It was initially believed that Th1 cells did not produce the factors necessary to induce this effect. Yet, when IFN-γ effects were blocked in the Th1-induced airway inflammation, mucus was readily induced, indicating that all the necessary signals for mucus induction were provided in the respiratory tract in Th1 inflammation [67]. The ability of Th1 cells to stimulate mucus metaplasia was due to IL-13 production, but could only be observed when IFN-γ responses were blocked. IFN-γ could inhibit mucus metaplasia even in the presence of high levels of Th2 cytokines, as was shown in studies of mixed Th1 and Th2 inflammation, in which there was partial inhibition of mucus metaplasia. Thus, IFN-γ inhibited mucus by inhibiting an IL-13-dependent pathway.

The molecular mechanisms by which IFN-γ inhibits mucus are not currently defined. IFN-γ was shown to inhibit IL-4-induced Stat6 phosphorylation and to increase the decay of IL-4-induced genes in cultured airway epithelial cells [68]. This indicates IFN-γ inhibits Th2-induced responses in epithelial cells through multiple pathways. IFN-γ also promotes resolution of mucus metaplasia. Following a Th2 inflammatory response in which mucus metaplasia was induced, IFN-γ stimulated goblet cell apoptosis via Bax-and caspase-dependent mechanisms [69, 70]. Thus, IFN-γ appears to have dual roles in the inhibition of goblet cell development and loss. This carefully regulated process of limiting mucus suggests that excess mucus hinders Th1 immunity, but such an effect has not been shown.

Therapy for Mucus Hypersecretion

Mucus hypersecretion in asthma results from persistent Th2 inflammation. This immune response appears to serve no positive function and only leads to pathology. Thus, blockade of excess mucus should improve patient symptoms without untoward consequences. Inhaled steroids are often sufficient to quell both inflammation and mucus production in asthma, but the effects may take days to be fully active. In patients controlled on inhaled steroids there is often a swift increase in mucus production during an exacerbation of the disease. Chronic mucus production is common in poorly controlled severe asthmatics. Inhibitors of IL-13, TNF-α, EGFR, and PKC offer potential new solutions to control mucus. Given the morbidity associated with mucus hyperproduction in asthma, it will be important to define how these new therapies influence goblet cell metaplasia and mucus secretion.

Acknowledgements The author would like to thank Dr. Robert Homer for contribution to the figures.

References

1. Osler W (1901) Principles and Practice of Medicine. New York: D. Appleton. pp. 628–629.
2. Huber HC, and Kossler, KK (1922) The pathology of bronchial asthma. Arch Int Med 30:689–760.

3. Hogg JC, Macklem, PT, and Thurlbeck, WM (1968) Site and nature of airway obstruction in chronic obstructive lung disease. N Engl J Med 278:1355–1360.

4. Moreno RH, Hogg, JC, and Pare, PD (1986) Mechanics of airway narrowing. Am Rev Respir Dis 133:1171–1180.

5. James A, and Carroll, N (1995) Theoretical effects of mucus gland discharge on airway resistance in asthma. Chest 107:110S.

6. Rose MC, and Voynow, JA (2006) Respiratory tract mucin genes and mucin glycoproteins in health and disease. Physiol Rev 86:245–278.

7. Perez-Vilar J (2007) Mucin granule intraluminal organization. Am J Respir Cell Mol Biol 36:183–190.

8. Groneberg DA, Eynott, PR, Lim, S, Oates, T, Wu, R, Carlstedt, I, Roberts, P, McCann, B, Nicholson, AG, Harrison, BD, et al. (2002) Expression of respiratory mucins in fatal status asthmaticus and mild asthma. Histopathology 40:367–373.

9. Ordonez CL, Khashayar, R, Wong, HH, Ferrando, R, Wu, R, Hyde, DM, Hotchkiss, JA, Zhang, Y, Novikov, A, Dolganov, G, et al. (2001) Mild and moderate asthma is associated with airway goblet cell hyperplasia and abnormalities in mucin gene expression. Am J Respir Crit Care Med 163:517–523.

10. Rogers DF (2004) Airway mucus hypersecretion in asthma: an undervalued pathology? Curr Opin Pharmacol 4:241–250.

11. Martin LD, Rochelle, LG, Fischer, BM, Krunkosky, TM, and Adler, KB (1997) Airway epithelium as an effector of inflammation: molecular regulation of secondary mediators. Eur Respir J 10:2139–2146.

12. Li Y, Martin, LD, Spizz, G, and Adler, KB (2001) MARCKS protein is a key molecule regulating mucin secretion by human airway epithelial cells in vitro. J Biol Chem 276:40982–40990.

13. Singer M, Martin, LD, Vargaftig, BB, Park, J, Gruber, AD, Li, Y, and Adler, KB (2004) A MARCKS-related peptide blocks mucus hypersecretion in a mouse model of asthma. Nat Med 10:193–196.

14. Shimura S, Andoh, Y, Haraguchi, M, and Shirato, K (1996) Continuity of airway goblet cells and intraluminal mucus in the airways of patients with bronchial asthma. Eur Respir J 9:1395–1401.

15. Aikawa T, Shimura, S, Sasaki, H, Ebina, M, and Takishima, T (1992) Marked goblet cell hyperplasia with mucus accumulation in the airways of patients who died of severe acute asthma attack. Chest 101:916–921.

16. Carroll NG, Mutavdzic, S, and James, AL (2002) Increased mast cells and neutrophils in submucosal mucous glands and mucus plugging in patients with asthma. Thorax 57:677–682.

17. Reader JR, Tepper, JS, Schelegle, ES, Aldrich, MC, Putney, LF, Pfeiffer, JW, and Hyde, DM (2003) Pathogenesis of mucous cell metaplasia in a murine asthma model. Am J Pathol 162:2069–2078.

18. Tyner JW, Kim, EY, Ide, K, Pelletier, MR, Roswit, WT, Morton, JD, Bataile, JT, Patel, AC, Patterson, A, Castro, M, et al. (2006) Blocking airway mucous cell metaplasia by inhibiting EGFR anti-apoptosis and IL-13 transdifferentiation signals. J Clin Invest 116:309–321.

19. Evans CM, Williams, OW, Tuvim, MJ, Nigam, R, Mixides, GP, Blackburn, MR, DeMayo, FJ, Burns, AR, Smith, C, Reynolds, SD, et al. (2004) Mucin is produced by clara cells in the proximal airways of antigen-challenged mice. Am J Respir Cell Mol Biol 31:382–394.

20. Hayashi T, Ishii, A, Nakai, S, and Hasegawa, K (2004) Ultrastructure of goblet-cell metaplasia from Clara cell in the allergic asthmatic airway inflammation in a mouse model of asthma in vivo. Virchows Arch 444:66–73.

21. Ollerenshaw S, and Woolcock, AJ (1992) Characteristics of the inflammation in biopsies from large airways of subjects with asthma and subjects with chronic airflow limitation. Am Rev Respir Dis 145:922–927.

22. Bentley AM, Meng, Q, Robinson, DS, Hamid, Q, Kay, AB, and Durham, SR (1993) Increases in activated T lymphocytes, eosinophils, and cytokine mRNA expression for interleukin-5 and

granulocyte/macrophage colony-stimulating factor in bronchial biopsies after allergen inhalation challenge in atopic asthmatics. Am J Respir Cell Mol Biol 8:35–42.

23. Robinson DS, Hamid, Q, Ying, S, Tsicopoulos, A, Barkans, J, Bentley, AM, Corrigan, C, Durham, SR, and Kay, AB (1992) Predominant TH2-like bronchoalveolar T-lymphocyte population in atopic asthma. New Engl J Med 326:298–304.

24. Cohn L, Elias, JA, and Chupp, GL (2004) Asthma: mechanisms of disease persistence and progression. Annu Rev Immunol 22:789–815.

25. Bradley BL, Azzawi, M, Jacobson, M, Assoufi, B, Collins, JV, Irani, AM, Schwartz, LB, Durham, SR, Jeffery, PK, and Kay, AB (1991) Eosinophils, T-lymphocytes, mast cells, neutrophils, and macrophages in bronchial biopsy specimens from atopic subjects with asthma: comparison with biopsy specimens from atopic subjects without asthma and normal control subjects and relationship to bronchial hyperresponsiveness. J Allergy Clin Immunol 88:661–674.

26. Tanizaki Y, Kitani, H, Okazaki, M, Mifune, T, Mitsunobu, F, and Kimura, I (1993) Mucus hypersecretion and eosinophils in bronchoalveolar lavage fluid in adult patients with bronchial asthma. J Asthma 30:257–262.

27. Cohn L, Homer, RJ, Marinov, A, Rankin, J, and Bottomly, K (1997) Induction of airway mucus production By T helper 2 (Th2) cells: a critical role for interleukin 4 in cell recruitment but not mucus production. J Exp Med 186:1737–1747.

28. Corry DB, Folkesson, HG, Warnock, ML, Erle, DJ, Matthay, MA, Wiener-Kronish, JP, and Locksley, RM (1996) Interleukin 4, but not interleukin 5 or eosinophils, is required in a murine model of acute airway hyperreactivity [see comments] [published erratum appears in J Exp Med 1997 May 5;185(9):1715]. J Exp Med 183:109–117.

29. Gavett SH, Chen, X, Finkelman, F, and Wills-Karp, M (1994) Depletion of murine CD4 + T lymphocytes prevents antigen-induced airway hyperreactivity and pulmonary eosinophilia. Am J Respir Cell Mol Biol 10:587–593.

30. Lee JJ, McGarry, MP, Farmer, SC, Denzler, KL, Larson, KA, Carrigan, PE, Brenneise, IE, Horton, MA, Haczku, A, Gelfand, EW, et al. (1997) Interleukin-5 expression in the lung epithelium of transgenic mice leads to pulmonary changes pathognomonic of asthma. J Exp Med 185:2143–2156.

31. Rankin JA, Picarella, DE, Geba, GP, Temann, A, Prasad, B, DiCosimo, B, Tarallo, A, Stripp, B, Whitsett, J, and Flavell, RA (1996) Phenotypic and physiologic characterization of transgenic mice expressing interleukin 4 in the lung: lymphocytic and eosinophilic inflammation without airway hyperreactivity. Proc Nat Acad Sci U S A 93:7821–7825.

32. Zhu Z, Homer, R, Wang, Z, Chen, Q, Geba, G, Wang, J, Zhang, Y, and Elias, J (1999) Transgenic expression of IL-13 in murine lung causes airway inflammation, mucus hypersecretion, subendothelial fibrosis, eotaxin production and airways hyperresponsiveness to methacholine. J Clin Invest 103:779–788.

33. Temann UA, Prasad, B, Gallup, MW, Basbaum, C, Ho, SB, Flavell, RA, and Rankin, JA (1997) A novel role for murine IL-4 in vivo: induction of MUC5AC gene expression and mucin hypersecretion. Am J Respir Cell Mol Biol 16:471–478.

34. Humbles AA, Lloyd, CM, McMillan, SJ, Friend, DS, Xanthou, G, McKenna, EE, Ghiran, S, Gerard, NP, Yu, C, Orkin, SH, et al. (2004) A critical role for eosinophils in allergic airways remodeling. Science 305:1776–1779.

35. Lee JJ, Dimina, D, Macias, MP, Ochkur, SI, McGarry, MP, O'Neill, KR, Protheroe, C, Pero, R, Nguyen, T, Cormier, SA, et al. (2004) Defining a link with asthma in mice congenitally deficient in eosinophils. Science 305:1773–1776.

36. Cohn L, Homer, RJ, MacLeod, H, Mohrs, M, Brombacher, F, and Bottomly, K (1999) Th2-induced airway mucus production is dependent on IL-4Ralpha, but not on eosinophils. J Immunol 162:6178–6183.

37. Grunig G, Warnock, M, Wakil, AE, Venkayya, R, Brombacher, F, Rennick, DM, Sheppard, D, Mohrs, M, Donaldson, DD, Locksley, RM, et al. (1998) Requirement for IL-13 independently of IL-4 in experimental asthma [see comments]. Science 282:2261–2263.

38. Wills-Karp M, Luyimbazi, J, Xu, X, Schofield, B, Neben, TY, Karp, CL, and Donaldson, DD (1998) Interleukin-13: central mediator of allergic asthma. Science 282:2258–2261.
39. Whittaker L, Niu, N, Temann, UA, Stoddard, A, Flavell, RA, Ray, A, Homer, RJ, and Cohn, L (2002) Interleukin-13 mediates a fundamental pathway for airway epithelial mucus induced by CD4 T cells and interleukin-9. Am J Respir Cell Mol Biol 27:593–602.
40. Mattes J, Yang, M, Siqueira, A, Clark, K, MacKenzie, J, McKenzie, AN, Webb, DC, Matthaei, KI, and Foster, PS (2001) IL-13 induces airways hyperreactivity independently of the IL-4R alpha chain in the allergic lung. J Immunol 167:1683–1692.
41. Walter DM, McIntire, JJ, Berry, G, McKenzie, AN, Donaldson, DD, DeKruyff, RH, and Umetsu, DT (2001) Critical role for IL-13 in the development of allergen-induced airway hyperreactivity. J Immunol 167:4668–4675.
42. Justice JP, Crosby, J, Borchers, MT, Tomkinson, A, Lee, JJ, and Lee, NA (2002) CD4(+) T cell-dependent airway mucus production occurs in response to IL-5 expression in lung. Am J Physiol Lung Cell Mol Physiol 282:L1066–L1074.
43. Temann UA, Ray, P, and Flavell, RA (2002) Pulmonary overexpression of IL-9 induces Th2 cytokine expression, leading to immune pathology. J Clin Invest 109:29–39.
44. Temann UA, Laouar, Y, Eynon, EE, Homer, R, and Flavell, RA (2007) IL9 leads to airway inflammation by inducing IL13 expression in airway epithelial cells. Int Immunol 19:1–10.
45. Kuperman DA, Huang, X, Nguyenvu, L, Holscher, C, Brombacher, F, and Erle, DJ (2005) IL-4 receptor signaling in Clara cells is required for allergen-induced mucus production. J Immunol 175:3746–3752.
46. Kuperman DA, Huang, X, Koth, LL, Chang, GH, Dolganov, GM, Zhu, Z, Elias, JA, Sheppard, D, and Erle, DJ (2002) Direct effects of interleukin-13 on epithelial cells cause airway hyperreactivity and mucus overproduction in asthma. Nat Med 8:885–889.
47. Atherton HC, Jones, G, and Danahay, H (2003) IL-13-induced changes in the goblet cell density of human bronchial epithelial cell cultures: MAP kinase and phosphatidylinositol 3-kinase regulation. Am J Physiol Lung Cell Mol Physiol 285:L730–L739.
48. Dabbagh K, Takeyama, K, Lee, HM, Ueki, IF, Lausier, JA, and Nadel, JA (1999) IL-4 induces mucin gene expression and goblet cell metaplasia In vitro and In vivo [in process citation]. J Immunol 162:6233–6237.
49. Kondo M, Tamaoki, J, Takeyama, K, Isono, K, Kawatani, K, Izumo, T, and Nagai, A (2006) Elimination of IL-13 reverses established goblet cell metaplasia into ciliated epithelia in airway epithelial cell culture. Allergol Int 55:329–336.
50. Hackel PO, Zwick, E, Prenzel, N, and Ullrich, A (1999) Epidermal growth factor receptors: critical mediators of multiple receptor pathways. Curr Opin Cell Biol 11:184–189.
51. Burgel PR, and Nadel, JA (2004) Roles of epidermal growth factor receptor activation in epithelial cell repair and mucin production in airway epithelium. Thorax 59:992–996.
52. Takeyama K, Dabbagh, K, Jeong Shim, J, Dao-Pick, T, Ueki, IF, and Nadel, JA (2000) Oxidative stress causes mucin synthesis via transactivation of epidermal growth factor receptor: role of neutrophils. J Immunol 164:1546–1552.
53. Takeyama K, Dabbagh, K, Lee, HM, Agusti, C, Lausier, JA, Ueki, IF, Grattan, KM, and Nadel, JA (1999) Epidermal growth factor system regulates mucin production in airways. Proc Natl Acad Sci U S A 96:3081–3086.
54. Takeyama K, Fahy, JV, and Nadel, JA (2001) Relationship of epidermal growth factor receptors to goblet cell production in human bronchi. Am J Respir Crit Care Med 163:511–516.
55. Zhen G, Park, SW, Nguyenvu, LT, Rodriguez, MW, Barbeau, R, Paquet, AC, and Erle, DJ (2007) IL-13 and epidermal growth factor receptor have critical but distinct roles in epithelial cell mucin production. Am J Respir Cell Mol Biol 36:244–253.
56. Danahay H, Atherton, H, Jones, G, Bridges, RJ, and Poll, CT (2002) Interleukin-13 induces a hypersecretory ion transport phenotype in human bronchial epithelial cells. Am J Physiol Lung Cell Mol Physiol 282:L226–L236.
57. Kouznetsova I, Chwieralski, CE, Balder, R, Hinz, M, Braun, A, Krug, N, and Hoffmann, W (2007) Induced trefoil factor family 1 expression by trans-differentiating Clara cells in a murine asthma model. Am J Respir Cell Mol Biol 36:286–295.

58. Yasuo M, Fujimoto, K, Tanabe, T, Yaegashi, H, Tsushima, K, Takasuna, K, Koike, T, Yamaya, M, and Nikaido, T (2006) Relationship between calcium-activated chloride channel 1 and MUC5AC in goblet cell hyperplasia induced by interleukin-13 in human bronchial epithelial cells. Respiration 73:347–359.

59. Shim JJ, Dabbagh, K, Ueki, IF, Dao-Pick, T, Burgel, PR, Takeyama, K, Tam, DC, and Nadel, JA (2001) IL-13 induces mucin production by stimulating epidermal growth factor receptors and by activating neutrophils. Am J Physiol Lung Cell Mol Physiol 280:L134–L140.

60. Wan H, Kaestner, KH, Ang, SL, Ikegami, M, Finkelman, FD, Stahlman, MT, Fulkerson, PC, Rothenberg, ME, and Whitsett, JA (2004) Foxa2 regulates alveolarization and goblet cell hyperplasia. Development 131:953–964.

61. Wan H, Xu, Y, Ikegami, M, Stahlman, MT, Kaestner, KH, Ang, SL, and Whitsett, JA (2004) Foxa2 is required for transition to air breathing at birth. Proc Natl Acad Sci U S A 101:14449–14454.

62. Homer RJ, Zhu, Z, Cohn, L, Lee, CG, White, WI, Chen, S, and Elias, JA (2006) Differential expression of chitinases identify subsets of murine airway epithelial cells in allergic inflammation. Am J Physiol Lung Cell Mol Physiol 291:L502–L511.

63. Park KS, Korfhagen, TR, Bruno, MD, Kitzmiller, JA, Wan, H, Wert, SE, Khurana Hershey, GK, Chen, G, and Whitsett, JA (2007) SPDEF regulates goblet cell hyperplasia in the airway epithelium. J Clin Invest 117:978–988.

64. Whiting PJ (2003) The GABAA receptor gene family: new opportunities for drug development. Curr Opin Drug Discov Devel 6:648–657.

65. Xiang YY, Wang, S, Liu, M, Hirota, JA, Li, J, Ju, W, Fan, Y, Kelly, MM, Ye, B, Orser, B, et al. (2007) A GABAergic system in airway epithelium is essential for mucus overproduction in asthma. Nat Med 13:862–867.

66. Young HW, Williams, OW, Chandra, D, Bellinghausen, LK, Perez, G, Suarez, A, Tuvim, MJ, Roy, MG, Alexander, SN, Moghaddam, SJ, et al. (2007) Central role of Muc5ac expression in mucous metaplasia and its regulation by conserved 5' elements. Am J Respir Cell Mol Biol 37:273–290.

67. Cohn L, Homer, RJ, Niu, N, and Bottomly, K (1999) T helper 1 cells and interferon gamma regulate allergic airway inflammation and mucus production. J Exp Med 190:1309–1318.

68. Heller NM, Matsukura, S, Georas, SN, Boothby, MR, Rothman, PB, Stellato, C, and Schleimer, RP (2004) Interferon-gamma inhibits STAT6 signal transduction and gene expression in human airway epithelial cells. Am J Respir Cell Mol Biol 31:573–582.

69. Shi ZO, Fischer, MJ, De Sanctis, GT, Schuyler, MR, and Tesfaigzi, Y (2002) IFN-gamma, but not Fas, mediates reduction of allergen-induced mucous cell metaplasia by inducing apoptosis. J Immunol 168:4764–4771.

70. Tesfaigzi Y, Fischer, MJ, Daheshia, M, Green, FH, De Sanctis, GT, and Wilder, JA (2002) Bax is crucial for IFN-gamma-induced resolution of allergen-induced mucus cell metaplasia. J Immunol 169:5919–5925.

Mechanisms of Cough in Asthma
and Allergic Airway Disease

Kevin M. White, Michael S. Tankersley, and Pramod S. Kelkar

Introduction

Cough is a common symptom in medicine, accounting for the second most frequent reason for a visit to a physician in the United States behind only a "general medical examination" [1]. The allergist is uniquely suited to be comfortable with the evaluation of a patient with cough. Several diseases allergists evaluate and treat are manifested by the presence of a cough. In addition, diseases allergists treat (e.g. asthma and rhinitis) may be complicated by a cough from another diagnosis and allergists must have a methodical approach to such patients. Allergists also evaluate adults and children who have unique characteristics that must be individually considered in the evaluation of a chronic cough. This chapter aims to discuss the cough reflex, its association with various diseases of concern to the allergist, and an approach to the evaluation and treatment of the patient with a chronic cough.

Anatomy and Physiology of the Normal Cough Reflex

Cough is a respiratory reflex that clears secretions and foreign matter from the airway. The exact neuronal pathways are still under debate [2, 3]. The cough reflex is stimulated by neuronal receptors that have terminal fibers between ciliated cells of the respiratory epithelium. These sensory nerve fibers are located from the nasopharynx to the terminal bronchioles [4, 5]. Three principal neuronal subtypes of the vagus nerve are thought to be responsible for initiating the cough reflex arc: C-fibers, rapidly adapting stretch receptors, and slowly adapting stretch receptors [2, 6]. These neuronal subtypes differ based on myelination, conduction velocity, and response to mechanical or chemical stimulation.

K.M. White (✉) and M.S. Tankersley
Department of Allergy/Immunology, Wilford Hall Medical Center, 59th MDOS/SGO5A
2200 Bergquist Dr. Ste 1, Lackland AFB, TX 78236, USA

P.S. Kelkar
Allergy and Asthma Care, PA 12000 Elm Creek Blvd, #200, Maple Grove, MN 55369, USA

R. Pawankar et al. (eds.), *Allergy Frontiers: Clinical Manifestations*,   187
DOI: 10.1007/978-4-431-88317-3_12, © Springer 2009

Neuronal Receptors

C-fibers make up the majority of pulmonary vagal afferents. They have been found in lung parenchyma and in the airway wall [6]. They are unmyelinated, relatively insensitive to mechanical stimuli and quite sensitive to chemical stimuli such as capsaicin (the active chemical compound in chili peppers), and inflammatory mediators such as histamine, bradykinin, prostaglandins and substance P [6, 7]. The C-fiber response to capsaicin is mediated by the type 1 vanilloid receptor (transient receptor potential vanilloid-1 or TRPV-1) [8–10]. This is a recently described receptor that responds to noxious stimuli, including capsaicin and bradykinin [11]. Rapidly adapting stretch receptors (RARs) terminate predominantly beneath intrapulmonary airways [2, 12–14]. They are myelinated, conduct rapidly, and are stimulated primarily by changes in airway mechanical properties such as lung inflation and compliance [2, 13]. Thus, they may result in cough by mechanical stimulation, such as the probing of respiratory mucosa. Slowly adapting stretch receptors (SARs) are a neuronal subtype that terminate beneath the respiratory epithelium of the intrapulmonary airways [2]. Like RARs, SARs are myelinated, conduct rapidly, and are sensitive to mechanical forces. They are thought to be the fibers responsible for triggering expiration when the lungs are inflated [15]. Activation of the SARs thus leads to central inhibition of respiration. Animal research suggests that inhibition of SAR activity may decrease cough [16].

Stimulation for the cough reflex can occur outside of the airway. The auricular branch of the vagus nerve (Arnold's nerve) innervates the external auditory meatus and stimulation (by hair, cerumen, foreign body, or tumor) may result in a cough [17]. A distal tracheo-esophageal reflex has also been demonstrated in patients with chronic cough from gastroesophageal reflux disease (GERD) [18]. This reflex is thought to be vagally mediated as with other cough reflexes [19] and likely connects to the afferent fibers previously discussed.

Central Pathways

Extra- and intrathoracic vagal afferent fibers terminate primarily in the nucleus of the solitary tract located in the brainstem [7]. There are separate termination regions within the brainstem for each of the major afferent neuronal subtypes mentioned above. An efferent signal is generated that travels down the vagus, phrenic, and spinal motor nerves to expiratory muscles to produce cough. The signal results in closure of the vocal cords, followed by the build up of intrathoracic pressure, then a release of high velocity expiratory air. Vigorous coughing can generate intrathoracic pressures of up to 300 mmHg and expiratory air velocity of 500 miles an hour [20]. Central control of the cough reflex is demonstrated by voluntary suppression of cough, similar in concept to the voluntary control over urination.

The Cough Reflex: Clinical Considerations

Several general comments can be made about factors that affect the cough reflex. Adult women have a more sensitive cough reflex when assessed by capsaicin challenge [21, 22] whereas in children, this gender difference does not exist [23]. There is no ethnic difference in cough sensitivity between Caucasians, Indians (from the Indian subcontinent) and Chinese [22]. Children have been demonstrated to have a change in cough reflex as they age [23]. Common causes of acute cough such as upper respiratory infections (URIs) have been shown to be associated with increased cough sensitivity when assessed with capsaicin [24–26]. As an important iatrogenic cause of chronic cough, ACE inhibitors increase the sensitivity of the cough reflex [27, 28].

Studies have demonstrated increased cough sensitivity in patients with chronic cough from a variety of causes when compared to normal controls. The mechanism for most causes is attributed to airway inflammation. Recent data indicates that the airways of patients with chronic cough of undetermined etiology may have a similar histologic appearance to patients with known etiology [20]. In patients with chronic cough, whether airway inflammation precedes the cough or the cough precedes airway inflammation is not known.

Cough and Allergic Disease

Post Nasal Drip Syndrome/Upper Airway Cough Syndrome

In 2006, the ACCP proposed a change in terminology from post-nasal drip syndrome to upper airway cough syndrome (UACS). UACS encompasses many diagnoses in the upper respiratory tract, including allergic rhinitis, non-allergic rhinitis, post-infectious (post-viral) cough, sinusitis, and anatomic abnormalities of the nose and sinuses. All of these diagnoses are a potential cause of mucosal secretions that drain into the posterior pharynx [29, 30]. In most studies of referral patient with cough, UACS is common, occurring in up to 87% of patients [31] and often between 20% to 40% [29, 30, 32, 33]. In the study of UACS and cough, there has often not been a clinical differentiation between allergic and non-allergic rhinitis [24, 25, 29] and allergic rhinitis as a subset of UACS is rare when reported [28]. When specifically studied, there is evidence both for [24, 35, 36], and against [37, 38], increased cough sensitivity in patients with allergic rhinitis.

Asthma

Asthma is characterized by chronic and/or recurrent respiratory symptoms associated with reversible airflow obstruction and airway inflammation. One of the cardinal symptoms is cough. Cough in asthma is thought to be caused by stimulation of airway sensory nerves by inflammation [6]. Patients with both asthma and chronic obstructive pulmonary disease (COPD) have been shown to have a heightened cough sensitivity when compared to controls [39]. Patients have an increased cough sensitivity even when their asthma is well controlled [40, 41]. Chronic cough was first reported to be a sole manifestation of asthma in 1979 by Corrao et al [42]. There have since been several reports of similar clinical presentations [29, 30]. Cough-variant asthma accounts for 24–29% of diagnoses for chronic cough in adult nonsmokers when assessed in referral populations [30–32]. Cough-variant asthma has been reported in children [43–46], however, the majority of children with isolated chronic cough have not been found to have asthma [47].

Eosinophilic Bronchitis

Eosinophilic bronchitis is a recently described pulmonary entity [48] found in a subset of patients with chronic cough. It has two important similarities with asthma: the presence of an eosinophilic airway infiltrate and its response to corticosteroid treatment. It causes chronic cough without evidence of variable airflow obstruction or bronchial hyperreactivity. Like asthma patients eosinophilic bronchitis patients have basement membrane thickening and elevated levels of exhaled nitric oxide reflective of airway eosinophilia [49]. By definition patients have sputum eosinophilia >3% [50]. This diagnosis has not been described in children [47]. It has been reported to account for 10–13% [51, 52] and up to 30% [53] of patients being evaluated in a referral center for chronic cough. A similar entity called atopic cough has been reported in Japan [54]. It shares the clinical characteristics of chronic nonproductive cough, sputum eosinophilia, and lack of bronchial hyperresponsiveness. In contrast to eosinophilic bronchitis, atopic cough has eosinophilia only in the upper airway and may not respond to inhaled corticoseroids [55].

The relation, if any, of eosinophilic bronchitis to asthma is not known. In a series of 52 patients followed for at least 1 year (follow-up was available for only 32), 3 (9%) developed asthma, 5 (16%) developed fixed airflow obstruction without asthma, and 21 (66%) had persistent symptoms [56]. In a series of 82 patients with atopic cough followed for a median of 4.8 years, only one developed asthma [55].

Gastroesophageal Reflux Disease

Gastroesophageal reflux disease (GERD) is the passage of acidic contents into the esophagus through the lower esophageal sphincter causing a variety of symptoms. GERD occurs in approximately 25% of Western populations [57] and has several extraesophageal manifestations that are of interest to the allergist. These include cough, wheeze, hoarseness, throat clearing and globus sensation. GERD is an important disease in patients with asthma. Asthmatics have been shown to have significantly decreased lower esophageal sphincter pressures and more frequent reflux episodes when compared to controls [58]. When interviewed, asthmatics report a higher prevalence of reflux symptoms – 71% complained of "heartburn" compared to 51% of controls in one study [59]. GERD has been demonstrated to be one of the most common causes of chronic cough in adults accounting for 10–25% of cases [29–33, 60]. In children, studies have shown that GERD is an uncommon cause of chronic cough [61] and has been more difficult to prove as the cause of cough [47].

The mechanism for GERD causing chronic cough is not known with certainty. Microaspiration from proximal esophageal reflux has been suspected as a mechanism, but has not been consistently demonstrated using distal and proximal pH probes in patients with chronic cough [62, 63]. A significant number of patients with GERD and associated chronic cough have no gastroesophageal symptoms [19] and some patients only have gastroesophageal symptoms after developing chronic cough [64]. Chronic cough may occur in the presence of non-acid refluxate [65–67].

Laryngopharyngeal Reflux

Laryngopharyngeal reflux (LPR) is the presence of gastric refluxate past the upper esophageal sphincter into the laryngopharynx causing inflammation. Symptoms often include hoarseness, throat clearing, globus sensation, and cough. It is suspected when the patient has hoarseness as part of their presenting symptoms, when inflammation is visualized in the posterior larynx with endoscopy and confirmed when medical treatment of reflux is successful in ameliorating symptoms. Dual pH probe may not be as helpful for diagnosing LPR as for GERD, there may be a role for esophageal impedance monitoring in assessing difficult cases [68]. LPR is initially approached and treated similarly to cough from GERD [69–72].

Idiopathic Cough

There is a distinct group of patients noted among cough referral clinics for which a diagnosis is not found. These patients are often perimenopausal females whose cough followed anURI and during a recent review it was hypothesized that there may be a hormonal influence on the cough reflex [73]. As more causes of chronic cough are discovered, such as eosinophilic bronchitis and non-acid GERD, the number of patients with idiopathic cough may decrease.

Evaluation of Patients with Chronic Cough

Adults

Multiple studies over the last 25 years have established that the three most common causes of chronic cough in a referral population of adults are UACS, cough-variant asthma, and GERD [29–33, 60]. These diagnoses each account for approximately 25% of cases, however up to 60% of patients may have multiple causes for their cough [33]. Most studies on chronic cough examined the adult patient with a chronic unexplained non-productive cough. They were immunocompetent nonsmokers (usually) with normal chest radiographs and normal baseline spirometry. If patients had sputum production [33] or abnormal chest radiograph findings [60], they were more likely to have structural lung disease, but they were still *more* likely to have those top three diagnoses accounting for their cough.

Determining where to start in the evaluation of chronic cough can be difficult. Clinical signs and symptoms for common diseases mentioned above may be absent or misleading [34]. In the adult with chronic cough, "ruling out" a diagnosis usually requires empiric therapy or some level of investigation. Table 1 lists the most common diagnoses for chronic cough in the adult. An extensive list of all disorders that can cause chronic cough in adults is beyond the scope of this review. This section will focus on the evaluation of chronic cough in the population that is likely to be referred to an allergist.

When the clinician approaches the adult with chronic cough, it is important to systematically evaluate for the common causes of cough mentioned above. Clinical findings may be minimal and it is imperative to use empiric treatment as a diagnostic tool. If the patient is immunocompromised, infectious causes and malignancy should be evaluated for as well as the common causes of cough. The clinician

Table 1 Common causes of chronic cough in adults

Cough-variant asthma
UACS
Allergic rhinitis
Non-allergic rhinitis (e.g. vasomotor rhinitis)
Chronic sinusitis
Post-infectious cough
GERD
LPR
Eosinophilic bronchitis
Tobacco use
Environmental/occupational exposure
ACE inhibitor use
Chronic bronchitis

UACS, upper airway cough syndrome; GERD, gastroesophageal reflux disease; LPR, laryngopharyngeal reflux

needs to elicit a clinical symptom or finding that will give them a starting point for the evaluation. Examples may be post nasal drip (UACS), a feeling of distaste in the mouth after meals (GERD/LPR) or coughing with exercise (asthma). Two common exacerbating factors for cough are tobacco smoke and ACE inhibitors. Tobacco smoke increases the prevalence of cough [74] and smoking cessation leads to short term increase in cough reflex sensitivity [75]. ACE inhibitors have been associated with cough in prospective studies in up to 3% of patients [76], and angiotensin receptor blockers are equivalent therapeutically in many cases without the associated risk of cough. Post-infectious cough should be suspected when an URI precedes the cough, is often self-limited, and can be treated as UACS. Chronic sputum production raises the likelihood of chronic bronchitis or bronchiectasis. The physical exam should focus on all aspects of the cardiopulmonary system and should include evaluating for nasal polyps, drainage in the posterior pharynx, and pulmonary abnormalities such as wheezing, rales, and fine crackles in the bases that may indicate fibrotic lung disease. Rhinoscopy may reveal anatomic obstruction, tumor, nasal polyps, or edema of the vocal cords and posterior pharynx in patients with LPR [68]. Spirometry is recommended for all patients to assess for obstructive lung disease. If obstruction is seen, reversibility should be assessed by administering a bronchodilator. It is recommended to obtain a baseline chest radiograph in adults presenting for evaluation of chronic cough to assess for parenchymal disease or anatomic causes of cough. In adults where the suspicion for malignancy is higher, for example in a chronic tobacco smoker or immunocompromised patient, chest computed tomography (CT) may be warranted due to the superiority of CT in evaluating for early cancerous lesions [77].

If there is evidence from the initial evaluation that the patient may have UACS or GERD, empiric treatment should be given (see treatment section). If there is suspicion that the patient may have asthma, then a methacholine challenge may be performed if the patient did not have reversibility on spirometry. Appropriate treatment for asthma should be given if the methacholine challenge is positive. If the methacholine challenge is negative, asthma is unlikely, however the patient may still respond to an inhaled steroid for the treatment of eosinophilic bronchitis. If sputum evaluation for eosinophils (>3%) is unavailable, then the presumptive diagnosis of eosinophilic bronchitis is made with resolution of cough with inhaled steroid in a patient without bronchial hyperreactivity.

If the history and physical examination are unrevealing, it is recommended to treat empirically for UACS first. If unsuccessful, then evaluate for asthma with a methacholine challenge. If unrevealing, treat empirically for eosinophilic bronchitis. If still unsuccessful then treat empirically for GERD. If there is an incomplete clinical response during any step of the evaluation, that treatment should be continued and the evaluation continued as many patients will have more than one cause for cough. As the clinician follows this empiric treatment pathway a few items are worth noting. If treatment for symptomatic UACS is undertaken and incompletely successful, consideration should be given to chronic sinusitis or anatomic obstruction, and a sinus CT scan entertained to evaluate further. If treatment for symptomatic or asymptomatic GERD is undertaken and unsuccessful, and there is no other elicited cause for the chronic cough, then consideration should be given to a gastroenterology referral for further evaluation (e.g. a 24 h pH probe, esophageal endoscopy, or impedance testing if indicated). The treatment section of the text discusses specific treatments and duration of therapy for each diagnosis.

Children

The pediatric aspects of this guideline apply to patients <14 years of age in accordance with ACCP recommendations [47]. After this age, adult guidelines are more applicable. In children, there are fewer studies on chronic cough in general, and there is less evidence of an association with upper airway disease, asthma, and GERD [47, 78]. In children, empiric treatment for such entities should be limited because these entities are less common and the treatment may incur more side effects than with adults [79] including case reports of deaths in young children from cough medications [80].

For the clinician evaluating a child with chronic cough, often the predominant question is whether the child has asthma as the cause. This section will address some of the differences in children with chronic cough, and will focus on evaluating children with cough for allergic disease. A well-written review addresses the wide differential diagnosis of pediatric chronic cough and should be referenced if other diagnoses are considered [47].

One of the significant differences between children and adults is in the annual incidence of viral URIs. Children on average have three to six URIs per year whereas adults average two [81]. Up to 10% of children have cough 3 weeks after a URI [82, 83]. Another important consideration in evaluating the child with a chronic cough is how much coughing is normal or expected. Healthy children have been noted to cough on average of 11.3 times in 24 h when recorded [84]. Children with stable mild asthma have been reported to average 25.5 coughing episodes in a 24 h period [41].

Few prospective studies have looked at the etiology of chronic cough in children. A major difficulty in studying children is that disease prevalence varies with age. In a prospective study of 72 children with chronic cough, the most common causes in patients 0–18 months were aberrant innominate artery (28%), GERD (28%) and cough-variant asthma (25%). From 18 months to 6 years of age the most common causes were sinusitis (50%) and cough-variant asthma (27%). From 6 to 18 years of age the most common causes were cough variant asthma (45%), followed by psychogenic cough (32%) and sinusitis (27%). The diagnosis of cough variant asthma was made in these children by improvement of symptoms with bronchodilator or reversibility on spirometry [45]. In contrast to this study, a recent prospective cohort of 108 children (median age 2.6 years) evaluated in a referral center with >3 weeks of cough (median 6 months), a final diagnosis was obtained in 90.8% of patients [61]. In this study, persistent bacterial bronchitis was found in 43 patients (39.8%), bronchiectasis in 5%, and asthma in 4%. Twenty-two percent resolved without therapy. This study used an algorithm recommended for adults [85] and concluded that children require a more age-applicable diagnostic approach.

The main consideration for the allergist in evaluating children with chronic cough is the presence of asthma. As diagnostic methods are more limited in children, e.g. spirometry may not be feasible at a young age, the clinician must rely on patient and parental history as well as studies of outcomes of children with chronic cough. In a study of 127 preschoolers with recurrent cough followed for 3 years, 56% became symptom free, 7.2% developed wheeze and 36.8% reported persistent cough. The patients with chronic cough were no more likely to be atopic than controls, and had almost half the prevalence of atopy than children who wheezed (24–27% versus 44% respectively) [86]. This is in agreement with other studies that have shown that most children with chronic isolated cough improve when followed over time [87]. Nocturnal cough is often attributed to asthma, however, in a questionnaire study of 5,321 children with nocturnal cough followed for 2 years, children with cough were no more likely than controls to be diagnosed with asthma over time [88]. An evaluation of 607 children with persistent nocturnal cough found that the presence of a nocturnal cough alone was a poor predictor of the presence of asthma [89]. These studies found that in a child with cough, without atopy they were not more likely to have asthma than controls.

Another method of evaluating a child with chronic cough for asthma who is unable to perform spirometry is to prescribe an empiric trial of inhaled steroids. Two randomized double-blind placebo controlled studies have examined the utility of this approach. A randomized, double-blind, placebo-controlled study in 43 pediatric patients with chronic cough found that 70% of those on beclomethasone diproprionate 200 µg twice daily for 4–5 weeks had improvement in cough frequency but so did 45% of those given placebo [90]. Another randomized, double-blind, placebo-controlled study evaluated a group of pediatric patients with chronic nocturnal cough and found that 71% of patients with high dose inhaled fluticasone improved after 2 weeks compared to 35% in the placebo group [91]. These studies underscore the high rate of improvement with placebo. Even if patients improve with therapy, many children with chronic cough simply improve with time. If considered, it is recommended to give a trial of moderate dose inhaled steroids for 2–4 weeks to assess for clinical response. If the child responds, the inhaled steroid should be stopped to observe the cough reappearance to confirm the effect. It is important to realize when giving a trial of inhaled steroids that if the child does not respond, it is likely that the reason they failed is that they do not have the diagnosis of asthma rather than they did not receive a high enough dose of inhaled steroid. Reconsideration of the differential diagnosis is appropriate at this point.

Treatment of Chronic Cough

In this section comments will be made on the treatment of UACS, asthma, eosinophilic bronchitis, and GERD. As there have been no randomized studies in children on the treatment of these three entities with respect to cough, extrapolation will be necessary, when appropriate, from adult data.

UACS

The regimen that has been used with success in adults for undifferentiated rhinitis causing post-nasal drainage has been the combination of a first-generation antihistamine with a long-acting decongestant. In several studies the antihistamine utilized has been dexbrompheniramine maleate [29, 30]. Azatadine has also been used [31]. Cough may start to improve in 1 week [31] but often take 7–10 weeks for full resolution [30, 31]. In most studies, if the initial treatment with the combination mentioned above is unsuccessful or partially successful, a trial of therapy for chronic sinusitis was undertaken, usually with a topical decongestant (e.g. a short course of oxymetazoline), often nasal steroids and occasionally empiric antibiotics for sinusitis.

Second-generation antihistamines have yielded limited and conflicting results in the treatment of chronic cough. Loratadine demonstrated reduction in cough in a small randomized double-blind crossover study of patients with unexplained cough [92], but fexofenadine was not found to decrease cough sensitivity in patients with a URI assessed with capsaicin [93]. Intranasal steroids have been evaluated specifically for cough by one large randomized double-blind placebo-controlled study and shown to decrease cough scores compared to placebo [94].

Asthma/Cough-Variant Asthma

Diagnostic and therapeutic trials for asthma have ranged from using a beta-agonist regularly for 1–2 weeks to see if it improves symptoms to a week of oral steroids at 1 mg/kg. If either is successful, inhaled glucocorticoids are then given to control symptoms. A reasonable approach is to prescribe a moderate to high dose inhaled glucocorticoid for 1 month and then reassess the diagnostic and/or therapeutic goal.

Eosinophilic Bronchitis

Eosinophilic bronchitis responds to medium dosed inhaled steroids [52, 95, 96]. The treatment should be viewed as similar to the treatment of asthma.

GERD

Randomized placebo-controlled blinded trials of twice-daily omeprazole at 40 mg in patients with cough have demonstrated benefit as soon as 2 weeks [97] but it may take up to 8 weeks for benefit [98]. A retrospective analysis of patients with chronic cough due either solely or partially to GERD found that once daily PPI therapy with or without the addition of a prokinetic was successful in 44 (79%) out of 56 patients [99]. These studies suggest 2–8 weeks of a moderate to high dose PPI up to twice daily as a therapeutic/diagnostic trial. If no benefit is seen from two PPIs for at least total of 8 weeks or from the addition of an antimotility agent to a PPI for total of 8 weeks of treatment, then the physician should either consider alternative diagnoses or seek assistance from gastroenterology. Further investigations then should include pH monitoring and possible impedance monitoring if clinically applicable. It is important to stress the importance of taking the PPI correctly – e.g. taking it 30 min prior to meals for maximum efficacy.

In children, there are no randomized controlled trials regarding the use of PPIs in the treatment of chronic cough. As this diagnosis is not as well substantiated as the cause of isolated cough in children, there is no uniform approach other than considering the data presented for adults. Guidelines exist in the diagnosis and treatment of GERD in children, which can be referenced if this diagnosis is considered [100].

Conclusion

Chronic cough is associated with an increase in cough reflex sensitivity, thought to be from airway inflammation. Chronic cough may be the main symptom of allergic disease or may be from a confounding diagnosis in a patient with allergic rhinitis or asthma. There is a wealth of evidence that UACS, asthma, and GERD are the most common causes of chronic cough in the adult population and should be evaluated and empirically treated in a stepwise fashion in order to identify the correct diagnosis. When approaching the child with chronic cough, the clinician should keep in mind that an isolated cough does not necessarily make the diagnosis of asthma more likely than in children without cough. If a trial of inhaled steroids fails to control the cough in a child, other diagnoses should be seriously considered. Clinicians should be comfortable with the initial evaluation and treatment of GERD in adults as it is a common cause of cough and is more common in asthmatics than in the general population.

References

1. Schappert SM (1997) Ambulatory care visits of physician offices, hospital outpatient departments and emergency departments: United States: 1995. Vital Health Stat 13:1–38
2. Canning BJ (2006) Anatomy and neurophysiology of the cough reflex. Chest 129:33S–47S
3. Widdicombe JG (1996) Sensory neurophysiology of the cough reflex. J Allergy Clin Immunol 98:S84–S90
4. Widdicombe JG (1954) The site of pulmonary stretch receptors in the cat. J Physiol 125:336–351
5. Widdicombe JG (1982) Pulmonary and respiratory tract receptors. J Exp Biol 100: 41–57

6. Widdicombe JG (2003) Overview of neural pathways in allergy and asthma. Pulm Pharmacol Ther 16:23–30
7. Kubin L, Alheid GF, Zuperku EJ, McCrimmon DR (2006) Central pathways of pulmonary and lower airway vagal afferents. J Appl Physiol 101:618–627
8. Morice AH, Geppetti P (2004) Cough 5: the type 1 vanilloid receptor: a sensory receptor for cough. Thorax 59:257–258
9. Mitchell JE, Campbell AP, New NE, Sadofsky LR, Mulrennan SA, Compton SJ, Morice AH (2005) Expression and characterization of the intracellular vanilloid receptor (TRPV1) in bronchi from patients with chronic cough. Exp Lung Res 31:295–306
10. Groneberg DA, Niimi A, Dinh QT, Cosio B, Hew M, Fischer A, Chung KF (2004) Increased expression of transient receptor potential vanilloid-1 in airway nerves of chronic cough. Am J Respir Crit Care Med 170:1276–1280
11. Carr MJ, Kollarik M, Meeker SN, Undem BJ (2003) A role for TRPV1 in bradykinin-induced excitation of vagal airway afferent nerve terminals. J Pharmacol Exp Ther 304:1275–1279
12. Bergren DR, Sampson SR (1982) Characterization of intrapulmonary, rapidly adapting receptors of guinea pigs. Respir Physiol 47:83–95
13. Jonzon A, Pisarria TE, Coleridge JC, Coleridge HM (1986) Rapidly adapting receptor activity in dogs is inversely related to lung compliance. J Appl Physiol 61:1980–1987
14. Canning BJ, Reynolds SM, Mazzone SB (2001) Multiple mechanisms of reflex bronchospasm in guinea pigs. J Appl Physiol 91:2642–2653
15. Ho CY, Gu Q, Lin YS, Lee LY (2001) Sensitivity of vagal afferent endings to chemical irritants in the rat lung. Respir Physiol 127:113–124
16. Hanacek J, Davies A, Widdicombe JG (1984) Influence of lung stretch receptors on the cough reflex in rabbits. Respiration 45:161–168
17. Todisco T (1982) The oto-respiratory reflex. Respiration 43:354–358
18. Ing AJ, Ngu MC, Breslin ABX (1994) Pathogenesis of chronic persistent cough associated with gastro-esophageal reflux. Am J Respir Crit Care Med 149:160–167
19. Ing AJ (2004) Cough and gastro-oesophageal reflux disease. Pulm Pharmacol Ther 17:403–413
20. Irwin RS, Ownbey R, Cagle PT, Baker S, Fraire AE (2006) Interpreting the histopathology of chronic cough, a prospective, controlled, comparative study. Chest 130:362–370
21. Dicpinigaitis PV, Rauf K (1998) The influence of gender on cough reflex sensitivity. Chest 113:1319–1321
22. Dicpinigaitis PV, Allusson VR, Baldanti A, Nalamati JR (2001) Ethnic and gender differences in cough reflex sensitivity. Respiration 68:480–482
23. Chang AB, Phelan PD, Sawyer SM, Del Brocco S, Robertson CF (1997) Cough sensitivity in children with asthma, recurrent cough and cystic fibrosis. Arch Dis Child 77:331–334
24. Plevkova J, Varechova S, Brozmanova M, Tatar M (2006) Testing of cough reflex sensitivity in children suffering from allergic rhinitis and common cold. J Physiol Pharmacol 57 Suppl 4:289–296
25. O'Connell F, Thomas VE, Studham JM, Pride NB, Fuller RW (1996) Capsaicin cough sensitivity increases during upper respiratory infection. Respir Med 90:279–286
26. O'Connell F, Thomas VE, Pride NB, Fuller RW (1994) Capsaicin cough sensitivity decreases with successful treatment of chronic cough. Am J Respir Crit Care Med 150:374–380
27. Morice AH, Lowry R, Brown MJ, Higenbottam T (1987) Angiotensin-converting enzyme and the cough reflex. Lancet 2(8568): 1116–1118
28. Bucca C, Rolla G, Pinna G, Oliva A, Bugiani M (1990) Hyperresponsiveness of the extrathoracic airway in patients with captopril-induced cough. Chest 98:1133–1137
29. Irwin RS, Corrao WM, Pratter MR (1981) Chronic persistent cough in the adult: the spectrum and frequency of causes and successful outcome of specific therapy. Am Rev Respir Dis 123:413–417
30. Irwin RS, Curley FJ, French CL (1990) Chronic cough: the spectrum and frequency of causes, key components of the diagnostic evaluation, and outcome of specific therapy. Am Rev Respir Dis 141:640–647

31. Pratter MR, Bartter T, Akers S, DuBois J (1993) An algorithmic approach to chronic cough. Ann Intern Med 119:977–983
32. McGarvey LP, Heaney LG, Lawson JT, Johnston BT, Scally CM, Ennis M, Shepherd DR, MacMahon J (1998) Evaluation and outcome of patients with chronic non-productive cough using a comprehensive diagnostic protocol. Thorax 53:738–743
33. Smyrnios NA, Irwin RS, Curley FJ (1995) Chronic cough with a history of excessive sputum production; The spectrum and frequency of causes, key components of the diagnostic evaluation, and outcome of specific therapy. Chest 108:991–997
34. Mello CJ, Irwin RS, Curley FJ (1996) Predictive values of the character, timing and complications of chronic cough in diagnosing its cause. Arch Intern Med 156:997–1003
35. Weinfeld D, Ternesten-Hasseus E, Lowhagan O, Millqvist E (2002) Capsaicin cough sensitivity in allergic asthmatic patients increases during the birch pollen season. Ann Allergy Asthma Immunol 89:419–424
36. Pecova R, Vrlik M, Tatar M (2005) Cough sensitivity in allergic rhinitis. J Physiol Pharmacol 56(Suppl 4):171–178
37. Hara J, Fujimura M, Myou S, Furusho S, Abo M, Oribe Y, Ohkura N, Herai Y, Sone T, Waseda Y, Yasui M, Kasahara K (2006) Eosinophilic inflammation, remodeling of lower airway, bronchial responsiveness and cough reflex sensitivity in non-asthmatic subjects with nasal allergy. Int Arch Allergy Immunol 140:327–333
38. Tatar M, Petriskova J, Zucha J, Pecova R, Hutka Z, Raffajova J, Brozmanova M (2006) Induced sputum eosinophils, bronchial reactivity, and cough sensitivity in subjects with allergic rhinitis. J Physiol Pharmacol 56(Suppl 4):227–236
39. Doherty MJ, Mister R, Pearson MG, Calverley PM (2000) Capsaicin responsiveness and cough in asthma and chronic obstructive pulmonary disease. Thorax 55:643–649
40. Li AM, Lex C, Zacharasiewicz A, Wong E, Erin E, Hansel T, Wilson NM, Bush A (2003) Cough frequency in children with stable asthma: correlation with lung function, exhaled nitric oxide and sputum eosinophil count. Thorax 58:974–978
41. Li AM, Tsang TW, Chan DF, Lam HS, So HK, Sung RY, Fok TF (2006) Cough frequency in children with mild asthma correlates with sputum neutrophil count. Thorax 61:747–750
42. Corrao WM, Braman SS, Irwin RS (1979) Chronic cough as the sole presenting manifestation of bronchial asthma. N Engl J Med 300:633–637
43. Cloutier MM, Loughlin GM (1981) Chronic cough in children: a manifestation of airway hyperreactivity. Pediatrics 67:6–12
44. Hannaway PJ, Hopper GD (1982) Cough variant asthma in children. JAMA 247:206–208
45. Holinger LD, Sanders AD (1991) Chronic cough in infants and children: an update. Laryngoscope 101:596–605
46. Todokoro M, Mochizuki H, Tokuyama K, Morikawa A (2003) Childhood cough variant asthma and its relationship to classic asthma. Ann Allergy Asthma Immunol 90:652–659
47. Chang AB, Glomb WB (2006) Guidelines for evaluating chronic cough in pediatrics. Chest 129:260S–283S
48. Gibson PG, Dolovich J, Denburg J, Ramsdale EH, Hargreave FE (1989) Chronic cough: eosinophilic bronchitis without asthma. Lancet 1:1346–1348
49. Brightling CE, Symon FA, Birring SS, Bradding P, Wardlaw AJ, Pavord ID (2003) Comparison of airway immunopathology of eosinophilic bronchitis and asthma. Thorax 58:528–532
50. Brightling CE (2006) Chronic cough due to nonasthmatic eosinophilic bronchitis ACCP evidence-based clinical practice guidelines. Chest 129:116S–121S
51. Carney IK, Gibson PG, Murree-Allen K, Saltos N, Olson LG, Hensley MJ (1997) A systematic evaluation of mechanisms in chronic cough. Am J Respir Crit Care Med 156:211–216
52. Brightling CE, Ward R, Goh KL, Wardlaw AJ, Pavord ID (1999) Eosinophilic bronchitis is an important cause of chronic cough. Am J Respir Crit Care Med 160:406–410
53. Ayik SO, Basoglu OK, Erdinc M, Bor S, Veral A, Bilgen C (2003) Eosinophilic bronchitis as a cause of chronic cough. Respir Med 97:695–701
54. Fujimura M, Sakamoto S, Matsuda T (1992) Bronchodilator-resistive cough in atopic patients: bronchial reversibility and hyperresponsiveness. Intern Med 31:447–452

55. Fujimura M, Ogawa H, Nishizawa Y, Nishi K (2003) Comparison of atopic cough with cough variant asthma: is atopic cough a precursor to asthma? Thorax 58:14–18
56. Berry MA, Hargadon B, McKenna S, Shaw D, Green RH, Brightling CE, Wardlaw AJ, Pavord ID (2005) Observational study of the natural history of eosinophilic bronchitis. Clin Exp Allergy 35:598–601
57. Moayyedi P, Talley NJ (2006) Gastro-oesophageal reflux disease. Lancet 367:2086–2100
58. Sontag SJ, O'Connell S, Khandelwal S, Miller T, Nemchausky B, Schnell TG, Serlovsky R (1990) Most asthmatics have gastroesophageal reflux with or without bronchodilator therapy. Gastroenterology 99:613–620
59. Sontag SJ, O'Connell S, Miller TQ, Bernsen M, Seidel J (2004) Asthmatics have more nocturnal gasping and reflux symptoms than nonasthmatics, and they are related to bedtime eating. Am J Gastroenterol 99:789–796
60. Kastelik JA, Aziz I, Ojoo JC, Thompson RH, Redington AE, Morice AH (2005) Investigation and management of chronic cough using a probability-based algorithm. Eur Respir J 25:235–243
61. Marchant JM, Master IB, Taylor SM, Cox NC, Seymour GJ, Chang AB (2006) Evaluation and outcome of young children with chronic cough. Chest 129:1132–1141
62. Paterson WG, Murat BW (1994) Combined ambulatory esophageal manometry and dual pH-metry in evaluation of patients with chronic unexplained cough. Dig Dis Sci 39:1117–1125
63. Gastral OL, Castell JA, Castell DO (1994) Frequency and site of gastroesophageal reflux in patients with chest symptoms: studies using proximal and distal pH monitoring. Chest 106:1793–1796
64. Laukka MA, Cameron AJ, Schei AJ (1994) Gastroesophageal reflux and chronic cough: which comes first? J Clin Gastroenterol 19:100–104
65. Irwin RS, Zawacki JK, Wilson MM, French CT, Callery MP (2002) Chronic cough due to gastroesophageal reflux disease; failure to resolve despite total/near-total elimination of esophageal acid. Chest 121:1132–1140
66. Mainie I, Tutuian R, Agrawal A, Adams D, Castell DO (2006) Combined multichannel intra-luminal impedance-pH monitoring to select patients with persistent gastro-oesophageal reflux for laparoscopic Nissen fundoplication. Br J Surg 93:1483–1487
67. Tutuian R, Mainie I, Agrawal A, Adams D, Castell DO (2006) Nonacid reflux in patients with chronic cough on acid-suppressive therapy. Chest 130:386–391
68. Ford CN (2005) Evaluation and management of laryngopharyngeal reflux. JAMA 294:1534–1540
69. Noordzij JP, Khidr A, Evans BA, Desper E, Mittal RK, Reibel JF Levine PA (2001) Evaluation of omeprazole in the treatment of reflux laryngitis: a prospective, placebo-controlled, randomized, double-blind study. Laryngoscope 111:2147–2151
70. Issing WJ, Karkos PD, Perreas K, Folwaczny C, Reichel O (2004) Dual-probe 24 hour ambulatory pH monitoring for diagnosis of laryngopharyngeal reflux. J Laryngol Otol 118:845–848
71. Wo JM, Grist WJ, Gussack G, Delgaudio JM, Waring JP (1997) Empiric trial of high-dose omeprazole in patients with posterior laryngitis: a prospective study. Am J Gastroenterol 92:2160–2165
72. Williams RB, Szczesniak MM, Maclean JC, Brake HM, Cole IE, Cook IJ (2004) Predictors of outcome in an open label, therapeutic trial of high-dose omeprazole in laryngitis. Am J Gastroenterol 99:777–785
73. McGarvey LPA (2005) Idiopathic chronic cough: a real disease or a failure of diagnosis? Cough 1:9
74. Janson C, Chinn S, Jarvis D, Burney P (2001) Determinants of cough in young adults participating in the European Community Respiratory Health Survey. Eur Respir J 18:647–654
75. Dicpinigaitis PV (2003) Cough reflex sensitivity in cigarette smokers. Chest 123:685–688
76. Dicpinigaitis PV (2006) Angiotensin-converting enzyme inhibitor-induced cough: ACCP evidence-based clinical practice guidelines. Chest 129(Suppl 1):169S–173S.
77. Patz EF Jr, Goodman PC, Bepler G (2000) Screening for lung cancer. N Engl J Med 343:1627–1633

78. Thomson F, Masters IB, Chang AB (2002) Persistent cough in children and the overuse of medications. J Paediatr Child Health 38:578–581
79. Kelly LF (2004) Pediatric cough and cold preparations. Pediatr Rev 25:115–123
80. Srinivasan A, Budnitz D, Shehab N (2007) Infant deaths associated with cough and cold medications – two states 2005. MMWR 56:1–4
81. Monto AS (2002) Epidemiology of viral respiratory infections. Am J Med 112(6A):4S–12S
82. Hay AD, Wilson AD (2002) The natural history of acute cough in children aged 0–4 years in primary care: a systematic review. Br J Gen Pract 52:401–409
83. Hay AD, Wilson AD, Fahey T, Peters TJ (2003) The duration of acute cough in pre-school children presenting to primary care: a prospective cohort study. Fam Pract 20:696–705
84. Munyard P, Bush A (1996) How much coughing is normal? Arch Dis Child 74:531–534
85. Irwin, RS, Boulet, LP, Cloutier, MM, Fuller R, Gold PM, Hoffstein V, Ing AJ, McCool FD, O'Byrne P, Poe RH, Prakash UB, Pratter MR, Rubin BK (1998) Managing cough as a defense mechanism and as a symptom: a consensus panel report of the American College of Chest Physicians. Chest 114(Suppl):133S–181S
86. Brooke AM, Lambert PC, Burton PR, Clarke C, Luyt DK, Simpson H (1995) The natural history of respiratory symptoms in preschool children. Am J Respir Crit Care Med 152:1872–1878
87. Chang AB, Asher MI (2001) A review of cough in children. J Asthma 38:299–309
88. Powell CV, Primhak RA (1996) Stability of respiratory symptoms in unlabelled wheezy illness and nocturnal cough. Arch Dis Child 75:385–391
89. Ninan TK, Macdonald L, Russell G (1995) Persistent nocturnal cough in childhood: a population based study. Arch Dis Child 73:403–407
90. Chang AB, Phelan PD, Carlin JB (1998) A randomized, placebo controlled trial of inhaled salbutamol and beclomethasone for recurrent cough. Arch Dis Child 79:6–11
91. Davies M, Fuller P, Picciotto A, McKenzie SA (1999) Persistent nocturnal cough: randomized controlled trial of high dose inhaled corticosteroid. Arch Dis Child 81:38–44
92. Tanaka S, Hirata K, Kurihara N, Yoshikawa J, Takeda T (1996) Effect of loratadine, an H1 antihistamine, on induced cough in non-asthmatic patients with chronic cough. Thorax 51:810–814
93. Dicpinigaitis PV, Gayle YE (2003) Effect of the second-generation antihistamine, fexofenadine, on cough reflex sensitivity and pulmonary function. Br J Clin Pharmacol 56:501–504
94. Gawchik S, Goldstein S, Prenner B, John A (2003) Relief of cough and nasal symptoms associated with allergic rhinitis by mometasone furoate nasal spray. Ann Allergy Asthma Immunol 90:416–421
95. Brightling CE, Ward R, Wardlaw AJ, Pavord ID (2000) Airway inflammation, airway responsiveness and cough before and after inhaled budesonide in patients with eosinophilic bronchitis. Eur Respir J 15:682–686
96. Gibson PG, Hargreave FE, Girgis-Gabardo A, Morris M, Denburg JA, Dolovich J (1995) Chronic cough with eosinophilic bronchitis: examination for variable airflow obstruction and response to corticosteroid. Clin Exp Allergy 25:127–132
97. Ours TM, Kavuru MS, Schilz RJ, Richter JE (1999) A prospective evaluation of oesophageal testing and a double blind, randomized study of omeprazole in a diagnostic and therapeutic algorithm for chronic cough. Am J Gastroenterol 94:3131–3138
98. Kiljander TO, Salomaa ERM, Hietanen EK, Terho EO (2000) Chronic cough and gastro-oesophageal reflux: a double-blind placebo controlled study with omeprazole. Eur Respir J 16:633–638
99. Poe RH, Kallay MC (2003) Chronic cough and gastroesophageal reflux disease. Experience with specific therapy for diagnosis and treatment. Chest 123:679–684
100. Rudolph CD, Mazur LJ, Liptak GS, Baker RD, Boyle JT, Colletti RB, Gerson WT, Werlin SL (2001) Guidelines for evaluation and treatment of gastroesophageal reflux in infants and children: recommendations of the North American Society for Pediatric Gastroenterology and Nutrition. J Pediatr Gastroenterol Nutr 32(Suppl 2):S1–S31

Airway Hyperresponsiveness: Inflammatory Mechanisms and Clinical Aspects

Salman Siddiqui, Fay Hollins, and Christopher Brightling

Introduction

The global initiative for asthma (GINA) [1] guidelines define the disease as a chronic inflammatory airway disorder, characterised by symptoms (e.g., cough, wheeze) and airway hyperresponsiveness (AHR). AHR is a fundamental feature of the asthma paradigm and is characterised by the capacity of the airway to narrow, in response to a host of direct and indirect stimuli to the airway smooth muscle (ASM). Direct challenge agents such as histamine and methacholine act via receptors located on ASM, involved in the regulation of static airway calibre. Indirect agents such as cold air [2], adenosine [3], mannitol [4] and exercise [5] induce bronchoconstriction by the release of mediators from resident airway cells. One of the first clinical descriptions of AHR was provided by Curry et al. [6], who demonstrated that nebulised, intramuscular and intravenous histamine could cause a significant reduction in the vital capacity of patients with symptomatic asthma. AHR has since emerged as a powerful tool in the management of asthma [1] and to define the asthma phenotype in both clinical and epidemiological studies.

In this chapter we shall summarise the current standardised clinical methods to assess AHR, the clinical utility of airway challenge in the diagnosis and management of asthma and the potential mechanisms that drive the development of AHR.

S. Siddiqui, F. Hollins, and C. Brightling
Institute for Lung Health, Department of Infection, Inflammation and Immunity,
University of Leicester, Leicester, UK

C. Brightling (✉)
Department of Respiratory Medicine, University Hospitals of Leicester, Groby Road,
Leicester, LE3 9QP, UK
e-mail: ceb17@le.ac.uk

R. Pawankar et al. (eds.), *Allergy Frontiers: Clinical Manifestations*,
DOI: 10.1007/978-4-431-88317-3_13, © Springer 2009

Assessment of Airway Hyperresponsiveness in Clinical Practice

Direct Airway Challenge Testing in Clinical Practice

The most commonly available direct challenge agents in clinical practice are methacholine and histamine. Both agents produce similar degrees of bronchoconstriction; however, methacholine is generally favoured because histamine is associated with more systemic side effects (headache, flushing and hoarseness). In addition, AHR measurements may be less reproducible when using histamine [7]. Methacholine challenge can be used in a wide range of situations, however, there are a number of important absolute contraindications (severe airflow limitation, $FEV_1 < 50\%$ predicted or <1.0l, heart attack/stroke within the last 3 months, uncontrolled hypertension, known aortic aneurysm). It is also important that patients refrain from taking drugs that can reduce AHR prior to the study (e.g., long-acting bronchodilators, 24 h prior to testing).

The most commonly advocated dosing protocols are continuous nebulisation during tidal breathing and five breaths of a fixed duration, using a dosimeter at the beginning of deep inhalation. The 2-min tidal breathing method delivers approximately twice the volume (90 vs 45 µl) at each methacholine concentration, compared to the five-breath dosimeter method; this is due primarily to differences in the method of inhalation. Both the lower dose and the potential bronchoprotection, induced by deep inhalations, can contribute to a reduced response with the dosimeter compared to the tidal breathing method. Therefore, recent studies have favoured the tidal breathing method [8–10]. A variety of different dosing protocols based upon serial doubling doses of methacholine (0.031–16 mg/g tidal breathing and 0.0625–6 mg/ml dosimeter) have been proposed. Dosing protocols may be shortened by quadrupling dosing with the dosimeter or starting with higher concentrations of methacholine; 1 mg/ml, missing doubling doses if <5% fall in FEV_1 with the tidal breathing method; if the clinical suspicion of asthma is low. Fewer concentrations have been used by many investigators without any apparent increase in risk of severe bronchospasm [11, 12]. Perhaps the only caveat to this rule is in children, who may develop severe bronchoconstriction with a shortened protocol, because of the increased dose: weight distribution.

Change in FEV_1 is the primary outcome measure for methacholine challenge testing. Spirometry should meet the American Thoracic Society (ATS) guidelines [13] and care should be taken to obtain high-quality baseline FEV_1 measurements to avoid false-positive or false-negative results. The provocation concentration to cause a 20% fall in FEV_1 from baseline or post-diluent (PC_{20}) is commonly used to summarise the results. In patients who are unable to perform acceptable spirometry manoeuvres, other outcome measures such as measurement of airway conductance (sGaw) using body plethysmography [14], transcutaneous oxygen tension (Ptc_{O2}) [15] and forced oscillation or impulse techniques [16] have been advocated. Forced inspiratory vital capacity may be a useful endpoint in patients with suspected vocal cord dysfunction, which may be revealed as a spontaneous or methacholine challenge testing-induced limitation of a forced inspiratory flow resulting in a plateau in the flow on the FIVC curves [17].

Interpretation of PC_{20} in Clinical Practice

PC_{20} can be derived by plotting the change in FEV_1 as a percentage of the baseline or post-diluent value against the log_{10} methacholine concentration using the equation below [18, 19].

$$PC_{20} = \text{antilog log } C_1 + (\log C_2 - \log C_1)(20 - R_1)(R_2 - R_1)$$

where

C_1 = second to last methacholine concentration
C_2 = final concentration of methacholine causing a $\geq 20\%$ fall in FEV_1
R_1 = percent fall in FEV_1 after C_1
R_2 = percent fall in FEV_1 after C_2

However, a number of studies have demonstrated that non-linear models are better at deriving PC_{20} values between doubling doses of methacholine than simple linear models [20, 21].

Challenge results are often defined categorically. AHR is considered to be present when the ratio of PC_{20} to histamine or methacholine is <8 mg/ml. However, AHR to methacholine and histamine is unimodally and log normally distributed and the continuity of this normal distribution leads to diagnostic uncertainty when trying to define a 'normal response'.

PC_{20} values of >16 mg/ml make it highly unlikely that a patient has asthma, even if the pre-test clinical probability is relatively high [22, 23]. In contrast if the PC_{20} is <1 mg/ml the diagnosis of asthma is highly likely even with a relatively low pre-test clinical probability. In this setting the specificity and positive predictive value of asthma approaches 100% [24], in contrast to a relatively poor sensitivity [22]. However, in patients with intermediate PC_{20} values between 1–16 mg/ml there is much more diagnostic uncertainty. For example the positive predictive value of a histamine PC_{20} < 8 mg/ml for the current asthma symptoms is <50% [22]. Therefore, perhaps the best clinical utility of methacholine/histamine challenge is its negative predictive value at >16 mg/ml. The only caveats to this rule are patients who develop transient AHR in response to allergen exposure [25] or occupational sensitizers [26] and are removed from exposure at the time of challenge testing. Further diagnostic confusion arises in the presence of fixed airflow limitation. Patients with COPD also demonstrate AHR to histamine and methacholine [27–30]. Therefore direct challenge bronchoprovocation lacks the specificity to detect asthma in the presence of airflow limitation.

The repeatability over a short term for methacholine challenge is ±1.5 doubling doses [31–40]. Recent evidence does not support the notion that tachyphylaxis occurs with methacholine if the challenge is repeated within 24 h, and repeatability within a single day is within one doubling dose [41].

Indirect Airway Challenge Testing in Clinical Practice

There are a variety of important pharmacological differences between direct and indirect agents. There is relatively weak association between methacholine AHR and indirect challenge-induced AHR, presumably reflecting the differing pathways by which these two forms of challenges regulate ASM contraction. Indirect challenge AHR occurs due to a wide range of inflammatory mediators and can be prevented by pre-treatment with cromomes, showing evidence of significant tachyphylaxis that leads to a refractory period during which subjects are refractory to other indirect challenges [42]. Furthermore, AHR, due to the indirect challenge, may reflect airway inflammation more closely than the direct challenge and reflect acute changes induced by airway inflammation or after treatment with inhaled corticosteroids.

Exercise challenge tests are useful in distinguishing patients who may have breathlessness associated with exertion due to asthma. Such a diagnosis cannot be made with methacholine challenge. The exercise challenge is more specific than direct challenges in the differentiation of asthmatics from normal subjects. Furthermore, in children, exercise-induced bronchoconstriction is a useful clinical tool in distinguishing asthma from other disorders that cause non-specific AHR (bronchiectasis, cystic fibrosis, ciliary dyskinesia and obliterative bronchiolitis). The recommendations for conducting an exercise test have been described in detail by the ATS [43] and European Respiratory Society (ERS) [19], and are similar. In brief, subjects should exercise for 6–8 min, breathing dry air at an intensity to raise minute ventilation to 14 times above the FEV_1 or for the heart rate to achieve 90% of the maximal, in the last 4 min of exercise.

Adenosine 5′-monophosphate (AMP) has emerged as a useful pharmacological challenge agent [44]. One of the major pharmacological effects of AMP is the release of histamine from primed mast cells, as evidenced by an increase in the histamine release in Bronchoalveolar lavage (BAL) and plasma after AMP-induced bronchoconstriction [45, 46], and further evidence to support this notion comes from the observation that the concentration of AMP causing the FEV_1 to drop by 20% (PC_{20}) is inhibited up to 80% by pre-treatment with antihistamines [47]. PC_{20} AMP improves to a larger extent with the use of inhaled corticosteroids than PC_{20} methacholine [48], and reflects more closely the extent of airway inflammation due to asthma than PC_{20} methacholine [49]. PC_{20}AMP in combination with other markers of airway inflammation may be useful in delineating patients with asthma in whom the dose of inhaled corticosteroids can be reduced successfully without deterioration in asthma control [50].

The final group of indirect challenge agents that have gained popularity in clinical practice are the osmotic agents, hypertonic (4.5%) saline and mannitol. Osmotic agents can be used to assess the likelihood of asthma control after reduction of inhaled corticosteroids and the severity of asthma [51, 52]. In severe asthma, further evidence of the intimacy of an association between the indirect challenge and airway inflammation comes from a study by In't Veen et al., who demonstrated that hypertonic saline, in contrast to methacholine, could detect the AHR induced during exacerbations caused by steroid withdrawal and associated eosinophilic inflammation [53]. As expected responsiveness to mannitol predicts responsiveness to hypertonic saline and also seems to be highly specific as a diagnostic tool for asthma in patients who are corticosteroid naïve [54]. Mannitol challenge offers promise, primarily due to the convenience, as it is administered via a capsule-based delivery device that could easily be adapted to the outpatient clinical setting. Furthermore it is likely that a clinical understanding of mannitol will deepen as experience with inhaled insulin increases; as mannitol is used as the carrier agent in inhaled insulin preparations. One advantage of hypertonic saline is that it can be combined with induced sputum to assess airway inflammation.

The underlying cause of AHR is unclear. In asthma, AHR may be related to changes in ASM mass or function, the geometry of the airway wall or airway inflammation. Each of these possibilities will be considered in turn, but it is important to note that within an individual a combination of these may co-exist.

Airway Hyperresponsiveness: An Innate Defect of Airway Smooth Muscle

The view that ASM is altered in asthma and that it is a critical determinant in the development of AHR is both longstanding and contentious. Early attempts to prove that the ASM from asthmatics is hypercontractile have met with little success, in that the opportunities to conduct contractile studies on asthma-derived muscle are rare and the results of the few studies that do exist vary from demonstrating increased or decreased contractility, decreased relaxation or no clear differences [55–59].

More recently, Ma et al. demonstrated that ASM freshly dissociated from bronchial biopsies had both increased velocity of contraction and maximal contraction [60]. Differences in the rates of ASM shortening are likely to be important, as these are implicated in counteracting the relaxing effects of deep inspiration [61, 62], and contribute to a greater extent in maximal airway narrowing [63–65]. ASM has been shown to exhibit length adaptation with recovery of contractile force as the muscle length changes; which is likely to be related to the adaptability of the contractile filaments and cytoskeleton, and helps to maintain optimum contractile protein overlap [66, 67] and orientation [68, 69]. The adaptation of contractile filaments is likely to involve changes in both the number of filaments in a series and in parallel.

The plasticity of contractile filaments is exhibited on a macroscale by the entire smooth muscle cell; which is in a constant state of structural fluidity and adaptation in response to the non-thermal agitation of the cytoskeleton, such that the cell behaves like soft glass [70]. Loss of adaptation may be fundamental to the aberrant ASM function in asthma. The reversal of bronchodilatation to deep inspiration would establish a condition in which the ASM remains continually shortened [71, 72], raising the possibility of contractile filament rearrangement and muscle length adaptation at shorter lengths [73].

In cultured ASM bundles from rabbits, chronic shortening of the bundle was found to be associated with increased passive stiffness and partial loss of the ability of the muscle to adapt when returned to its *in situ* length [74]. Indeed, these phenomena could provide an explanation for the enhanced airway reactivity of the Fisher inbred rat strain, wherein increased cytoskeletal remodelling was observed in cultured ASM from Fisher compared with Lewis rat strains [75]. There was therefore emerging evidence to support the view that ASM contractility was altered in asthma. For these changes in ASM mechanics to occur in asthma it was likely that there were differences in the fundamental mechanisms controlling ASM contraction.

Contraction of ASM is dependent upon activation of actin and myosin cross-bridges and the phosphorylation of the myosin light chain by myosin light chain kinase. This process is controlled by the interaction between calcium-excitation coupling and calcium sensitivity [76]. The mechanisms involved in this process are summarised in Fig. 1. Recent studies suggest that the calcium homeostasis of ASM from asthmatics may be abnormal, with increased cytosolic calcium and increased spontaneous calcium oscillations in asthmatic ASM [77, 78]. The mechanisms driving this aberrant Ca^{2+} signalling are under investigation and may reveal fundamental differences between ASM in health and disease. A similar process is evident in the Fisher rat strain in which calcium mobilisation is up-regulated in response to increased IP3 expression and altered PKC regulation [79]. In human disease, calcium sensitivity is also heightened in ASM with increased expression of myosin light chain kinase reported in freshly dispersed primary cells [60] and in ASM-bundles in bronchial biopsies [80]. This increase in calcium sensitivity together with an alteration in the control of intracellular calcium would be predicted to contribute to the abnormal ASM mechanics observed in asthma.

Therefore, the body of evidence is now swinging in favour of the view that the phenotype of ASM in asthma is fundamentally altered. Changes in calcium home-ostasis and calcium sensitivity in ASM from asthmatics provide an explanation for the increased velocity and maximal contraction. This in turns modifies ASM mechanics with ASM-shortening, exaggerated airway narrowing and inhibition of bronchial dilatation in response to deep inspiration. Importantly, these mechanisms do not occur in isolation, but are compounded by airway inflammation and remodelling.

In addition to its altered contractile phenotype ASM from asthmatics exhibits changes in its secretory and proliferative capacity [81]. ASM in asthma may also be

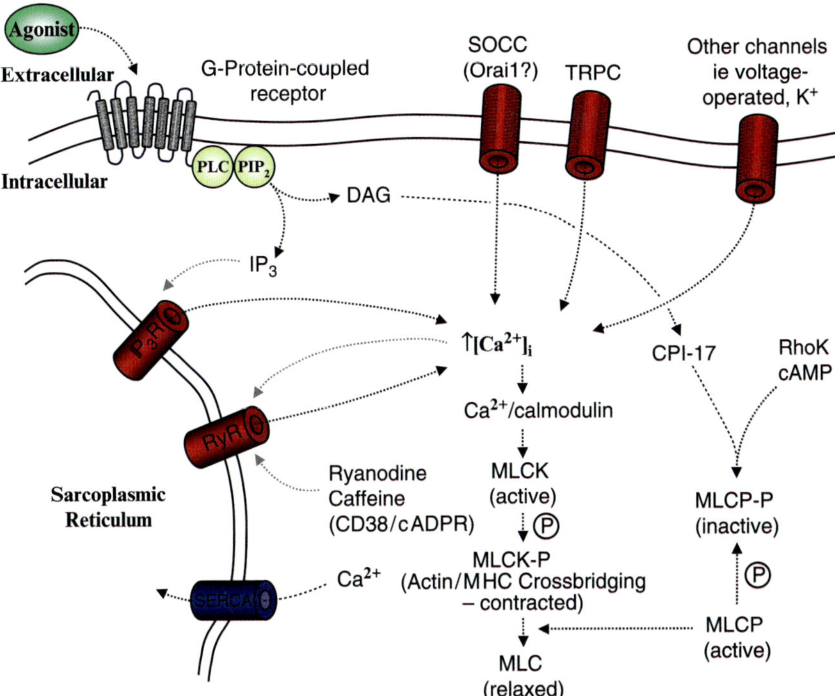

Fig. 1 Mechanisms involved in coupling ASM contraction with calcium excitation and sensitivity ASM contraction is dependent upon activation of actin and myosin cross-bridges and the phosphorylation of myosin light chain (MLC) by MLCK. This process is under the tight regulation of calcium sensitivity and calcium excitation. Calcium sensitivity reflects the balance between MLCK and MLC phosphatase (P) and can be modulated by a number of mechanisms including RhoKinase and cAMP; the latter up-regulated in response to activation of Gs-coupled receptors, by agents such as β-agonists. Calcium excitation, that is, the concentration of the free cytosolic calcium $[Ca^{2+}]_i$ is controlled by the influx/efflux of calcium from the intracellular store (sarcoplasmic reticulum) and extracellularly. In response to an agonist, for example,histamine via Gq-protein coupled receptors PIP_2 is converted by phospholipase (PL)C to IP3 and DAG. IP_3 activates the IP_3 receptor (IP_3R) on the sarcoplasmic reticulum and leads to a release of intracellular stores. This in turn activates the influx of extracellular calcium probably via store operated calcium channels (SOCC) (possibly via interactions between STIM-1 and Orai1), which can amplify the response, after activation of calcium homeostasis is restored by calcium pumps such as sarcoplasmic reticulum ATPase (SERCA). Importantly other potential mechanisms, some of which are shown, can modulate intracellular calcium concentration and modify the calcium sensitivity. Hence, it is important to note that this figure does not completely capture the complexity of the mechanisms involved (reviewed in [64] and [76])

intrinsically resistant to the anti-proliferative effects of inhaled corticosteroids due to an absence of C/EBP alpha, a complex of the glucocorticoid receptor enhancer binding protein [82]. In concert these changes are also likely to contribute to the development of airway remodelling and AHR via recruitment of inflammatory cells to the ASM-bundle, matrix deposition and ASM hyperplasia.

AHR: A Reflection of Altered Airway Geometry/Remodelling

Airway remodelling is a central feature of asthma and refers to the changes in the structural components of the airway wall. The major features of airway remodelling include epithelial cell fragility, goblet cell hyperplasia, matrix deposition, myofibroblast hyperplasia, increased ASM mass and angiogenesis [80, 83]. Studies of human disease have illustrated that some of the features of remodelling can occur early in the disease, in particular epithelial loss and basement membrane thickening [84]. Several studies have shown correlations with most of the features of remodelling and AHR in univariate analysis [80, 85], but whether these reflect causality or an epiphenomenon is unclear. Perhaps the most compelling is the association between ASM mass and AHR. Biopsy studies of asthma have consistently demonstrated an increase in the percentage of ASM mass compared to healthy subjects [86–88] due to a combination of ASM hyperplasia [89] and hypertrophy [80]. Mathematical modelling studies suggest that an increase in the content of ASM mass, irrespective of hypertrophy or hyperplasia, will increase the potential for airway narrowing [90]. In support of this view detailed bronchoscopic studies have attempted to define the relationship between airway dysfunction and features of remodelling; with ASM mass the feature most closely associated with airflow obstruction. However, to date, no study has used a similar approach to unravel the association between AHR and remodelling.

The relationship between remodelling and AHR is complex. Indeed, paradoxically some features of remodelling may protect the airway from remodelling. The beneficial effects include the potential of the airway to resist dynamic compression due to increased airway wall stiffness as a consequence of increased airway wall thickness, the theoretical attenuation of contraction by deposition of the matrix around the ASM cells [62], thus providing an elastic impedance [63] and the potential increased elastic load on the muscle, as a result of the distortion and folding of thickened remodelled tissue that occurs with ASM contraction [91]. Conversely, the structural changes of remodelling can have significant deleterious effects on airway resistance. Hyperplasia of the mucus-secreting goblet cells will contribute to luminal narrowing. An ASM layer of greater volume will narrow the airway lumen more than a lesser volume [92, 93]. Furthermore, mathematical models have predicted that an increase in the volume of the airway wall on the luminal side of the smooth muscle layer will greatly increase the effect of ASM contraction in narrowing the lumen of an airway [92, 94, 95]. Whereas, thickening of the outer adventitial wall may uncouple the airway from parenchymal elastic recoil forces and thus augment the ability of the wall to contract [96].

Imaging studies using computed tomography have been particularly informative of the global effects of airway wall thickening upon airway function. Niimi et al. have demonstrated that the sensitivity (the initial rise in airway resistance during methacholine challenge) of airways to constrict to methacholine in asthma is directly associated with eosinophil airway inflammation. In contrast thickening of the airway wall in proximal airways was associated with reduced airway reactivity (the slope of the methacholine dose response airway resistance curve) [97]. Remodelling of the airway wall may therefore protect against the development of AHR. In contrast Beigelman-Aubry et al. failed to demonstrate any difference in the cross-section airway calibre (airways > 4 mm² in size) on CT or lung attenuation, before and after methacholine and after inhaled salbutamol, in patients with mild intermittent asthma. However, the degree of air trapping on expiratory CT scans did increase significantly after methacholine challenge suggesting that the site of airflow resistance in asthma was in the small airways beyond the current resolving power of a conventional CT [98]. A previous imaging study by Goldin et al. had confirmed that small airways, 2–5 mm² in calibre, were the main sites of airflow limitation after methacholine challenge, in asthma [99]. We have demonstrated that proximal airway narrowing is a feature of asthma and airway wall thickness and is associated with AHR. Dilatation of the airway lumen is a feature in patients with non-asthmatic eosinophilic bronchitis (see later in chapter for detailed description of this disease), a condition characterised by cough and eosinophilic airway inflammation in the absence of AHR, which may be a mechanism that protects this group of patients from AHR [100].

Taken together, the findings are consistent with a fact that the sum effect of airway remodelling changes in asthma is a greater degree of airway narrowing, which results in increased airway resistance. However, to date, the literature on the relationship between AHR and remodelling is less clear. Importantly, remodelling is a dynamic process and one possible explanation for the apparent inconsistency in reports is the likelihood that in the early stages of the disease, components of airway remodelling exacerbate AHR, but as the disease becomes progressive some of the features of remodelling may protect against AHR. Therefore, longitudinal studies combining CT and parallel analysis of airway compartments in endobronchial biopsies before and after treatments, which modulate airway inflammation and/or airway wall remodeling, are required, to establish which components of the remodelling process are associated with AHR in asthma.

Airway Hyperresponsiveness: A Consequence of Airway Inflammation

A variety of allergen challenge studies have linked AHR with allergic airway inflammation and the late asthmatic response (LAR), and allergen challenge has been associated with eosinophilic airway inflammation in BAL and induced sputum [101–107]. However, the extent to which the increased bronchial reactivity, seen after allergen challenge and in animal models, is related to the AHR seen in clinical disease, is debatable. Despite intensive research over the last 20 years the extent to which AHR is caused by, or interacts with, airway inflammation and especially eosinophilic inflammation remains contentious. AHR and eosinophilic inflammation generally occurred together. In early bronchoscopy studies although there was a clear association between AHR and airway eosinophilia there was little evidence of a correlation between the severity of the AHR and the number of BAL eosinophils [108]. Similarly in a study by Foresi et al. on 15 asthmatics and 30 patients with seasonal allergic rhinitis, a good correlation was seen between sputum eosinophils and AHR, but this was skewed by the inclusion of patients with seasonal rhinitis without asthma. In a much larger study of 71 asthmatics no relationship was seen between sputum eosinophilia and AHR although the eosinophil count did inversely correlate with lung function. Some studies have seen a correlation. For example Jatakanon et al. found a weak inverse correlation ($r = -0.4$) between the sputum eosinophil count and AHR in 35 stable asthmatics, taking only $\beta2$ agonists [109]. In our own experience of over 200 stable asthmatics attending our routine outpatient clinics (46% atopic and 44% taking inhaled steroids), there was no relationship between log sputum eosinophil count and log PC_{20} in the whole group. However, there was a significant although weak inverse correlation in the atopic group ($r = -0.3$, $p < 0.01$) in both patients taking inhaled steroids and those on β_2 agonists alone [110]. Therefore, a number of studies have demonstrated modest associations of AHR to methacholine with eosinophilic airway inflammation in BAL [103, 111], and indirect AHR has been shown to correlate more closely with airway inflammation [49, 112].

Current evidence supports the idea that AHR and eosinophilic airway inflammation are not independently regulated, but closely interrelated, a view supported by a factor analysis undertaken by Rosi et al., of 99 mild asthmatics [113]. This would predict that in a cross-section of patients, for a given degree of inflammation, marked differences in AHR could result. This is consistent with the observation that eosinophilic inflammation can occur without AHR as in non-asthmatic eosinophilic bronchitis and marked AHR can occur in the context of minimal airway eosinophilia, non-eosinophilic asthma. However, inhaled corticosteroids [48] and allergen avoidance [114] have been shown to improve both AHR and airway inflammation, which suggests that within an individual, changes in AHR may mirror changes in eosinophilic airway inflammation to the extent that airway inflammation could be used longitudinally to guide asthma management.

Non-asthmatic Eosinophilic Bronchitis

Non-asthmatic eosinophilic bronchitis (EB) is a condition of unknown aetiology in which patients present with a chronic, minimally productive cough, and are found to have airway eosinophilia (>3% in sputum), but without wheeze, shortness of breath, variable airflow obstruction or AHR [115]. It has been found in 13% of the patients who have presented with cough [116]. The natural history of the disease is unclear, although in some cases persistent airflow obstruction may occur [117, 118]. While EB is interesting in its own right, it has a particular significance in offering clues as to why eosinophilic airway inflammation in some, but not all individuals, leads to asthma.

We have investigated the immunopathology of EB in comparison with that of asthma, and have confirmed that EB is characterised by submucosal eosinophilic inflammation, subepithelial thickening of the collagen layer [119, 120] and increased vascularity [85]. The expression of T-cell activation and of chemokine receptors and T-cell cytokines is also similar to those in asthma, with both showing a Th2 pattern of T-cell activation [121]. Indeed, the only immunopathological difference we observed between the two conditions was infiltration of the ASM by mast cells in asthmatics (Fig. 2), with increased expression of IL-13, but not in patients with EB or in normal subjects [119, 122]. Table 1 summarises the difference in immunopathology between asthma and EB. There was also a significant correlation between the number of mast cells in the ASM and AHR. This was despite the observation that the overall numbers of mast cells in the airway lamina propria in the three groups was the same, and our previous demonstration that EB was characterised by increased amounts of histamine and prostaglandin D_2 in the sputum, suggesting the presence of activated mast cells in the epithelium [123]. Strikingly, there was no infiltration of the ASM by eosinophils or T cells in asthma or EB.

Importantly, in addition to mast cell infiltration into the ASM bundle recent CT studies show that the airway wall is thickened and the lumen narrowed in asthma

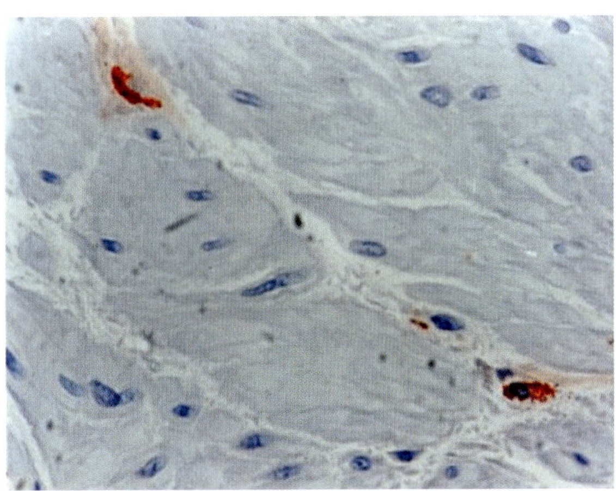

Fig. 2 Mast cell localization to the ASM bundle in asthma Photomicrograph of mast cells (stained red) in an ASM-bundle from a bronchial biopsy taken from an asthmatic (×400)

Table 1 Comparative immunopathology of asthma and non-asthmatic eosinophilic bronchitis

	Asthma	Non-asthmatic eosinophilic bronchitis
Mast cells in ASM	++	--
Increased IL-13 expression in the airway subepithelium	++	--
Increased IL-13 expression in peripheral blood	++	--
Vascular remodelling	++	++
Reticular basement membrane thickening	++	++
Increased ASM mass/matrix deposition	++	??
Proximal and distal airway wall thickening on HRCT	++	--
Evidence of small airways disease on HRCT	++	++

ASM, Airway smooth muscle; IL-13, interleukin-13; HRCT, high resolution computed tomography

compared with EB [100, 124]. This suggests that changes in the airway wall geometry, in asthma, perhaps influenced by interactions between ASM and mast cells, may also contribute to the disordered airway physiology.

Non-Eosinophilic Asthma: AHR Remains Despite the Absence of Eosinophilic Airway Inflammation

Non-eosinophilic asthma (NEA) is defined by clinical symptoms of asthma and AHR in the absence of sputum eosinophilia [125, 126], defined by a sputum eosinophil count of <1.01% (95th centile value of a healthy population). Non-eosinophilic inflammation extends across the entire spectrum of asthma severity and the phenotype is unlikely to be simply related to corticosteroid treatment [127–130]. Corticosteroids appear to have limited efficacy in NEA [129]. A recent double-blind, placebo-controlled, cross-over trial [131] of inhaled mometasone, 400 µg once daily, in eosinophilic asthma (EA) versus NEA, demonstrated that patients with EA had a significant 5.5-doubling dose improvement in methacholine PC_{20} after 8 weeks of mometasone, compared to placebo versus a 0.5 doubling dose improvement in patients with NEA. A parallel pathological analysis of endobronchial biopsies revealed that patients with EA had increased submuscosal tissue eosinophilia and thicker lamina reticularis and reticular basement membranes, compared to patients without EA. Interestingly the number of mast cells within the ASM did not differ between the two groups, but was significantly greater than in the matched healthy controls, again suggesting that mast cell smooth muscle myositis is a defining feature of the asthma phenotype.

From this evidence in EB and NEA, it is therefore the localisation of mast cells within the ASM-bundle that is implicated in causing bronchoconstriction and AHR.

Mast Cells in the Airway Smooth Muscle: Fundamental to the Pathogenesis of AHR in Asthma

In asthma the ASM-bundle is infiltrated by mast cells, predominately of the chymase-positive phenotype [119, 132–137]. Mast cell-ASM interactions in asthma are summarised in Fig. 3. Mast cells adhere avidly to ASM in part via a tumour suppressor in lung cancer-1 (TSLC-1) heterophilic adhesion molecule and in part via an unidentified Ca^{2+} independent pathway [138]. The mast cell number correlated inversely with AHR [119] and positively with the bronchoconstrictor response to deep inspiration [139], suggesting that mast cell-ASM cell interactions are likely to be central in the development of the disordered physiology in asthma. One post-mortem study of fatal and non-fatal asthma has shown that there was a marked increase in mast cell degranulation in the ASM-bundle in both the large and small airways [140] and another demonstrated that increased numbers of mast

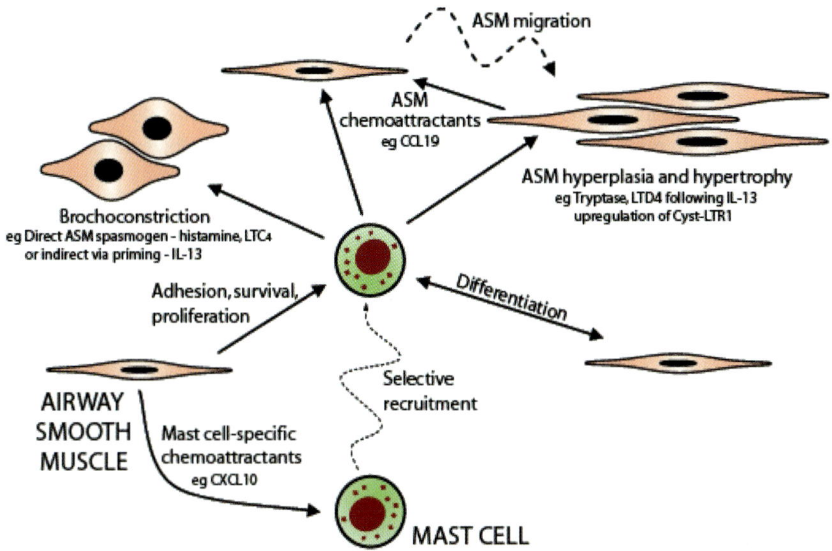

Fig. 3 Mast cell-ASM interactions Mast cells are recruited to the ASM under the influence of ASM-derived chemoattractants and adhere to the ASM. In the ASM-bundle there is an appropriate environment to support mast cell survival, and the cells interact resulting in cellular differentiation, ASM hyperplasia, recruitment of ASM progenitors and ASM contraction, either directly or indirectly (see text for details)

cells (degranulated and intact) were associated with increased ASM shortening in fatal asthma [141].

Activation of inflammatory cells within the ASM-bundle would be predicted to have important consequences on ASM function. Following mast cell degranulation the mediators histamine, PGD_2 and LTC_4 are released, which are all potent agonists for ASM contraction [142]. Mast cell cytokines may further contribute to AHR. The mast cells in the ASM-bundles in asthma, but not in COPD, express IL-13 [143]. IL-13 has been shown to attenuate relaxation to β-agonists and augment contractility to acetylcholine [144, 145]. Similarly, the mast cell protease may be important in modulating ASM contractility and AHR [146, 147].

The interactions between inflammatory cells and ASM cells may have more long-term consequences. Mast cells co-cultured with ASM promote ASM differentiation with increased α-smooth muscle actin expression [148]. Similarly, mast cell differentiation towards the chymase-positive phenotype, observed within the ASM-bundle, may be mediated by mast cell-ASM interactions. Increased ASM mass is a well-established feature of asthma [86]. A number of mast cell mediators including histamine [149], tryptase [150] and LTD_4 [151], promote ASM proliferation. Alternatively increased ASM mass may be a consequence of the recruitment of ASM progenitors. This view is supported by the increased number of fibrocytes that migrate into the airway following allergen challenge [152]. Recent evidence suggests that ASM migration towards the ASM-bundle is mediated by the activation of CCR7 by ASM- and mast cell-derived CCL19 [153].

Therefore mast cell interactions with ASM in asthma are likely to be important in the development of AHR and may play a critical role in the development of increased ASM mass and the development of fixed airflow obstruction seen in severe disease.

Modulating AHR: Pharmacological and Non-pharmacological Treatment

A variety of anti-inflammatory agents have been utilised to modulate AHR in asthma. Corticosteroids cause marked eosinopenia when given orally and both oral and topical corticosteroids reduce the tissue eosinophilia in a dose-dependent manner [154]. The evidence that corticosteroids reduce eosinophil counts in asthma is consistent. For example 6 days of treatment with oral cortciosteroids reduced the sputum eosinophil count and eosinophilic cationic protein (ECP) level in 24 asthmatics from 14% to 1%, whereas, no change was observed in the placebo group. Moreover the increase in peak flow associated with steroid treatment correlated with the fall in eosinophil count [155]. Oral prednisolone caused a fall in the sputum eosinophil count and ECP level in patients with severe exacerbations of their disease. The improvement in sputum eosinophils and ECP levels correlated with improvement in lung function [156]. In a bronchial biopsy study of 10 asthmatics, treatment with 2,000 µg of beclomethasone dipropionate for 6 weeks resulted in an improvement in lung function, symptoms, AHR and a reduction in markers of inflammation, including the eosinophil count [157]. Inhaled budesonide resulted in a fall in eosinophil counts, which correlated with the improvement in AHR in 14 asthmatics [158]. Oral prednisolone given for 2 weeks caused a significant fall in eosinophil counts, which was not seen in the placebo limb of the study [159]. In all these studies, comparable effects were also seen on mast cell and T cell counts emphasising the broad spectrum of anti-inflammatory actions of corticosteroids.

In contrast to corticosteroids, a specific blockade of mediators including histamine [160], leukotrienes [161], IgE [162], and cytokines IL-5 [163, 164], IL-4 [165, 166], IFN-γ [167] and IL-12 [168], has generally proven to have a weak and often negligible effect upon AHR in asthma. Most notably anti-IL-5, in an allergen challenge study of the antibodies, has been well tolerated and effective in reducing the peripheral blood and to a lesser extent sputum eosinophilia, but no effect has been seen on either the early or late response, or on the severity of AHR in these very mild subjects [163]. One notable exception is inhibition of TNF-α [169], Berry demonstrated a 3.5 doubling dose improvement in PC_{20} methcholine with Entanercept in refractory asthma and a parallel reduction in peripheral blood TNF activity in patients with the largest magnitude of improvement in methacholine responsiveness. Therefore, the success of targeted anti-cytokine therapy may be limited to patients who have evidence of specific up-regulation of cytokine axes.

Whether modulation in other cytokines implicated in AHR such as IL-13 leads to improvement in AHR is unknown, and results of studies in progress are eagerly awaited.

A promising and emerging non-pharmacological approach has been the use of bronchial thermoplasty to selectively target the proximal airway wall with a heat signal in asthma. Studies examining the effects of bronchial thermoplasty in adult asthma suggest that targeting the remodelling of proximal airways by heating the airway and selectively reducing the airway smooth muscle mass does have an impact upon AHR in the short-term and improves the health-related quality of life [170, 171].

Targeted Therapy in Asthma Directed by AHR

Biomarkers have been used to direct anti-inflammatory treatment in asthma. The most notable success has been with sputum eosinophil counts where three studies have consistently demonstrated improvements in symptoms, AHR and exacerbation eosinophil-based strategy [172–174]. Similar approaches have been attempted using AHR to direct therapy. Sont et al. compared a management strategy aimed at reducing AHR in mild-to-moderate persistent adult asthma compared to the usual clinical guideline-based practice. Patients treated in the AHR reduction group had a significant reduction in mild exacerbations over a 2-year period compared to the guideline group and a significant improvement in FEV_1 [175]. Similarly, a recent study in the Netherlands in asthmatic children with moderate atopic asthma assessed whether a treatment strategy based upon AHR was superior to a symptom-based strategy at improving lung function and symptom-free days. After 2 years there was no evidence of any improvement in the symptom-free days between the two treatment strategies; however pre-bronchodilator FEV_1 was greater in the AHR management group. Interestingly the improvement in FEV_1 was explained by gradual deterioration in lung function in a subgroup of children with low symptom scores, suggesting that an AHR-based strategy might preserve lung function decline in asthmatics who had discordance of symptoms and physiology and were poor perceivers of their asthma control [176].

The use of AHR to direct therapy is therefore less successful than sputum eosinophil counts. Indirect challenges such as mannitol may more closely reflect inflammation, and studies are underway to assess the utility of this measure in directing treatment in asthma.

Conclusions

Finally, it must be borne in mind that asthma is characterised by a variety of distinct disease domains in a multi-dimensional umbrella (symptoms, physiology, AHR, atopy, inflammation), and these domains are often dissociated and the expression of individual asthma may be biased towards some but not all of the domains [177]. For example some patients with asthma are non-atopic, have fixed airflow obstruction, but do not have eosinophilic airway inflammation and have limited evidence of AHR or bronchodilator reversibility; in contrast to others who have the classical model of atopic asthma with eosinophilic, corticosteroid-responsive asthma, marked AHR and bronchodilator reversibility. Therefore, although AHR is a key feature of asthma, we need to be cognizant of its limitations as it fails to completely define or capture the complexity of the disease within an individual.

Thus, AHR has a clinical utility in combination with other measures in the diagnosis of asthma and potentially to direct therapy. Recent studies have given us a real opportunity to unravel the relationship between AHR, airway inflammation and remodelling, and have given prominence to the role of mast cell-ASM interactions. However, the challenge for clinicians in the future is to be able to understand the mechanisms driving AHR in an individual asthmatic, and to select the specific therapy appropriate to normalise airway function.

References

1. Global Initiative for Asthma Guidelines (2007) Available from: http://www.ginasthma.com
2. O'Byrne PM, Ryan G, Morris M, McCormack D, Jones NL, Morse JL, et al. (1982) Asthma induced by cold air and its relation to nonspecific bronchial responsiveness to methacholine. Am. Rev. Respir. Dis. 125:281–285.
3. Holgate ST, Mann JS, Cushley MJ (1984) Adenosine as a bronchoconstrictor mediator in asthma and its antagonism by methylxanthines. J. Allergy Clin. Immunol. 74:302–306.
4. Anderson SD, Brannan J, Spring J, Spalding N, Rodwell LT, Chan K, et al. (1997) A new method for bronchial-provocation testing in asthmatic subjects using a dry powder of mannitol. Am. J. Respir. Crit. Care Med. 156:758–765.
5. McFadden ER, Jr, Gilbert IA (1994) Exercise-induced asthma. N. Engl. J. Med. 330: 1362–1367.
6. Curry JJ (1946) The action of histamine on the respiratory tract in normal and asthmatic subjects. J. Clin. Invest. 25:785–791.
7. Juniper EF, Frith PA, Dunnett C, Cockcroft DW, Hargreave FE (1978) Reproducibility and comparison of responses to inhaled histamine and methacholine. Thorax 33:705–710.
8. Allen ND, Davis BE, Hurst TS, Cockcroft DW (2005) Difference between dosimeter and tidal breathing methacholine challenge: contributions of dose and deep inspiration bronchoprotection. Chest 128:4018–4023.
9. Cockcroft DW, Davis BE, Todd DC, Smycniuk AJ (2005) Methacholine challenge: comparison of two methods. Chest 127:839–844.
10. Cockcroft DW, Davis BE (2006) The bronchoprotective effect of inhaling methacholine by using total lung capacity inspirations has a marked influence on the interpretation of the test result. J. Allergy Clin. Immunol. 117:1244–1248.
11. Parker CD, Bilbo RE, Reed CE (1965) Methacholine aerosol as a test for bronchial asthma. Arch. Intern. Med. 115:452–458.
12. Kremer AM, Pal TM, Oldenziel M, Kerkhof M, de Monchy JG, Rijcken B (1995) Use and safety of a shortened histamine challenge test in an occupational study. Eur. Respir. J. 8:737–741.
13. Standardization of spirometry (2007) Am. J. Respir. Crit. Care Med. 152:1107–1136.
14. Cockcroft DW, Berscheid BA (1983) Measurement of responsiveness to inhaled histamine: comparison of FEV1 and Sgaw. Ann. Allergy 51:374–377.

15. van Broekhoven P, Hop WC, Rasser E, de Jongste JC, Kerrebijn KF (1991) Comparison of FEV1 and transcutaneous oxygen tension in the measurement of airway responsiveness to methacholine. Pediatr. Pulmonol. 11:254–258.
16. Wilson NM, Bridge P, Phagoo SB, Silverman M (1995) The measurement of methacholine responsiveness in 5 year old children: three methods compared. Eur. Respir. J. 8:364–370.
17. Christopher KL, Wood RP, Eckert RC, Blager FB, Raney RA, Souhrada JF (1983) Vocal-cord dysfunction presenting as asthma. N. Engl. J. Med. 308:1566–7150.
18. Eiser NM, Kerrebjjn KF, Quanjer PJ (1983) Guidelines for standardization of bronchial challenges with (nonspecific) bronchoconstrictor agents. Bull. Eur. Physiopathol. Respir. 19:495–514.
19. Sterk PJ, Fabbri LM, Quanjer PH, Cockcroft DW, O'Byrne PM, Anderson SD, et al. (1993) Airway responsiveness. Standardized challenge testing with pharmacological, physical and sensitizing stimuli in adults. Report Working Party Standardization of Lung Function Tests, European Community for Steel and Coal. Official Statement of the European Respiratory Society. Eur. Respir. J. (Suppl 16):53–83.
20. Verlato G, Cervcri I, Villani A, Pasquetto M, Ferrari M, Fanfulla F, et al. (1996) Evaluation of methacholine dose-response curves by linear and exponential mathematical models: goodness-of-fit and validity of extrapolation. Eur. Respir. J. 9:506–511.
21. Cockcroft DW, Murdock KY, Mink JT (1983) Determination of histamine PC20. Comparison of linear and logarithmic interpolation. Chest 84:505–506.
22. Cockcroft DW, Murdock KY, Berscheid BA, Gore BP (1992) Sensitivity and specificity of histamine PC20 determination in a random selection of young college students. J. Allergy Clin. Immunol. 89:23–30.
23. Gilbert R, Auchincloss JH, Jr (1990) Post-test probability of asthma following methacholine challenge. Chest 97:562–565.
24. Juniper EF, Cockcroft DW, Hargreave FE (1994) Histamine and methacholine inhalaltion tests: tidal breathing method-laboratory procedure and standardisation. Lund, Astra Draco.
25. Boulet LP, Cartier A, Thomson NC, Roberts RS, Dolovich J, Hargreave FE (1983) Asthma and increases in nonallergic bronchial responsiveness from seasonal pollen exposure. J. Allergy Clin. Immunol. 71:399–406.
26. Hargreave FE, Ramsdale EH, Pugsley SO (1984) Occupational asthma without bronchial hyperresponsiveness. Am. Rev. Respir. Dis. 130:513–515.
27. Ramsdell JW, Nachtwey FJ, Moser KM (1982) Bronchial hyperreactivity in chronic obstructive bronchitis. Am. Rev. Respir. Dis. 126:829–832.
28. Ramsdale EH, Roberts RS, Morris MM, Hargreave FE (1985) Differences in responsiveness to hyperventilation and methacholine in asthma and chronic bronchitis. Thorax 40:422–426.
29. Ramsdale EH, Morris MM, Roberts RS, Hargreave FE (1984) Bronchial responsiveness to methacholine in chronic bronchitis: relationship to airflow obstruction and cold air responsiveness. Thorax 39:912–918.
30. Verma VK, Cockcroft DW, Dosman JA (1988) Airway responsiveness to inhaled histamine in chronic obstructive airways disease: chronic bronchitis vs emphysema. Chest 94:457–461.
31. Ryan G, Dolovich MB, Roberts RS, Frith PA, Juniper EF, Hargreave FE, et al. (1981) Standardization of inhalation provocation tests: two techniques of aerosol generation and inhalation compared. Am. Rev. Respir. Dis. 123:195–199.
32. Yan K, Salome C, Woolcock AJ (1983) Rapid method for measurement of bronchial responsiveness. Thorax 38:760–765.
33. Knox AJ, Wisniewski A, Cooper S, Tattersfield AE (1991) A comparison of the Yan and a dosimeter method for methacholine challenge in experienced and inexperienced subjects. Eur. Respir. J. 4:497–502.
34. Peat JK, Salome CM, Bauman A, Toelle BG, Wachinger SL, Woolcock AJ (1991) Repeatability of histamine bronchial challenge and comparability with methacholine bronchial challenge in a population of Australian school children. Am. Rev. Respir. Dis. 144:338–343.
35. Dehaut P, Rachiele A, Martin RR, Malo JL (1983) Histamine dose-response curves in asthma: reproducibility and sensitivity of different indices to assess response. Thorax 38:516–522.

36. Chinn S, Britton JR, Burney PG, Tattersfield AE, Papacosta AO (1987) Estimation and repeatability of the response to inhaled histamine in a community survey. Thorax 42:45–52.
37. Weiss ME, Wheeler B, Eggleston P, Adkinson NF, Jr (1989) A protocol for performing reproducible methacholine inhalation tests in children with moderate to severe asthma. Am. Rev. Respir. Dis. 139:67–72.
38. Boulet LP, Morin D, Turcotte H (1990) Variations of airway responsiveness to methacholine and exercise in asthmatic and normal subjects over a 12-month period. Clin. Invest. Med. 13:60–66.
39. Balzano G, Delli CI, Gallo C, Cocco G, Melillo G (1989) Intrasubject between-day variability of PD20 methacholine assessed by the dosimeter inhalation test. Chest 95:1239–1243.
40. Josephs LK, Gregg I, Mullee MA, Campbell MJ, Holgate ST (1992) A longitudinal study of baseline FEV1 and bronchial responsiveness in patients with asthma. Eur. Respir. J. 5:32–39.
41. Cockcroft DW, Davis BE (2005) Lack of tachyphylaxis to methacholine at 24 h. Chest 128:1248–1251.
42. Van Schoor J, Joos GF, Pauwels RA (2000) Indirect bronchial hyperresponsiveness in asthma: mechanisms, pharmacology and implications for clinical research. Eur. Respir. J. 16:514–533.
43. Guidelines for Methacholine and Exercise Challenge Testing (1999) Am. J. Respir. Crit. Care Med. 161:309–329.
44. Cushley MJ, Tattersfield AE, Holgate ST (2004) Inhaled adenosine and guanosine on airway resistance in normal and asthmatic subjects (Reprinted from Br. J. Clin. Pharmacol. 15:161–165, 1983). Br. J. Clin. Pharmacol. 58:S751–S755.
45. Phillips GD, Ng WH, Church MK, Holgate ST (1989) The response of plasma histamine to bronchoprovocation with methacholine, adenosine 5′-monophosphate, and allergen in atopic nonasthmatic subjects. Am. Rev. Respir. Dis. 141:9–13.
46. Polosa R, Ng WH, Crimi N, Vancheri C, Holgate ST, Church MK, et al. (1995) Release of mast-cell-derived mediators after endobronchial adenosine challenge in asthma. Am. J. Respir. Crit. Care Med. 151:624–629.
47. Phillips GD, Holgate ST (1989) The effect of oral terfenadine alone and in combination with flurbiprofen on the bronchoconstrictor response to inhaled adenosine 5-monophosphate in nonatopic asthma. Am. Rev. Respir. Dis. 139:463–469.
48. Meijer RJ, Kerstjens HA, Arends LR, Kauffman HF, Koeter GH, Postma DS (1999) Effects of inhaled fluticasone and oral prednisolone on clinical and inflammatory parameters in patients with asthma. Thorax 54:894–899.
49. van den BM, Meijer RJ, Kerstjens HA, de Reus DM, Koeter GH, Kauffman HF, et al. (2001) PC(20) adenosine 5′-monophosphate is more closely associated with airway inflammation in asthma than PC(20) methacholine. Am. J. Respir. Crit. Care Med. 163:1546–1550.
50. Prieto L, Uixera S, Gutierrez V, Bruno L (2002) Modifications of airway responsiveness to adenosine 5′-monophosphate and exhaled nitric oxide concentrations after the pollen season in subjects with pollen-induced rhinitis. Chest 122:940–947.
51. Rodwell LT, Anderson SD, Seale JP (1992) Inhaled steroids modify bronchial responses to hyperosmolar saline. Eur. Respir. J. 5:953–962.
52. Leuppi JD, Salome CM, Jenkins CR, Anderson SD, Xuan W, Marks GB, et al. (2001) Predictive markers of asthma exacerbation during stepwise dose reduction of inhaled corticosteroids. Am. J. Respir. Crit. Care Med. 163:406–412.
53. in't Veen JC, Smits HH, Hiemstra PS, Zwinderman AE, Sterk PJ, Bel EH (1999) Lung function and sputum characteristics of patients with severe asthma during an induced exacerbation by double-blind steroid withdrawal. Am. J. Respir. Crit. Care Med. 160:93–99.
54. Brannan JD, Anderson SD, Perry CP, Freed-Martens R, Lassig AR, Charlton B (2005) The safety and efficacy of inhaled dry powder mannitol as a bronchial provocation test for airway hyperresponsiveness: a phase 3 comparison study with hypertonic (4.5%) saline. Respir. Res. 6:144.
55. Seow CY, Schellenberg RR, Pare PD (1998) Structural and functional changes in the airway smooth muscle of asthmatic subjects. Am. J. Respir. Crit. Care Med. 158(5 Pt 3): S179–S186.

56. Whicker SD, Armour CL, Black JL (1988) Responsiveness of bronchial smooth muscle from asthmatic patients to relaxant and contractile agonists. Pulm. Pharmacol. 1:25–31.
57. Bai TR (1991) Abnormalities in airway smooth muscle in fatal asthma: a comparison between trachea and bronchus. Am. Rev. Respir. Dis. 143:441–443.
58. Bai TR (1990) Abnormalities in airway smooth muscle in fatal asthma. Am. Rev. Respir. Dis. 141:552–557.
59. Goldie RG, Spina D, Henry PJ, Lulich KM, Paterson JW (1986) In vitro responsiveness of human asthmatic bronchus to carbachol, histamine, beta-adrenoceptor agonists and theophylline. Br. J. Clin. Pharmacol. 22:669–676.
60. Ma X, Cheng Z, Kong H, Wang Y, Unruh H, Stephens NL, et al. (2002) Changes in biophysical and biochemical properties of single bronchial smooth muscle cells from asthmatic subjects. Am. J. Physiol. Lung Cell Mol. Physiol. 283:L1181–L1189.
61. Jackson AC, Murphy MM, Rassulo J, Celli BR, Ingram RH, Jr (2004) Deep breath reversal and exponential return of methacholine-induced obstruction in asthmatic and nonasthmatic subjects. J. Appl. Physiol. 96:137–142.
62. Skloot G, Permutt S, Togias A (1995) Airway hyperresponsiveness in asthma: a problem of limited smooth muscle relaxation with inspiration. J. Clin. Invest. 96:2393–2403.
63. O'Byrne PM, Inman MD (2003) Airway hyperresponsiveness. Chest 123:411S–416S.
64. Gil FR, Lauzon AM (2007) Smooth muscle molecular mechanics in airway hyperresponsiveness and asthma. Can. J. Physiol. Pharmacol. 85:133–140.
65. Stephens NL, Li W, Jiang H, Unruh H, Ma X (2003) The biophysics of asthmatic airway smooth muscle. Respir. Physiol. Neurobiol. 137:125–140.
66. Seow CY (2005) Myosin filament assembly in an ever-changing myofilament lattice of smooth muscle. Am. J. Physiol. Cell Physiol. 289:C1363–C1368.
67. Gunst SJ, Wu MF (2001) Selected contribution: plasticity of airway smooth muscle stiffness and extensibility: role of length-adaptive mechanisms. J. Appl. Physiol. 90:741–749.
68. Gunst SJ, Meiss RA, Wu MF, Rowe M (1995) Mechanisms for the mechanical plasticity of tracheal smooth muscle. Am. J. Physiol. 268:C1267–C1276.
69. Gunst SJ, Wu MF, Smith DD (1993) Contraction history modulates isotonic shortening velocity in smooth muscle. Am. J. Physiol. 265:C467–C476.
70. Bursac P, Lenormand G, Fabry B, Oliver M, Weitz DA, Viasnoff V, et al. (2005) Cytoskeletal remodelling and slow dynamics in the living. Cell Nat. Mater. 4:557–561.
71. Wang L, Pare PD, Seow CY (2001) Selected contribution: effect of chronic passive length change on airway smooth muscle length-tension relationship. J. Appl. Physiol. 90:734–740.
72. Silberstein J, Hai CM (2002) Dynamics of length-force relations in airway smooth muscle. Respir. Physiol. Neurobiol. 132:205–221.
73. Bai TR, Bates JH, Brusasco V, Camoretti-Mercado B, Chitano P, Deng LH, et al. (2004) On the terminology for describing the length-force relationship and its changes in airway smooth muscle. J. Appl. Physiol. 97:2029–2034.
74. Naghshin J, Wang L, Pare PD, Seow CY (2003) Adaptation to chronic length change in explanted airway smooth muscle. J. Appl. Physiol. 95:448–453.
75. An SS, Fabry B, Trepat X, Wang N, Fredberg JJ (2006) Do biophysical properties of the airway smooth muscle in culture predict airway hyperresponsiveness? Am. J. Respir. Cell Mol. Biol. 35:55–64.
76. An SS, Bai TR, Bates JH, Black JL, Brown RH, Brusasco V, et al. (2007) Airway smooth muscle dynamics: a common pathway of airway obstruction in asthma. Eur. Respir. J. 29:834–860.
77. Hollins F, Saunders D, Kaur D, Sutcliffe A, Challiss RAJ, Bradding P, Brightling CE (2007) Human airway smooth muscle activation. Clin. Exp. Allergy 37:1881(abstract).
78. Mahn K, Hirst SJ, McVicker CG, Snelkov VA, Kanabar V, Simcock DE, O'Connor BJ, Lee TH (2006) Calcium signaling in asthmatic airway smooth muscle is abnormal. Proc. Am. Thorac. Soc. A772.
79. Tao FC, Tolloczko B, Eidelman DH, Martin JG (1999) Enhanced Ca(2+) mobilization in airway smooth muscle contributes to airway hyperresponsiveness in an inbred strain of rat. Am. J. Respir. Crit. Care Med. 160:446–453.

80. Benayoun L, Druilhe A, Dombret MC, Aubier M, Pretolani M (2003) Airway structural alterations selectively associated with severe asthma. Am. J. Respir. Crit. Care Med. 167:1360–1368.
81. Oliver BG, Black JL (2006) Airway smooth muscle and asthma. Allergol. Int. 55:215–223.
82. Roth M, Johnson PR, Borger P, Bihl MP, Rudiger JJ, King GG, et al. (2004) Dysfunctional interaction of C/EBPalpha and the glucocorticoid receptor in asthmatic bronchial smooth-muscle cells. N. Engl. J. Med. 351:560–574.
83. Davies DE, Wicks J, Powell RM, Puddicombe SM, Holgate ST (2003) Airway remodeling in asthma: new insights. J. Allergy Clin. Immunol. 111:215–225.
84. Barbato A, Turato G, Baraldo S, Bazzan E, Calabrese F, Panizzolo C, et al. (2006) Epithelial damage and angiogenesis in the airways of children with asthma. Am. J. Respir. Crit. Care Med. 174:975–981.
85. Siddiqui S, Sutcliffe A, Shikotra A, Woodman L, Doe C, McKenna S, Wardlaw AJ, Bradding P, Pavord I, and Brightling CE (2007) Vascular remodelling is a feature of asthma and non-asthmatic eosinophilic bronchitis. J. Allergy Clin. Immunol. 120(4): 813–819.
86. Carroll N, Elliot J, Morton A, James A (1993) The structure of large and small airways in nonfatal and fatal asthma. Am. Rev. Respir. Dis. 147:405–410.
87. Ebina M, Takahashi T, Chiba T, Motomiya M (1993) Cellular hypertrophy and hyperplasia of airway smooth muscles underlying bronchial asthma. A 3-D morphometric study. Am. Rev. Respir. Dis. 148:720–726.
88. Kuwano K, Bosken CH, Pare PD, Bai TR, Wiggs BR, Hogg JC (1993) Small airways dimensions in asthma and in chronic obstructive pulmonary disease. Am. Rev. Respir. Dis. 148:1220–1225.
89. Woodruff PG, Dolganov GM, Ferrando RE, Donnelly S, Hays SR, Solberg OD, et al. (2004) Hyperplasia of smooth muscle in mild to moderate asthma without changes in cell size or gene expression. Am. J. Respir. Crit. Care Med. 169:1001–1006.
90. Lambert RK, Wiggs BR, Kuwano K, Hogg JC, Pare PD (1993) Functional significance of increased airway smooth muscle in asthma and COPD. J. Appl. Physiol. 74:2771–2781.
91. McParland BE, Macklem PT, Pare PD (2003) Airway wall remodeling: friend or foe? J. Appl. Physiol. 95:426–434.
92. Moreno RH, Hogg JC, Pare PD (1986) Mechanics of airway narrowing. Am. Rev. Respir. Dis. 133:1171–1180.
93. Wiggs BR, Bosken C, Pare PD, James A, Hogg JC (1992) A model of airway narrowing in asthma and in chronic obstructive pulmonary-disease. Am. Rev. Respir. Dis. 145:1251–1258.
94. Wiggs BR, Hrousis CA, Drazen JM, Kamm RD (1997) On the mechanism of mucosal folding in normal and asthmatic airways. J. Appl. Physiol. 83:1814–1821.
95. James AL, Pare PD, Hogg JC (1989) The mechanics of airway narrowing in asthma. Am. Rev. Respir. Dis. 139:242–246.
96. Macklem PT (1995) Theoretical basis of airway instability: Roger S. Mitchell lecture. Chest 107:87S–88S.
97. Niimi A, Matsumoto H, Takemura M, Ueda T, Chin K, Mishima M (2003) Relationship of airway wall thickness to airway sensitivity and airway reactivity in asthma. Am. J. Respir. Crit. Care Med. 168:983–988.
98. Beigelman-Aubry C, Capderou A, Grenier PA, Straus C, Becquemin MH, Similowski T, et al. (2002) Mild intermittent asthma: CT assessment of bronchial cross-sectional area and lung attenuation at controlled lung volume. Radiology 223:181–187.
99. Goldin JG, McNitt-Gray MF, Sorenson SM, Johnson TD, Dauphinee B, Kleerup EC, et al. (1998) Airway hyperreactivity: assessment with helical thin-section CT. Radiology 208:321–329.
100. Siddiqui S, Cruse G, Haldar P, McKenna S, Monteiro W, Bradding P, Wardlaw AJ, Pavord ID, Entwisle J, Brightling CE. Differences in airway wall geometry of the apical bronchus in asthma and non asthmatic eosinophilic bronchitis. Proc. Am. Thorac. Soc. A332.

101. Altounyan RE (1964) Variation of drug action on airway obstruction in man. Thorax 19:406–415.
102. Cartier A, Thomson NC, Frith PA, Roberts R, Hargreave FE (1982) Allergen-induced increase in bronchial responsiveness to histamine: relationship to the late asthmatic response and change in airway calibre. J. Allergy Clin. Immunol. 170:170–177.
103. De Monchy JG, Kauffman HF, Venge P, Koeter GH, Jansen HM, Sluiter HJ, et al. (1985) Bronchoalveolar eosinophilia during allergen-induced late asthmatic reactions. Am. Rev. Respir. Dis. 131:373–376.
104. Metzger WJ, Richerson HB, Worden K, Monick M, Hunninghake GW (1986) Bronchoalveolar lavage of allergic asthmatic patients following allergen bronchoprovocation. Chest 89:477–483.
105. Fabbri LM, Boschetto P, Zocca E, Milani G, Pivirotto F, Plebani M, et al. (1987) Bronchoalveolar neutrophilia during late asthmatic reactions induced by toluene diisocyanate. Am. Rev. Respir. Dis. 136:36–42.
106. Flint KC, Leung KB, Hudspith BN, Brostoff J, Pearce FL, Johnson NM (1985) Bronchoalveolar mast cells in extrinsic asthma: a mechanism for the initiation of antigen specific Bronchoconstriction. Br. Med. J. 291:923–926.
107. Pin I, Freitag AP, O'Byrne PM, Girgis-Gabardo A, Watson RM, Dolovich J, et al. (1992) Changes in the cellular profile of induced sputum after allergen-induced asthmatic responses. Am. Rev. Respir. Dis. 145:1265–1269.
108. Wardlaw AJ, Dunnette S, Gleich GJ, Collins JV, Kay AB (1988) Eosinophils and mast cells in bronchoalveolar lavage in subjects with mild asthma. Relationship to bronchial hyper-reactivity. Am. Rev. Respir. Dis. 137:62–69.
109. Jatakanon A, Lim S, Kharitonov SA, Chung KF, Barnes PJ (1998) Correlation between exhaled nitric oxide, sputum eosinophils, and methacholine responsiveness in patients with mild asthma. Thorax 53:91–95.
110. Green RH, Brightling CE, Woltmann G, Parker D, Wardlaw AJ, Pavord ID (2002) Analysis of induced sputum in adults with asthma: identification of subgroup with isolated sputum neutrophilia and poor response to inhaled corticosteroids. Thorax 57:875–879.
111. Wardlaw AJ, Dunnette S, Gleich GJ, Collins JV, Kay AB (1988) Eosinophils and mast cells in bronchoalveolar lavage in subjects with mild asthma. Relationship to bronchial hyper-reactivity. Am. Rev. Respir. Dis. 137:62–69.
112. Polosa R, Renaud L, Cacciola R, Prosperini G, Crimi N, Djukanovic R (1998) Sputum eosinophilia is more closely associated with airway responsiveness to bradykinin than methacholine in asthma. Eur. Respir. J. 12:551–556.
113. Rosi E, Ronchi MC, Grazzini M, Duranti R, Scano G (1999) Sputum analysis, bronchial hyperresponsiveness, and airway function in asthma: results of a factor analysis. J. Allergy Clin. Immunol. 103:232–237.
114. van Velzen E, van den Bos JW, Benckhuijsen JA, van Essel T, de Bruijn R, Aalbers R (1996) Effect of allergen avoidance at high altitude on direct and indirect bronchial hyper-responsiveness and markers of inflammation in children with allergic asthma. Thorax 51:582–584.
115. Gibson PG, Dolovich J, Denburg J, Ramsdale EH, Hargreave FE (1989) Chronic cough: eosinophilic bronchitis without asthma. Lancet 1:1346–1348.
116. Brightling CE, Ward R, Goh KL, Wardlaw AJ, Pavord ID (1999) Eosinophilic bronchitis is an important cause of chronic cough. Am. J. Respir. Crit. Care Med. 160:406–410.
117. Berry MA, Hargadon B, McKenna S, Shaw D, Green RH, Brightling CE, et al. (2005) Observational study of the natural history of eosinophilic bronchitis. Clin. Exp. Allergy 35:598–601.
118. Brightling CE, Woltmann G, Wardlaw AJ, Pavord ID (1999) Development of irreversible airflow obstruction in a patient with eosinophilic bronchitis without asthma. Eur. Respir. J. 314:1228–1230.
119. Brightling CE, Bradding P, Symon FA, Holgate ST, Wardlaw AJ, Pavord ID (2002) Mast-cell infiltration of airway smooth muscle in asthma. N. Engl. J. Med. 346:1699–7105.

120. Brightling CE, Symon FA, Birring SS, Bradding P, Wardlaw AJ, Pavord ID (2003) Comparison of airway immunopathology of eosinophilic bronchitis and asthma. Thorax 58:528–532.

121. Brightling CE, Symon FA, Birring SS, Bradding P, Pavord ID, Wardlaw AJ (2002) T(H)2 cytokine expression in bronchoalveolar lavage fluid T lymphocytes and bronchial submucosa is a feature of asthma and eosinophilic bronchitis. J. Allergy Clin. Immunol. 110: 899–905.

122. Berry MA, Parker D, Neale N, Woodman L, Morgan A, Monk P, et al. (2004) Sputum and bronchial submucosal IL-13 expression in asthma and eosinophilic bronchitis. J. Allergy Clin. Immunol. 114:1106–1109.

123. Brightling CE, Ward R, Woltmann G, Bradding P, Sheller JR, Dworski R, et al. (2000) Induced sputum inflammatory mediator concentrations in eosinophilic bronchitis and asthma. Am. J. Respir. Crit. Care Med. 162:878–882.

124. Park SW, Park JS, Lee YM, Lee JH, Jang AS, Kim DJ, et al. (2005) Differences in radiological/HRCT findings in eosinophilic bronchitis compared to asthma: implication for bronchial responsiveness. Thorax 61:41–47.

125. O'Donnell RA, Frew AJ (2002) Is there more than one inflammatory phenotype in asthma. Thorax 57:566–568.

126. Douwes J, Gibson P, Pekkanen J, Pearce N (2002) Non-eosinophilic asthma: importance and possible mechanisms. Thorax 57:643–648.

127. Gibson PG, Simpson JL, Saltos N (2001) Heterogeneity of airway inflammation in persistent asthma: evidence of neutrophilic inflammation and increased sputum interleukin-8. Chest 119:1329–1336.

128. Wenzel SE, Schwartz LB, Langmack EL, Halliday JL, Trudeau JB, Gibbs RL, et al. (1999) Evidence that severe asthma can be divided pathologically into two inflammatory subtypes with distinct physiologic and clinical characteristics. Am. J. Respir. Crit. Care Med. 160:1001–1008.

129. Pavord ID, Brightling CE, Woltmann G, Wardlaw AJ (1999) Non-eosinophilic corticosteroid unresponsive asthma. Lancet 353:2213–2214.

130. Godon P, Boulet LP, Malo JL, Cartier A, Lemiere C (2002) Assessment and evaluation of symptomatic steroid-naive asthmatics without sputum eosinophilia and their response to inhaled corticosteroids. Eur. Respir. J. 20:1364–1369.

131. Berry MA, Morgan A, Shaw DE, Parker D, Green RH, Brightling CE, et al. (2007) Pathological features and inhaled corticosteroid response of eosinophilic and non-eosinophilic asthma. Thorax 62:1043–1049.

132. Koshino T, Teshima S, Fukushima N, Takaishi T, Hirai K, Miyamoto Y, et al. (1993) Identification of basophils by immunohistochemistry in the airways of post-mortem cases of fatal asthma. Clin. Exp. Allergy 23:919–925.

133. Amin K, Janson C, Boman G, Venge P (2005) The extracellular deposition of mast cell products is increased in hypertrophic airways smooth muscles in allergic asthma but not in nonallergic asthma. Allergy 60:1241–1247.

134. Ammit AJ, Bekir SS, Johnson PR, Hughes JM, Armour CL, Black JL (1997) Mast cell numbers are increased in the smooth muscle of human sensitized isolated bronchi. Am. J. Respir. Crit. Care Med. 155:1123–1129.

135. El Shazly A, Berger P, Girodet PO, Ousova O, Fayon M, Vernejoux JM, et al. (2006) Fraktalkine produced by airway smooth muscle cells contributes to mast cell recruitment in asthma. J. Immunol. 176:1860–1868.

136. Berger P, Girodet PO, Begueret H, Ousova O, Perng DW, Marthan R, et al. (2003) Tryptase-stimulated human airway smooth muscle cells induce cytokine synthesis and mast cell chemotaxis. FASEB J. 17:2139–2141.

137. Begueret H, Berger P, Vernejoux JM, Dubuisson L, Marthan R, Tunon-de-Lara JM (2007) Inflammation of bronchial smooth muscle in allergic asthma. Thorax 62:8–15.

138. Yang W, Kaur D, Okayama Y, Ito A, Wardlaw AJ, Brightling CE, et al. (2006) Human lung mast cells adhere to human airway smooth muscle, in part, via tumor suppressor in lung cancer-1. J. Immunol. 176:1238–1243.

139. Slats AM, Janssen K, van Schadewijk A, van der Plas DT, Schot R, van den Aardweg JG, et al. (2007) Bronchial inflammation and airway responses to deep inspiration in asthma and COPD. Am. J. Respir. Crit. Care Med. (in press).
140. Carroll NG, Mutavdzic S, James AL (2002) Distribution and degranulation of airway mast cells in normal and asthmatic subjects. Eur. Respir. J. 19:879–885.
141. Chen FH, Samson KT, Miura K, Ueno K, Odajima Y, Shougo T, et al. (2004) Airway remodeling: a comparison between fatal and nonfatal asthma. J. Asthma 41:631–638.
142. Brightling CE, Bradding P, Pavord ID, Wardlaw AJ (2003) New insights into the role of the mast cell in asthma. Clin. Exp. Allergy 33:550–556.
143. Saha S, Neale N, Berry M, May R, Monk R, Bradding P, Wardlaw AJ, Pavord ID, Brightling CE (2006) Interleukin-13 + cells are increased in the airway smooth muscle bundle of asthmatics but not COPD. Proc. Am. Thorac. Soc. A29.
144. Laporte JC, Moore PE, Baraldo S, Jouvin MH, Church TL, Schwartzman IN, et al. (2001) Direct effects of interleukin-13 on signalling pathways for physiological responses in cultured human airway smooth muscle cells. Am. J. Respir. Crit. Care Med. 164:141–148.
145. Grunstein MM, Hakonarson H, Leiter J, Chen M, Whelan R, Grunstein JS, et al. (2002) IL-13-dependent autocrine signaling mediates altered responsiveness of IgE-sensitized airway smooth muscle. Am. J. Physiol. Lung Cell Mol. Physiol. 282:L520–L528.
146. Johnson PR, Ammit AJ, Carlin SM, Armour CL, Caughey GH, Black JL (1997) Mast cell tryptase potentiates histamine-induced contraction in human sensitized bronchus. Eur. Respir. J. 10:38–43.
147. Berger P, Walls AF, Marthan R, Tunon-de-Lara JM (1998) Immunoglobulin E-induced passive sensitization of human airways: an immunohistochemical Study. Am. J. Respir. Crit. Care Med. 157:610–616.
148. Woodman L, Kaur D, Sutcliffe A, Bradding P, Brightling CE (2005) α-smooth muscle actin expression by human airway smooth muscle cells is upregulated in co-culture with mast cells. Thorax 60: ii118.
149. Panettieri RA, Yadvish PA, Kelly AM, Rubinstein NA, Kotlikoff MI (1990) Histamine stimulates proliferation of airway smooth muscle and induces c-fos expression. Am. J. Physiol. 259:L365–L371.
150. Berger P, Perng DW, Thabrew H, Compton SJ, Cairns JA, McEuen AR, et al. (2001) Tryptase and agonists of PAR-2 induce the proliferation of human airway smooth muscle cells. J. Appl. Physiol. 9:1372–1379.
151. Espinosa K, Bosse Y, Stankova J, Rola-Pleszczynski M (2003) CysLT1 receptor upregulation by TGF-beta and IL-13 is associated with bronchial smooth muscle cell proliferation in response to LTD4. J. Allergy Clin. Immunol. 111:1032–10440.
152. Schmidt M, Sun G, Stacey MA, Mori L, Mattoli S (2003) Identification of circulating fibrocytes as precursors of bronchial myofibroblasts in asthma. J. Immunol. 171:380–389.
153. Kaur D, Saunders R, Berger P, Siddiqui S, Woodman L, Wardlaw A, et al. (2006) Airway smooth muscle and mast cell-derived CC chemokine ligand 19 mediate airway smooth muscle migration in asthma. Am. J. Respir. Crit. Care Med. 174:1179–1188.
154. Wardlaw AJ, Brightling C, Green R, Woltmann G, Pavord I (2000) Eosinophils in asthma and other allergic diseases. Br. Med. Bull. 56:985–1003.
155. Claman DM, Boushey HA, Liu J, Wong H, Fahy JV (1994) Analysis of induced sputum to examine the effects of prednisone on airway inflammation in asthmatic subjects. J. Allergy Clin. Immunol. 94:861–869.
156. Pizzichini MM, Pizzichini E, Clelland L, Efthimiadis A, Mahony J, Dolovich J, et al. (1997) Sputum in severe exacerbations of asthma: kinetics of inflammatory indices after prednisone treatment. Am. J. Respir. Crit. Care Med. 155:1501–1508.
157. Djukanovic R, Wilson JW, Britten KM, Wilson SJ, Walls AF, Roche WR, et al. (1992) Effect of an inhaled corticosteroid on airway inflammation and symptoms in asthma. Am. Rev. Respir. Dis. 145:669–674.
158. Lim S, Jatakanon A, John M, Gilbey T, O'Connor BJ, Chung KF, et al. (1999) Effect of inhaled budesonide on lung function and airway inflammation assessment by various inflammatory markers in mild asthma. Am. J. Respir. Crit. Care Med. 159:22–30.

159. Bentley AM, Hamid Q, Robinson DS, Schotman E, Meng Q, Assoufi B, et al. (1996) Prednisolone treatment in asthma. Reduction in the numbers of eosinophils, T cells, tryptase-only positive mast cells, and modulation of IL-4, IL-5, and interferon-gamma cytokine gene expression within the bronchial mucosa. Am. J. Respir. Crit. Care Med. 153:551–556.

160. Aubier M, Neukirch C, Peiffer C, Melac M (2001) Effect of cetirizine on bronchial hyper-responsiveness in patients with seasonal allergic rhinitis and asthma. Allergy 56:35–42.

161. Hamilton A, Faiferman I, Stober P, Watson RM, O'Byrne PM (1998) Pranlukast, a cysteinyl leukotriene receptor antagonist, attenuates allergen-induced early- and late-phase bronchoconstriction and airway hyperresponsiveness in asthmatic subjects. J. Allergy Clin. Immunol. 102:177–183.

162. Boulet LP, Chapman KR, Cote J, Kalra S, Bhagat R, Swystun VA, et al. (1997) Inhibitory effects of an anti-IgE antibody E25 on allergen-induced early asthmatic response. Am. J. Respir. Crit. Care Med. 155:1835–1840.

163. Leckie MJ, ten Brinke A, Khan J, Diamant Z, O'Connor BJ, Walls CM, et al. (2000) Effects of an interleukin-5 blocking monoclonal antibody on eosinophils, airway hyper-responsiveness, and the late asthmatic response. Lancet 35:2144–2148.

164. Kips JC, O'Connor BJ, Langley SJ, Woodcock A, Kerstjens HA, Postma DS, et al. (2003) Effect of SCH55700, a humanized anti-human interleukin-5 antibody, in severe persistent asthma: a pilot study. Am. J. Respir. Crit. Care Med. 167:1655–1659.

165. Borish LC, Nelson HS, Corren J, Bensch G, Busse WW, Whitmore JB, et al. (2001) Efficacy of soluble IL-4 receptor for the treatment of adults with asthma. J. Allergy Clin. Immunol. 107:963–970.

166. Borish LC, Nelson HS, Lanz MJ, Claussen L, Whitmore JB, Agosti JM, et al. (1999) Interleukin-4 receptor in moderate atopic asthma. A phase I/II randomized, placebo-controlled trial. Am. J. Respir. Crit. Care Med. 160:1816–1823.

167. Boguniewicz M, Schneider LC, Milgrom H, Newell D, Kelly N, Tam P, et al. (1993) Treatment of steroid-dependent asthma with recombinant interferon-gamma. Clin. Exp. Allergy 23:785–790.

168. Bryan SA, O'Connor BJ, Matti S, Leckie MJ, Kanabar V, Khan J, et al. (2000) Effects of recombinant human interleukin-12 on eosinophils, airway hyper-responsiveness, and the late asthmatic response. Lancet 356:2149–2153.

169. Berry MA, Hargadon B, Shelley M, Parker D, Shaw DE, Green RH, et al. (2006) Evidence of a role of tumor necrosis factor alpha in refractory asthma. N. Engl. J. Med. 354:697–708.

170. Cox G, Miller JD, McWilliams A, FitzGerald JM, Lam S (2006) Bronchial thermoplasty for asthma. Am. J. Respir. Crit. Care Med. 173:965–969.

171. Cox G, Thomson NC, Rubin AS, Niven RM, Corris PA, Siersted HC, et al. (2007) Asthma control during the year after bronchial thermoplasty. N. Engl. J. Med. 356:1327–1337.

172. Green RH, Brightling CE, McKenna S, Hargadon B, Parker D, Bradding P, et al. (2002) Asthma exacerbations and sputum eosinophil counts: a randomised controlled trial. Lancet 360:1715–1721.

173. Jayaram L, Pizzichini MM, Cook RJ, Boulet LP, Lemiere C, Pizzichini E, et al. (2006) Determining asthma treatment by monitoring sputum cell counts: effect on exacerbations. Eur. Respir. J. 27:483–494.

174. Chlumsky J, Striz I, Terl M, Vondracek J (2006) Strategy aimed at reduction of sputum eosinophils decreases exacerbation rate in patients with asthma. J. Int. Med. Res. 34:129–139.

175. Sont JK, Willems LN, Bel EH, van Krieken JH, Vandenbroucke JP, Sterk PJ (1999) Clinical control and histopathologic outcome of asthma when using airway hyperresponsiveness as an additional guide to long-term treatment. The AMPUL Study Group. Am. J. Respir. Crit. Care Med. 159:1043–1051.

176. Nuijsink M, Hop WC, Sterk PJ, Duiverman EJ, de Jongste JC (2007) Long-term asthma treatment guided by airway hyperresponsiveness in children: a randomized controlled trial. Eur. Respir. J 30:457–466.

177. Wardlaw AJ, Silverman M, Siva R, Pavord ID, Green R (2005) Multi-dimensional phenotyping: towards a new taxonomy for airway disease. Clin. Exp. Allergy 35:1254–1262.

Mechanisms of Nocturnal Asthma

Krzysztof Kowal and Lawrence Du Buske

Overview

Nocturnal asthma can be defined as a nighttime exacerbation of asthma symptoms, which is associated with decreased lung function and increased bronchial hyper-responsiveness, inflammation and need for medication. In patients with nocturnal asthma diurnal changes in forced expiratory volume during the first second (FEV_1) or peak expiratory flow rate (PEFR) are greater than 15% [1]. The presence of nocturnal symptoms leads to awakening and sleep deprivation, which in turn results in impaired quality of life but is also associated with increased asthma severity, morbidity, and mortality. The great majority of fatal events in asthma are preceded by nocturnal deterioration of lung function [2]. As many as 70% of deaths from asthma occur during the nighttime hours with the majority of respiratory arrests and sudden deaths occurring between midnight and 8 AM [2, 3]. In a study evaluating 3,129 patients with nocturnal asthma, 94% of dyspneic episodes were reported between 10 PM and 7 AM with the greatest frequency around 4 AM [4] (Fig. 1).

Nocturnal symptoms are frequently experienced by asthma patients, but in routine clinical practice they seem to be under-diagnosed and therefore under-treated [5]. The prevalence of any nocturnal symptoms in asthma patients is high, ranging from 60–80%, however symptoms occurring regularly every night are encountered in less than 50% of asthma patients [5, 6]. In the first large study including 7,729 patients with asthma nocturnal symptoms occurring at least once per week were reported by 74%, at least three times per week by 64%, and every night by 40% of patients [5]. A recent large cross-sectional study evaluated 13,493 asthma patients in a primary care setting [6]. In that population 60% of patients had nocturnal symptoms. Interestingly in the subgroup of patients who declared

K. Kowal
Medical University of Bialystok, Sklodowskiej-Curie 24a, 15-276 Bialystok, Poland
e-mail: kowalkmd@umwb.edu.pl

L.M. Du Buske
Brigham and Women's Hospital, Harvard Medical School, 75 Francis Street, Boston, MA 02115, USA
e-mail: ldubuske@aol.com

R. Pawankar et al. (eds.), *Allergy Frontiers: Clinical Manifestations,*
DOI: 10.1007/978-4-431-88317-3_14, © Springer 2009

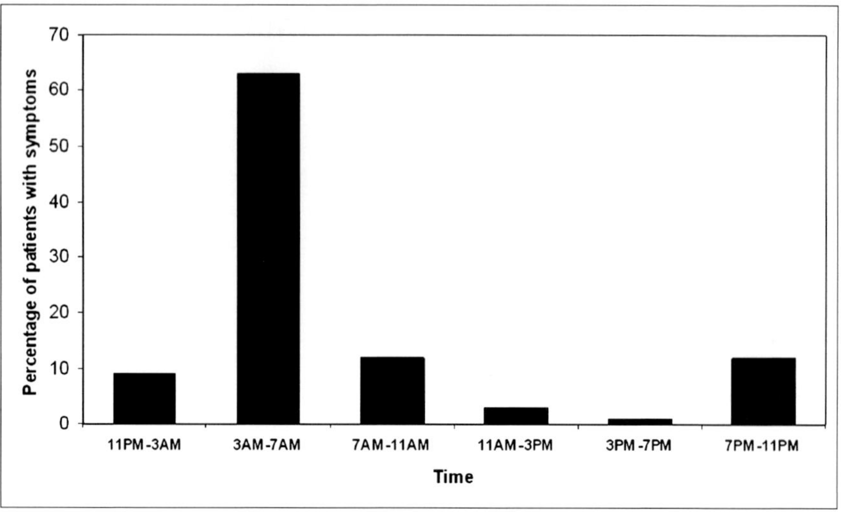

Fig. 1 Timing of dyspneic episodes in asthma

having no nocturnal symptoms, the symptoms were detected by the physician in 42% of cases. Children seem to experience nocturnal asthma symptoms less frequently than adults do [7–9]. However, the symptoms not only significantly affect school attendance and school performance of those children but also lead to increased number of missed work days of their parents [7–9]. The importance of nocturnal asthma symptoms as an indicator of poor asthma control has been appreciated in several guidelines for asthma management including the National Asthma Education and Prevention Program (NAEPP) and the Global Initiative for Asthma (GINA) [1, 10]. Understanding the mechanisms responsible for nocturnal asthma exacerbation may help in appropriate adjustment of asthma treatment and the search for new possible therapeutic strategies.

Lung Function in Health

Even in healthy subjects evident circadian changes in respiratory function have been demonstrated [11]. Those changes are mild and include decreased pulmonary ventilation with a concomitant increase in arterial carbon dioxide (CO_2) content and a fall of pulmonary function such as FEV_1 or PEFR [11–13]. They seem to be predominantly driven by endogenous circadian rhythms as sleep deprivation fails to cause a significant change in the evaluated variables [12, 13]. In healthy subjects, diurnal changes in lung function results are of small amplitude usually below 10%. In one study, the best lung function occurred at 4 PM, while the worst at 4 AM, with a peak-to-trough difference of approximately 8% [14]. Those values are of statistical, but not clinical, significance as they are not associated with any detectable changes in bronchial reactivity, cellular composition of bronchial mucosa, or significant differences in production of inflammatory mediators within the lungs [12, 13]. They do however follow the pattern of changes in general metabolism as reflected by plasma cortisol and epinephrine levels or body temperature [12]. Other physiological effects associated with decreased metabolism at night such as decreased sympathetic and increased parasympathetic nervous function may also participate in increased nocturnal airway resistance in healthy subjects.

Mechanisms of Nocturnal Impairment of Lung Function in Asthmatics

Several mechanisms have been implicated in the pathophysiology of nocturnal symptoms in asthmatic patients. Those include: (1) endogenous circadian rhythm disturbances including cycles of endogenous corticosteroids, sympathetic tone and parasympathetic activity and their effects on airway function and inflammatory processes; (2) concomitant disorders such as gastroesophageal reflux disease (GERD), rhinosinusitis, or obstructive sleep apnea (OSA); (3) behavioral factors such as changes in activity, posture, meals, or sleep; or (4) environment factors such as change in ambient temperature, light exposure or allergen exposure [15–20].

Changes in bronchial resistance resemble the diurnal pattern seen in healthy subjects, although the variations in flow rate are much greater, with at least 15% decrease of FEV_1 or PEFR occurring at night usually reaching nadir around 4 AM [1] (Fig. 2). In some patients the peak-to-trough swing may be as high as 50% [14]. In asthmatic patients, the lower airway resistance increases during the night starting from midnight to 6 AM, and the basic circadian rhythm is independent of sleep [21]. However, the resistance increases further while asleep indicating the existence of sleep related amplification of lower airway resistance in asthma patients [21] (Fig. 3). Interestingly, as mentioned above, diurnal changes in airway resistance in healthy controls are totally sleep independent [12, 13, 21]. Examination of the relationship between sleep stages and nocturnal asthma episodes fails to reveal a consistent relationship of a specific sleep stage to enhanced risk of nocturnal asthma [22]. Thus, it would seem unlikely that the rapid eye movement (REM) sleep associated with dreaming is the major cause of nocturnal asthma awakenings. Moreover, brief sleep interruption with 15 min of exercise did not alter the continuous fall of PEFR throughout the night in asthmatic patients [23]. Another factor which can be associated with nocturnal fall of lung function is the recumbent position. No such association, however, was demonstrated in asthma patients [24]. Finally, a possible relation of solar time on the changes in airway resistance has been studied [25]. Studies of workers who rapidly change from day to night to day work shift demonstrated that the circadian rhythm of airway resistance functions according to a period of sleep (rest) rather than clock hour [25].

A circadian change in bronchial reactivity occurs in parallel to the change in PEFR. This change in reactivity of the airways is proportionate to the circadian

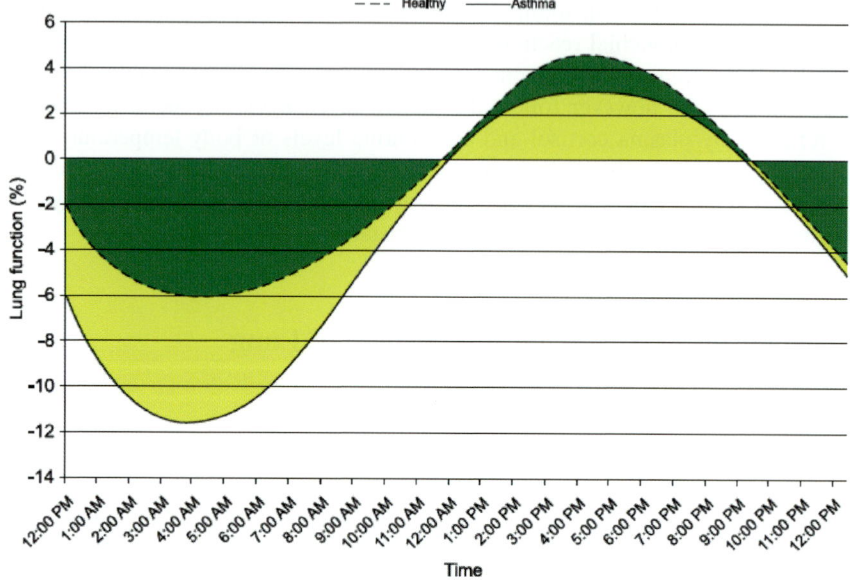

Fig. 2 The circadian variation of lung function in subject with asthma and healthy controls

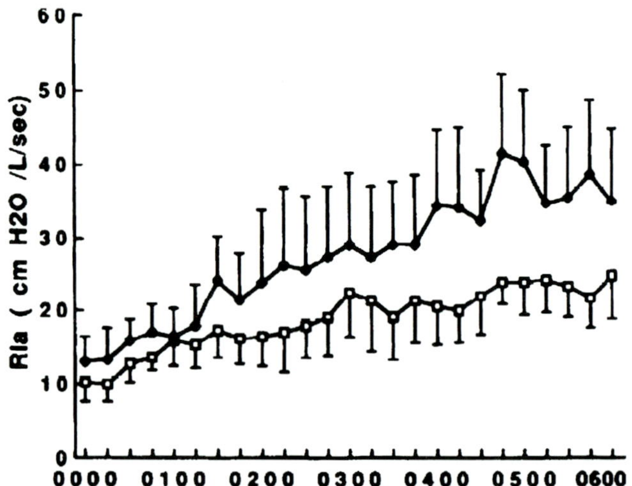

Fig. 3 Lower airway resistance (RIa) in asthmatic subjects, from midnight to 6:00 A.M. when awake (dots) or asleep (squares). (Reproduced from [21] with permission)

change in airflow so the greater the nocturnal fall of PEFR, the greater the circadian change of bronchial hyperreactivity [26] (Fig. 4). Even if one segregates those asthmatic patients clearly having nocturnal symptoms from asthmatics without nocturnal symptoms, one sees that those asthmatics not cognizant of nocturnal symptoms

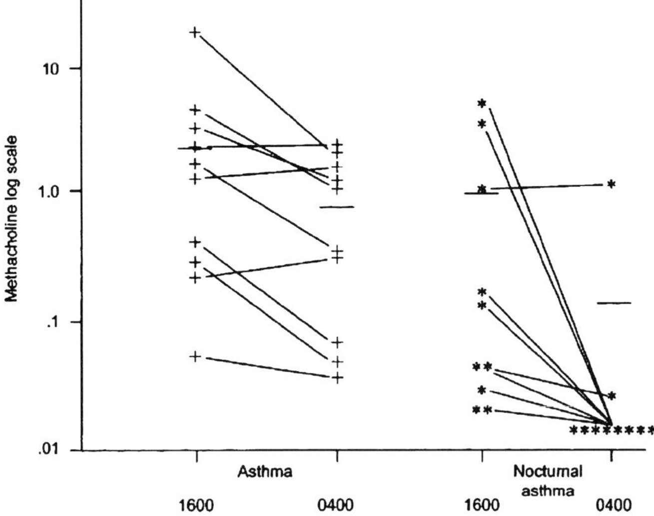

Fig. 4 The circadian variation in bronchial reactivity between 4:00 P.M. and 4:00 A.M. in contro land nocturnal asthmatics (horizontal lines represent mean values). (Reproduced from [26] with permission)

still demonstrate heightened airway reactivity to methacholine challenge at 4 AM compared with 4 PM [26]. Moreover, there is also an association between diurnal changes in PEFR and bronchial reactivity to histamine tested between 12 AM and 5 PM [27]. Patients having greater diurnal variability of PEFR are characterized by greater bronchial reactivity to histamine measured in the afternoon [27]. Interestingly, those patients with greater circadian PEFR variability responded also with greater improvement of FEV_1 to inhaled bronchodilator [27]. In a study comparing bronchial reactivity to direct and indirect stimuli in asthmatic patients with and without nocturnal fall of airflow, significant difference between those groups was demonstrated in bronchial reactivity to adenosine monophosphate (AMP) but not to metacholine [28]. Patients with nocturnal airflow limitation were more sensitive to AMP than those without nocturnal airflow limitation [28]. Moreover, as compared to measurements performed at 4 PM, at 4 AM in subjects with circadian PEFR variation greater than 15%, the bronchial responsiveness to AMP increased much more that to methacholine [28]. Interestingly, the circadian change in bronchial reactivity to AMP, but not to methacholine, was significantly related to the circadian changes in PEFR [28]. This suggests that mast cell activation rather than primary changes in smooth muscle cell contraction plays a predominant role in the nocturnal airway obstruction and indicates the important role of inflammation in the development of nocturnal airflow limitation.

In several studies which evaluated exhaled nitric oxide (ENO) concentration in asthmatic patients, the patients who reported nocturnal symptoms had significantly greater ENO concentration than those without nocturnal symptoms [29–32]. The increased ENO output seen in nocturnal asthma patients seem to predominantly derive from distal airways and alveolar compartment [29]. In two studies the circadian changes of ENO concentration were evaluated [31, 32]. In one study the presence of nocturnal symptoms in asthmatic patients was associated with increased ENO concentration in the exhaled air measured both at day and night, but no clear circadian fluctuations of ENO concentration was demonstrated [31]. However, significant increase in ENO concentration at 4 AM as compared to 4 PM levels was demonstrated in nocturnal asthma patients but not in non-nocturnal asthmatics or healthy controls [31]. The increase in ENO concentration at 4 AM corresponded with the nadir of FEV_1 [31]. In the second study, significant circadian changes in ENO concentration were demonstrated in nocturnal asthma patients [32]. Paradoxically, the concentration of ENO decreased along with the nocturnal fall of lung function [32]. The decrease in ENO levels may reflect the impaired endogenous production of NO, which may participate in the pathogenesis of nocturnal asthma. Nitric oxide possess strong bronchodilatory properties and therefore nocturnal fall of ENO concentration may reflect important chronobiological defect in the endogenous production and/or increased disposition of NO which could play a role in nocturnal asthma exacerbations. On the other hand, the fall of ENO level at night in nocturnal asthma patients may depend on the nocturnal bronchoconstriction as the levels of ENO depend on airway flow [33]. This may be the case as only in nocturnal asthma patients, but not in non-nocturnal asthma patients, significant increase in ENO concentration after inhalation of a bronchodilator was demonstrated [32].

The possible association between the circadian rhythm and the development of airway inflammation was evaluated using bronchial allergen challenge model [34]. Exposure to inhaled allergen in the morning with a dose which produces an early asthmatic reaction (EAR) leads to delayed bronchospasm (late asthmatic reaction – LAR) 3–8 h later in approximately half of the patients. The tendency to develop a LAR is enhanced by increasing the dose of the allergen that is inhaled. The time of day of an inhalant allergen challenge is also critical to development of the LAR [34]. Interestingly, when the same asthmatics are challenged with the same allergen dose in the evening, all but one developed a LAR [34]. The pathophysiology of the EAR and LAR appear quite different. The EAR is dominated by mast cell-derived mediators of bronchospasm including preformed mast cell secretory granule components such as histamine and also the newly generated lipid-derived mediators such as cysteinyl leukotrienes (cysLTs) and prostaglandin D_2 (PGD_2), which may augment bronchospastic responses. The LAR involves a complex interaction of inflammatory cells including eosinophils, neutrophils, basophils, macrophages, and lymphocytes and a wide array of inflammatory mediators including cysLTs, reactive oxygen species, and an assortment of cytokines derived from multiple cellular sources. This mechanistic difference between the EAR and the LAR makes the highly inflammatory late response an ideal candidate for significant modulation by chronobiologic fluctuations in endogenous factors that modulate inflammatory cell activity.

In summary, in patients with nocturnal asthma, strong association exists between circadian variations in airway resistance clinically measured as drop in PEFR or FEV_1, bronchial hyperreactivity and airway inflammation. Moreover, circadian rhythm seems to predispose to the development of airway inflammation and subsequently deterioration of airway function.

Asthma is characterized by the presence of airway inflammation and increased intensity of airway inflammation is associated with loss of asthma control and appearance of symptoms. Several authors, therefore, have attempted to search for unique features of inflammatory response in nocturnal asthma patients and for possible modulation of the inflammatory response by the circadian rhythm. The results of those studies demonstrated that in patients who experience nocturnal symptoms, the fall of lung function at night is accompanied by significant increase in intensity of airway inflammation as demonstrated by increased numbers of eosinophils and neutrophils in the airways at night [26, 35–42]. The changes are not dependent on the sleep pattern because the sleep pattern and sleep staging were similar in those with and without nocturnal symptoms [26]. Interestingly, circadian variations in intensity of the inflammatory response could be demonstrated not only in the lungs but also in the peripheral blood [26, 35, 36]. The peak number of circulating eosinophils, however is observed around midnight but not at the time of the greatest fall in lung function – at 4 AM [35]. That rise in the number of eosinophils in the peripheral blood may participate in the pathology of nocturnal symptoms as they seem to precede the increase in the number of eosinophils in the airway tissue. Nevertheless, in patients with nocturnal airflow limitation the number of circulating eosinophils at 4 AM is significantly greater than at 4 PM [35, 36]. In patients with nocturnal symptoms, but not in those without nocturnal symptoms, the increased number of circulating eosinophils in the early morning hours is associated with significant increase in the number of low-density eosinophils [37]. Importantly, it was the number of low density eosinophils but not total number of eosinophils which correlated with nocturnal fall of FEV_1 [37]. Low density eosinophils represent a population of eosinophils with greater proinflammatory potential. Increased number of circulating low density eosinophils is encountered in asthmatic patients during the LAR. Those observations suggest the existence of similar mechanisms which are responsible for airflow limitation during the LAR and nocturnal asthma. In addition to eosinophils, altered platelet function and increased platelet activation was observed in nocturnal asthma patients at 4 AM [38].

Application and bronchoscopy with bronchoalveolar lavage (BAL) and endobronchial and transbronchial biopsies allowed for studying the inflammation in the airways. In several studies BAL fluid was used for evaluation of airway inflammation in nocturnal asthma patients [36, 39–45]. Cytological evaluation of BAL fluid demonstrated, in nocturnal asthma patients, increased numbers of eosinophils and lymphocytes and greater level of eosinophil cationic protein (ECP) in BAL samples obtained at 4 AM compared with 4 PM [39]. No such differences could be demonstrated in the group of control subjects [39]. Similarly, in a study comparing asthmatic patients with and without nocturnal symptoms, increased numbers of eosinophils, lymphocytes, and neutrophils in BAL fluid were demonstrated in samples obtained at 4 AM in comparison with samples obtained at 4 PM only in the former group [40]. Interestingly, separate evaluation of asthmatics with more severe asthma who did not report nocturnal symptoms did not demonstrate increase in the number of inflammatory cells in BAL at 4 AM indicating that nocturnal deterioration of lung function is not simply related to the disease severity [40]. Moreover, performed in several patients, BAL fluid analysis after bronchoconstriction in response to histamine at 4 PM revealed no changes in cellular BAL components indicating that this is not bronchoconstriction per se which is associated with inflammatory response in the airways [40]. Cytological evaluation of BAL fluid samples obtained from nocturnal asthma patients at 4 AM and 4 PM demonstrated significantly greater number of lymphocytes with increased percentage of CD4 + cells at the former than at the latter time point [36]. The FEV_1 at 4 AM was inversely correlated with the number of lymphocytes and CD4 + cells in the BAL fluid. Moreover, stimulated with phytohemagluttinin (PHA) cells derived form BAL fluid released interleukin-5 (IL-5) and the secretion of IL-5 correlated with BAL eosinophilia [36]. This study demonstrated that circadian changes in lung function are associated with an influx of CD4 + cells to the lungs and potential of those cells to release cytokine which increase eosinophil survival and activates eosinophils (IL-5) [35]. Two other studies, which evaluated in BAL fluid cellular composition and some soluble markers of mast cells and eosinophil activation failed to demonstrate circadian changes in the studied parameters in nocturnal asthmatics [41, 42]. However, they found in BAL fluid more activated alveolar macrophages and increased levels of PGD_2 in nocturnal asthmatics in comparison with non-nocturnal asthmatics suggesting that the former suffered from more severe asthma [41, 42]. On the other hand circadian changes in superoxide anion generation by air-space cells has been demonstrated [43]. The superoxide anion production was significantly greater at 4 AM than at 4 PM in patients with nocturnal asthma symptoms, and the level of superoxide anion generation at 4 AM was significantly greater in nocturnal asthma patients than in patients without nocturnal symptoms [43]. Moreover, circadian changes of IL-1 beta concentration has been demonstrated in BAL fluid in nocturnal asthma patients [44]. In asthmatics with nocturnal airflow obstruction, the concentration of IL-1 beta in BAL fluid was significantly greater at 4 AM than at 4 PM [44]. Altogether these data indicate that both in peripheral blood and in the lungs increased intensity of inflammation is observed in nocturnal asthma patients. Furthermore, in those patients at least some of the inflammatory cells and mediators undergo circadian changes with the maximum activation found in the early morning hours, which corresponds to the nadir in lung function.

In order to evaluate the predominant localization of the characteristic for nocturnal asthma circadian changes in the inflammatory process in the lungs, Kraft et al. compared endobronchial and transbronchial biopsies from nocturnal and non-nocturnal asthmatics obtained at 4 PM and at 4 AM [45–47]. Significant increase in the number of inflammatory cells including eosinophils, macrophages and lymphocytes was demonstrated at 4 AM only in transbronchial biopsies derived from nocturnal asthma patients [45, 46]. The nighttime significant eosinophil influx was seen only in the small airways (less than 2 mm diameter) and the surrounding alveolar tissue [45, 46] (Fig. 5). The eosinophilic inflammation in the biopsies derived from larger airways did not demonstrate significant circadian differences in both nocturnal and non-nocturnal asthmatics. The association between distal airway eosinophilic inflammation and nocturnal symptoms was further strengthened by demonstration of strong correlation between the change in the number of alveolar

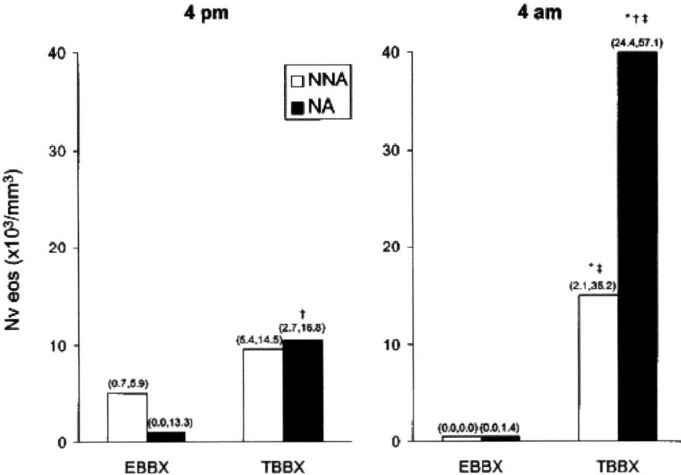

Fig. 5 The number per volume (Nv) of eosinophils (eos) in the nocturnal asthma (NA) and non-nocturnal asthma (NNA) groups in the endobronchial (airway tissue, EBBX) and transbronchial (alveolar tissue, TBBX) biopsies at 4:00 A.M. and 4:00 P.M. Values are expressed as medians with 25-75 interquartile range in the parentheses above each bar *†‡ p≤0.05. (Reproduced from [45] with permission)

eosinophils and the nocturnal fall in FEV_1. Macrophages and CD4 + lymphocytes infiltrations followed the pattern described for eosinophils, and in nocturnal asthma patients at 4 AM they migrated predominantly to the alveolar compartment [45, 46]. Similarly, as with eosinophils, the number of CD4 + cells detected at 4 AM in the peripheral lung tissue correlated significantly with the fall in FEV_1 in nocturnal asthma patients. Subsequent study by the same group supported the earlier findings concerning peripheral localization of the predominant inflammatory changes in the lungs of nocturnal asthma patients by evaluation of changes in airway resistance associated with nocturnal symptoms [47]. It was elevated peripheral airway resistance which distinguished nocturnal asthma patients from non-nocturnal asthmatics and healthy subjects [47]. Moreover, only in nocturnal asthma patients but not in non-nocturnal asthma patients or healthy subjects significant further increase in peripheral airway resistance was found at 4 AM in comparison with 4 PM values [47]. Those studies emphasize the role of peripheral airways and alveolar tissue in the development of nocturnal symptoms in asthmatic patients.

The mechanisms responsible for circadian variations in intensity of inflammation in asthma patients who suffer form nocturnal symptoms have been studied for years. Circadian variation in exposure to exogenous stimuli such as allergen or environmental tobacco smoke have been associated with nocturnal worsening of asthma [48]. In particular, high levels of house dust mite allergen in mattresses and exposure to environmental tobacco smoke were linked with increased circadian PEFR amplitude [48]. Other studies focused on circadian changes in endogenous factors such as neural activity, hormone secretion including adrenal – pituitary axis, melatonin, secretion of inflammatory mediators, and differences in the sensitivity of target cells.

It has been suggested that circadian changes in secretion of cortisol and epinephrine, two hormones which have strong anti-inflammatory and anti-asthma effects may participate in the development of nocturnal airway obstruction [49, 50]. Plasma concentrations of epinephrine and cortisol reach the lowest concentration at night which corresponds to the nadir of PEFR in asthmatic patients [49]. Moreover, in asthma patients the nadir of the plasma epinephrine level is associated with the peak in histamine plasma level [49, 50]. However, no significant differences in the circadian variations of cortisol or epinephrine concentrations have been demonstrated between nocturnal and non-nocturnal asthma patients [49, 50]. Similar plasma epinephrine and cortisol circadian changes are also seen in healthy subjects [49, 50]. It seems therefore that circulated hormone levels is not related to the airway limitation in nocturnal asthma patients. It cannot be excluded however, that secretion of those anti-inflammatory hormones at the levels detected in nocturnal asthma patients may be not adequate to extinguish increasing inflammatory response at night. This is supported by significantly greater plasma corticotropin levels in the morning hours observed in nocturnal asthma patients in comparison with non-nocturnal asthma patients or healthy subjects [51]. This morning rise in plasma corticotropin is not accompanied in nocturnal asthma patients by the adequate increase in cortisol level [51]. Interestingly several investigators demonstrated suboptimal response of target cells to cortisol or epinephrine [49, 50, 52, 53]. In vitro studies demonstrated that for the inhibition of lymphocyte proliferation by dexamethasone or hydrocortisone, approximately tenfold greater concentration of those steroids were required when peripheral blood mononuclear cells were collected from nocturnal asthma patients at 4 AM when compared with inhibition of cells collected at 4 PM [52]. No such circadian difference was seen when cells from non-nocturnal asthma patients or healthy subjects were used for inhibition assay [52]. Interestingly, when cells from BAL were used for inhibition studies, no circadian differences in inhibition of lymphocyte proliferation by dexamethasone were demonstrated in nocturnal asthma patients [53]. Significant differences in circadian suppression by dexamethasone of mediator release by BAL macrophages were demonstrated [53]. The secretion of IL-8 and tumor necrosis factor alpha (TNF-α) was less suppressed by dexamethasone when the cells were obtained at 4 AM in comparison to 4 PM [53]. In non-nocturnal asthma, dexamethasone suppressed those cytokine release by macrophages equally at both time points. The resistance to corticosteroids is caused by increased expression of glucocorticoid receptor beta (GRβ) at night in nocturnal asthma patients [53]. The GRβ is a splice variant of GR, which competes with GRα in binding corticosteroids but GRβ in contrast to GRα signals poorly after binding corticosteroids. Interestingly, increased expression of IL-13 at night by nocturnal asthma patients is responsible for increased expression of GRβ [53]. The circadian variation in IL-13 expression by BAL cells was observed in asthmatic patients with, but not without, nocturnal airflow limitation [53]. Experiments with in vitro inhibition of IL-13 resulted in decreased expression of GRβ [53].

Decreased response to epinephrine has also been suggested in nocturnal asthma. Polymorphonuclear leukocytes obtained from nocturnal asthma patients at 4 AM responded to isoproterenol with significantly lower production of cAMP than those obtained from non-nocturnal asthma patients or from healthy controls [49, 50]. This may result from lower affinity of beta 2-adrenergic receptors [50]. A genetic background for a defective beta 2-adrenergic receptor function in nocturnal asthma has been proposed [54]. The single nucleotide polymorphism in the coding region of the beta 2-adrenergic receptor gene results in the substitution of glycine at the position 16 for arginine. The polymorphic variant containing glycine is more susceptible for agonist dependent down-regulation of beta 2-adrenergic receptor. In one study, nocturnal asthma was associated with homozygosity for glycine at the position 16 of the beta 2-adrenergic receptor [54].

It seems that although in nocturnal asthma circadian changes in plasma levels of cortisol and epinephrine, hormones which exert anti-inflammatory and anti-asthma effects, are not altered. The responsiveness of the target tissues cells to those hormones may play a role in the development of nocturnal airway obstruction.

The potential effect of increased vagal tone in the development of nocturnal symptoms comes primarily from a study based on pharmacological intervention [55]. Morrison et al. evaluated, in a placebo controlled study, the effect of intravenous atropine on PEFR at 4 AM and 4 PM in patients with nocturnal asthma [55]. The improvement of PEFR after atropine was seen at both time points, but was significantly greater at 4 AM. The circadian variations which existed after placebo treatment were almost completely abolished after atropine [55]. This study supports the role of increased parasympathetic tone in the development of nocturnal airway obstruction.

Plasma levels of histamine, a mast cell and basophil product, which possesses strong bronchoconstricting properties, vary in a circadian rhythm [56]. The plasma histamine concentration peaks in the early morning hours, and the highest plasma histamine levels coincide with the greatest bronchoconstriction [56]. There is no evidence however that circadian changes in plasma histamine concentration are different in patients with and without nocturnal symptoms [49, 56]. It cannot be excluded that increased responsiveness to circulating histamine at night may play a role in the pathogenesis of nocturnal asthma. Antagonists of histamine receptors are not effective in asthma indicating that this possibility is unlikely.

Finally, melatonin, secretion of which is strongly associated with regulation of circadian homeostasis, has been implicated in the pathophysiology of nocturnal asthma. Melatonin has pro-inflammatory properties. Serum melatonin levels are elevated in patients with nocturnal asthma and the level of melatonin inversely correlates lung function in nocturnal asthma patients at night [57]. Melatonin induces secretion of pro-inflammatory cytokines from peripheral blood mononuclear cells and therefore can participate in the amplification of airway inflammation in nocturnal asthma patients [57, 58].

Concomitant diseases such as Gastroesophageal Reflux Disease (GERD), chronic rhinitis or Obstructive Sleep Apnea (OSA) have been proposed to aggravate nocturnal asthma symptoms. In a large cross-sectional study of 2,661 individuals, GERD was associated with nocturnal asthma symptoms, peak flow variability, and objectively diagnosed asthma as compared with individuals without GERD [59]. In Obstructive Sleep Aphex (OSA) patients, upper airway obstruction at night might cause reflex bronchoconstriction, and recurrent upper airway obstruction has been reported to cause bronchoconstriction [60]. Application of nasal continuous positive airway pressure (CPAP) improves daytime and nighttime PEFR, symptoms, and usage of medications, but only in nocturnal asthma patients with OSA [61].

Therapeutic Consequences

The therapy of nocturnal asthma is first directed at correcting those factors that may be identified as causative of asthma exacerbations. Those include avoidance of exposure to allergens and irritants and correction of concomitant diseases such as GERD or upper respiratory tract diseases. Upper respiratory tract is often affected in asthmatic patients. Rhinitis symptoms such as nasal obstruction shift the predominant pattern of breathing from nasal to oral. When the air is inhaled by mouth it is not appropriately conditioned and therefore it may dry and cool the bronchial mucosa. In fact, mechanical dilation of the nostrils with improved nasal breathing reduces nocturnal asthma symptoms [62]. The patients manifesting clinically significant gastroesophageal reflux may benefit from H_2 antagonists or proton pomp inhibitor therapy, however a meta-analysis of clinical trials of the treatment of GERD in patients with nocturnal asthma produced equivocal results [63]. Nevertheless, empiric treatment of GERD should be considered in patients with significant nocturnal symptoms who respond sub-optimally to anti-asthma therapy.

Pharmacologic Therapy of Nocturnal Asthma

Currently used for asthma treatment, inhaled and oral regimens can be optimized to ensure maximal efficacy overnight by changing the timing of the dosage of such medications and selecting optimal delivery systems.

Beta Adrenergic Agonist Therapy

Selective beta 2-adrenergic receptor agonists are the most effective symptomatic therapy in asthma (GINA). In patients with mild decrease in lung function at night, some improvement in lung function could be demonstrated using inhaled short acting beta agonists such as albuterol or fenoterol. Unfortunately, the bronchodilatory effect of those medications lasts less than 4 h, therefore their action is restricted to symptomatic application at night rather than prophylactic therapy of nocturnal symptoms. In patients with nocturnal asthma, beta 2-adrenergic receptor function decreases overnight, therefore higher doses of beta 2-agonsits are likely to be needed for symptom relief as well as for protective (prophylactic) therapy.

Sustained release preparations of albuterol and terbutaline have improved symptoms of nocturnal asthma in many patients [64, 65]. Similarly, good improvement in nocturnal symptoms is achieved using oral long-acting beta 2-agonist (LABA) bambuterol 20 mg taken once daily in moderate to severe asthma patients [66, 67]. However, oral therapy seems to be associated with greater frequency of side effects than application of new inhaled LABAs such as salmeterol or formoterol. In a study comparing inhaled salmeterol with oral slow-release terbutaline in nocturnal asthma patients, side effects were reported in 16% of patients treated with salmeterol as compared to 29% treated with slow-release terbutaline [68]. The frequency of side effects with inhaled formoterol in the treatment of nocturnal asthma did not differ from that seen in patients treated with albuterol [69, 70]. Both formoterol and salmeterol are the most effective therapy in preventing nocturnal symptoms in patients with asthma [69, 71–76]. The effective protection against nocturnal airflow limitation was demonstrated in mild, moderate and severe asthmatics who experienced nocturnal symptoms and who were treated with different doses of anti-inflammatory medications [71–76] (Fig. 5). Symptomatic improvement after application of LABA in patients with nocturnal asthma symptoms is not associated with improvement of airway inflammation index [77]. Inhaled LABA given together with inhaled corticosteroids therefore should be considered as the agents of choice for symptomatic management of nocturnal asthma patients who have nocturnal airflow limitation despite appropriate anti-inflammatory therapy and other preventive measurements such as environmental control and treatment of concomitant conditions such as OSA or GERD [78].

Theophylline Therapy

A number of investigations have noted that specific theophylline preparations may be uniquely effective in treatment of nocturnal asthma. Sustained-release theophylline preparations administered twice daily or once daily decreased nocturnal symptoms in asthmatic children in comparison with placebo [79, 80]. To optimize the therapy of nocturnal asthma, the level of theophylline must be maximal during the time that airflow reaches its nadir, generally between midnight and 4 AM. Use of control-release theophylline preparation, which is given once daily at supper, provides maximal theophylline concentrations between 3 and 5 AM, producing theophylline blood levels between 16 and 18 mcg/ml [81]. Extended release theophylline improves lung function and nocturnal symptoms in asthmatic patients treated with and without inhaled corticosteroids [82–86]. In contrast to beta 2-agonists during theophylline therapy significant anti-inflammatory effect was demonstrated [84].

Anticholinergic Therapy

Anticholinergic agents may be of some use in nocturnal asthma to combat nocturnal increase in vagal tone. In one study, intravenous atropine administered at day and at night improved daytime and nighttime PEFR and almost totally abolished circadian variation in PEFR [55]. This indicates that increased vagal tone may be particularly important in triggering symptoms at night in nocturnal asthma patients.

It seems that higher bedtime doses of ipratropium bromide may improve overnight reductions in peak flow. This drug unfortunately does not have sustained efficacy overnight [87, 88]. Tiotropium bromide, a novel inhaled anticholinergic agent with a long duration of action, seems to be promising in therapy of nocturnal asthma patients. The prolonged bronchodilator response and protection against metacholine challenge suggests that at once daily dosing, tiotropium may be useful in the treatment of nocturnal asthma [89]. Further studies are warranted to define the clinical utility of tiotropium in asthma therapy.

Corticosteroid Therapy

Appreciation of the chronopathology of nocturnal asthma with circadian variation in lung inflammation, particularly located at the distal airways and alveolar space has caused reevaluation of the most appropriate regimens of anti-inflammatory therapy. Because large increases in morning corticosteroid dosages typically increase corticosteroid-related adverse effects more than therapeutic effects, changing the timing of oral corticosteroid dosing to administration in the afternoon, generally about 3 PM should be considered [90]. The afternoon dosing of corticosteroids not only significantly improves nocturnal lung function, including a 65% increase in PEFR, but also significantly reduces the level of blood eosinophils through the night and early morning hours and consequently induces a generalized decrease in inflammatory cells appearing in BAL at 4 AM [90]. No such improvement occurs in early morning inflammatory cell infiltrates in the lungs of patients who are given corticosteroids at 8 AM or 8 PM, despite changes in blood eosinophil counts induced by these alternate times of corticosteroid dosing [90].

Inhaled corticosteroids (ICS) are the most commonly used anti-inflammatory agents for asthma. They seem to act rapidly and effectively in steroid naïve moderate nocturnal asthma [91]. A single dose of ICS (beclomethasone 1,000 mcg or fluticasone 1,000 mcg) reduced the fall in FEV_1 in patients with nocturnal asthma when administered at 4 PM indicating that appropriate timing of ICS dosing is also important to increase efficacy of ICS in nocturnal asthma patients [91]. However, in patients already treated with budesonide 200 mcg bid who experience nocturnal symptoms, even fourfold increase of budesonide dose is not effective in reduction of nocturnal symptoms [73]. Possibly not only escalation of the daily dose but changes in timing of ICS dosing might have increased their efficacy in preventing nocturnal symptoms. Two studies evaluated chronotherapy with ICS [92, 93]. In nocturnal asthma patients, Pincus et al. compared efficacy of triamcinolone administered either 800 mcg as a single dose at 3 PM or 200 mcg four times daily. The PEFR and FEV_1 improved equally in both groups. In a follow-up study two time points of triamcinolone dosing at 8 AM or 5:30 PM were compared. The investigators concluded that the optimal time to deliver ICS is between 3 PM and 5:30 PM. In yet another study, inhaled beclomethasone 400 mcg four times a day has been reported to improve symptoms of nocturnal asthma in only about half of the patients receiving such treatment [94]. The potential explanation for this low efficacy of ICS in preventing nocturnal deterioration of airflow in asthmatic patients may be explained by the low penetration of currently used formulations to distal airways and alveolar space. In fact, the predominant circadian changes in intensity of inflammation index are observed in the distal airways and alveolar compartment [45–47]. Usage of mometasone furoate is optimized with nocturnal dosing as a dosage (220 mcg), which is ineffective when given in the morning, has been shown to be effective in the evening, this evening dosage being as effective as twice this dosage given in either in the morning or given as a twice daily divided dosage. New formulations of inhaled corticosteroids, in which hydrofluoroalkane (HFA) is used as a propellant have an average particle size of 1.1 μm compared with up to 4.0 μm in currently used CFC (chlorofluorocarbon) aerosols [96]. Those HFA formulations are characterized by high pulmonary deposition, up to 68.3% in case of flunisolide [96]. In a study comparing CFC and HFA formulations of flunisolide, Corren et al. demonstrated that at one-third the dose of CFC flunisolide, the HFA flunisolide provided similar improvement in pulmonary function versus placebo [97]. The outcome values for all secondary efficacy measures, including nocturnal awakenings, were numerically superior in patients receiving HFA flunisolide compared with the CFC formulation [97]. Similarly, improved asthma control has been achieved using beclomethasone HFA formulations in comparison to fluticasone and budesonide delivered using dry powder devices [98].

Leukotriene Modifier Therapy

Leukotrienes are proinflammatory mediators and are increased at night in patients with nocturnal asthma [99]. Therapy with 5-lipoxygenase inhibitor in nocturnal asthmatic patients resulted in decreased leukotriene production which correlated with decreased peripheral blood eosinophilia and improvement in the morning FEV_1 [100]. Similarly, cysLT receptor antagonist montelukast when given as an evening dosage improves nighttime symptoms in asthmatic patients treated with and without ICS [101, 102].

Combined Therapy

As mentioned above, escalation of the ICS dose is not a good therapeutic strategy in patients who are already treated with low-moderate doses of ICS and experience nocturnal symptoms [73]. On the contrary in the same large study, formoterol added to either low or high dose of budesonide caused further improvement of nocturnal symptoms and consumption of rescue medications [73]. During the last few years combination formulations containing formoterol with budesonide or salmeterol with fluticasone in one inhaler have been introduced to asthma therapy. Six weeks therapy with combination of salmeterol (250 mcg) and fluticasone (50 mcg) in nocturnal asthma patients more efficiently improved bronchial reactivity to AMP than salmeterol or fluticasone used alone [103]. In another study evaluating moderate-to-severe asthma, salmeterol/fluticasone (50/250 mcg) twice daily administered in a single device was at least as effective as an approximately threefold higher microgram corticosteroid dose of budesonide (800 mcg) twice daily given concurrently with formoterol (12 mcg) twice daily in terms of reducing nights with symptoms and nighttime awakenings [104]. Adjusting the maintenance dosing of budesonide/formoterol in a single inhaler allows to achieve similar efficacy in reduction of nighttime symptoms as using a fixed maintenance dose [105]. The adjustable maintenance dosing was associated with significantly lower consumption of the medication [105]. Further studies are needed to clarify the role of combination medications in the treatment of nocturnal asthma.

References

1. National Asthma Education and Prevention Program, Expert panel report 2; guidelines for diagnosis and prevention of asthma. Publication No 97–405. Bethesda, MD: National Institute of Health; April 1997.
2. Hetzel MR, Clark TJH, Braithwaite MA. Analysis of sudden deaths and ventilatory arrests in hospital. Br Med J 1977; 1: 808–11.
3. Cochrane GM, Clark TJH. A survey of asthma mortality in patients between ages 35 and 64 in the Greater London hospitals in 1971. Thorax 1975; 30: 300–5.
4. Dathlefsen U, Repgas R. Ein neues Terapieprinzip bei Nachtlichen Asthma. Klin Med 1985; 80: 44–7.
5. Raherison C, Abouelfath A, Le Gros V, Taytard A, Molimard M. Underdiagnosing of nocturnal symptoms in asthma in general practice. J Asthma 2006; 43: 199–202.
6. Turner-Warwick M. Epidemiology of nocturnal asthma. Am J Med 1988; 85 (Suppl 1B): 6–8.
7. Tomalak W, Elbousefi A, Kurzawa R, et al. Diurnal variations of respiratory system resistance and compliance derived from input impedance in asthmatic children. Respir Physiol 2000; 123: 101–8.
8. Diette GB, Markson L, Skinner EA, et al. Nocturnal asthma in children affects school performance, and parents' work attendance. Arch Pediatr Adolesc Med 2000; 154: 923–8.
9. Weersink EJM, van Zomeren EH, Koeter GH, et al. Treatment of nocturnal airway obstruction improves daytime cognitive performance in asthmatics. Am J Respr Crit Care Med 1997; 156: 1144–50.
10. Global Initiative for Asthma, 11/2006, WHO
11. Mortola JP. Breathing around the clock: an overview of the circadian pattern of respiration. Eur J Appl Physiol 2004; 91: 119–29.
12. Spengler CM, Shea SA. Endogenous circadian rhythm of pulmonary function in healthy humans. Am J Respir Crit Care Med 2000; 162: 1038–42.
13. Spengler CM, Czeisler CA, Shea SA. An endogenous circadian rhythm of respiratory control in humans. J Physiol 2000; 526: 683–94.
14. Hetzel MR, Clark TJH. Comparison of normal and asthmatic circadian rhythms in peak expiratory flow rate. Thorax 1980; 35: 732–8.
15. Shigemitsu H, Afshar K. Nocturnal asthma. Curr Opinion Pulm Med 2007; 13: 49–55.
16. Sutherland ER. Nocturnal asthma. J Allergy Clin Immunol 2005; 116: 1179–86.
17. Calhoun WJ. Nocturnal asthma. Chest 2003; 123: S399–S405.

18. Skloot GS. Nocturnal astma: mechanisms and management. Mt Sinai J Med 2002; 69: 140–7.
19. Di Stefano A, Lusuardi M, Braghiroli A, Donner CF. Nocturnal asthma: mechanisms and therapy. Lung 1997; 175: 53–61.
20. DuBuske LM. Asthma: diagnosis and management of nocturnal symptoms. Compr Ther 1994; 20: 628.
21. Ballard RD, Saathoff MC, Patel DK, Kelly PL, Martin RJ. Effect of sleep on nocturnal bronchoconstriction and ventilatory patterns in asthmatics. J Appl Physiol 1989; 67: 243–9.
22. Kales A, Beall GN, Bajor GR, et al. Sleep studies in asthmatic adults: relationship of attacks to sleep stage and time of night. J Allergy 1968; 41: 164–73.
23. Hetzel MR, Clark TJH. Does sleep cause nocturnal asthma? Thorax 1979; 34: 749–54.
24. Clark TJH, Hetzel MR. Diurnal variation in asthma. Br J Dis Chest 1977; 71: 87–92.
25. Bonjer FH. Physiological aspects of shift work. Proc Int Congr Occup Health 1960; 13: 848–51.
26. Martin RJ, Cicutto LC, Ballard RD. Factors related to the nocturnal worsening of asthma. Am Rev Respir Dis 1990; 141: 33–8.
27. Ryan G, Latimer KM, Dolovich J, Hargreave FE. Bronchial responsiveness to histamine: relationship to diurnal variation of peak flow rate, improvement after bronchodilator, and airway caliber. Thorax 1982; 37: 423–9.
28. Oosterhoff Y, Koeter GH, De Monchy JG, Postma DS. Circadian variation in airway responsiveness to metacholine, propranolol, and AMP in atopic asthmatic subjects. Am Rev Respir Dis 1993; 147: 512–7.
29. Lehtimaki L, Kankaanranta H, Saarelainen S, Turjanmaa V, Moilanen E. Increased alveolar nitric oxide concentration in asthmatic patients with nocturnal symptoms. Eur Respir J 2002; 20: 841–5.
30. Covar RA, Szefler SJ, Martin RJ, et al. Relations between exhaled nitric oxide and measures of disease activity among children with mild-to-moderate asthma. J Pediatr 2003; 142: 469–75.
31. ten Hacken NH, van der Vaart H, van der Mark TW, et al. Exhaled nitric oxide is higher both at day and night in subjects with nocturnal asthma. Am J Respir Crit Care Med 1998; 158: 902–7.
32. Georges G, Bartelson BB, Martin RJ, Silkoff PE. Circadian variation in exhaled nitric oxide in nocturnal asthma. J Asthma 1999; 36: 467–73.
33. Silkoff PE, McClean PA, Slutsky AS, et al. Exhaled nitric oxide and bronchial reactivity during and after inhaled beclomethasone in mild asthma. J Asthma 1998; 35: 473–9.
34. Mohiouddin AA, Martin RJ. Circadian basis of the late asthmatic response. Am Rev Respir Dis 1990; 142: 1153–7.
35. Bates ME, Clayton M, Calhoun W, et al. Relationship of plasma epinephrine and circulating eosinophils to nocturnal asthma. Am J Respir Crit Care Med 1994; 149: 667–72.
36. Kelly EAB, Houtman JJ, Jarjour NN. Inflammatory changes associated with circadian variation in pulmonary function in subjects with mild asthma. Clin Exp Allergy 2004; 34: 227–33.
37. Calhoun WJ, Bates ME, Schrader L, Sedgwick JB, Busse WW. Characteristics of peripheral blood eosinophils in patients with nocturnal asthma. Am Rev Respir Dis 1992; 145: 577–81.
38. Gresele P, Dottorini M, Selli ML, et al. Altered platelet function associated with the bronchial hyperresponsiveness accompanying nocturnal asthma. J Allergy Clin Immunol 1993; 91: 894–902.
39. Mackay TW, Wallace WAH, Howie SEM, et al. Role of inflammation in nocturnal asthma. Thorax 1994; 149: 667–72.
40. Martin RJ, Cicutto LC, Smith HR, Ballard RD, Szefler SJ. Airways inflammation in nocturnal asthma. Am Rev Respir Dis 1991; 143: 351–7.
41. Postma DS, Oosterhoff Y, van Aalderen WMC, et al. Inflammation in nocturnal asthma? 1994; 150: S83–6.

42. Oosterhoff Y, Hoogsteden HC, Rutgers B, Kauffman HF, Postma DS. Lymphocyte and macrophage activation in bronchoalveolar lavage fluid in nocturnal asthma. Am J Respir Crit Care Med 1995; 151: 75–81.
43. Jarjour NN, Busse WW, Calhoun WJ. Enhanced production of oxygen radicals in nocturnal asthma. Am Rev Respir Dis 1992; 146: 905–11.
44. Jarjour NN, Busse WW. Cytokines in bronchoalveolar lavage fluid of patients with nocturnal asthma. A J Respir Crit Care Med 1995; 152: 1474–7.
45. Kraft M, Djukanovic R, Wilson S, et al. Alveolar tissue inflammation in asthma. Am J Respir Crit Care Med 1996; 154: 1505–10.
46. Kraft M, Martin RJ, Wilson S, Djukanovic R, Holgate ST. Lymphocyte and eosinophil influx into alveolar tissue in nocturnal asthma. Am J Respir Crit Care Med 1999; 159: 228–34.
47. Kraft M, Pak J, Martin RJ, Kaminsky D, Irvin CG. Distal lung dysfunction at night in nocturnal asthma patients. Am J Respir Crit Care Med 2001; 163: 1551–6.
48. Meijer GG, Postma DS, van der Heide S, et al. Exogenous stimuli and circadian peak expiratory flow variation in allergic asthmatic children. Am J Respir Crit Care Med 1996; 153: 237–42.
49. Szefler SJ, Ando R, Cicutto LC, et al. Plasma histamine, epinephrine, cortisol, and leukocyte beta-adrenergic receptors in nocturnal asthma. Clin Pharmacol Ther 1991; 49: 59–68.
50. Haen E, Hauck R, Emslander HP, et al. Nocturnal asthma. Beta 2-adrenoreceptors on peripheral mononuclear leukocytes, cAMP- and cortisol-plasma concentrations. Chest 1991; 100: 1239–45.
51. Sutherland ER, Ellison MC, Kraft M, Martin RJ. Altered pituitary-adrenal interaction in nocturnal asthma. J Allergy Clin Immunol 2003; 112: 52–7.
52. Kraft M, Vianna E, Martin RJ, Leung DYM. Nocturnal asthma is associated with reduced glucocorticoid receptor (GR) binding affinity and decreased steroid responsiveness at night. J Allergy Clin Immunol 1999; 103: 66–71.
53. Kraft M, Hamid Q, Chrousos GP, Martin RJ, Leung DYM. Decreased steroid responsiveness at night in nocturnal asthma. Am J Respir Crit Care Med 2001; 163: 1219–25.
54. Turki J, Pak J, Green SA, et al. Genetic polymorphisms of the beta 2-adrenergic receptor in nocturnal asthma: evidence that Gly16 correlates with the nocturnal phenotype. J Clin Invest 1995; 95: 1635–41.
55. Morrison JF, Pearson SB, Dean HG. The parasympathetic nervous system in nocturnal asthma. BMJ 1988; 296: 1427–9.
56. Barnes P, FitzGerald G, Brown M, Dollery C. Nocturnal asthma and changes in circulating epinephrine, histamine and cortisol. N Engl J Med 1980; 303: 263–7.
57. Sutherland RE, Ellison MC, Kraft M, Martin RJ. Elevated serum melatonin is associated with the nocturnal worsening of asthma. J Allergy Clin Immunol 2003; 112: 513–7.
58. Sutherland ER, Martin RJ, Ellison MC, Kraft M. Immunomodulatory effect of melatonin in asthma. Am J Respir Crit Care Med 2002; 166: 1055–61.
59. Gislason T, Janson C, Vermeire P, et al. Respiratory symptoms and nocturnal gastroesophageal reflux: a population based survey of young adults in three European countries. Chest 2002; 121: 158–63.
60. Bohadana AB, Hannhart B, Teculescu DB. Nocturnal worsening of asthma and sleep-disorder breathing. J Asthma 2002; 39: 85–100.
61. Chan CS, Woolcock AJ, Sullivan CE. Nocturnal asthma: role of snoring and obstructive sleep apnea. Am Rev Respir Dis 1988; 137: 1502–4.
62. Petruson B, Theman K. Reduced nocturnal asthma by improved nasal breathing. Acta Otolaryngol 1996; 116: 490–2.
63. Gibson PG, Henry RL, Coughlan JL. Gastro-esophageal reflux treatment for asthma in adults and children. Cochrane Library 2005; 3.
64. Milledge JS, Morris J. A comparison of slow-release salbutamol with slow-release aminophyllin in nocturnal asthma. J Int Med Res 1979; 7: 106–10.
65. Postma DS, Koter GH, Mark TW, et al. The effects of oral slow-release terbutaline on circadian variation in spirometry and arterial blood gas levels in patients with chronic airflow obstruction. Chest 1985; 87: 653–7.

66. Wallaert B, Brun P, Ostinelli J, et al. A comparison of two long-acting beta-agonists, oral bambuterol and inhaled salmeterol, in the treatment of moderate to severe asthmatic patients with nocturnal symptoms. The French Bambuterol Study Group. Respir Med 1999; 93: 33–8.
67. Crompton GK, Ayres JG, Basran G, et al. Comparison of oral bambuterol and inhaled salmeterol in patients with symptomatic asthma and using inhaled corticosteroids. Am J Respir Crit Care Med 1999; 159: 824–8.
68. Brambilla C, Chastang C, Georges D, Bertin L. Salmeterol compared with slow-release terbutaline in nocturnal asthma. A multicenter, randomized, double-blind, double-dummy, sequential clinical trial. French Multicenter Study Group. Allergy 1994; 49: 421–6.
69. Bensch G, Lapidus RJ, Levine BE, et al. A randomized, 12-week, double-blind, placebo-controlled study comparing formoterol dry powder inhaled with albuterol metered-dose inhaler. Ann Allergy Asthma Immunol 2001; 86: 19–27.
70. Busse W, Levine B, Andriano K, Laveschia C, Yegen U. Efficacy, tolerability, and effect on asthma-related quality of life of formoterol bid via multidose dry powder inhaler and albuterol QID via metered dose inhaler in patients with persistent asthma: a multicenter, randomized, double-blind, double-dummy, placebo-controlled, parallel-group study. Clin Ther 2004; 26: 1587–98.
71. Maesen FP, Smeets JJ, Gubbelmans HL, Zweers PG. Formoterol in the treatment of nocturnal asthma. Chest 1990; 98: 866–70.
72. Faurschou P, Engel AM, Haanaes OC. Salmeterol in two different doses in the treatment of nocturnal bronchial asthma poorly controlled by other therapies. Allergy 1994; 49: 827–32.
73. Pauwels RA, Lofdahl CG, Postma DS, et al. Effect of inhaled formoterol and budesonide on exacerbations of asthma. Formoterol and Corticosteroids Establishing Therapy (FACET) International Study Group. N Engl J Med 1997; 337: 1405–11.
74. Norhaya MR, Yap TM, Zainudin BM. Addition of inhaled salmeterol to inhaled corticosteroids in patients with poorly controlled nocturnal asthma. Respirology 1999; 4: 77–81.
75. Ilowite J, Webb R, Friedman B, et al. Addition of montelukast or salmeterol to fluticasone for protection against asthma attacks: a randomized, double-blind, multicenter study. Ann Allergy Asthma Immunol 2004; 92: 641–8.
76. Lockey RF, DuBuske LM, Friedman B, et al. Nocturnal asthma: effect of salmeterol on quality of life and clinical outcomes. Chest 1999; 115: 666–73.
77. Kraft M, Wenzel SE, Bettinger CM, Martin RJ. The effect of salmeterol on nocturnal symptoms, airway function and inflammation in asthma. Chest 1997; 111: 1249–54.
78. Holimon TD, Chafin CC, Self TH. Nocturnal asthma uncontrolled by inhaled corticosteroids: theophylline or long-acting beta2 agonists? Drugs 2001; 61: 391–418.
79. Elias-Jones AC, Higenbottam TW, Barnes ND, et al. Sustained release theophylline in nocturnal asthma. Arch Dis Child 1984; 59: 1159–61.
80. Bose B, Cater JI, Clark RA. A once daily theophylline preparations in prevention of nocturnal symptoms in childhood asthma. Eur J Pediatr 1987; 146: 524–7.
81. Martin RJ, Cicutto LC, Ballard RD. Circadian variations in theophylline concentrations and the treatment of nocturnal asthma. Am Rev Respir Dis 1989; 139: 575–8.
82. Fairfax AJ, Clarke R, Chatterjee SS, et al. Controlled-release theophyllin in the treatment of nocturnal asthma. J Int Med Res 1990; 18: 273–81.
83. Rivington RN, Boulet LP, Cote J, et al. Efficacy of uniphyl, salbutamol, and their combination in asthmatic patients on high-dose inhaled steroids. Am J Respir Crit Care Med 1995; 151: 325–32.
84. Kraft M, Torvik JA, Trudeau JB, et al. Theophylline: potential anti-inflammatory effects in nocturnal asthma. J Allergy Clin Immunol 1996; 97: 1242–6.
85. Crescioli S, Carobbo AD, Maestrelli P, et al. Controlled-release theophylline inhibits early morning airway obstruction and hyperresponsiveness in asthmatic subjects. Ann Allergy Asthma Immunol 1996; 77: 106–10.
86. Grossman J. Multicenter comparison of once-daily uniphyl tablets administered in the morning or evening with baseline twice daily theophylline therapy in patients with nocturnal asthma. Am J Med 1988; 85: 11–3.

87. Cox ID, Hughes DTD, McDonnell KA. Ipratropium bromide in patients with nocturnal asthma. Postgrad Med J 1984; 60: 526–8.

88. Hughes DTD. The use of anticholinergic drugs in nocturnal asthma. Postgrad Med J 1987; 63 (Suppl): 47–51.

89. O'Connor BJ, Towse LJ, Barnes PJ. Prolonged effect of tiotropium bromide on metacholine induced bronchoconstriction in asthma. Am J Respir Crit Care Med 1996; 154: 876–80.

90. Beam WR, Weiner DE, Martin RJ. Timing of prednisone and alterations of airways inflammation in nocturnal asthma. Am Rev Respir Dis 1992; 146: 1524–30.

91. Frezza G, Terra-Filho J, Martinez JA, Vianna EO. Rapid effect of inhaled steroids on nocturnal worsening of asthma. Thorax 2003; 58: 632–3.

92. Pincus DJ, Szefler SJ, Ackerson LM, et al. Chronotherapy of asthma with inhaled steroids: the effect of dosage timing on drug efficacy. J Allergy Clin Immunol 1995; 95: 1172–78.

93. Pincus DJ, Humeston TR, Martin RJ. Further studies on chronotherapy of asthma with inhaled steroids: the effect of dosage timing on drug efficacy. J Allergy Clin Immunol 1997; 100: 771–4.

94. Horn CR, Clark TJH, Cochrane GM. Inhaled therapy reduces morning dips in asthma. Lancet 1984; I: 1143–5.

95. Leach CL. Improved delivery of inhaled steroids to the large and small airways. Respir Med 1998; 92 (Suppl A): 3–8.

96. Richards J, Hirst P, Pitcairn G, et al. Deposition and pharmacokinetics of flunisolide delivered from inhalers containing non-CFC and CFC propellants. J Aerosol Med 2001; 14: 197–208.

97. Corren J, Nelson H, Greos LS, et al. Effective control of asthma with hydrofluoroalkane flunisolide delivered as an extrafine aerolsol in asthma patients. Ann Allergy Asthma Immunol 2001; 87: 405–11.

98. Molimard M, Martinat Y, Rogeaux Y, et al. Improvement of asthma control with beclomethasone extrafine aerosol compared to fluticasone and budesonide. Respir Med 2005; 99: 770–8.

99. Bellia V, Bananno A, Cibella F, et al. Urinary leukotriene E4 in the assessment of nocturnal asthma. J Allergy Clin Immunol 1996; 97: 735–41.

100. Wenzel SE, Tradeau JB, Kaminsky DA, et al. Effect of 5-lipoxygenase inhibition on bronchoconstriction and airway inflammation in nocturnal asthma. Am J Respir Crit Care Med 1995; 152: 897–905.

101. Reiss TF, Chervinsky P, Dockhorn RJ, et al. Montelukast, a once-daily leukotriene receptor antagonist, in the treatment of chronic asthma: a multicenter, randomized, double-blind trial. Montelukast Clinical Research Study Group. Arch Intern Med 1998; 158: 1213–20.

102. Vaquerizo MJ, Casan P, Castillo J, et al. Effect of montelukast added to inhaled budesonide on control of mild to moderate asthma. Thorax 2003; 58: 204–10.

103. Weersink EJ, Douma RR, Postma DS, Koeter GH. Fluticasone propionate, salmeterol xinofate, and their combination in the treatment of nocturnal asthma. Am J Respir Crit Care Med 1997; 155: 1241–6.

104. Ringdal N, Chuchalin A, Chovan L, et al. Evaluation of different inhaled combination therapies (EDICT): a randomised, double-blind comparison of Seretide (50/250 mg bd Discus) vs. formoterol (12 mg bd) and budesonide (800 mg bd) given concurrently (both via Turbuhaler) in patients with moderate-to-severe asthma. Respir Med 2002; 96: 851–61.

105. Canonica GW, Castellani P, Cazzola M, et al. Adjustable maintenance dosing with budesonide/formoterol in a single inhaler provides effective asthma symptom control at a lower dose than fixed maintenance dosing. Pulm Pharmacol Ther 2004; 17: 239–47.

Severe Asthma in Adults: Pathology to Clinical Aspects

Kazuyuki Chibana and Sally Wenzel

Introduction

Severe asthma affects only a small percentage of the asthma population. However, these patients disproportionately consume health care resources related to asthma. Severe asthma remains poorly understood and frustrating to care for, partly because it is a heterogeneous disease. This heterogeneity likely has contributed to some of the inconsistent pathologic findings, and made the relationship to clinical outcomes more difficult to determine. In this review we will discuss the pathobiologic aspects of severe asthma, focusing on the relationship of severe asthma to phenotypes. We will then utilize these phenotypes to suggest a logical approach to the clinical evaluation and management of these patients.

Definition

To understand the pathobiology of severe asthma, a common definition must be agreed upon such that comparisons can be made across studies. Definitions of severe asthma have ranged from those defined purely by airway obstruction (often <60% predicted) on no anti-inflammatory therapy, with unclear relation to symptoms and exacerbations, to traditional guideline definitions, which include lung function and symptoms, all before treatment, and finally, various severe asthma network definitions that have generally incorporated treatment [1, 2]. Most recently, an international consensus conference of severe asthma experts suggested that the American Thoracic Society Workshop definition be adopted as the "preferred" definition of severe asthma [3]. This definition requires the patient to have had a physiologic diagnosis of asthma, have had complicating factors addressed, and to be on the current state-of-the-art care for asthma (high-dose corticosteroids (CS)). However, in addition to being on a high dose of inhaled or oral CS, two of

K. Chibana and S. Wenzel
Division of Pulmonary, Allergy and Critical Care Medicine, University of Pittsburg, Pittsburg, PA, USA

R. Pawankar et al. (eds.), *Allergy Frontiers: Clinical Manifestations*,
DOI: 10.1007/978-4-431-88317-3_15, © Springer 2009

seven additional minor criteria were required. The minor criteria included FEV1, symptoms, exacerbations and urgent care, deterioration with reduction in CS dose, history of near fatal events, and the use of one or more additional controller medications. This definition has recently been incorporated into the National Heart Lung and Blood Institute's (NHLBI) sponsored network, to study severe asthma (Severe Asthma Research Program (SARP)), and defines a group of patients with both frequent and high intensity health care utilization, despite being treated with the "gold standards" of asthma care today: CS, long-acting beta agonists, and/or leukotriene modifiers [4]. Although these definitions are a start, it is likely that ongoing objective investigations of severe asthma populations will markedly improve our ability to identify, study, and treat severe asthmatics.

Epidemiology

Close to 20 million Americans (6–7% of the population) currently have asthma (2003). Four thousand people died with asthma in the same year and reported asthma as the underlying cause of death [5]. Severe or refractory asthma likely afflicts a small percentage (likely <10%) of that asthma population although the exact percentage remains difficult to determine. In Japan, asthma may affect a slightly smaller percentage (3–4%) of the population. Despite that lower percentage, over 3,000 people died of asthma attacks in 2005, suggesting that the severity of asthma in Japan may be higher than in the United States [6]. However, treatment of asthma in the two countries differs as well.

Genetic Risk Factors Which May Contribute to the Pathobiology of Severe Asthma

Risk factors for asthma can be divided into genetic and environmental. From a genetic perspective, it has been difficult to implicate one gene, as asthma is a complex disease involving multiple genes. Furthermore, until recently, there have not been cohorts of sufficient size or well characterized enough to do meaningful studies. Despite this, mutations in both the promoter region of the IL-4 gene or the promoter/coding regions of the IL-4 receptor, some of which have been linked to loss of lung function, others to near-fatal events, have been identified [7–9]. These polymorphisms in the IL-4Rα have been replicated in the NHLBI SARP network, where single nucleotide polymorphisms (SNPs) in the coding region of the gene (exon 12) are linked to higher percentages of subjects with severe exacerbations and to lower lung function. These clinical and physiologic changes are also associated with pathologic changes, including higher tissue mast cells and IgE expression [10]. Interestingly, genes related to "non-Th2" factors have also been associated with asthma severity, including those for transforming growth factor (TGF)-ß1 and monocyte chemotactic protein (MCP)-1, both of which can promote fibrotic reactions [11, 12]. In addition, two small studies have suggested polymorphisms in ADAM-33, which are associated with a more rapid decline in lung function [13, 14].

Environmental Risk Factors Which May Contribute to the Pathobiology of Severe Asthma

Allergen exposure has long been described as an important environmental risk factor for asthma and severe asthma in particular, with the strongest data for house dust mite, cockroach, and alternaria exposures [15–17]. However, both the European and the US networks for severe asthma have reported a lower percentage of severe asthma subjects with atopy, by skin testing, as compared to milder asthmatics (85% in mild in SARP to 71% in severe asthmatics) [4]. This could imply that allergic responses must be combined with other factors, including prolonged and/or high-dose allergen exposure, to increase disease severity.

In addition, the age at onset of asthma may influence the level of allergic pathobiology observed in severe asthma populations. A recent study of 80 severe asthmatics found that nearly two thirds developed the disease before the age of 12 and one third developed asthma after age 12 (late onset) [18]. These two groups differed markedly in allergic responses, with 98% of early onset asthmatics demonstrating positive allergy skin tests, whereas, only 76% of late onset asthmatics had positive tests ($p = 0.007$). Seventy percent to 75% of early onset asthmatics answered that symptoms occurred most or all of the time to these stimuli, whereas, 40–50% of late onset asthmatics answered similarly. In addition, both a history of eczema and a family history of asthma were significantly more common in the early onset group. As up to one third of severe asthmatics appear to have developed the disease in adulthood, the lower level of atopy in severe asthma in general, may be partly explained by the lower level of atopic disease in this group. In general, the early-onset severe asthma group appears to be a remarkably homogeneous group, with strong genetic influences and the presence of allergic responses (similar to extrinsic asthma), while the late-onset disease group is a more heterogeneous group, with evidence of both the allergic and nonallergic disease.

Cigarette smoke is another environmental factor which may contribute to asthma severity. Past or current smoking asthmatics are more symptomatic, exacerbate more frequently and severely, and have a more rapid decline in lung function than nonsmoking asthmatics [19–22]. Aggressive efforts to discontinue tobacco consumption are necessary. Pathologically, sputum eosinophils appear to be diminished in smoking asthmatics, as compared to nonsmoking asthmatics, while neutrophils are increased [23]. Therefore, it is not clear how closely the pathogenesis of smoking-related severe asthma relates to the severe asthma arising in nonsmokers, or whether the pathology is more representative of chronic obstructive pulmonary disease. More studies are needed.

Severe asthma also develops in life-long nonsmokers. In these instances, infection could also contribute to severe disease, with respiratory syncytial virus infections and rhinovirus implicated in childhood, while pathogens like mycoplasma and chlamydia may play a role in adults [24–27]. Data from the SARP network also suggest that a history of pneumonia is an independent risk factor for the development of severe asthma [4]. Finally, occupational factors are likely to contribute and interact with allergic responses in asthma that arose or worsened in adulthood [28].

Pathobiologic Phenotypes

It has long been evident that variability exists in the clinical presentation of severe asthma. Numerous attempts at classifying potential phenotypes of asthma and severe asthma have been proposed, including eosinophilic asthma, noneosinophilic asthma, intrinsic/allergic versus extrinsic/nonallergic asthma, brittle versus stable airflow limitation, early versus late onset, and corticosteroid resistant versus not corticosteroid resistant [29].

Despite the likelihood that these phenotypes overlap, studies have generally tended to focus on one or the other without integrating the potential phenotypes. However, reasonable supporting evidence exists for the presence of —2–3 severe asthma phenotypes based on differences in the pathology of the disease (Fig. 1). Of these —2–3 pathologic phenotypes, there are likely to be additional immunologic factors (allergy, infection, obesity), which further modify these phenotypes.

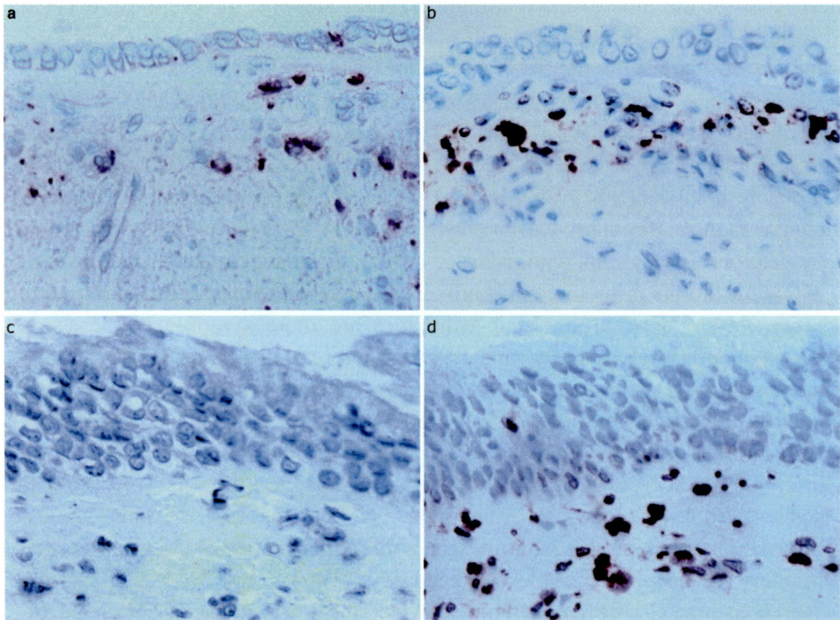

Fig. 1 EG2 (a) and neutrophil elastase (b) staining of tissue from an eosinophil (+) severe asthmatic. EG2 (c) and neutrophil elastase (d) staining of tissue from an eosinophil (−) severe asthmatic

(a) Eosinophilic phenotypes. Pathologic (large airway biopsy, bronchoalveolar lavage, and sputum) studies of severe asthma suggest that one half to two thirds of severe asthmatics have persistent large airway tissue eosinophils, despite continued high-dose systemic and inhaled steroids. The presence of eosinophils (as measured by sputum, lavage, biopsy, or perhaps to exhaled nitric oxide levels) appears to represent a phenotype of severe asthma with more symptoms, a greater likelihood of exacerbations and near fatal events, and greater airway obstruction (and reversibility) than the group without eosinophils [18, 30–32]. Defining an asthmatic (of any severity) as a eosinophilic may also depend on the compartment measured (sputum, lavage, or biopsy) and the threshold criteria used [33, 34]. Currently, evidence suggests sputum more commonly contains increased eosinophils as compared to tissue and may better discriminate severe asthma from milder forms of the disease [33]. While the reasons for these differences are not yet known, possibilities include tissue sampling issues, contribution from the distal airways missed in large airway biopsies, and the possibility that it is present in severe asthma, where eosinophils migrate more quickly from the tissue into the lumen.

Although eosinophils have been associated with Th2 immune processes, whether Th2 inflammation drives lung eosinophilia in severe asthma is not clear. IL-4 or IL-13 appears to be elevated in both atopic and nonatopic forms of mild asthma [35]. However, in severe eosinophilic asthma, despite concomitant increases in tissue CD3(+) lymphocytes, consistent increases in Th2 cytokines, commonly associated with asthmatic inflammation, including IL-4, IL-5, and IL-13, have not been reported [36, 37]. While these low levels may be secondary to high doses of CSs, the ongoing activity of the disease in these individuals, despite their low levels, brings into question their relative importance to severe asthma pathogenesis.

In contrast to the Th2 cytokines, however, severe asthmatics with persistent eosinophils have increased levels of the 15 lipoxygenase (LO) enzyme and its product, 15 hydroxyeicosatetraenoic acid (15-HETE), tissue expression of IgE bound to mast cells, as well as expression of the potent eosinophilic chemokine, eotaxin-3, in airway epithelial cells [38–41]. The very consistent increases in these enzymes, chemokines, and IgE, in the absence of increased Th2 cytokines are surprising, given the large body of evidence that Th2 cytokines, IL-4 and IL-13 upregulate these factors in vitro [42–44]. Whatever the reason, the increased tissue IgE expression in eosinophilic severe asthmatics may partly explain the increased tendency to exacerbations in this phenotype, as this expression appears to be an independent risk factor for severe exacerbations of asthma [40].

Several studies support a relationship between eosinophils and specific types of airway remodeling, including subepithelial basement membrane thickness [30, 45] (Fig. 2). The mechanisms for this increased fibrotic process are not clear, but are likely due to the production of the profibrotic factor, transforming growth factor (TGF)-ß (specifically TGF-ß2), by tissue eosinophils [46, 47]. In pathologic studies, eosinophils expressing TGF-ß are recognized to cluster just below the subepithelial basement membrane (SBM) [30].

There is also some evidence to suggest that the presence of eosinophils in severe asthma is related to either the shorter duration of the disease or the later age of onset

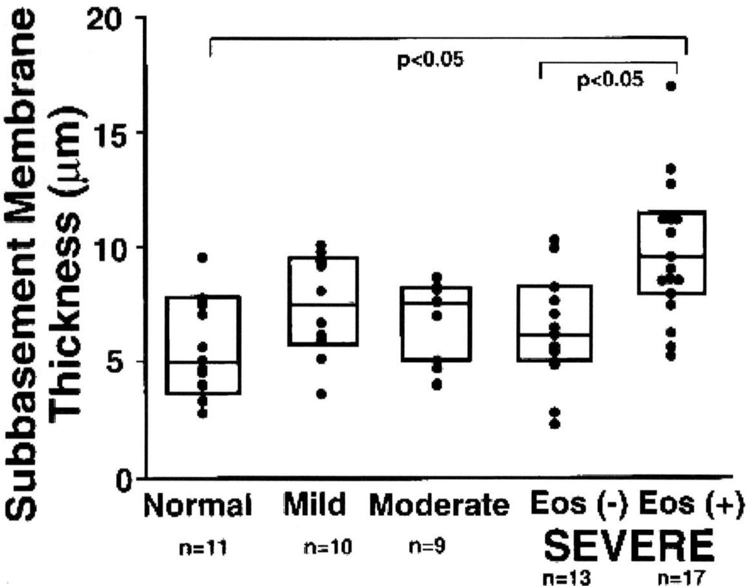

Fig. 2 Eosinophil (+) severe asthmatics had a significantly thicker SBM than normal control subjects or eosinophil (−) severe asthmatics. There were no significant differences between the eosinophil (+) severe asthmatics and the milder asthmatic control subjects (overall $p = 0.002$). All data expressed as median with interquartile range (These two figures are used by permission from reference Am J Respir Crit Care Med. 1999;160:1001–1008)

of the disease [18, 33]. As increases in eosinophlic inflammation are widely recognized in the phenotype of aspirin-sensitive asthma, which is well recognized to originate later in adulthood, this relationship to later onset, shorter duration disease might be expected [18].

(b) Non-eosinophilic phenotype. In addition to a prominent and increasingly well-defined eosinophilic group of severe asthmatics, there remains a large group of severe asthmatics with very little overall inflammation of the classic eosinophilic variety [34, 48]. Very little is understood about the pathogenesis of the disease in this group, as it is very likely a heterogeneous group, including individuals with prominent neutrophilic inflammation and those with very little inflammation. Possibilities for disease pathogenesis in this phenotype include the presence of localized distal lung inflammation not usually accessible by bronchoscopic studies, a nonmigratory cell-type inflammation (i.e., smooth muscle cells or epithelial cell-driven), residual neutrophilic inflammation in the presence of CS, or a manifestation of a totally different, perhaps more bronchiolitic disease.

Several studies have now suggested that in severe asthma, large airway inflammatory changes may be absent, while inflammation persists in the distal lung [49]. In particular, mast cells, specifically the chymase (+) phenotype, appear to persist in the distal lung, despite low levels in large airways [47]. Many additional studies of the distal lung are needed.

It is also possible that the lungs have been structurally altered to result in persistent clinical symptoms, but that inflammation, in the classic sense, is no longer present. In fact, studies by Benayoun and colleagues report that the primary differentiating factor between tissues from mild and severe asthmatics is not inflammation related, but rather, shows an increase in the amount of smooth muscle [50]. Finally, it is possible that a type of inflammation exists involving "nonclassic" inflammatory/asthma cells, particularly epithelial cells.

Obesity has also recently been associated with noneosinophilic asthma. The relationship to severe disease is less clear, but body mass index appears to be inversely related to exhaled NO levels, as a marker for eosinophilic inflammation [51].

Neutrophilic inflammation may also be seen in some individuals, in isolation or in the presence of eosinophils [30, 52]. This increase in neutrophils has been seen in sputum, lavage, and biopsy studies from severe/difficult asthmatics on high doses of inhaled/oral steroids [53, 54]. Neutrophilia also is more commonly seen in sputum than in biopsies perhaps because neutrophils are less likely to be tissue-resident cells. In fact, neutrophils, through expression of IL-8 and matrix metalloproteinases, may serve to open up the SBM to enhance eosinophilic migration into the lumen [55, 56].

The clinical implications for this neutrophilic inflammation are not clear. In some cases (likely more common in late onset disease) it may represent a "pathologically different disease" such as bronchiolitis obliterans or a variant thereof [57, 58]. Cigarette smoking asthmatics have been reported to have high neutrophil as opposed to eosinophil levels in the sputum [23]. This neutrophilia may also be the only "residual" inflammation left in the airways, with steroids having effectively reduced the eosinophils. Compared with patients with eosinophilic asthma, those with noneosinophilic, neutrophilic asthma are more likely to be female and nonatopic and to report the onset of symptoms in middle age [34].

Finally, steroids themselves have been reported to suppress neutrophil apoptosis, such that treatment of severe asthma may increase neutrophil numbers [59]. No study has evaluated the effect of corticosteroid therapy on the exacerbation frequency in noneosinophilic asthma. However, there is some evidence that it is diminished, because a longitudinal study of sputum-directed treatment in asthma showed that patients with persistently noneosinophilic sputum could reduce corticosteroid treatment without any increase in the frequency of asthma exacerbations over a period of 12 months [34].

The mechanisms for increased neutrophils are not yet clear. However, increases in IL-8 and LTB4 have been suggested, with a recent report suggesting CXCL5 (epithelial derived neutrophil chemoattactant-78), CXCR1, and 2 receptors are involved as well [52, 53, 60]. Whatever the underlying reason for increased neutrophils, their presence is associated with an increase in matrix metalloproteinase (MMP)-9 in BAL fluid and tissue (SBM), as well as lower lung function and air trapping on CT scans [56, 61]. The MMP-9 is specifically increased in a high molecular weight form associated with the neutrophil granular protein, lipocalin, believed to be poorly inhibited by the natural inhibitors of MMPs and tissue inhibitors of MMPs (TIMPs) [62]. In severe asthma, expression of this MMP-9 is also poorly inhibited by corticosteroids both *in vivo* in BAL fluid and *in vitro* in BAL cell supernatants [62].

Thus, at our current level of understanding, eosinophilic disease despite the lack of a strong connection with Th2 cytokines, or even allergic responses, still generally bears the footprint of a Th2 inflammatory process, with increased tissue IgE, 15 LO1, and eotaxin-3. Non-eosinophilic asthma is a much more heterogeneous process, some with no obvious migratory cell inflammation, some elements of remodeling, and/or prominent neutrophilic inflammation.

Evaluation of Severe Asthma

There are no validated algorithms to substantiate the most useful approach to the evaluation of severe asthma. However, it is rational to suggest that the approach should have at least three components: (1) confirmation that the disease is "asthma", (2) evaluation of confounding/exacerbating factors, and (3) evaluation of asthma phenotype. Under Category #1, *Confirmation*, appropriate tests include full pulmonary function tests (with reversibility testing, lung volumes, and diffusing capacity), chest CT scan, and perhaps most importantly, a standard methacholine challenge followed immediately by laryngoscopy when indicated, to look for paradoxical inspiratory closure of the vocal cords (vocal cord dysfunction) [63, 64]. These tests can be used to differentiate subtle changes related to interstitial diseases, mixed obstructive/restrictive diseases (hypersensitivity pneumonitis and sarcoidosis) as well as to evaluate for allergic bronchopulmonary aspergillosis, emphysema, bronchoilitis obliterans, and vocal cord dysfunction. It is likely that many studies of severe asthma often include a mix of subjects who, in fact, do not meet the strict criteria for "asthma" including reversible airflow limitation and/or bronchial hyperresponsiveness [4]. Under Category #2, *Confounding/exacerbating disease*, a pH probe to evaluate gastroesophageal reflux disease (GERD) (or, a trial of a proton pump inhibitor), a sinus CT to evaluate for surgically amenable disease, nasal/sinus polyps and fungal disease, an IgE level and allergen skin testing, a sleep study, and, when patients are on systemic steroids, an AM cortisol to evaluate compliance/adherence are helpful. Although this testing is specifically performed to uncover confounding diseases that may be treated to improve asthma, there are minimal data to confirm that this approach is valid [65, 66]. Finally, testing specific for Category #3, *Evaluation of phenotype*, likely the least proven, could potentially be highly beneficial. Categorization into early/allergic or late-onset disease can be made when appropriate questions are asked beyond "how long have you had asthma?" Additional helpful questions include those related to history of bronchitis or pneumonias in childhood and inability to keep up with physical activities in childhood, which may suggest that although a diagnosis was not made, the disease was present. Support for an early-onset or a late-onset *allergic* phenotype can be made by asking about symptoms related to allergen exposure, and performing allergy skin testing. Relationship to onset of disease after a respiratory infection, especially in adults, is also helpful, as are queries regarding aspirin sensitivity, as they may guide the approach to therapy. Evaluation for the presence or absence of eosinophilic inflammation can be done with sputum induction for eosinophils. As noted previously, sputum eosinophils may more robustly identify lung eosinophils than endobronchial biopsies and are certainly less invasive [33]. However, the procedure and processing are highly operator dependent and should only be done in qualified centers. Further, the actual threshold value for eosinophilic inflammation ranges from 2–3%, with few comparison studies to determine whether one is better than the other. Exhaled nitric oxide may be the easiest to obtain, and does bear some relation to tissue eosinophils. However, the relation to sputum eosinophils appears to be less [33, 67].

Treatment by Phenotype

Treatment of severe asthma remains highly problematic. Steroids remain the drug of choice, likely because of their broad and nonspecific effects. If a patient has not been on high-dose, high-potency inhaled corticosteroids, then a trial is certainly warranted [68]. However, substantial evidence now exists to suggest that severe asthmatics with persistent eosinophils respond better to increased doses of CSs than those patients without evidence of eosinophilia. Hence, in refractory patients, estimating the level of persistent eosinophilic inflammation before treating with more aggressive anti-inflammatory therapy would seem to be warranted. This "better" response to CS has been shown in both adult and pediatric studies [34]. In addition, monitoring eosinophils in sputum over time has been shown, in two studies, to decrease the number and intensity of asthma exacerbations, while not increasing the inhaled CS use [31, 69]. For reasons that remain unclear, systemic CSs also appear to be more beneficial than inhaled CSs in severe asthma. In fact, an injection of high dose (120 mg) triamcinolone was shown to have a significant impact on adult eosinophilic severe asthmatics, improving inflammation, lung function, and symptoms [70]. This injection of high dose steroids can also be helpful in determining the level of steroid responsiveness, while removing issues of compliance. Whether this improved response is due to high systemic levels of CSs or increased delivery to the distal lung is not known. However, a trial of the addition of an inhaled corticosteroid with smaller particle size and better peripheral distribution might also be indicated in these patients.

Treatment with a 5-lipoxygenase inhibitor (as opposed to a leukotriene receptor antagonist) can (anecdotally) be very helpful in patients with an aspirin sensitive/ eosinophilic phenotype. Whether specific eosinophil-targeted therapies, such as imitinib or mepolizumab (anti-IL-5) will have efficacy in this group awaits clinical trials. Finally, some of the previously described nonspecific anti-inflammatory therapies, such as cyclosporine and methotrexate, which have had modest and inconsistent results in the large population of severe asthmatics, have never been evaluated with a particular phenotype in mind [71, 72].

The noneosinophilic severe asthma group is a highly problematic group. Increasing steroids in this population is likely to have negative effects related to the systemic effects of CSs [73]. No other therapies have been specifically tried in this mixed population. In certain cases, antibiotics, particularly macrolide antibiotics, may be helpful [74]. The efficacy of anti-tumor necrosis factor therapy, broncho-thermoplasty, and 5-lipoxygenase inhibitors (or other drugs targeted at neutrophils) in this population is not known.

In the loosely defined phenotype of allergic asthma (asthma in the face of IgE > 30 and positive skin tests), anti-IgE therapy reduces hospitalizations in patients with moderate-to-severe allergic asthma, but their utility in very severe asthma (or "less allergic" asthma) is not clear [75]. Unfortunately, no additional biomarkers or phenotypes identify responders to this therapy.

Conclusions

The basic understanding of the pathobiology of severe asthma is only beginning to be elucidated. Although severe asthmatics share similarities, including consistencies in airway obstruction, reversibility, and hyperresponsiveness, the "disease" of severe asthma is likely made up of different phenotypes with eosinophilic and noneosinophilic inflammation best defined to date. Additionally, several subgroups may also exist. Studies of treatment of severe asthma, which target certain phenotypes, suggest this approach may lead to improved outcomes.

References

1. European Network for Understanding Mechanisms of Severe Asthma (2003) The ENFUMOSA cross-sectional European multicentre study of the clinical phenotype of chronic severe asthma. Eur Respir J. 22:470–477.
2. Wenzel SE, Fahy JV, Irvin CG, Peters SP, Spector S, and Szefler SJ (2000) Proceedings of the ATS workshop on refractory asthma - current understanding, recommendations and unanswered questions. Am J Respir Crit Care Med. 162:2341–2351.
3. Chanez P, Wenzel SE, Anderson GP, Anto JM, Bel EH, Boulet LP, Brightling CE, Busse WW, Castro M, Dahlen B, Dahlen SE, Fabbri LM, Holgate ST, Humbert M, Gaga M, Joos GF, Levy B, Rabe KF, Sterk PJ, Wilson SJ, Vachier I (2007) Severe asthma in adults: what are the important questions? J Allergy Clin Immunol. 119:1337–1348.
4. Moore WC, Bleecker ER, Curran-Everett D, Erzurum SC, Ameredes BT, Bacharier L, Calhoun WJ, Castro M, Chung KF, Clark MP, Dweik RA, Fitzpatrick AM, Gaston B, Hew M, Hussain I, Jarjour NN, Israel E, Levy BD, Murphy JR, Peters SP, Teague WG, Meyers DA, Busse WW, Wenzel SE; National Heart, Lung, Blood Institute's Severe Asthma Research Program (2007) Characterization of the severe asthma phenotype by the National Heart, Lung, and Blood Institute's Severe Asthma Research Program. J Allergy Clin Immunol. 119:405–413.
5. http://www.lungusa.org
6. http://www.mhlw.go.jp/toukei/saikin/hw/jinkou/geppo/nengai05/toukei5.html

7. Sandford AJ, Chagani T, Zhu S, Weir TD, Bai TR, Spinelli JJ, Fitzgerald JM, Behbehani NA, Tan WC, Pare PD (2000) Polymorphisms in the IL4, IL4Rα, and FCERIB genes and asthma severity. J Allergy Clin Immunol. 106:135–140.

8. Burchard EG, Silverman EK, Rosenwasser LJ, Borish L, Yandava C, Pillari A, Weiss ST, Hasday J, Lilly CM, Ford JG, Drazen JM (1999) Association between a sequence variant in the IL-4 gene promoter and FEV(1) in asthma. Am J Respir Crit Care Med. 160:919–922.

9. Rosa-Rosa L, Zimmermann N, Bernstein JA, Rothenberg ME, Khurana Hershey GK (1999) The R576 IL-4 receptor alpha allele correlates with asthma severity. J Allergy Clin Immunol. 104:1008–1014.

10. Wenzel SE, Balzar S, Ampleford E, Hawkins GA, Busse WW, Calhoun WJ, Castro M, Chung KF, Erzurum S, Gaston B, Israel E, Teague WG, Curran-Everett D, Meyers DA, Bleecker ER (2007) IL4R alpha mutations are associated with asthma exacerbations and mast cell/IgE expression. Am J Respir Crit Care Med. 175:570–576.

11. Pulleyn LJ, Newton R, Adcock IM, Barnes PJ (2001) TGF beta1 allele association with asthma severity. Hum Genet. 109:623–627.

12. Szalai C, Kozma GT, Nagy A, Bojszko A, Krikovszky D, Szabo T, Falus A (2001) Polymorphism in the gene regulatory region of MCP-1 is associated with asthma susceptibility and severity. J Allergy Clin Immunol. 108:375–381.

13. Jongepier H, Boezen HM, Dijkstra A, Howard TD, Vonk JM, Koppelman GH, Zheng SL, Meyers DA, Bleecker ER, Postma DS (2004) Polymorphisms of the ADAM33 gene are associated with accelerated lung function decline in asthma. Clin Exp Allergy. 34:757–760.

14. Simpson A, Maniatis N, Jury F, Cakebread JA, Lowe LA, Holgate ST, Woodcock A, Ollier WE, Collins A, Custovic A, Holloway JW, John SL (2005) Polymorphisms in a disintegrin and metalloprotease 33 (ADAM33) predict impaired early-life lung function. Am J Respir Crit Care Med. 172:55–60.

15. Squillace SP, Sporik RB, Rakes G, Couture N, Lawrence A, Merriam S, Zhang J, Platts-Mills AE (1997) Sensitization to dust mites as a dominant risk factor for asthma among adolescents living in central Virginia. Multiple regression analysis of a population-based study. Am J Respir Crit Care Med. 156:1760–1764.

16. Halonen M, Stern DA, Wright AL, Taussig LM, Martinez FD (1997) Alternaria as a major allergen for asthma in children raised in a desert environment. Am J Respir Crit Care Med. 155:1356–1361.

17. Rosenstreich DL, Eggleston P, Kattan M, Baker D, Slavin RG, Gergen P, Mitchell H, McNiff-Mortimer K, Lynn H, Ownby D, Malveaux F (1997) The role of cockroach allergy and exposure to cockroach allergen in causing morbidity among inner-city children with asthma. N Engl J Med. 336:1356–1363.

18. Miranda C, Busacker A, Balzar S, Trudeau J, Wenzel SE (2004) Distinguishing severe asthma phenotypes: role of age at onset and eosinophilic inflammation. J Allergy Clin Immunol. 113:101–108.

19. Ulrik CS, Lange P (1994) Decline of lung function in adults with bronchial asthma. Am J Respir Crit Care Med. 150:629–634.

20. Siroux V, Pin I, Oryszczyn MP, Le Moual N, Kauffmann F (2000) Relationships of active smoking to asthma and asthma severity in the EGEA study. Epidemiological study on the Genetics and Environment of Asthma. Eur Respir J. 15:470–477.

21. Silverman RA, Boudreaux ED, Woodruff PG, Clark S, Camargo CA Jr (2003) Cigarette smoking among asthmatic adults presenting to 64 emergency departments. Chest. 123:1472–1479.

22. Turner MO, Noertjojo K, Vedal S, Bai T, Crump S, Fitzgerald JM (1998) Risk factors for near-fatal asthma. A case-control study in hospitalized patients with asthma. Am J Respir Crit Care Med. 157:1804–1809.

23. Chalmers GW, MacLeod KJ, Thomson L, Little SA, McSharry C, Thomson NC (2001) Smoking and airway inflammation in patients with mild asthma. Chest. 120:1917–1922.

24. ten Brinke A, van Dissel JT, Sterk PJ, Zwinderman AH, Rabe KF, Bel EH (2001) Persistent airflow limitation in adult-onset nonatopic asthma is associated with serologic evidence of Chlamydia pneumoniae infection. J Allergy Clin Immunol. 107:449–454.

25. Kraft M, Cassell GH, Henson JE, Watson H, Williamson J, Marmion BP, Gaydos CA, Martin RJ (1998) Detection of Mycoplasma pneumoniae in the airways of adults with chronic asthma. Am J Respir Crit Care Med. 158:998–1001.
26. Wenzel SE, Gibbs RL, Lehr MV, Simoes EA (2002) Respiratory outcomes in high-risk children 7 to 10 years after prophylaxis with respiratory syncytial virus immune globulin. Am J Med. 112:627–633.
27. Gern JE, Brooks GD, Meyer P, Chang A, Shen K, Evans MD, Tisler C, Dasilva D, Roberg KA, Mikus LD, Rosenthal LA, Kirk CJ, Shult PA, Bhattacharya A, Li Z, Gangnon R, Lemanske RF Jr (2006) Bidirectional interactions between viral respiratory illnesses and cytokine responses in the first year of life. J Allergy Clin Immunol. 117:72–78.
28. Mapp CE, Boschetto P, Maestrelli P, Fabbri LM (2005) Occupational asthma. Am J Respir Crit Care Med. 172:280–305.
29. Wenzel SE (2006) Asthma: defining of the persistent adult phenotypes. Lancet. 368:804–813.
30. Wenzel SE, Schwartz LB, Langmack EL, Halliday JL, Trudeau JB, Gibbs RL, Chu HW (1999) Evidence that severe asthma can be divided pathologically into two inflammatory subtypes with distinct physiologic and clinical characteristics. Am J Respir Crit Care Med. 160:1001–1008.
31. Green RH, Brightling CE, McKenna S, Hargadon B, Parker D, Bradding P, Wardlaw AJ, Pavord ID (2002) Asthma exacerbations and sputum eosinophil counts: a randomised controlled trial. Lancet. 360:1715–1721.
32. ten Brinke A, de Lange C, Zwinderman AH, Rabe KF, Sterk PJ, Bel EH (2001) Sputum induction in severe asthma by a standardized protocol: predictors of excessive bronchoconstriction. Am J Respir Crit Care Med. 164:749–753.
33. Lemiere C, Ernst P, Olivenstein R, Yamauchi Y, Govindaraju K, Ludwig MS, Martin JG, Hamid Q (2006) Airway inflammation assessed by invasive and noninvasive means in severe asthma: eosinophilic and noneosinophilic phenotypes. J Allergy Clin Immunol. 118:1033–1039.
34. Haldar P, Pavord ID (2007) Noneosinophilic asthma: a distinct clinical and pathologic phenotype. J Allergy Clin Immunol. 119:1043–1052.
35. Humbert M, Durham SR, Kimmitt P, Powell N, Assoufi B, Pfister R, Menz G, Kay AB, Corrigan CJ (1997) Elevated expression of messenger ribonucleic acid encoding IL-13 in the bronchial mucosa of atopic and nonatopic subjects with asthma. J Allergy Clin Immunol. 99:657–665.
36. Truyen E, Coteur L, Dilissen E, Overbergh L, Dupont LJ, Ceuppens JL, Bullens DM (2006) Evaluation of airway inflammation by quantitative Th1/Th2 cytokine mRNA measurement in sputum of asthma patients. Thorax. 61:202–208.
37. Wenzel S, Balzar S, Chu HW, Cundall M (2005) The Phenotype of steroid dependent severe asthma in not associated with increased lung levels of Th2 cytokines. J World Allergy Org. Suppl 2:158–161.
38. Chu HW, Balzar S, Westcott JY, Trudeau JB, Sun Y, Conrad DJ, Wenzel SE (2002) Expression and activation of 15-lipoxygenase pathway in severe asthma: relationship to eosinophilic phenotype and collagen deposition. Clin Exp Allergy. 32:1558–1565.
39. Ferreira DS, Wescott JY, Trudeau JB, Wenzel SE (2005) The ratio of 15(S)-HETE/PGE2 in induced in eosinophil (+) severe asthmatics. Am J Respir Crit Care Med. A77.
40. Balzar S, Strand M, Rhodes D, Wenzel SE (2007) IgE expression pattern in lung: relation to systemic IgE and asthma phenotypes. J Allergy Clin Immunol. 119:855–862.
41. Trudeau JB, Chibana K, Wenzel SE (2007) Human bronchial epithelial cell expression of Eotaxin-3 mRNA is increased in severe asthma and correlates with lung function and exhaled nitric oxide. Am J Respir Crit Care Med. A837.
42. Shankaranarayanan P, Nigam S (2003) IL-4 induces apoptosis in A549 lung adenocarcinoma cells: evidence for the pivotal role of 15-hydroxyeicosatetraenoic acid binding to activated peroxisome proliferator-activated receptor gamma transcription factor. J Immunol. 170:887–894.

43. Bonnefoy JY, Shields J, Mermod JJ (1990) Inhibition of human interleukin 4-induced IgE synthesis by a subset of anti-CD23/Fc epsilon RII monoclonal antibodies. Eur J Immunol. 20:139–144.
44. Wenzel SE, Trudeau JB, Barnes S, Zhou X, Cundall M, Westcott JY, McCord K, Chu HW (2002) TGF-beta and IL-13 synergistically increase eotaxin-1 production in human airway fibroblasts. J Immunol. 169:4613–4619.
45. Flood-Page P, Menzies-Gow A, Phipps S, Ying S, Wangoo A, Ludwig MS, Barnes N, Robinson D, Kay AB (2003) Anti-IL-5 treatment reduces deposition of ECM proteins in the bronchial subepithelial basement membrane of mild atopic asthmatics. J Clin Invest. 112:1029–1036.
46. Minshall EM, Hamid QA (2000) Fibroblasts: a cell type central to eosinophil recruitment? Clin Exp Allergy. 30:301–303.
47. Balzar S, Chu HW, Strand M, Wenzel S (2005) Relationship of small airway chymase-positive mast cells and lung function in severe asthma. Am J Respir Crit Care Med. 171:431–439.
48. Jenkins HA, Cherniack R, Szefler SJ, Covar R, Gelfand EW, Spahn JD (2003) A comparison of the clinical characteristics of children and adults with severe asthma. Chest. 124:1318–1324.
49. Balzar S, Wenzel SE, Chu HW (2002) Transbronchial biopsy as a tool to evaluate small airways in asthma. Eur Respir J. 20:254–259.
50. Benayoun L, Druilhe A, Dombret MC, Aubier M, Pretolani M (2003) Airway structural alterations selectively associated with severe asthma. Am J Respir Crit Care Med. 167:1360–1368.
51. Komakula S, Khatri S, Mermis J, Savill S, Haque S, Rojas M, Brown L, Teague GW, Holguin F (2007) Body mass index is associated with reduced exhaled nitric oxide and higher exhaled 8-isoprostanes in asthmatics. Respir Res. 8:32.
52. Wenzel SE, Szefler SJ, Leung DY, Sloan SI, Rex MD, Martin RJ (1997) Bronchoscopic evaluation of severe asthma. Persistent inflammation associated with high dose glucocorticoids. Am J Respir Crit Care Med. 156:737–743.
53. Jatakanon A, Uasuf C, Maziak W, Lim S, Chung KF, Barnes PJ (1999) Neutrophilic inflammation in severe persistent asthma. Am J Respir Crit Care Med. 160:1532–1539.
54. Louis R, Lau LC, Bron AO, Roldaan AC, Radermecker M, Djukanovic R (2000) The relationship between airways inflammation and asthma severity. Am J Respir Crit Care Med. 161:9–16.
55. Kikuchi I, Kikuchi S, Kobayashi T, Hagiwara K, Sakamoto Y, Kanazawa M, Nagata M (2006) Eosinophil trans-basement membrane migration induced by interleukin-8 and neutrophils. Am J Respir Cell Mol Biol. 34:760–765.
56. Wenzel SE, Balzar S, Cundall M, Chu HW (2003) Subepithelial basement membrane immunoreactivity for matrix metalloproteinase 9: association with asthma severity, neutrophilic inflammation, and wound repair. J Allergy Clin Immunol. 111:1345–1352.
57. Jensen SP, Lynch DA, Brown KK, Wenzel SE, Newell JD (2002) High-resolution CT features of severe asthma and bronchiolitis obliterans. Clin Radiol. 57:1078–1085.
58. Holgate ST, Davies DE, Puddicombe S, Richter A, Lackie P, Lordan J, Howarth P (2003) Mechanisms of airway epithelial damage: epithelial-mesenchymal interactions in the pathogenesis of asthma. Eur Respir J. Suppl 44:24s–29s.
59. Cox G (1995) Glucocorticoid treatment inhibits apoptosis in human neutrophils. Separation of survival and activation outcomes. J Immunol. 154:4719–4725.
60. Qiu Y, Zhu J, Bandi V, Guntupalli KK, Jeffery PK (2007) Bronchial mucosal inflammation and upregulation of CXC chemoattractants and receptors in severe exacerbations of asthma. Thorax. 62:475–482.
61. Kotaru C, Wenzel SE, Castro M, Busse WW, Hoffman E, Everett D, Newell JD (2006) Air trapping on CT predicts severity of asthma, symptoms and ICU admissions. Am J Respir Crit Care Med. A16.
62. Cundall M, Sun Y, Miranda C, Trudeau JB, Barnes S, Wenzel SE (2003) Neutrophil-derived matrix metalloproteinase-9 is increased in severe asthma and poorly inhibited by glucocorticoids. J Allergy Clin Immunol. 112:1064–1071.

63. Perkins PJ, Morris MJ (2002) Vocal cord dysfunction induced by methacholine challenge testing. Chest. 122:1988–1993.
64. Thomas PS, Geddes DM, Barnes PJ (1999) Pseudo-steroid resistant asthma. Thorax. 54:352–356.
65. Reddel H, Jenkins C, Woolcock A (1999) Diurnal variability – time to change asthma guidelines? BMJ. 319:45–47.
66. Heaney LG, Conway E, Kelly C, Johnston BT, English C, Stevenson M, Gamble J (2003) Predictors of therapy resistant asthma: outcome of a systematic evaluation protocol. Thorax. 58:561–566.
67. Silkoff PE, Lent AM, Busacker AA, Katial RK, Balzar S, Strand M, Wenzel SE (2005) Exhaled nitric oxide identifies the persistent eosinophilic phenotype in severe refractory asthma. J Allergy Clin Immunol. 116:1249–1255.
68. Sher ER, Leung DY, Surs W, Kam JC, Zieg G, Kamada AK, Szefler SJ (1994) Steroid-resistant asthma. Cellular mechanisms contributing to inadequate response to glucocorticoid therapy. J Clin Invest. 93:33–39.
69. Jayaram L, Duong M, Pizzichini MM, Pizzichini E, Kamada D, Efthimiadis A, Hargreave FE (2005) Failure of montelukast to reduce sputum eosinophilia in high-dose corticosteroid-dependent asthma. Eur Respir J. 25:41–46.
70. ten Brinke A, Zwinderman AH, Sterk PJ, Rabe KF, Bel EH (2004) "Refractory" eosinophilic airway inflammation in severe asthma: effect of parenteral corticosteroids. Am J Respir Crit Care Med. 170:601–605.
71. Lock SH, Kay AB, Barnes NC (1996) Double-blind, placebo-controlled study of cyclosporin A as a corticosteroid-sparing agent in corticosteroid-dependent asthma. Am J Respir Crit Care Med. 153:509–514.
72. Erzurum SC, Leff JA, Cochran JE, Ackerson LM, Szefler SJ, Martin RJ, Cott GR (1991) Lack of benefit of methotrexate in severe, steroid-dependent asthma. A double-blind, placebo-controlled study. Ann Intern Med. 1991 Mar 1;114(5):353–360.
73. Green RH, Brightling CE, Woltmann G, Parker D, Wardlaw AJ, Pavord ID (2002) Analysis of induced sputum in adults with asthma: identification of subgroup with isolated sputum neutrophilia and poor response to inhaled corticosteroids. Thorax. 57:875–879.
74. Kraft M, Cassell GH, Pak J, Martin RJ (2002) Mycoplasma pneumoniae and Chlamydia pneumoniae in asthma: effect of clarithromycin. Chest. 121:1782–1788.
75. Holgate ST, Chuchalin AG, Hebert J, Lotvall J, Persson GB, Chung KF, Bousquet J, Kerstjens HA, Fox H, Thirlwell J, Cioppa GD; Omalizumab 011 (International Study Group) (2004) Efficacy and safety of a recombinant anti-immunoglobulin E antibody (omalizumab) in severe allergic asthma. Clin Exp Allergy. 34:632–638.

Exercise-Induced Asthma: Clinical Manifestations

Peter J. Helms

Whatever the cause, or causes, of the current high prevalence of asthma and wheezing illness in urbanized consumer societies, one of the features of the disease is that affected individuals often become more breathless than their unaffected peers, on exercise. Such symptoms will clearly have a greater impact on physically active individuals, including young children and athletes, than other more sedentary populations. The association of exercise with exacerbation of the disease has been known for centuries and amongst the early descriptions of this feature, Floyer, in 1698, noted that "all violent exercise makes the asthmatics to breathe short" [1]. Since Floyer's time a great deal has been discovered about this troublesome feature of asthma although the underlying mechanisms are still not completely understood.

Pathogenesis

McFadden and coworkers suggested that airway cooling and vasoconstriction due to respiratory heat loss was the probable cause of asthma-associated, exercise-induced bronchospasm (EIB) [2]. Through thermal mapping they demonstrated decreasing temperature from the upper trachea to the subsegmental bronchi with increasing ventilation, suggesting that cooling may cause bronchial obstruction by reflex stimulation of sensory receptors in the airway. Others suggested the mechanisms were reflex vasoconstriction followed by reactive hyperaemia and oedema. However, subsequent research has shown that vascular engorgement and bronchovascular hyperpermeability, at least in laboratory animals, persists for at least 24 h and that EIB does not develop with cooling and rewarming in the absence of hyperpnoea-induced airway drying [3, 4].

There is also evidence that mediator release from mast cells and other inflammatory cells occurs during the genesis of EIB [5]. For example, increased urinary

P.J. Helms (✉)
Department of Child Health, University of Aberdeen, Royal Aberdeen Children's Hospital, Westburn Road, Aberdeen, AB25 2ZG, UK
e-mail: p.j.helms@abdn.ac.uk

R. Pawankar et al. (eds.), *Allergy Frontiers: Clinical Manifestations*,
DOI: 10.1007/978-4-431-88317-3_16, © Springer 2009

levels of the mast cell mediator $9\alpha,11\beta$-prostaglandin F_2 have been reported after exercise [6], as have increased levels of LTE_4 [7], increased serum eosinophilic protein (ECP) and serum myeloperoxidase (MPO) [8].

During exercise, water vapour loss increases rapidly with increasing ventilation, particularly when inhaling cold air. This is hardly surprising as air at 37°C, fully saturated with water vapour contains 44 mg H_2O/L, whereas, at 22°C and 50% relative humidity this falls to 9.7 mg H_2O/l, and to 1.15 mg H_2O/l at −10°C and 50% relative humidity. Thus at the high ventilation rates associated with exercise, the potential for water to be lost from the lower airway is considerable, particularly in cool and dry environments. Exercise-induced mediator release is thought to be a consequence of changes in the osmolarity of airway lining fluid [9], and the mediators detected in sputum include histamine, tryptase and cysteinyl leukotrienes, with decrements in prostaglandin E_2 and thromboxane B_2 [10]. With respiratory heat loss both the direct effects of airway fluid and mediator release may work together to cause EIB, although airway cooling is not the entire answer to the problem as breathing hot dry air can also result in severe EIB [9, 11].

Testing for Exercise-Induced Bronchoconstriction

Although EIB has been found in 70–80% of individuals with established asthma [12], the widespread use of inhaled corticosteroids (ICS) needs to be accounted for in performing and interpreting formal exercise tests [13–15]. Although studies performed in the early 1970s led to the recommendation that a submaximal exercise load with heart rate at a level of 170 per min was required [16], the most recent American Thoracic Society (ATS) guidelines recommended an exercise load of 80–90% of the estimated maximum, at a relative humidity below 50% and an ambient temperature of 20–25°C [17]. As EIB was influenced by the humidity and temperature of inhaled air [18], cold air at −20°C had been used with significant improvements in test sensitivity and specificity [19]. Both European Respiratory Society (ERS) and ATS recommendations set a 10% reduction in FEV_1 as the diagnostic criterion for confirmation of EIB [17, 20].

More widely applicable, free range running tests, for identifying EIB have been suggested as alternatives to formal testing under controlled laboratory conditions [21, 22] although others have questioned the validity of such easily applied tests [23, 24]. However the problems with simpler and more widely applicable tests need to be balanced against the relevance of exercise in the controlled laboratory environment to exercise in the real world, where interaction with air pollution and other provoking agents in the natural environment can occur. Furthermore it may be possible to exclude true EIB in the majority by a comprehensive history and clinical examination [25]. However there are conditions including laryngeal dysfunction and the particular case of elite athletes where formal testing may be required.

Differential Diagnoses

Although breathlessness on moderate-to-severe exercise in otherwise healthy individuals and in athletes is commonly reported, many individuals referred with these symptoms are subsequently shown not to have asthma or significant EIB [26]. A not infrequent differential diagnosis is vocal cord dysfunction, which presents as a predominant inspiratory stridor during exercise and/or during periods of hyperventilation. This most commonly occurs in young females, is unresponsive to asthma therapy and is thought to be a consequence of large negative swings in intrathoracic pressures, reducing the calibre of the larynx during heavy exercise. An important differential diagnosis is paradoxical movement of the vocal cords with adduction during inspiration, which can be confirmed by direct fibreoptic laryngoscopy. Maximal inspiratory and expiratory flow volume loops may also help in establishing the diagnosis (Fig. 1).

Other less recognized causes include arterial hypoxemia [27] and swimming induced pulmonary oedema (SIPE) [28]. Arterial hypoxemia can occur during high levels of sustained exercise and is thought to be due to diffusion limitations and ventilation-perfusion inequalities [27] and may be demonstrable in up to 50% of elite endurance athletes [28–30]. Current explanation is, too rapid red blood cell transit time through the pulmonary capillaries. Although physical training improves muscle strength and endurance with increased cardiovascular capacity, improvements in the respiratory capacity are limited with little or no change in the pressure-generating capability of inspiratory muscles [31]. Thus asthma and EIB include a range of diagnoses, many of which can be identified by comprehensive clinical and physiological assessments (Table 1).

Although other chronic disorders including unrecognized heart disease should be considered, particularly if the level of symptoms seems disproportionate to the intensity of exercise, the most common explanations are either poor physical fitness or overtraining. These latter two explanations are more likely when the performance fails to meet the expectations of the athletes themselves, their parents or trainers.

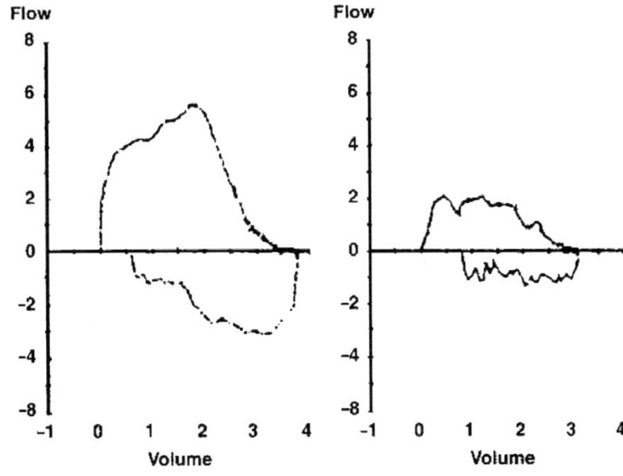

Fig. 1 Maximal expiratory and inspiratory flow volume curves from a young woman with laryngeal dysfunction. Left panel in basal unaffected state, right panel during an exercise/hyperventilation induced episode. Note the reduction in inspiratory and expiratory flows with the typical "saw tooth" pattern

Table 1 Differential diagnoses of exercise-induced breathlessness

Condition	Typical features
Exercise-induced asthma (EIA)	– Rapid onset
	– Improvement either spontaneously or after inhaled bronchodilator
	– >10% fall in FEV_1
Poor physical fitness	– High heart rate, low-grade exercise load
	– Muscular stiffness
Vocal cord dysfunction	– During maximum exertion or hyperventilation
	– Stridor and reduced flows during episodes
	– Unaffected by bronchodilator
Exercise hypoxemia	– In elite athletes during high intensity exercise
Swimming-induced pulmonary oedema (SIPE)	– Only during or soon after intense swimming
	– Fine crackles on auscultation
	– Hemoptysis
	– Reduced SaO_2
	– Restrictive lung function lasting up to 1 week
Chronic lung disease	– Reduced lung function
	– Features of disease
	– Desaturation on modest levels of exercise
Heart disease	– Related to underlying disorder

Management

Anti-inflammatory treatment with ICS is effective in reducing asthma-associated EIB and has maximal effects after 3–4 weeks of regular use [13]. ICS also enhances the protective effect of the inhaled β_2-agonists [13].

If long-acting inhaled β_2-agonists (LABA) are used, some tolerance (i.e., lack of effectiveness) can occur, a phenomenon not seen with the leukotreine receptor antagonist (LTRA) Montelukast [32], a potential advantage for the latter agent that needs to be balanced by the lack of protection of LTRA's in some subjects [33].

Cromones

Other strategies include the use of disodium cromoglycate (DSCG) and related nedocromil sodium [34], given immediately before exercise. The protection provided is thought to be due to inhibition of the prostaglandin release that occurs in response to the osmotic stimulus associated with airway drying [35].

β_2-Agonists

Short-acting inhaled β_2-agonists have an almost immediate effect upon EIB, with maximum protective effect 20 min after inhalation, with a subsequent reducing protection over the next 4 h [36]. The recommended inhaled doses are 200–400 µg of Salbutamol or 250–500 µg of Terbutaline. LABA Salmeterol provides protection from 30 min and up to 6–12 h following inhalation, whereas, LABA Formoterol has a similar long-lasting protective effect on EIB, with an onset of protective effect as rapid as Salbutamol or Terbutaline [37].

However it needs to be remembered that inhaled β_2-agonists do not entirely abolish EIB [38] and that regular use of LABAs may be associated with varying degrees of tolerance (loss of effect). Tolerance has been shown after 4 and 8 weeks of regular daily dosing of Salmeterol although less regular use (three times or less a week) does not appear to result in such tolerance [39, 40]. Consequently the regular daily use of LABAs for EIB alone should be discouraged.

Ipratropium Bromide

Ipratropium bromide may be effective against EIA in some but not all patients [41, 42] although it may have an additional protective effect when used together with an inhaled β_2-agonist [43].

Non-Pharmacological Options

Medication is not the only way to manage troublesome EIB as a type of physical activity, and environmental conditions need to be considered. The more humid and warmer the air, the less the chance of stimulating EIB, conditions most likely to be met in indoor sporting venues. Wearing a mask or face covering (i.e., a scarf) may help to warm and humidify outdoor air, but may not be appropriate or practical for high levels of intensive exercise. Physical activity on days of high air pollution should be avoided or minimized (early-morning activity may reduce exposure in some cities) and for individuals who are highly sensitive to pollen, intense activity should be restricted when pollen counts are high.

The refractory period of about 1 h post-exercise, during which subsequent exercise symptoms are reduced may also be used beneficially. Encouraging an athlete to exercise in several 2–3-min increments or "warm-ups", 10–20 min before the main activity, may induce a period of up to 1 h during which EIB is less likely to occur. However this approach is only likely to be relevant in those undertaking short bursts of high intensity exercise.

EIB and Asthma in Athletes

Several studies of asthma prevalence in athletes and its impacts on performance and management have been reported. Examples include the USA team at the Los Angeles 1984 Olympics, in which 67 of 597 participants were identified with

EIB or asthma. This did not appear to adversely affect their performance as 41 of these 67 went on to win medals [44]. Prevalences may also differ between sports with high rates in cyclists and none in divers and weight/lifters [45]. Usage of inhaled β_2-agonists appears to be greatest in endurance sports such as cycling, triathlon and swimming [46].

Asthma Medication and Sport

The significant prevalence of asthma and EIB reported by elite athletes has raised understandable concerns that some of the high levels of reporting may not be due to asthma at all, but rather due to the breathlessness associated with extreme exercise [47].

Although athletes with established asthma can and do perform well in high level competition, as reviewed above, concerns remain about the balance that must be struck between controlling symptoms and the theoretical potential for improving physical performance. Of all the medicines used to control asthma most of the attention has focused on Beta$_2$ agonists, purportedly used to control symptoms, which may be used to seek ergogenic advantage [47, 48]. No systemic administration of Beta$_2$ agonists is allowed in competitive sport, whereas, administration by inhalation is allowed in asthmatics, but not healthy athletes. Other asthma medicines including theophylline, ipratropium bromide, leukotriene antagonists, cromones, antihistamines and topical steroids for eczema and rhinoconjunctivitis are not subject to restriction.

Inhaled steroids (ICS) can be used by athletes with asthma after application for a therapeutic use exemption (TUE) to responsible sports organizations, such as, the world anti-doping agency (WADA), the international Olympic association (IOC) medical commission or other recognized international sports associations. Few well-conducted studies have been performed assessing the possible performance-enhancing effect of ICS in healthy athletes although the evidence is that in well-trained, healthy athletes there are no measurable improvements in performance [49].

Regulation with regard to inhaled β_2-agonists vary between sporting bodies with the IOC and the International. Association of Athletic Federations (IAAF) requires evidence of the current bronchial hyperresponsiveness (BHR) and reversibility. Other organizations such as WADA have less stringent requirements although all bodies require a physician's diagnosis of asthma as a minimum. Inhaled β_2-agonists such as formoterol and salmeterol have systemic effects upon heart rate, diastolic blood pressure and plasma glucose and potassium concentrations [50], and for this group of drugs the possibility of enhanced performance in healthy athletes is especially important and has been extensively studied. Beta$_2$ agonists can, theoretically, promote muscle anabolism and increase metabolism of lipids and carbohydrate [51–53], although in short-term studies and at conventional doses of inhaled Beta$_2$ agonists, no such advantages have been demonstrated [48].

Many studies of varying design and quality have been performed with both systemic and inhaled β_2-agonists and the evidence is overwhelming that inhaled β_2-agonists do not improve athletic performance in healthy athletes [54].

Conclusions

Whereas levels of physical activity appear to be on a decline in urbanized, consumer societies, exercise-induced bronchospasm (EIB) continues to be a common complaint in individuals with asthma and a concern for athletes and their medical attendants.

The general decline of physical activity in the general population alongside little change or marginal increase in energy input and the resultant increase in obesity is also relevant to any discussion about exercise and asthma. In this regard it appears that on one hand low levels of physical activity, reduced physical fitness and associated obesity may contribute to the severity and persistence of asthma [55], while on the other regular exercise and the associated increased physical fitness, might reduce the risk of persistent disease [56].

All these issues come together in the real and perceived associations between asthma and EIB. On the one hand, exercise is good thing, whereas, on the other, it may provoke unpleasant symptoms of airflow obstruction in the presence of established asthma, particularly in individuals exercising at very high intensity. Furthermore in elite athletes the diagnosis has the potential of being used to justify the abuse of asthma medication, Beta$_2$ agonists in particular.

Set against these concerns it needs to be remembered that EIB may be a feature of poorly controlled disease requiring a greater intensity of prophylactic treatment including inhaled corticosteroids, long-acting Beta agonists and/or leukotriene receptor antagonists [57]. EIB and asthma may also be overdiagnosed unless confirmed by careful clinical assessment and formal exercise testing [25, 58].

Health care professionals and the general public would benefit from a better understanding of the relevance of EIB. A distinction should be drawn between the provocation of airflow obstruction as a cause of breathlessness and other common causes interpreted as EIB, such as, poor physical fitness, laryngeal dysfunction or in the case of athletes, the high demands of exercise itself.

References

1. Floyer J (1698) A treatise of the asthma. London: R. Wilkins and W. Innes.
2. Gilbert IA, McFadden ER, Jr. (1992) Airway cooling and rewarming. The second reaction sequence in exercise-induced asthma. J Clin Invest 90:699–704.
3. Freed AN, Kelly LJ, Menkes HA (1987) Airflow-induced bronchospasm. Imbalance between airway cooling and airway drying? Am Rev Respir Dis 13:595–9.
4. Freed AN, Omori C, Schofield BH, Mitzner W (1994) Dry air-induced mucosal cell injury and bronchovascular leakage in canine peripheral airways. Am J Respir Cell Mol Biol 11:724–32.

5. Lee TH, Nagakura T, Papageorgiou N, Cromwell O, Ikura Y, Kay AB (1994) Mediators in exercise-induced asthma. J Allergy Clin Immunol 73:634–9.
6. O'Sullivan S, Rooquet A, Dahlén B, Larsen F, Eklund A, Kumlin M, et al. (1998) Evidence for mast cell activation during exercise-induced bronchoconstriction. Eur Respir J 12:345–50.
7. Reiss TF, Hill JB, Harman E, Zhang J, Tanaka WK, Bronsky E, et al. (1997) Increased urinary excretion of LTE4 after exercise and attenuation of exercise-induced bronchospasm by montelukast, a cysteinyl leukotriene receptor antagonist. Thorax 52:1030–5.
8. Rønsen O, Hem E, Edvardsen E, Halvorsen R, Carlsen KH (1995) Changes in airways inflammatory markers during high intensity training in elite cross country skiers. Eur Respir J 8:473s.
9. Anderson SD, Daviskas E (2000) The mechanism of exercise-induced asthma is. J Allergy Clin Immunol 106:453–9.
10. Hallstrand TS, Moody MW, Wurfel MM, Schwartz LB, Henderson WR, Jr., Aitken ML (2005) Inflammatory basis of exercise-induced bronchoconstriction. Am J Respir Crit Care Med 172:679–86.
11. Anderson SD, Schoeffel RE, Black JL, Daviskas E (1985) Airway cooling as the stimulus to exercise-induced asthma: a re-evaluation. Eur Respir J 67:20–30.
12. Lee TH, Anderson SD (1985) Heterogeneity of mechanisms in exercise-induced asthma. Thorax 40:481–7.
13. Henriksen JM, Dahl R (1983) Effects of inhaled budesonide alone and in combination with low-dose terbutaline in children with exercise-induced asthma. Am Rev Respir Dis 128:993–7.
14. Waalkens HJ, van Essen-Zandvliet EE, Gerritsen J, Duiverman EJKK, Knol K (1993) The effect of an inhaled corticosteroid (budesonide) on exercise- induced asthma in children. Dutch CNSLD Study Group. Eur Respir J 6:652–6.
15. Jonasson G, Carlsen KH, Hultquist C (2000) Low-dose budesonide improves exercise-induced bronchospasm in schoolchildren. Pediatr Allergy Immunol 11:120–5.
16. Silverman M, Anderson SD (1972) Standardization of exercise tests in asthmatic children. Arch Dis Child 47:882–9.
17. Crapo RO, Casaburi R, Coates AL, Enright PL, Hankinson JL, Irvin CG, et al. (2000) Guidelines for methacholine and exercise challenge testing-1999. Am J Respir Crit Care Med 161:309–29.
18. Amirav I, Dowdeswell RJ, Plit M (1986) Respiratory heat loss in exercise-induced asthma. Measurement and clinical application. S Afr Med J 69:227–32.
19. Carlsen KH, Engh G, Mørk M, Schrøder E (1998) Cold air inhalation and exercise-induced bronchoconstriction in relationship to metacholine bronchial responsiveness. Different patterns in asthmatic children and children with other chronic lung diseases. Respir Med 92:308–15.
20. Sterk PJ, Fabbri LM, Quanjer PH, Cockcroft DW, O'Byrne PM, Anderson SD, et al. (1993) Airway responsiveness. Standardized challenge testing with pharmacological, physical and sensitizing stimuli in adults. Eur Respir J Suppl 16:53–83.
21. Tsanakas JN, Milner RDG, Bannister OM, Boon AW (1988) Free running asthma screening test. Arch Dis Child 63:261–5.
22. Williams D, Bruton J, Wilson I (1993) Screening a state middle school for asthma using the free running asthma screening test. Arch Dis Child 69:667–9.
23. Ninan TK, Russell G (1993) Is exercise testing useful in a community based asthma survey? Thorax 48:1218–21.
24. Powell CVE, White RD, Primhak RA (1996) Longitudinal study of free running exercise challenge: reproducibility. Arch Dis Child 74:108–14.
25. Seear M, Wensley D, West N (2005) How accurate is the diagnosis of exercise induced asthma amongst Vancouver school children? Arch Dis Child 90: 898–902.
26. Stensrud T, Carlsen KH (2004) Exercise induced bronchoconstriction among athletes. Am J Respir Crit Care Med 169:A694.
27. Powers SK, Williams J (1987) Exercise-induced hypoxaemia in highly trained athletes. Sports Med 4:46–53.
28. Adir Y, Shupak A, Gil A, Peled N, Keynan Y, Domachevsky L, et al. (2004) Swimming-induced pulmonary edema: clinical presentation and serial lung function. Chest 126:394–9.

29. Powers SK, Dodd S, Lawler J, Landry G, Kirtley M, McKnight T, et al. (1988) Incidence of exercise induced hypoxemia in elite endurance athletes at sea level. Eur J Appl Physiol Occup Physiol 58:298–302.
30. Powers SK, Martin D, Cicale M, Collop N, Huang D, Criswell D (1992) Exercise-induced hypoxemia in athletes: role of inadequate hyperventilation. Eur J Appl Physiol Occup Physiol 65:37–42.
31. Dempsey JA, Johnson BD, Saupe KW (1990) Adaptations and limitations in the pulmonary system during exercise. Chest 97:81S–87S.
32. Villaran C, O'Neill SJ, Helbling A, Van Noord JA, Lee TH, Chuchalin AG, et al. (1999) Montelukast versus salmeterol in patients with asthma and exercise-induced bronchoconstriction. J Allergy Clin Immunol 104:547–53.
33. de Benedictis FM, del Giudice MM, Forenza N, Decimo F, de BD, Capristo A (2006) Lack of tolerance to the protective effect of montelukast in exercise-induced bronchoconstriction in children. Eur Respir J 28:291–5.
34. Kelly K, Spooner CH, Rowe BH (2000) Nedocromil sodium vs. sodium cromoglycate for preventing exercise-induced bronchoconstriction in asthmatics. Cochrane Database Syst Rev 4:CD002731.
35. Brannan JD, Gulliksson M, Anderson SD, Chew N, Seale JP, Kumlin M (2006) Inhibition of mast cell PGD2 release protects against mannitol-induced airway narrowing. Eur Respir J 27:944–50.
36. Shapiro GG, Kemp JP, DeJong R, Chapko M, Bierman CW, Altman LCFC, et al. (1990) Effects of albuterol and procaterol on exercise-induced asthma. Ann Allerg 65:273–6.
37. Boner AL, Spezia E, Piovesan P, Chiocca E, Maiocchi G (1994) Inhaled formoterol in the prevention of exercise-induced bronchoconstriction in asthmatic children. Am J Respir Crit Care Med 149:935–9.
38. Carlsen KH, Røksund O, Olsholt K, Njå F, Leegaard J, Bratten G (1995) Overnight protection by inhaled salmeterol on exercise-induced asthma in children. Eur Respir J 8:1852–5.
39. Davis BE, Reid JK, Cockcroft DW (2003) Formoterol thrice weekly does not result in the development of tolerance to bronchoprotection. Can Respir J 10:23–6.
40. Anderson SD, Caillaud C, Brannan JD (2006) Beta2-agonists and exercise-induced asthma. Clin Rev Allergy Immunol (2–3):163–80.
41. Boner AL, Vallone G, De SG (1989) Effect of inhaled ipratropium bromide on methacholine and exercise provocation in asthmatic children. Pediatr Pulmonol 6:81–5.
42. Boulet LP, Turcotte H, Tennina S (1989) Comparative efficacy of salbutamol, ipratropium, and cromoglycate in the prevention of bronchospasm induced by exercise and hyperosmolar challenges. J Allergy Clin Immunol 83:882–7.
43. Greenough A, Yuksel B, Everett L, Price JF (1993) Inhaled ipratropium bromide and terbutaline in asthmatic children. Respir Med 87:111–4.
44. Voy RO (1986) The U.S. Olympic Committee experience with exercise-induced bronchospasm, 1984. Med Sci Sports Exerc 18:328–30.
45. Weiler JM, Layton T, Hunt M (1998) Asthma in United States Olympic athletes who participated in the 1996 Summer Games. J Allergy Clin Immunol 102:722–6.
46. Fitch KD (2006) Beta2-agonists at the Olympic Games. Clin Rev Allergy Immunol 31:259–68.
47. Cummiskey J (2001) Exercise-induced asthma: an overview. Am J Med Sci 322:200–3.
48. Goubault C, Perault MC, Leleu E, Bouquet S, Legros P, Vandel B, et al. (2001) Effects of inhaled salbutamol in exercising non-asthmatic athletes. Thorax 56:675–9.
49. Papalia SM (1996) Aspects of inhaled budesonide use in asthma and exercise. Department of Human Movement, University of Western Australia.
50. Guhan AR, Cooper S, Oborne J, Lewis S, Bennett J, Tattersfield AE (2000) Systemic effects of formoterol and salmeterol: a dose-response comparison in healthy subjects. Thorax 55:650–6.
51. Lafontan M, Berlan M, Prud'hon M (1988) Les agonistes beta-adrénergiques. Mécanismes d'actio: lipomobilisation et anabolisme. Reprod Nutr Develop 28:61–122.
52. Price AH, Clissold SP (1989) Salbutamol in the 1980's. A reappraisal of its clinical efficacy. Drugs 38:77–122.

53. Martineau L, Horan MAS, Rothwell NJ, et al. (1992) Salbutamol, a β_2 adrenoceptor agonist, increases skeletal muscle strength in young men. Clin Sci 83:615–621.
54. Carlsen KH, Anderson SD, Bjermer L, Bonini S, Brusasco V, Canonica W, Cummiskey J, Del Giacco SR, Delgado L, Drobnic F, Haahtela T, Larsson K, Palange P, Popov T, van Cauwenberge P (2008) Treatment of exrecise-induced asthma, respiratory and allergic disorders in sports and the relationship to doping: Allergy 63:492–505.
55. Weiss ST, Shore S (2004) Obesity and asthma: directions for research. Am J Respir Crit Care Med 169:963–8.
56. Rasmussen F, Lambrechtsen J, Siersted HC, Hansen HS, Hansen NC (2000) Low physical fitness in childhood is associated with the development of asthma in young adulthood: the Odense schoolchild study. Eur Respir J 16:866–70.
57. British Thoracic Society (2003) British guideline on the management of asthma. Thorax 58 Suppl 1:i1–i94.
58. Hallstrand TS, Curtis JR, Koepsell TD, Martin DP, Schoene RB, Sullivan SD, et al. (2002) Effectiveness of screening examinations to detect unrecognized exercise-induced broncho-constriction. J Pediatr 141:343–8.

Aspirin-Sensitive Asthma

Andrzej Szczeklik, Ewa Nizankowska-Mogilnicka, and Marek Sanak

Introduction

Most people tolerate aspirin and other nonsteroidal anti-inflammatory drugs (NSAID) well. Asthmatics, however, are exception. First reports on the attacks of bronchoconstriction following aspirin ingestion appeared over a hundred years ago, shortly after introduction of aspirin into therapy. It took several decades to realize that aspirin-induced asthma (AIA), as it started to be addressed, constitutes a clear-cut clinical syndrome. Some of the mechanisms operating in the syndrome have been clarified, but its origin still awaits the explanation. Within the last years a few reviews on AIA were published [1–5]. In this paper we, therefore, concentrate on the most recent findings, following presentation of the basic data.

Definition

Aspirin-induced asthma (AIA) is a distinct clinical syndrome of intractable inflammation in both the upper and lower respiratory tract, which is characterized by chronic eosinophilic rhinosinusitis with nasal polyposis and asthma. Aspirin and other NSAIDs that inhibit cyclooxygenase-1 (COX-1) exacerbate this condition. At the biochemical level profound alterations in arachidonic acid metabolism are characteristic. The disease runs a protracted course, even if COX-1 inhibitors are avoided, and about half of the patients require systemic corticosteroids to control their rhinosinusitis and asthma. Since exposure to aspirin does not initiate the underlying inflammatory disease, this syndrome is increasingly referred to as: aspirin-exacerbated respiratory disease (AERD).

A. Szczeklik (✉), E. Nizankowska-Mogilnicka and M. Sanak
Department of Medicine, Jagiellonian University School of Medicine,
8 Skawinska Str., 31-066 Cracow, Poland
e-mail: mmszczek@cyf-kr.edu.pl

R. Pawankar et al. (eds.), *Allergy Frontiers: Clinical Manifestations*,
DOI: 10.1007/978-4-431-88317-3_17, © Springer 2009

Prevalence

The prevalence of aspirin hypersensitivity in general population ranges from 0.6% to 2.5%, while in asthmatics, according to large questionnaire surveys, it varies from 4.3% to 11% [1]. Following a meta-analysis of 15 studies using oral aspirin challenges to diagnose AIA, Jenkins et al. found that prevalence of AIA reached 21% (CI 14–29%) [6]. In patients with chronic hyperplastic eosinophilic sinusitis (CHES) and nasal polyposis, the prevalence of aspirin hypersensitivity reaches 30–40% [1, 7]. AIA is quite rare in pre-school children and teenagers. Ibuprofen, the most frequently prescribed analgesic in North America, caused bronchospastic reactions in 2% of children during oral challenges [8].

Many asthmatic subjects may not be aware of their hypersensitivity, because rather than aspirin they use paracetamol. Underdiagnosis of AIA may also stem from the lack of routine diagnostic aspirin challenges as even many allergy and pulmonary specialists seem to be afraid of carrying out these tests. In most studies AIA is more frequent in female than in male subjects [9, 10], but racial or ethnic predilection was not identified. In 1–6% of cases of AIA the family history of aspirin hypersensitivity is positive [9, 10].

Natural History and Presentation

Rhinorrhoea and nasal congestion are usually the first symptoms of AIA. They appear on the average at the age of 30 years [9, 10], and are related to an upper respiratory tract infection – common cold. Perhaps a viral infection may initiate the vicious circle of inflammatory events leading to AIA in genetically susceptible subjects [11]. Two to four years later asthma is diagnosed and often, about the same time, the first unexpected adverse clinical reactions following aspirin or other NSAID appear in these patients who previously tolerated analgesic very well.

The "classic" adverse reaction to aspirin includes: bronchospasm of varying severity, accompanied by rhinorhea, nasal congestion, sneezing, ocular "injection," and lacrimation. Many patients experience skin rush and erythrema of the head and neck which should not be confounded with aspirin-induced urticaria. The severity of hypersensitivity reactions to aspirin or other NSAIDs could range from isolated rhinitis to life-threatening anaphylactic reactions, or even death. Rare patients following aspirin ingestion manifest nausea, stomach cramps, or myocardial ischemia [12].

Almost half of AIA patients suffer from severe type of asthma. Asthma runs a protracted course despite avoidance of aspirin and other NSAID. Recent report indicated that [13] patients with multiple exacerbations of asthma suffered more frequently from AIA and required more frequent hospitalizations. Aspirin hypersensitivity is strongly associated with a near-fatal asthma [14].

When the adult subjects with AIA (n = 459) were compared with asthmatics tolerating aspirin well (n = 2,848) [15], the former had significantly lower mean postbronchodilator percent predicted FEV_1, and were more likely to have: severe asthma, bronchial intubation, a steroid burst in the previous 3 months, and a high dose of inhaled corticosteroids. Thus, aspirin sensitivity is associated with increased asthma severity, it carries a substantial risk to a patient and probably leads to remodeling of both the upper and lower airways.

Positive skin-prick tests to common aeroallergens are found in 34–64% of AIA patients [10, 16]. Elevated sputum and blood eosinophil counts are frequent. Many patients have typical symptoms of eosinophilic sinusitis and nasal polyps fill all sinuses (pansinusitis); not rarely the destructed bone structures are seen on CT scans. Loss of smell is very frequent. Nasal polyps are characterized by rapid regrowth resulting in multiple sinus surgeries [10].

Cross-Reactions with Aspirin and NSAIDs

Patients with AIA are also hypersensitive to all NSAIDs that preferentially inhibit COX-1 [17–20].

Acetaminophen is a weak inhibitor of COX-1 and therefore is regarded as a relatively safe alternative for majority patients suffering from AIA, but in doses not exceeding 500–1,000 mg. In a study of Jenkins et al. [6] less than 2% of asthmatics were sensitive to both aspirin and acetaminophen.

Preferential COX-2 inhibitors, meloxicam and nimesulide, are usually well tolerated by majority of patients with AIA when given at low doses. However, higher doses could elicit bronchospastic reactions [21–24]. On the contrary, highly selective COX-2 inhibitors – coxibs (rofecoxib, celecoxib, valdecoxib, etoricoxib, parecoxib, and lumiracoxib) were found to be well tolerated in series of the placebo-controlled clinical trials [25–31]. However, in rare patients, very sensitive to aspirin, even coxibs may provoke hypersensitive reactions [32–37]. Occasionally, these unusual reactions may be IgE-mediated.

Pathogenesis

The onset of AIA is slow and nonspecific. In most cases it reminds of a protracted viral respiratory infection. Thus, a viral origin of the disease was proposed [11]. Although initial symptoms are similar to a common cold they tend to persist and progress. Human rhinoviruses (HRV) have been the suspect pathogen, because they are the leading cause of infections of the upper respiratory tract. Rhinoviral infection was recently demonstrated to affect the lower airways [38]. Deficiency in antiviral response was proposed to explain delayed clearance of HRV. It seems a characteristic feature for asthmatic bronchial epithelia, since Peng et al. [39] demonstrated inadequate interferon-beta response to HRV14 caused by inhibition of interferon regulatory factor-3. A broader consequence of inappropriate signaling by this transcription factor is a tolerance to a double strand RNA, which normally elicits antiviral response mediated by NF-κB and interferons. This phenotype permissive for HRV was further characterized by Wark et al. [40] who found that HRV infection of primary bronchial epithelia results in a diminished production of interferon-beta. Moreover, Contoli et al. [41] observed a similarly decreased induction of the novel interferon-lambda family. Because deficit in the interferon-lambda antiviral activity was not specific for HRV infection, and was detectable following bacterial enterotoxin, these findings suggest an error in innate immunity, which can contribute to the inflammatory process in AIA.

Genetic Studies

Many studies have been published recently on candidate genes in AIA. It has to be stressed, that the disease is acquired and sometimes self-limited. Thus, a genetic susceptibility may rather correspond to the risk of disease providing an appropriate triggering event happened, possibly a persistent pathogen infection.

Within the immune system genes, studies on a genetic variability of human leucocytes antigens class II revealed genetic association of AIA with HLA-DRB1 locus allele *0301. This observation was replicated in two ethnically distant populations of Slavians and Koreans [42, 43].

In the immune system transforming growth factor-β can be released by regulatory T lymphocytes and inhibit response of effector cells. Recently, Kim et al. [44] described a genetic association between promoter polymorphism of *TGFβ1* and rhinosinusitis in AIA patients. Along with HLA, *TGFβ1* variants may represent susceptibility genes for the disease.

Prostaglandins

The mechanism underlying precipitation of asthmatic attacks by aspirin is nonallergic [17]. It consists in pharmacological inhibition of cyclooxygenase (COX) of arachidonic acid. Cross-reactivity between NSAIDs can be explained not by a different chemical structure of drugs, but by their relative affinity to COX-1 isoenzyme.

Generally, tolerance of NSAIDs which preferably inhibit inducible COX-2 is much better in susceptible patients [45]. Unusual sensitivity of COX-1 to the pharmacological inhibition, which characterizes AIA, remains unexplained. Expression of COX-2 was found decreased using mRNA and protein studies of nasal mucosa and the bronchial fibroblasts [46–48], but no difference in COX-1 levels were observed.

In vitro studies of peripheral blood leukocytes revealed other peculiarities of arachidonic acid metabolism in AIA. When exposed to aspirin or other NSAIDs, the cells release much more 15-hydoxyeicosatetraenoic acid. Importance of this finding in pathogenesis is unknown, but this observation was proposed to be useful in diagnosis [49, 50].

In most cells, the main product of cyclooxygenase pathway is prostaglandin E_2 (PGE_2). Biological action of this prostanoid varies with its cellular receptors. Type 1 receptor (EP1) is activatory because of phospholipase C and inositol triphosphate/diacylglycerol coupling. Type 2 and 4 receptors (EP2 and EP4) increase cyclic AMP, while type 3 receptor (EP3) inhibits adenylate cyclase. Due to its abundance in inflammatory cells, EP2 was studied in AIA [51]. It can inhibit release of cysteinyl leukotrienes from activated mast cells [52] in a PGE_2 dependent relation.

Interestingly, PGE_2 can decrease 15-HETE production *in vitro* as evidenced by a non specific EP2/EP3 receptors agonist misoprostol [49].

In a genomic study encompassing several possible candidate genes of arachidonic acid pathways, EP2 gene polymorphisms of a regulatory region of the gene (*PTGER2*) were associated with AIA [53]. Moreover, in immunochemistry studies, infiltrating inflammatory cells of aspirin-sensitive patients had lower expression of EP2 receptor [51].

Leukotrienes

Cysteinyl leukotrienes are produced from arachidonic acid by 5-lipoxygenase, the enzyme abundant in granulocytes. However, only limited types of cells can express leukotriene C_4 synthase, an enzyme controlling production of cysteinyl leukotrienes. AIA is characterized by a marked increase of production of cysteinyl leukotrienes. The end metabolite, leukotriene E_4 is distinctly elevated in urine, and it further increases also in nasal exudate or bronchoalveolar lavage fluid, following challenge with aspirin in a time dependent manner [54–59]. Recently, an increased urinary excretion of leukotriene B_4 metabolite was also described in aspirin-sensitive patients [60]. Thus, 5-lipoxygenase pathway seems upregulated in the disease.

The cellular source for cysteinyl leukotrienes in AIA patients are eosinophils and mast cells. Bronchial biopsies in these patients demonstrate an increased expression of leukotriene C_4 synthase [61]. Within the regulatory region of the leukotriene C_4 synthase gene, a common genetic variant ($A_{-444} > C$) was demonstrated to cause increased expression of the enzyme, although this association characterized severe asthma in general [62]. Other variants of genes participating in the lipoxygenase pathway were studied in aspirin hypersensitivity [63–66]; these associations await replication in other populations.

Common inflammatory mechanism of mast cells and eosinophils can be involved in AIA independently from allergic sensitization [67]. In many studies, mast cells were pointed out as the main source of inflammatory mediators during exposure to aspirin. Mast cells specifically produce prostaglandin D_2 [68], which along with tryptase, increases following the precipitation of symptoms [54]. A baseline urinary excretion of LTE$_4$ is increased in AIA patients to the level which significantly differ it from aspirin-tolerant asthmatics [69]. Cysteinyl leukotrienes are produced by airways mucosa. Reducing hyperplastic rhinosinusitis by surgery can substantially decrease the level of cysteinyl leukotrienes metabolite in urine [70].

Among two subtypes of cysteinyl leukotrienes receptors, CysLT1 receptor is a predominant one in respiratory and inflammatory cells, including eosinophils, mast cells, lymphocytes, macrophages, and neutrophils. Upregulation of CysLT1 was observed quite specifically in patients with AIA [71]. Similarly, increased expression of the other subtype-CysLT2 was described by Corrigan et al. [72] on inflammatory cells. Decreased abundance of CysLT1 receptor has been proposed as a mechanism explaining aspirin desensitization [71].

Lipoxins

Lipoxins are another class of arachidonic acid derivatives affected by NSAIDs, and altered in AIA patients. Due to a transcellular biosynthesis, lipoxins are generated by infiltrating cells and may help to resolve inflammation. Aspirin, by inhibition of COX-1, can trigger production of 15-epi-lipoxin A$_4$ with more potent anti-inflammatory properties. AIA patients have decreased capacity for lipoxin biosynthesis. This was observed mostly *in vitro* using peripheral blood granulocytes [49, 73, 74].

Alterations in eicosanoids metabolism, though more profound in AIA, were also described in patients tolerant to aspirin, mostly with severe asthma. Probably these mechanisms are common to all patients with severe asthma. Increased production of cysteinyl leukotrienes and diminished biosynthesis of lipoxins was reported in such subjects [75].

Genetic variability can contribute to upregulation of the lipoxygenase pathway only partially. Promoter variants of 5-lipoxygensae gene (*ALOX5*) and leukotriene C4 synthase (*LTC4S*) were associated with severe asthma [76]. As common mechanisms of inflammation are not unique for aspirin hypersensitivity, the identification of a triggering mechanism for aspirin-triggered bronchospasm can help in management of this disease. Recently, a comprehensive evaluation of cysteinyl leukotrienes and PGE$_2$ metabolites in aspirin-sensitive patients resulted in quite unexpected conclusions [77]. Although urinary LTE$_4$ excretion followed well known pattern of increase following aspirin challenge in sensitive patients, no changes were noted in the two end-metabolites of PGE$_2$. Quite paradoxically, the same metabolites were suppressed by a similar dose of aspirin in aspirin-tolerant patients or healthy controls. Moreover, a selective COX-2 inhibitor, celecoxib, decreased PGE$_2$ urinary metabolites regardless of aspirin hypersensitivity. It seems that COX-1 inhibition, which is an essence of NSAIDs intolerance in aspirin-sensitive patients, is totally masked if a systemic biosynthesis of PGE$_2$ is considered. These observations further support profound abnormalities in eicosanoids balance, which is characteristic for AIA.

Diagnosis of Aspirin Hypersensitivity

Diagnosis of aspirin hypersensitivity provides the patient with a comprehensive list of analgesics that must be avoided because of the high risk of adverse, sometimes life-threatening reactions; it also indicates which NSAIDs can be usually taken safely. Although history of hypersensitivity reactions, as well as typical clinical presentation of AIA, may rise a suspicion of aspirin hypersensitivity, the diagnosis can be definitely established only through provocation tests with aspirin. There is no reliable *in vitro* diagnostic test, although studies are in progress [50, 78]. There are four types of provocation challenges with aspirin: oral, inhalational (bronchial), nasal, and intravenous [79–85].

Oral, inhalation, and intravenous aspirin challenges have to be carried out under the direct supervision of a physician and technicians skilled in performing provocation tests. Emergency resuscitative equipment should be readily available. Patients should have an intravenous line attached, and asthmatics must be in a stable clinical condition. Baseline FEV_1 should be at least 70% of the predicted value. Aspirin challenge should be always preceded by a placebo challenge.

The oral challenge tests with aspirin were started in the early 1970s in Poland [17, 18] and than introduced into clinical practice in many other countries. The oral route mimics natural exposure and the challenge procedure does not require special equipment, except spirometry. There exist various protocols of oral challenges. The EAACI/GA2LEN [85] guideline uses four exponentially increasing doses of aspirin (27, 44, 117, and 312 mg) at 1.5–2 h intervals until a cumulative dose of 500 mg is reached. If a patient with a strong suspicion of aspirin hypersensitivity shows no reaction after administration of a cumulative dose of 500 mg, another capsule containing 500 mg of aspirin should be administered 1.5–2 h following the preceding dose; the cumulative dose in that case will be equivalent to 1,000 mg of aspirin.

FEV_1 is measured before each consecutive dose of aspirin and subsequently every 30 min, i.e. at 30, 60 and 90 (120) min thereafter. The challenge is interrupted, if a decrease in $FEV_1 \geq 20\%$ of baseline occurs (a positive reaction), or when the maximum cumulative dose of aspirin (1,000 mg) is reached without a fall in $FEV_1 \geq 20\%$ and the symptoms of aspirin hypersensitivity do not appear (a negative reaction). The test is also regarded as positive when severe extrabronchial symptoms (e.g. very severe nasal congestion, profound rhinorrhea, etc.) of aspirin hypersensitivity appear. Recently it was found that the severity of the history of aspirin/NSAID-induced asthma attack was not predictive of severity of bronchospasm during oral aspirin challenge [86].

In inhalational (bronchial) challenge, lysine-aspirin is administered by a dosimeter-controlled jet-nebuliser. The detailed protocol of the test has been recently published [85]. This challenge, more frequently used in Europe, is safer and faster to carry out than the oral test, although it is slightly less sensitive. Treatment of adverse respiratory reactions due to oral and bronchial aspirin challenges has been reviewed in detail elsewhere [7, 85].

Nasal aspirin challenges with lysine-aspirin [80, 82] or rarely ketorolac solutions [87] are less frequently performed. Evaluation of the nasal responses following instillation of 16 mg of aspirin into the nostrils (as lysine-aspirin solution) could be based on nasal symptoms scores, rhinomanometry, acoustic rhinometry, or peak nasal inspiratory flow (PNIF). These test do not produce systemic reactions and are recommended particularly for those asthmatics in whom oral or inhalation tests are contraindicated because of the asthma severity. As the negative predictive value is lower than in the other two tests, a negative nasal challenge should be followed, whenever possible, by the oral or inhalational test.

Intravenous tests with lysine-aspirin (administration increasing doses of aspirin every 30 min: 12.5, 25, 50, 100, and 200 mg) are used preferentially in Japan [67, 88].

Prevention and Treatment

When diagnosis of AIA is confirmed, the patients must not use aspirin or any other NSAIDs inhibiting COX-1; their education is of great importance. All AIA patients should receive a list of drugs which are contraindicated and also the list of drugs that could be well tolerated. Acetaminophen, meloxicam, nimesulide, coxibs, and codeine are optimal preferential choice for acute pain. As mentioned earlier, meloxicam, nimesulide, and coxibs are usually well tolerated by AIA patients, although a small degree of residual COX-1 inhibition displayed by these compounds may be enough to trigger hypersensitive reactions when they are used at higher doses. Therefore, when administering these drugs, it is safer to administer the first dose in physician's office or to carry out a short challenge test.

Treatment of AIA should follow international guidelines (GINA 2006 revised). The patients need often intensive therapy to control their symptoms; frequently high doses of inhaled corticosteroids and oral corticosteroids are necessary. In the AIANE (European Network on Aspirin-Induced Asthma) study, more than 50% of AIA patients were on chronic oral and inhaled corticotherapy [9, 89]. Similarly, in the US, in a study involving 300 AIA patients, systemic corticosteroids were used as short courses in 134 (45%) and on a daily basis in 95 (32%) patients [10].

The discovery of antileukotrienes, such as montelukast, zafirlukast, pranlukast (cys-LT$_1$ receptor inhibitors), or zileuton (5-LOX inhibitor) provided a new opportunity for treatment of AIA. In the Polish–Swedish, double-blind placebo-controlled study, the clinical efficacy of zileuton in AIA was well documented as an add-on treatment [90]. Positive therapeutic effects were also obtained with montelukast [91]. Against expectations, however, AIA patients seem not to respond better to leukotriene receptor antagonists than aspirin-tolerant asthmatics. The treatment success with these drugs was only significantly better in the carriers of the variant C allele of LTC$_4$S [92–94] and HLA-DPB1*0301 marker [95]. In mild or moderate atopic asthmatics with concomitant hypersensitivity to aspirin, allergen avoidance and immunotherapy could be considered. Anti-IgE treatment with omalizumab could be useful in severe cases of AIA with atopic trait.

The aspirin-sensitive eosinophilic rhinosinusitis is particularly difficult to treat. High doses of intranasal corticosteroids on long-term are indicated [96]. Extended courses of broad-spectrum antibiotics are administered during acute bacterial infections. Some patients with severe nasal obstruction could require 1- to 3-week burst of systemic corticosteroids to control their symptoms ("medical polypectomy"). An additional relief could be obtained with oral and nasal decongestants and antihistamines.

In many patients nasal patency can be restored only through surgery. Usually functional endoscopic sinus surgery must be carried out ("pansinus surgery") [97, 98]. The subjective success rate for nasal symptoms after "pansinus surgery" could reach 80%, but the benefits of this procedure are short-lived, since the polyps almost always recur. Reoperation for nasal polyps is frequently required every 3 years in AIA patients [10]. However, a retrospective analysis published recently, showed long-term postoperative improvement of asthma in 94% of patients subjected to sinus surgery [99]. In a recent randomized prospective study comparing surgical vs medical therapy of chronic rhinosinusitis and concomitant asthma, overall asthma control was better maintained after medical therapy as evidenced by an increase in FEV_1 and decrease in exhaled nitric oxide [100].

One of the treatment options is chronic desensitization to aspirin. AIA patients can be desensitized to ASA or NSAID using a protocol that requires 1–3 days inpatient treatment and continuous daily ASA ingestion (600–1,200 mg) to maintain the desensitized state [101]. Desensitization is utilized in some centers for treatment of refractory AIA patients with predominant symptoms of chronic sinusitis and recurrent nasal polyps requiring repeated polypectomies [101, 102]. It should be also considered in patients with AERD controlled only with unacceptably high doses of systemic corticosteroids and in patients who require NSAIDs for treatment of other diseases, particularly ischaemic heart disease [103, 104]. The detailed data concerning aspirin desensitization has been reviewed recently elsewhere [101–107] and the rapid desensitization protocols for patients with cardiovascular disease and aspirin hypersensitivity have been published very recently [108].

The study using topical lysine-aspirin (nasal administration) did not reveal any significant clinical benefit of this procedure as compared to placebo [109].

References

1. Szczeklik A, Sanak M (2006) The broken balance in aspirin hypersensitivity. Eur J Pharmacol 533:145–155.
2. Stevenson DD, Szczeklik A (2006) Clinical and pathologic perspectives on aspirin sensitivity and asthma. J Allergy Clin Immunol 118:773–786.
3. Kowalski M, Makowska JS (2006) Aspirin-exacerbated respiratory disease. An update on diagnosis and management. Allergy Clin Immunol Int – J World Allergy Org 18:140–149.
4. Szczeklik A, Nizankowska-Mogilnicka E, Sanak M (2007) Hypersensitivity to aspirin and other NSAIDs: mechanisms, clinical presentation and management. In: Pichler WJ (ed) Drug Hypersensitivity. Basel, Switzerland, Karger, pp. 340–351.

5. Wenzel SE (2006) Asthma: defining of the persistent adult phenotypes. Lancet 368: 804–813.
6. Jenkins C, Costello J, Hodge L (2004) Systematic review of prevalence of aspirin-induced asthma and its implications for clinical practice. BMJ 328:434–437.
7. Szczeklik A, Nizankowska Mogilnicka E, Sanak M (2008) Hypersensitivity to aspirin and non-steroidal anti-inflammatory drugs. In: Adkinson NF, Busse W, Bodnner BS, Holgate ST, Simons FER, Lemanslec RF (eds) Middleton's Allergy: Principles and practice. 7th Ed. Mosby Inc, Elsevier, London, pp.1227–1243.
8. Debley JS, Carter ER, Gibson RL, Rosenfeld M, Redding GJ (2005) The prevalence of ibuprofen-sensitive asthma in children: a randomized controlled bronchoprovocations challenge study. J Pediatr 147:233–238.
9. Szczeklik A, Nizankowska E, Duplaga M (2000) Natural history of aspirin-induced asthma. AIANE investigators. European network on aspirin-induced asthma. Eur Respir J 16:432–436.
10. Berges-Gimeno M, Simon RA, Stevenson DD (2002) The natural history and clinical characteristics of aspirin exacerbated respiratory disease. Ann Allergy Asthma Immunol 89:474–478.
11. Szczeklik A (1988) Aspirin-induced asthma as a viral disease. Clin Allergy 18:15–20.
12. Szczeklik A, Nizankowska E, Mastalerz L, Bochenek G (2002) Myocardial ischemia possibly mediated by cysteinyl leukotrienes. J Allergy Clin Immunol 109:572–573.
13. Koga T, Oshita Y, Kamimura T, Koga H, Aizawa H (2006) Characterisation of patients with frequent exacerbation of asthma. Respir Med 100:273–278.
14. Yoshimine F, Hasegawa T, Suzuki E, Terada M, Koya T, Kondoh A, Arakawa M, Yoshizawa H, Gejyo F (2005) Contribution of aspirin-intolerant asthma to near fatal asthma based on a questionnaire survey in Niigata Prefecture, Japan. Respirology 10:477–484.
15. Mascia K, Haselkorn T, Deniz YM, Miller DP, Bleecker ER, Borish L for the TENOR Study Group (2005) Aspirin sensitivity and severity of asthma: evidence for irreversible airway obstruction in patients with severe or difficult-to-treat asthma. J Allergy Clin Immunol 116:970–975.
16. Bochenek G, Nizankowska E, Szczeklik A (1996) The atopy trait in hypersensitivity to non-steroidal anti-inflammatory drugs. Allergy 51:16–23.
17. Szczeklik A, Gryglewski RJ, Czerniawska-Mysik G (1975) Relationship of inhibition of prostaglandin biosynthesis by analgesics to asthma attacks in aspirin-sensitive patients. Br Med J 1:67–60.
18. Szczeklik A, Gryglewski RJ, Czerniawska-Mysik G (1977) Clinical patterns of hypersensitivity to nonsteroidal anti-inflammatory drugs and their pathogenesis. J Allergy Clin Immunol 60:276–284.
19. Mathison DA, Stevenson DD (1979) Hypersensitivity to non-steroidal anti-inflammatory drugs: indications and methods for oral challenge. J Allergy Clin Immunol 64:669–674.
20. Czerniawska-Mysik G, Szczeklik A (1981) Idiosyncrasy to pyrazolone drugs. Allergy 36:381–384.
21. Asero R (2000) Multiple sensitivities to NSAIDs. Allergy 55:893–894.
22. Quaratino D, Romano A, Di Fonso M, Papa G, Perrone MR, D'Ambrosio FP, Venuti A (2000) Tolerability of meloxicam in patients with histories of adverse reactions to nonsteroidal anti-inflammatory drugs. Ann Allergy Asthma Immunol 84:613–617.
23. Bavbek S, Celik G, Ozer F, Mungan D, Misirligil Z (2004) Safety of selective COX-2 inhibitors in aspirin/NSAID intolerant patients: comparison of nimesulide, meloxicam and rofecoxib. J Asthma 41:67–75.
24. Bavbek S, Dursun AB, Dursun E, Eryilmaz A, Misirligil Z (2007) Safety of meloxicam in aspirin-hypersensitive patients with asthma and/or nasal polyps. A challenge-proven study. Int Arch Allergy Immunol 142:64–69.
25. Yoshida S, Ishizaki Y, Onuma K, Shoji T, Nakagawa H, Amayasu H (2000) Selective cyclo-oxygenase 2 inhibitor in pateints with aspirin-induced asthma. J Allergy Clin Immunol 106:1201–1202.

26. Stevenson DD, Simon RA (2001) Lack of cross-reactivity between rofecoxib and aspirin in aspirin-sensitive patients with asthma. J Allergy Clin Immunol 108:47–51.

27. Szczeklik A, Nizankowska E, Bochenek G, Nagraba K, Mejza F, Swierczynska M (2001) Safety of a specific COX-2 inhibitor in aspirin-induced asthma. Clin Exp Allergy 31:219–225.

28. Woessner KM, Simon RA, Stevenson DD (2002) The safety of celecoxib in aspirin exacerbated respiratory disease. Arthritis and Rheumatism 46:2201–2206.

29. Gyllfors P, Bochenek G, Overholt J, Drupka D, Kumlin M, Sheller J, Nizankowska E, Isakson PC, Mejza F, Lefkowith JB, Dahlén SE, Szczeklik A, Murray JJ, Dahlén B (2003) Biochemical and clinical evidence that aspirin-intolerant asthmatic subjects tolerate the cyclooxygenase-2 selective analgetic drug celecoxib. J Allergy Clin Immunol 111:1116–1121.

30. El Miedany Y, Youssef S, Ahmed I, El Gaafary M (2006) Safety of etoricoxib, a specific cyclooxygenase-2 inhibitor, in asthmatic patients with aspirin-exacerbated respiratory disease. Ann Allergy Asthma Immunol 97:105–109.

31. Viola M, Quaratino D, Volpetti S, Gaeta F, Romano A (2006) Parecoxib tolerability in patients with hypersensitivity to nonsteroidal anti-inflammatory drugs. J Allergy Clin Immunol 117: 1189–1190.

32. Levy MB, Fink JN (2001) Anaphylaxis to celecoxib. Ann Allergy Asthma Immunol 87: 72–73.

33. Murr D, Bocquet H, Lelouet H, Fischer RM, Revuz J, Cosnes A (2003) Adverse cutaneous reaction to celecoxib: 6 cases. Ann Dermatol Venereol 130:519–521.

34. Passero M (2003) Cyclooxygenase-2 inhibitors in aspirin sensitive asthma. Chest 123: 2155–2156.

35. Baldassarre S, Schandene L, Choufani G, Michils A (2006) Asthma attacks induced by low doses of celecoxib, aspirin and acetaminophen. J Allergy Clin Immunol 117:215–217.

36. Mastalerz L, Sanak M, Gawlewicz A, Gielicz A, Faber J, Szczeklik A (2006) Different eicosanoid profile of the hypersensitivtiy reactions triggered by aspirin and celecoxib in a patient with sinusitis, asthma and urticaria. J Allergy Clin Immunol 118:957–958.

37. Morais-Almeida M, Marinho S, Rosa S, Gaspar A, Rosado-Pinto JE (2006) Multiple drug intolerance including etoricoxib. Allergy 61:144–145.

38. Woś M, Sanak M, Burchell L, Mosser A, Soja J, Olechnowicz H, Szczeklik A, Busse W (2008) Rhinovirus infection in lower airways of asthmatic patients. J Allergy Clin Immunol 117:S314.

39. Peng T, Kotla S, Bumgarner RE, Gustin KE (2006) Human rhinovirus attenuates the type I interferon response by disrupting activation of interferon regulatory factor 3. J Virol 80:5021–5031.

40. Wark PA, Johnston SL, Bucchieri F, Powell R, Puddicombe S, Laza-Stnca V, Holgate ST, Davies DE (2005) Asthmatic bronchial epithelial cells have a deficient immune response to infection with rhinovirus. J Exp Med 21:937–947.

41. Contoli M, Message SD, Laza-Stanc V, Edwards MR, Wark PAB, Bartlett NW, Kebadze T, Mallia P, Stanciu LA, Parker HL, Slater L, Lewis-Antes A, Kon OM, Holgate ST, Davies DE, Kotenko SV, Papi A, Johnston SL (2006) Role of deficient type III interferon-lambda production in asthma exacerbations. Nat Med 12:1023–1026.

42. Dekker JW, Niżankowska E, Schmitz-Schumann M, Pile K, Bochenek G, Dyczek A, Cookson WO, Szczeklik A (1997) Aspirin-induced asthma and HLA-DRB1 and HLA-DPB1 genotypes. Clin Exp Allergy 27:574–577.

43. Choi JH, Lee KW, Oh HB, Lee KJ, Suh YJ, Park CS, Park HS (2004) HLA association in aspirin-intolerant asthma: DPB1*0301 as a strong marker in a Korean population. J Allergy Clin Immunol 113:562–564.

44. Kim SH, Park HS, Holloway JW, Shin HD, Park CS (2007) Association between a TGFβ1 promoter polymorphism and rhinosinusitis in aspirin-intolerant asthmatic patients. Resp Med 101:490–495.

45. Szczeklik A, Sanak M (2002) The role of COX-1 and COX-2 in asthma pathogenesis and its significance in the use of selective inhibitors. Clin Exp Allergy 32:339–342.

46. Picado C, Fernandez-Morata JC, Roc-Ferrer J, Fuentes M, Xaubet A, Mullol J (1999) Cyclooxygenase-2 mRNA is downexpressed in nasal polyps from aspirin-sensitive asthmatics. Am J Respir Crit Care Med 160:291–296.
47. Kowalski ML, Pawliczak R, Wozniak J, Sluda M, Poniatowska J, Iwaszkiewicz T, et al. (2000) Differential metabolism of arachidonic acid in nasal polyp epithelial cells cultured from aspirin-sensitive and aspirin-tolerant patients. Am J Respir Crit Care Med 161:391–398.
48. Pierzchalska M, Szabo Z, Sanak M, Soja J, Szczeklik A (2003) Deficient prostaglandin E2 production by bronchial fibroblasts of asthmatic patients, with special reference to aspirin-induced asthma. J Allergy Clin Immunol 111:1041–1048.
49. Kowalski ML, Ptasinska A, Bienkiewicz B, Pawliczak R, DuBuske L (2003) Differential effects of aspirin and misoprostol on 15-hydroxyecosatetraenoic acid generation by leukocytes from aspirin-sensitive asthmatic patients. J Allergy Clin Immunol 112:505–512.
50. Kowalski ML, Ptasinska A, Jedrzejczak M, Bienkiewicz B, Grzegorczyk J, Pawliczak R, DuBuske L (2005) Aspirin-triggered 15-HETE generation in peripheral blood leukocytes is a specific and sensitive Aspirin-Sensitive Patients Identification Test (ASPITest). Allergy 60:1139–1145.
51. Ying S, Meng Q, Scadding G, Parikh A, Corrigan CJ, Lee TH (2006) Aspirin-sensitive rhinosinusitis is associated with reduced E-prostanoid 2 receptor expression on nasal mucosal inflammatory cells. J Allergy Clin Immunol 117:312–318.
52. Celik G, Bavbek S, Misirligi Z, Melli M (2001) Release of cysteinyl leukotrienes with aspirin stimulation and the effect of prostaglandin E2 on this release from peripheral blood leucocytes in aspirin-induced asthmatic patients. Clin Exp Allergy 31:1615–1622.
53. Jinnai M, Sakagani T, Sekigawa T, Kakihara M, Nakajima T, Yoshud K, Goto S, Hasegawa T, Koshino T, Hasegawa Y, Inoue H, Suzuki N, Sano Y, Inoue I (2004) Polymorphisms in the prostaglandin E2 receptor subtype 2 confer susceptibility to aspirin-intolerant asthma: a candidate gene approach. Hum Mol Genet 13:3203–3217.
54. Sładek K, Szczekilk A (1993) Cysteinyl leukotrienes overproduction and mast cell activation in aspirin-provoked bronchospasm in asthma. Eur Respir J 6:39–399.
55. Sładek K, Dworski R, Soja J, Sheller JR, Niżankowska E, Oates JA, Szczeklik A (1994) Eicosanoids in bronchoalveolar lavage fluid of aspirin-intolerant patients with asthma after aspirin challenge. Am J Respir Crit Care Med 149:940–946.
56. Sanak M, Sampson AP (1999) Biosynthesis of cysteinyl leucotrienes in aspirin-intolerant asthma. Clin Exp All 29:306–316.
57. Antczak A, Montuschi P, Kharitonov S, Górski P, Barnes PJ (2002) Increased exhaled cysteinyl-leukotrienes and 8-isoprostane in aspirin-induced asthma. Am J Respir Crit Care Med 2002 166:301–306.
58. Obase Y, Shimoda T, Tomari SY, Mitsuta K, Kawano T, Matsuse H, Kohno S (2002) Effects of pranlukast on chemical mediators in induce sputum on provocation tests in atopic and aspirin-intolerant asthmatic patients. Chest 121:143–150.
59. Świerczyńska M, Niżankowska-Mogilnicka E, Zarychta J, Gielicz A, Szczeklik A (2003) Nasal versus bronchial and nasal response to oral aspirin challenge: clinical and biochemical differences between patients with aspirin-induced asthma/rhinitis. J Allergy Clin Immunol 112:995–1001.
60. Mita H, Turikisawa N, Yamada T, Taniguchi M (2007) Quantification of leukotriene B4 glucuronide in human urine. Prostagland Lipid Mediat 83:42–49.
61. Cowburn AS, Sładek K, Soja J, Adamek L, Niżankowska E, Szczeklik A, Lam BK, Penrose JF, Austen FK, Holgate ST, Sampson AP (1998) Overexpression of leukotriene C4 synthase in bronchial biopsies from patients with aspirin intolerant asthma. J Clin Invest 101:834–846.
62. Sanak M, Pierzchalska M, Bazan-Socha S, Szczeklik A (2000a) Enhanced expression of the leukotriene C4 synthase due to overactive transcription of an allelic variant associated with aspirin-intolerant asthma. Am J Respir Cell Mol Biol 23:290–296.
63. Kim SH, Bae JS, Suh CH, Nahm DH, Holloway JW, Park HS (2005a, 2005b) Polymorphism of tandem repeat in promoter of 5-lipoxygenase in ASA-intolerant asthma: a positive association with airway hyperresponsiveness. Allergy 60:760–765.

64. Kim SH, Choi JH, Park HS, Holloway JW, Lee SK, Shin HD (2005b) Association of thromboxane A2 receptor gene polymorphism with phenotype of acetyl salicylic acid-intolerant asthma. Clin Exp Allergy 35:585–590.

65. Kim SH, Oh JM, Kim YS, Palmer LJ, Suh CH, Nahm DH, Park HS (2006) Cysteinyl leukotriene receptor 1 promoter polymorphism is associated with aspirin-intolerant asthma in males. Clin Exp Allergy 36:433–439.

66. Park JS, Chang HS, Park CS, Lee YM, Choi JH, Park HS, Kim LH, Park BL, Choi YH, Shin HD (2005) Association analysis of cysteinyl-leukotriene receptor 2 (CYSLTR2) polymorphism with aspirin-intolerant asthma. Pharmacogenet Genomics 20:232–236.

67. Mita H, Endoh S, Kudoh M, Kawagishi Y, Kobayashi M, Taniguchi M, Akiyama K (2001) Possible involvement of mast-cell activation in aspirin provocation of aspirin-induced asthma. Allergy 56:106–1067.

68. Bochenek G, Nagraba K, Niżankowska E, Szczeklik A (2003) A controlled study of 9alpha,11beta-PGF2 (a prostaglandin D2 metabolite) in plasma and urine of patients with bronchial asthma and healthy controls after aspirin challenge. J Allergy Clin Immunol 111:743–749.

69. Sanak M, Kiełbasa B, Bochenek G, Szczeklik A (2004) Exhaled eicosanoids following oral aspirin challge in asthmatic patients. Clin Exp Allergy 34:1899–1904.

70. Higashi N, Taniguchi M, Mita H, Kawagishi Y, Ishi T, Higashi A, Osame M, Akiyama K (2004) Clinical features of asthmatic patients with increased urinary leukotriene E4 excretion (hyperleukotrienuria): involvement of chronic hyperplastic rhinosinusitis with nasal polyposis. J Allergy Clin Immunol 113:277–283.

71. Sousa AR, Parikhs A, Scadding G, Corrigan CJ, Lee TH (2002) Leukotriene-receptor expression on nasal mucosal inflammatory cells in aspirin-sensitive rhinosinusitis. N Engl J Med 347:1493–1499.

72. Corrigan C, Mallet K, Ying S, Roberts D, Parikh A, Scadding G, Lee T (2005) Expression of the cysteinyl leukotriene receptors cysLT1 and cysLT2 in aspirin-sensitive and aspirin-tolerant chronic rhinosinusitis. J Allergy Clin Immunol 115:316–322.

73. Sanak M, Levy BD, Clish CB, Chiang N, Gronert K, Mastalerz L, Serhan CN, Szczeklik A (2000b) Apirin-tolerant asthmatics generate more lipoxins than aspirin-intolerant asthmatics. Eur Respir J 16:44–49.

74. Perez-Novo CA, Watelet JB, Clayes C, Van Cauvenberge P, Bachert C (2005) Prostaglandin, leukotriene and lipoxin balance in chronic rhinosinusitis with and without nasal polyposis. J Allergy Clin Immunol 115:1189–1196.

75. Levy BD, Bonnns C, Silverman ES, Palmer LJ, Marigowda G, Israel E (2005) Diminished lipoxin biosynthesis in severe asthma. Am J Respir Crit Care Med 172:824–830.

76. Choi JH, Park HS, Oh HB, Lee JH, Suh YJ, Park CS, Shin HD (2004) Leukotriene-related gene polymorphisms in ASA-intolerant asthma: an association with a haplotype of 5-lipoxygene. Hum Genet 114:337–344.

77. Mastalerz L, Sanak M, Gawlewicz-Mroczka A, Ćmiel A, Gielicz A, Szczeklik A (2008) Prostaglandin E2 systemic production in patients with asthma with and without aspirin hypersensitivity. Thorax 63:27–34.

78. Gamboa P, Sanz ML, Caballero MR, Urrutia I, Antépara I, Esparza R, de Weck AL (2004) The flow-cytometric determination of basophil activation by aspirin and other non-steroidal anti-inflammatory drugs (NSAIDs) is useful for in vitro diagnosis of the NSAID hypersensitivity syndrome. Clin Exp Allergy 34:1448–1457.

79. Dahlen B, Zetterstrom O (1990) Comparison of bronchial and per oral provocation with aspirin in aspirin-sensitive asthmatics. Eur Respir J 3:527–534.

80. Milewski M, Mastalerz L, Nizankowska E, Szczeklik A (1998) Nasal provocation test with lysine-aspirin for diagnosis of aspirin-sensitive asthma. J Allergy Clin Immunol 101:581–586.

81. Nizankowska E, Bestynska-Krypel A, Cmiel A, Szczeklik A (2000) Oral and bronchial provocation tests with aspirin for diagnosis of aspirin-induced asthma. Eur Respir J 15:863–869.

82. Alonso-Llamazares A, Martinez-Cocera C, Dominguez-Ortega J, Robledo-Echarren T, Cimarra-Alvarez M, Mesa del Castillo M (2002) Nasal provocation test (NPT) with aspirin: a sensitive and safe method to diagnose aspirin-induced asthma. Allergy 57:632–635.

83. Stevenson DD, Simon RR, Zuraw BL (2003) Sensitivity to aspirin and NSAIDs. In: Adkinson NJ, Yunginger JW, Busse WW, Bochner BS, Holgate ST, Simon FE (eds) Allergy Principles and Practice, 6th edn. CV Mosby, Middleton, Philadelphia, PA, pp. 1695–1710.

84. Mita H, Higashi N, Taniguchi M, Higashi A, Akiyama K (2004) Increase in urinary leukotriene B4 glucuronide concentration in patients with aspirin-intolerant asthma after intravenous aspirin challenge. Clin Exp Allergy 34:1262–1269.

85. Nizankowska-Mogilnicka E, Bochenek G, Mastalerz L, Swierczynska M, Picado C, Scadding G, Kowalski ML, Setkowicz M, Ring J, Brockow K, Bachert C, Wöhrl S, Dahlén B, Szczeklik A (2007) EAACI/GA2LEN guideline: aspirin provocation tests for diagnosis of aspirin hypersensitivity. Allergy 62(10):1111–1118.

86. Williams AN, Simon RA, Woessner KM, Stevenson DD (2007) The relationship between historical aspirin-induced asthma and severity of asthma induced during oral aspirin challenges. J Allergy Clin Immunol 120(2):273–277.

87. White AA, Bigby T, Stevenson DD (2006) Intranasal ketorolac challenge for the diagnosis of aspirin exacerbated respiratory disease. Ann Allergy Asthma Immunol 97:190–195.

88. Mita H, Higashi N, Taniguchi M, Higashi A, Akiyama K (2004) Increase in urinary leukotriene B4 glucuronide concentration in patients with aspirin-intolerant asthma after intravenous aspirin challenge. Clin Exp Allergy 34:1262–1269.

89. Nizankowska E, Duplaga M, Bochenek G, Szczeklik A on behalf of the AIANE project (1998) Clinical course of aspirin-induced asthma, results of AIANE. In: Szczeklik A, Gryglewski R, Vane J (eds) Eicosanoids, Aspirin and Asthma. Marcel Dekker, New York, pp. 451–472.

90. Dahlén B, Nizankowska E, Szczeklik A, Zetterström O, Bochenek G, Kumlin M, Mastalerz L, Pinis G, Swanson LJ, Boodhoo TI, Wright S, Dubé LM, Dahlén SE (1998) Benefits from adding the 5-lipoxygenase inhibitor zileuton to conventional therapy in aspirin-intolerant asthmatics. Am J Respir Crit Care Med 157:1187–1194.

91. Micheletto C, Tognella S, Visconti M, Pomari C, Trevisan F, Dal Negro RW (2004) Montelukast 10 mg improves nasal function and nasal response to aspirin in ASA-sensitive asthmatics: a controlled study vs placebo. Allergy 59:289–294.

92. Sampson AP, Siddiqui S, Buchanan D, Howarth PH, Holgate ST, Holloway JW, Sayers I (2000) Variant LTC(4) synthase allele modifies cysteinyl leukotriene synthesis in eosinophils and predicts clinical response to zafirlukast. Thorax 55(Suppl):S28–S31.

93. Asano K, Shiomi T, Hasegawa N, Nakamura H, Kudo H, Matsuzaki T, Hakuno H, Fukunaga K, Suzuki Y, Kanazawa M, Yamaguchi K (2002) Leukotriene C_4 synthase gene A(-444)C polymorphism and clinical response to an LT(1) antagonist, pranlukast, in Japanese patients with moderate asthma. Pharmacogenetics 12:565–570.

94. Mastalerz L, Nizankowska E, Sanak M, Mejza F, Pierzchalska M, Bazan-Socha S, Bestynska-Krypel A, Cmiel A, Szczeklik A (2002) Clinical and genetic features underlying the response of patients with bronchial asthma to treatment with a leukotriene receptor antagonist. Eur J Clin Invest 32:949–955.

95. Park HE, Kim SH, Sampson AP, Lee KW, Park CS (2004) The HLA-DPB1*0301 marker might predict the requirement for leukotriene receptor antagonist in patients with aspirin-intolerant asthma. J Allergy Clin Immunol 114:688–689.

96. Aukema AA, Mulder PG, Fokkens WJ (2005) Treatment of nasal polyposis and chronic rhinosinusitis with fluticasone propionate nasal drops reduces need for sinus surgery. JACI 115:1017–1023.

97. Jankowski R, Pigret D, Decroocq F (1997) Comparison of functional results after ethmoidectomy and nasalization for diffuse and severe nasal polyposis. Acta Otolaryngol (Stockh) 117:601–608.

98. Hosemann W (2000) Surgical treatment of nasal polyposis in patients with aspirin intolerance. Thorax 55:87–90.

99. Loehrl TA, Ferre RM, Toohill RJ, Smith TL (2006) Long-term asthma outcomes after endoscopic sinus surgery in aspirin triad patients. Am J Otolaryngol 27:154–160.

100. Ragab S, Scadding GK, Lund VJ, Saleh H (2006) Treatment of chronic rhinosinusitis and its effects on asthma. Eur Respir J 28:68–74.
101. Stevenson DD (2003) Aspirin desensitization in patients with AERD. Clin Rev Allergy Immunol 24:159–168.
102. Stevenson DD, Simon RA (2006) Selection of patients for aspirin desensitization treatment. J Allergy Clin Immunol 118:801–804.
103. Gollapudi RR, Teirstein PS, Stevenson DD, Simon RA (2004) Aspirin sensitivity: implications for patients with coronary artery disease. JAMA 292:3017–3023.
104. Silberman S, Neukirch-Stoop C, Steg PG (2005) Rapid desensitization procedure for patients with aspirin hypersensitivity undergoing coronary stenting. Am J Cardiol 95:509–510.
105. Macy E, Bernstein JA, Castells MC, Gawchik SM, Lee TH, Settipane RA, Simon RA, Wald J, Woessner KM; Aspirin Desensitization Joint Task Force (2007) Aspirin challenge and desensitization for aspirin-exacerbated respiratory disease: a practice paper. Ann Allergy Asthma Immunol 98:172–174.
106. Pfaar O, Klimek L (2006) Aspirin desensitization in aspirin intolerance: update on current standards and recent improvements. Curr Opin Allergy Clin Immunol 6:161–166.
107. Lee JY, Simon RA, Stevenson DD (2007) Selection of aspirin dosages for aspirin desensitization treatment in patients with aspirin-exacerbated respiratory disease. J Allergy Clin Immunol 119:157–164.
108. Page NA, Schroeder WS (2007) Rapid desensitization protocols for patients with cardiovascular disease and aspirin hypersensitivity in an era of dual antiplatelet therapy. Ann Pharmacother 41:61–67.
109. Parikh AA, Scadding GK (2005) Intranasal lysine-aspirin in aspirin-sensitive nasal polyposis: a controlled trial. Laryngoscope 115:1385–1390.

Airway Remodeling in Asthma and Therapeutic Implications

Tari Haahtela

Introduction

Asthma is a chronic, inflammatory condition of the lower airways characterized by largely reversible airflow obstruction, airway hyperresponsiveness, and episodic respiratory symptoms, including wheezing, productive cough, and sensations of breathlessness and chest tightness [1]. Asthma is also regarded as a local manifestation of a systemic inflammatory process.

Patients with asthma demonstrate a spectrum of clinical symptoms and, likewise, of inflammatory changes. The inflammatory processes cause, or are parallel with variable patterns of airway wall structural changes, so called remodeling, as well as differences in the extent of remodeling (Table 1). These changes include goblet cell metaplasia (their numbers increase first), bronchial mucous gland enlargement (excess production of mucus), epithelial shedding or denudation (as a result of toxic proteins released especially by eosinophils), thickening of the subepithelial structures like reticular basement membrane (maybe to prevent inflammatory cells to intrude epithelium from deeper tissue), increased smooth muscle mass (hyperplasia), angiogenesis or neovasculature (chronic attraction of inflammatory cells from the vasculature), and many alterations in extracellular matrix [2]. These changes involve both large and small airways, but the individual variation is large.

Chronic inflammation causes tissue injury, which is partly repaired between inflammatory exacerbations. Remodeling is developed during the cycle of injury and repair and gradually affects lung function. Remodeling seems to be the cause of more or less persistent airway hyperresponsiveness and fixed airway obstruction.

The functional effects of different features or airway remodeling, are, however, not known. This is a challenge to treatment, which ideally should prevent any permanent structural changes in the airways. There are indications that early anti-inflammatory treatment, especially with inhaled corticosteroids, is clinically beneficial and improves the outcome, but little is known on how and to what extent

T. Haahtela (✉)
Professor of Clinical Allergology, Skin and Allergy Hospital, Helsinki University Central Hospital, PO Box 160, 00029 HUS, Finland

R. Pawankar et al. (eds.), *Allergy Frontiers: Clinical Manifestations*,
DOI: 10.1007/978-4-431-88317-3_18, © Springer 2009

Table 1 Characteristics of airway structural changes (remodeling). As a consequence of these changes bronchial obstruction may become partially irreversibe and resistant to treatment. In the majority of asthmatics the structural changes are small and do not essentially affect long-term lung function. In a minority asthma runs a severe course and lung function may rapidly deteriorate

Goblet cell metaplasia, their numbers increase first

Bronchial mucous gland enlargement, excess production of mucus

Epithelial shedding or denudation

Thickening of the subepithelial structures like reticular basement membrane

Increased smooth muscle mass, hyperplasia

Angiogenesis or neovasculature, chronic attraction of inflammatory cells from the vasculature

Alterations in extracellular matrix

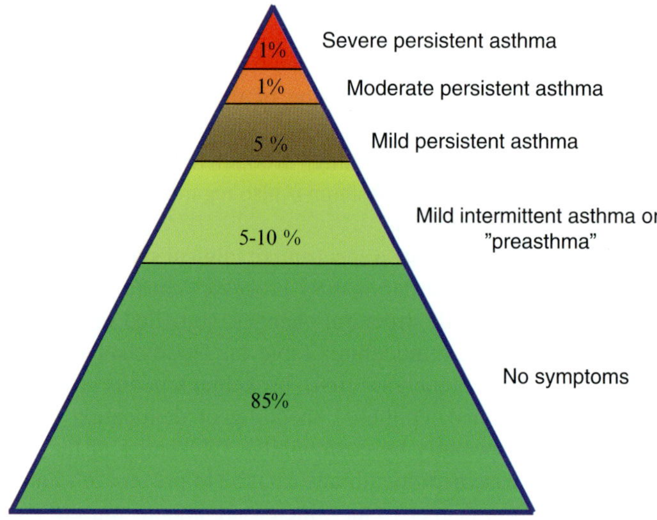

Fig. 1 At the population level, most of asthma is mild and do not significantly disable patients (estimate made in the Finnish population).

such treatment really inhibits structural changes? What component of remodeling is affected, and how should we monitor the effects?

Cellular and molecular pathways involved in remodeling are poorly understood, and do not give apparent targets to new type of drugs. Increase in airway smooth muscle mass is taking place in chronic asthma, and may be most promising target to new innovations. At the moment, detecting asthmatic inflammation early and intervening immediately give patients the best chance to maintain good lung function and live a normal life.

At the population level, most of asthma (70–80%) is mild and does not significantly disable patients (Fig. 1). Clinically significant and progressive remodeling takes place in the minority of patients, but they should be in special focus and carefully followed. They may be severely incapacitated, and also cause most of the costs (medication, emergencies, hospitalizations and other health care use, disability, deaths).

Inflammation and Remodeling in Asthma

Both inflammation and structural changes (remodeling) occur in the tracheobronchial tree of patients with asthma. Persistent, eosinophilic inflammation seems to be a prerequisite for the development of remodeling, which is supported by some animal experimental evidence [3]. In humans, it is not fully established which comes first: chronic inflammation or remodeling? [4–8]. Knowing this would help to determine the optimal 'window of opportunity' for prevention of disease progression. Moreover, this knowledge might help to predict which preschool 'wheezers' will go on to develop asthma.

Measuring airway function (e.g. forced expiratory volume in 1 s, FEV_1) gives indirect information of the long-term airway inflammation and structural changes, but is not the tool to detect early inflammatory processes. They can be present even in patients with normal lung function but with symptoms indicative of asthma [9]. On the other hand, symptomatic infants, who have reversible airflow obstruction (i.e., asthma by functional definition) may not show either bronchial tissue eosinophilia or remodeling (Fig. 2) [5].

The pathological structural changes of the airways are already present and maximal in severely asthmatic school children [4], indicating that changes began earlier. The changes, which are not apparent in infants, may begin already between the ages of 1 and 3 years; tissue eosinophilia and reticular basement membrane thickening

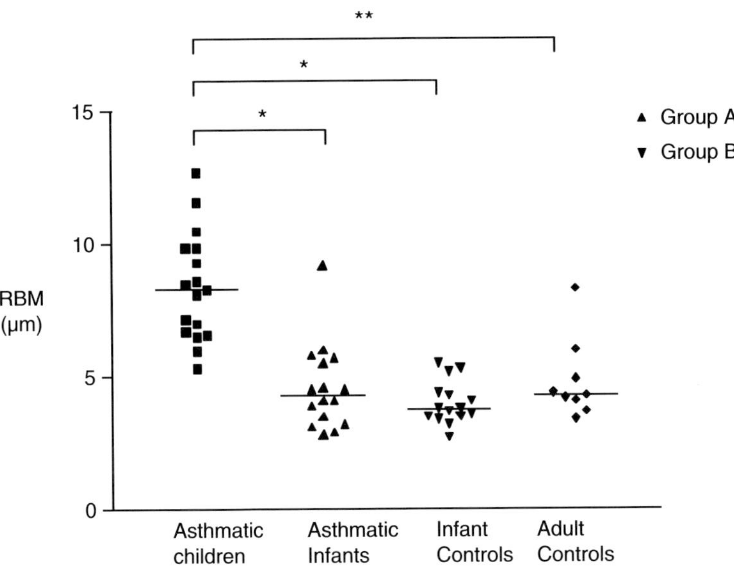

Fig. 2 Thickness of reticular basement membrane in school-aged children, asthmatic infants, and in healthy infants and adults. In asthmatic infants basement membrane is still mostly normal but clearly thickened in older asthmatic children (From Ref. [5] with permission)

are positively associated [7]. The new evidence indicates that the characteristic pathological features of asthma in adults and school-aged children develop between this age window of 1 and 3 years, a time when intervention may modify the natural history of asthma [8].

Chronic inflammation and remodeling contribute to airway wall thickening, which narrows the airway lumen and increases resistance to airflow. Airway secretions also contribute to the air flow limitation in asthma, and increase in amount and viscosity of the secretions plays a crucial role especially in acute, life-threatening exacerbations [10].

Increased vascularity and expression of vascular endothelial growth factor are features of the asthmatic airway, but little is known of their contribution to airway remodeling. Recently, Siddiqui et al. [11] showed that vascular remodeling is a feature of asthma, and is inversely correlated with postbronchodilator FEV1 indicating a role in airflow obstruction.

Inflammation

Lymphocytic inflammation enriched by eosinophils is characteristic of the bronchi in both asthmatic adults and school children. Along with increasing disease severity, neutrophils are playing an increasing role, and the inflammation may involve all lower airways, including the small airways (airways 2 mm or smaller in diameter) [12].

About 80% of childhood and 50% of adult asthma is allergic (i.e., IgE associated). The cellular pattern of inflammation is, however, rather similar in allergic and non-allergic asthma. In the latter, the triggers of eosinophilic inflammation are poorly known, but are probably microbes or microbial components. In allergic asthma, inhaled allergens penetrate the mucociliary lining and enter the airway epithelium either via the tight junctions that surround the apical zone of bronchial epithelial cells, or by direct uptake by the cells per se. Allergens are presented to mast cells, and cross-linking of allergen specific mast cell surface IgE causes release of mediators such as histamine and leukotrienes. They increase vascular permeability, and initiate a cascade of recruitment of more inflammatory cells and further release of pro-inflammatory mediators.

In asthma, chronic inflammation is driven by the CD4 or T-helper lymphocyte, producing key regulatory cytokines such as interleukin-5 (IL-5) and IL-4 [13]. Partly in response to IL-5, eosinophils, originating in the bone marrow, are released into the circulation, resulting in a blood eosinophilia. Eosinophils are then selectively retained at endothelial surfaces of bronchial vessels by IL-4-induced upregulation of adhesive molecules. This is followed by transmigration of eosinophils to the tissue and up into the mucosa as a result of further response to chemoattractants released by structural and immune elements. Activated eosinophils release highly toxic granules, the evolutionary function of which has probably been killing the potentially dangerous invader. Especially in allergic asthma this immune function is working inappropriately as allergens, like pollens, are not a real threat. Eosinophil derivatives damage the surface epithelial cells, loosening their attachments and resulting in shedding of cells into the airway lumen, where they admix with eosinophils, neutrophils and mucus.

Eosinophil chemoattractants include eotaxin, macrophage/monocyte chemotactic protein 4 (MCP4), RANTES (regulated upon activation, normal T-lymphocyte expressed), and cysteinyl leukotrienes (cysLT) among others [14]. They act on distinct cell surface receptors (e.g. CC chemokine receptor 3 [CCR3] and $cysLT_1$) present on the eosinophil, but not exclusively so. As far as leukotrienes are concerned, challenge with leukotriene E_4 (LTE_4) results in greatly increased numbers of eosinophils in the bronchial wall [14]. A recent study used the molecular techniques of *in situ* hybridization and immunohistochemistry to localize cells that express either the mRNA or the protein for the $cysLT_1$ receptor, respectively [15]. The receptor appears to be present on a variety of bronchial inflammatory cells in addition to the eosinophil, including neutrophils, mast cells, macrophages, B lymphocytes, and plasma cells. The study also demonstrated that the numbers of inflammatory cells expressing the $cysLT_1$ receptor are increased, by comparison with normal healthy nonsmokers, in nonsmoking patients with mild, stable asthma and that there is a further, significant increase among patients experiencing a severe exacerbation of asthma leading to hospitalization [15].

Allergen challenge causes inflammation, but it is interesting that in dual responders (early and late-phase reaction) with asthma the increase in the number of airway wall inflammatory cells resolves in 7 days, whereas the increases in airway hyperresponsiveness and markers or remodeling persist [16].

Remodeling

Remodeling is defined as a change in structure that is inappropriate to the maintenance of normal airway function [2, 13]. Some features of remodeling are evident, even in newly diagnosed or mild asthma and is characterized by epithelial fragility and reticular basement membrane thickening [17] (Fig. 3). With increasing severity of asthma, the changes are more pronounced and clear: increases of airway smooth muscle mass, vascularity, numbers of fibroblasts, and interstitial collagen, as well as mucous gland hypertrophy [13]. These changes appear to be greatest in the larger, more proximal airways.

Thickening of the reticular basement membrane occurs early in asthma, even before diagnosis, and is detected in children with mild asthma [6]. In school children between the ages of 6 and 16 with severe asthma it is already maximally thickened but there is no significant association between its thickness and age or symptom duration [4]. These changes appear in preschool wheezy children by the age of 29 months [7]. Bourdin et al. [18] showed recently, that reticular basement thickness is a hallmark of severe asthma, but not of mild asthma or COPD.

Airway smooth muscle surrounds the airways as two opposing helices, i.e., a geodesic pattern. Thus, as muscle shortens, it not only constricts but also tends to shorten the airway against an elastic load. There are at least three possible mechanisms of smooth muscle mass enlargement in asthma: (1) myocyte hypertrophy, (2) myocyte hyperplasia due to cell division and proliferation, or (3) myocyte de-differentiation

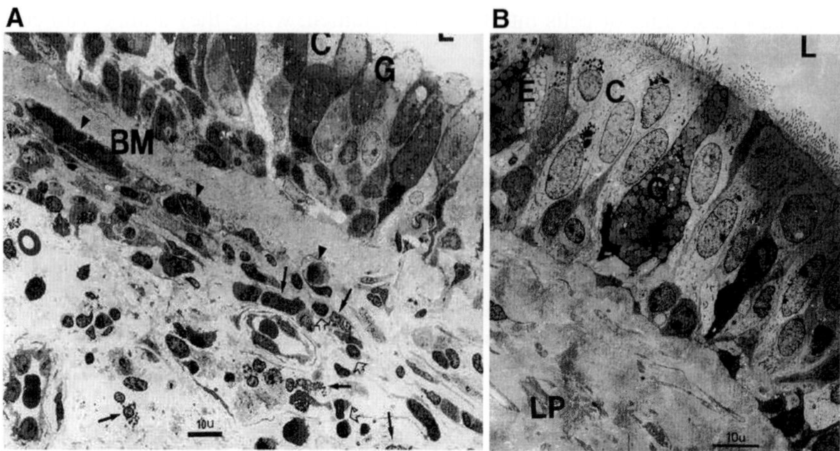

Fig. 3 A. General morphological features of a large airway in a patient with newly detected asthma. The basement membrane (BM) is slightly thickened. The epithelium exhibits goblet cell (G) hyperplasia and their number is increased. The number of ciliated cells (C) is decreased. Numerous capillaries (arrows) are located beneath the basement membrane, and some inflammatory cells penetrate the basement membrane. Eosinophils (closed arrows) and lymphocytes (open arrows) are in lamina propria indicating ongoing inflammation. B. For comparison the airways of a healthy subject showing normal pseudostratified columnar epithelium (E) with ciliated epithelial cells (C) and a few goblet cells (G). No inflammatory cells in lamina propria. Transmission electron microscopy (From Ref. [17] with permission)

and migration across the mucosa in the form of myofibroblasts, or fibromyocytes. It is speculated that these may then re-differentiate to form new blocks of smooth muscle that come to lie just below (external to) the epithelium [13].

Recently, greater numbers of mast cells have been found located within bronchial smooth muscle of patients with asthma than in those with eosinophilic bronchitis. Patients with eosinophilic bronchitis, which is probably more common than thought, do also show airway eosinophilia and remodeling but do not clinically fulfill the functional criteria of asthma, i.e. reversible airway obstruction. The difference in smooth muscle mast cell number that discriminates between these conditions has led to the hypothesis that the infiltration of airway smooth muscle by mast cells is responsible for the disordered airway function characteristic of asthma. Thus, asthma would be the result of a mast cell myositis [19]. The mast cell mediators, such as tryptase and cytokines, can modulate airway smooth muscle cell function Mast cells contribute to multiple features of chronic asthma in mast cell deficient mice, and they play an important role in tissue remodeling [20].

It is likely, however, that asthma and eosinophilic bronchitis are not really distinctly separate entities, but reflect disease severity and genetic polymorphisms; genetic disposition of the individual to develop bronchial hyperresponsiveness. Nevertheless, these data highlight an important point, namely localization of inflammatory cells to different tissue compartments rather than their overall number per se.

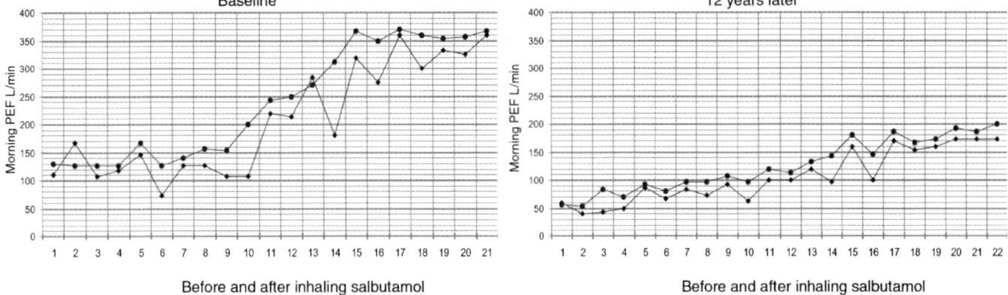

Fig. 4 Development of a mostly irreversible airway obstruction due to remodeling in a non-smoking young man with severe asthma during 12 years. The patient was hospitalized because of an asthma attack and gained relatively normal peak expiratory flow during two weeks' treatment (left). He was hospitalized again 12 years later, but his peak expiratory level remained in a low level in spite of intensive treatment (right)

Severe asthma is characterized by a degree of fixed airflow obstruction, which is probably caused by increase in smooth muscle leading to hyperresponsiveness as well as by a more general airway wall remodeling (Fig. 4). Holgate et al. [21] suggest that aberrant epithelial-mesenchymal communication leads to chronic wound scenario with activation of the epithelial-mesenchymal trophic unit, epithelial damage, the laying on of new matrix, and greater involvement of neutrophils.

Interactions Between Asthma and Rhinitis

Asthma and rhinitis are often considered to be clinical manifestations of the same condition, the chronic allergic respiratory syndrome [22–24].

Remodeling in the nose in persistent allergic (eosinophilic) rhinitis appears to be less extensive than that in the lower airways [25, 26]. The differences in remodeling between upper and lower airways include: (1) the secretory activity of smooth muscle cells present in bronchi but not in the nose, and (2) the differences in embryologic origins of bronchi and nose [25].

Bronchial hyperresponsiveness is common in people with allergic rhinitis, even if they have no symptoms of asthma, and bronchial inflammation can result from nasal allergen challenge in patients with rhinitis but not obvious asthma [27]. Conversely, patients with asthma can have eosinophilic infiltration of their nasal mucosa without reporting the symptoms of rhinitis [22, 23]. Moreover, segmental bronchial provocation in patients with rhinitis but not asthma can induce nasal inflammation [28, 29]. However, not all patients with asthma have rhinitis and not all patients with rhinitis have asthma. Genetic differences contribute to this discrepancy, for example, certain haplotypes of GPR 154 gene predispose the individual to IgE-mediated rhinitis but not asthma [30].

Airway inflammation is manifestation of a systemic immune response, and nasal inflammation propagates systemically to the bronchial mucosa or vice versa, through so called "systemic cross-talk", which works via effects of mediators and inflammatory cells on bone marrow [31].

Evaluating of Airway Inflammation

Several techniques are available, but not really widely performed in clinical practice, for evaluating inflammation in the airways in both clinical and research settings.

Peripheral blood eosinophilia is sometimes present in asthma and reflects the presence of systemic inflammation but is an insensitive measure. The patient may have full blown asthma without signs of blood eosinophilia.

Induced sputum samples can be used to study inflammatory cell numbers and soluble inflammatory markers [9, 32]. Measurement of biological markers in the airways can be made before and after provocation with allergen, pharmacological, or physical agents in order to study the dynamics of the inflammatory responses to such challenges. Induced sputum is slightly invasive, when the patient inhales hypertonic saline, which causes cough and sometimes mild bronchoconstriction. The method is still mostly used for research, because a lot of laboratory work is needed to handle the sample, and to make biomarker analyses as well as cell differentiation.

Measuring fractional concentration of exhaled nitric oxide (FENO) is at the moment the most useful and handy method to assess airway inflammation in diagnostic work or to monitor the effects of anti-inflammatory therapy, even in children [33–37]. With the newly launched hand-held devices the measurement is also available for office practice.

Finally, the airways can be investigated by fiberoscopy [38, 39], which is used to collect endobronchial biopsies or brushings as well as bronchoalveolar lavage. Biopsy permits histopathological, immunohistological, and molecular examination of respiratory mucosa. Bronchoscopy has obvious limitations of being invasive and not feasible outside of special clinics.

Effects of Treatment on Remodeling

In patients with asthma, inhalation of corticosteroids (ICS) reduces bronchial inflammation in days or weeks (Table 2). Whether ICS can affect airway remodeling, e.g. reduce reticular basement membrane (RBM) thickening, is difficult to study, and only a few trials have tried to address the problem. Sterk et al. [40] observed that 2-year treatment of persistent asthma with ICS, dose adjusted according to hyperreactivity measurements, was able to decrease RBM thickening. Ward et al. [41] also suggested that ICS produce reductions in reticular basement membrane

Table 2 Some options to halt asthmatic inflammation and possibly airway remodeling. Many of the treatments are in an experimental stage

- Inhaled corticosteroids – early and effective treatment still best option
- Leukotriene antagonists – useful to control inflammation, some in vitro evidence indicate potential to inhibit remodeling
- IgE blockade (e.g. omalizumab) – beneficial in severe asthma, effect on remodeling to be shown
- TNF-alpha blockade (monoclonal antibodies) – improvement in airway hyperresponsiveness
- Doxycyclin (aerosol) – some inhibition of remodeling in a mouse model
- CpG oligonucleotids – some inhibition of remodeling in a mouse model
- Toll-like receptor-7/8 ligand S28463 – some inhibition of remodeling in a mouse model
- Bronchial thermoplasty – may reduce airway smooth muscle mass

thickening after about 1 year. Thus, it seems that only an intensive treatment over longer periods might have a measurable effect on RBM. Nevertheless, ICS may prevent airway remodeling in the first place if given early in the course of disease. A Korean group developed a mouse model of airway remodeling including smooth muscle thickening, and showed that intranasal administration of fluticasone can modulate remodeling of smooth muscle via regulation of TGF-beta1 production and active signaling [42].

Steroid-resistant asthma is rare, but may be a key to understand factors predisposing to remodeling. Goleva et al. [43] observed, that impaired bronchodilator reversibility in patients with steroid-resistant asthma is associated with a shift in MMP-g/TIMP-1 ratio caused by inability of steroids to enhance TIMP-1 production, potentially promoting proteolytic activity in the airways.

Treatment with leukotriene antagonists, montelukast or pranlukast, reduces peripheral eosinophil counts, eosinophils in induced sputum or reduces bronchial inflammation in endobronchial biopsies [44, 45]. There is in vitro evidence from isolates and cultures of human airway smooth muscle that leukotrienes enhance myocyte proliferation and migration, processes that can be attenuated by LTRA [46–48].

Other options to prevent or modulate airway remodeling certainly will appear. Doxycycline administered by aerosols has decreased allergen-induced airway inflammation and hyperresponsivenss and inhibited development of bronchial remodeling in a mouse model by modulation of cytokines production and matrix metalloproteinase activity [49].

Again in a mouse model, CpG oligonucleotides has prevented not only acute allergic inflammation but also reduced markers (airway hyperresponsiveness, subepithelial collagen deposition, goblet cell hyperplasia) of airway remodeling that develop after chronic allergen exposure [50]. The clinical relevance of these observations is not known.

One of the Toll-like receptor-7/8 ligands, the synthetic compound S28463 (resquimod, R-848) inhibits acute allergic reaction in mice, but was also recently shown to prevent goblet cell hyperplasia and increase in airway smooth muscle mass [51]. Chronic severe asthma is accompanied by a marked increase in tumor necrosis factor alpha production. TNF blockade with monoclonal antibodies has produced improvement in symptoms as well as in airway hyperresponsiveness.

In severe allergic asthma blockade of IgE with omalizumab confers marked clinical benefit [52], but effects on airway remodeling are to be shown. The same applies to TNF-alpha as a therapeutic target of severe asthma [53].

Bronchial thermoplasty is a bronchoscopic procedure to reduce the mass of airway smooth muscle and attenuate bronchoconstriction. Cox et al. [54] examined the effect of bronchial thermoplasty on the control of moderate or severe persistent asthma during 1 year. Mild exacerbations were slightly reduced in actively treated patients compared with a control group. Patients stopped using long-acting beeta-2-agonists during the trial. The procedure itself may increase risk of hospitalisation. It is too early to recommend this treatment, but it may increase asthma control in carefully selected, severely ill patients with changes of airway wall structures.

Early Treatment with Emphasis on ICS

Asthma is a syndrome, which has been difficult to define in precision. Asthma is an "umbrella" diagnosis, characterized clinically by reversible bronchial obstruction, but it covers several genotypes in terms of factors affecting disease severity or responses to treatments and drugs. At the population level most of asthma is intermittent or mild (70–80%), and these patients are probably not facing any significant lung function loss over time even regardless their treatment. More attention should be paid on the mild end of the asthma spectrum, to the majority of patients to estimate better the clinical impact of remodeling and lung function loss over time. Unnecessary or even harmful over-treatment may otherwise occur. Strategies to treat mild asthma are not well based on evidence, neither in children nor adults. How intensive should the initial treatment be? For how long it should go on, in children and adults? When is intermittent treatment sufficient, and for how long should the treatment periods take? If treatment is altogether stopped by the patient, what is the risk for disease escalation?

But there are the "decliners", those patients (estimates range from 20% to 30% of asthmatics) in whom significant irreversible airway obstruction develops over time. Is the possible "slowing down" effect of ICS seen more readily in them? Recent 10-year observational data from Denmark indicate that may be the case [55]. In a general population sample treatment of asthma with ICS was associated with a less steep decline in FEV1 of 18 mL/year compared with patients not receiving this treatment ($p = 0.01$).

The clinical benefits of early treatment with anti-inflammatory therapy for persistent-type, but still mostly mild asthma were shown in studies in the early 1990s [56, 57]. The first results in the mid-1990s also indicated that delays in initiating ICS therapy may lead to an impaired functional response [57]. However, the study was not designed to study the effect of the delay at the first place. The non-randomized studies by Agertoft and Pedersen [58] and Selroos et al. [59] pointed, nevertheless, to the same direction: delay was harmful. However, the prospective CAMP study questioned the benefit of inhaled corticosteroids on children lung function, but as no significant FEV1 decline was seen in the placebo group, treatment effect was difficult to demonstrate [60].

It is probable that we will never get the ultimate answer to the question: do ICS alter the long-term functional (natural) course, and remodeling, of asthma? Length of the follow-up required, ethical considerations and costs will prevent that. These doubts should not, however, hinder us to use the most effective treatment and use it early enough. The results of O'Byrne et al. [61] and Lange et al. [55] reassure our current practice of preventing all asthma events with regular use of ICS – the dose can vary – in patients who have symptoms on most days.

Most asthma drug studies have been accomplished in patients with moderate persistent asthma (to have room for improvement and possibility to show treatment differences), and the results are often carelessly generalized to whole asthmatic population. Along with better options to measure not only lung function but the inflammatory component of asthma [9, 62], the early and often milder stages of the disease, when lung function is still mostly preserved, can be better addressed.

In 1994, the Finnish asthma program was established to reduce morbidity of asthma in Finland with a focus on early detection and treatment of inflammation, as implemented by a network of asthma-responsible doctors, nurses, and pharmacists. While this program has not halted the increase of asthma in Finland, disability pensions and the number of hospital bed days for asthma and deaths from asthma have greatly decreased over the past 10 years [63]. This outcome can be attributed mainly to early and more effective use of anti-inflammatory medication.

Most patients get free of symptoms if treated early and effectively with ICS alone. If the clinical result is suboptimal, there are arguments that favor the combined use of ICS and an LTRA to strengthen the anti-inflammatory therapy: (1) Leukotriene levels in induced sputum remain increased in patients with asthma receiving ICS, suggesting that corticosteroids do not fully suppress leukotriene production [64], (2) The addition of the LTRA montelukast improves clinical endpoints [65, 66].

For patients with comorbid rhinitis and asthma (80% of patients with persistent asthma have rhinitis), effective management of rhinitis may improve the co-existing asthma [67].

The World Allergy Organization (WAO) has published Guidelines for the Prevention of Allergy and Allergic Asthma [68]. WAO/WHO guidelines emphasize the need to treat the underlying inflammatory process as early as possible. ICS responsive inflammatory changes are already present in the mildest forms (intermittent) asthma [69]. The guidelines also recommend treating allergic rhinitis to prevent the development of asthma.

Conclusions

In asthma the relationships of airway inflammation, remodeling and lung function are becoming better understood; they are consecutive but also parallel phenomenon, which vary largely both in severity and timing between individuals. Anti-inflammatory therapy, ICS (supplemented by leucotriene antagonists or even small dose of theophylline) still remains the best option for the vast majority of patients to improve asthma control. The inflammatory element of asthma can be detected more readily than before by measuring exhaled NO, or examining cells and soluble markers in induced sputum. Increased airway responsiveness is a surrogate marker of inflammation and seems to reflect development of structural changes in the airways. Persistently increased bronchial responsiveness means remodeling and is partly resistant to therapy. Several studies have the same message: in moderate to severe asthma it is not enough to adjust anti-inflammatory treatment according to symptoms and lung function (e.g. PEF-follow-up). Exacerbation rate is reduced, if more direct inflammatory markers – exhaled NO, sputum eosinophils or hyperresponsiveness – are employed to guide treatment. New modes on anti-inflammatory therapy have emerged, but are still mostly in an experimental stage. Anti-IgE – and anti-TNFalpha-therapies hold best promise, but their effect on halting airway remodeling in severe disease is not known. Regular long-acting β_2-agonists are used if anti-inflammatory therapy fails to control the disease, as indicated by increasing daily requirement for short-acting β_2-agonist. Their effect on airway remodeling is not known. Given the similarity that exists between the patterns of inflammation in asthma and allergic rhinitis, treatment should focus on the entire airway rather than only a part, as well as the skin (inflammation in atopic eczema) as necessary. Asthma, rhinitis (and atopic eczema) are also regarded as local manifestations of a systemic inflammatory process [70].

References

1. Bousquet J, Jeffery PK, Busse WW, Johnson M, Vignola AM. Asthma. From bronchoconstriction to airways inflammation and remodeling. *Am J Respir Crit Care Med* 2000, 161(5):1720–1745.
2. Mauad T, Bel EH, Sterk PJ. Asthma therapy and airway remodeling. J Allergy Clin Immunol 2007, 120:997–1009.
3. Humbles AA, Lloyd CM, McMillan SJ, Friend DS, Xanthou G, McKenna EE, Ghiran S, Gerard NP, Yu C, Orkin SH et al. A critical role for eosinophils in allergic airways remodeling. *Science* 2004, 305(5691):1776–1779.
4. Payne DN, Rogers AV, Adelroth E, Bandi V, Guntupalli KK, Bush A, Jeffery PK. Early thickening of the reticular basement membrane in children with difficult asthma. *Am J Respir Crit Care Med* 2003, 167(1):78–82.
5. Saglani S, Malmstrom K, Pelkonen AS, Malmberg LP, Lindahl H, Kajosaari M, Turpeinen M, Rogers AV, Payne DN, Bush A et al. Airway remodeling and inflammation in symptomatic infants with reversible airflow obstruction. *Am J Respir Crit Care Med* 2005, 171(7):722–727.
6. Barbato A, Turato G, Baraldo S, Bazzan E, Calabrese F, Tura M, Zuin R, Beghe B, Maestrelli P, Fabbri LM et al. Airway inflammation in childhood asthma. *Am J Respir Crit Care Med* 2003, 168(7):798–803.
7. Saglani S, Payne DN, Nicholson AG, Jeffery PK, Bush A. Thickening of the epithelial reticular basement membrane in pre-school children with troublesome wheeze. *American Thoracic Society 2005*; *San Diego, CA* 2005: A515.
8. Saglani S, Payne DN, Zhu J, Wang Z, Nicholson AG, Bush A, Jeffery PK. Early detection of airway remodeling and eosinophilic inflammation in preschool wheezers. *Am J Respir Crit Care Med* 2007, 176:858–864.

9. Rytila P, Metso T, Heikkinen K, Saarelainen P, Helenius IJ, Haahtela T. Airway inflammation in patients with symptoms suggesting asthma but with normal lung function. *Eur Respir J* 2000, 16(5):824–830.

10. Bai TR, Cooper J, Koelmeyer T, Pare PD, Weir TD. The effect of age and duration of disease on airway structure in fatal asthma. *Am J Respir Crit Care Med* 2000, 162(2 Pt 1): 663–669.

11. Siddiqui S, Sutcliffe A, Shikotra A, Woodman L, Doe C, McKenna S, Wardlaw A, Bradding P, Pavord I, Brightling CE. Vascular remodeling is a feature of asthma and nonasthmatic eosinophilic bronchitis. *J Allergy Clin Immunol* 2007, 120:813–819.

12. Balzar S, Wenzel SE, Chu HW. Transbronchial biopsy as a tool to evaluate small airways in asthma. *Eur Respir J* 2002, 20(2):254–259.

13. Jeffery PK. Remodeling and inflammation of bronchi in asthma and chronic obstructive pulmonary disease. *Proc Am Thorac Soc* 2004, 1(3):176–183.

14. Laitinen LA, Laitinen A, Haahtela T, Vilkka V, Spur BW, Lee TH. Leukotriene E4 and granulocytic infiltration into asthmatic airways. *Lancet* 1993, 341(8851):989–990.

15. Zhu J, Qiu YS, Figueroa DJ, Bandi V, Galczenski H, Hamada K, Guntupalli KK, Evans JF, Jeffery PK. Localization and upregulation of cysteinyl leukotriene-1 receptor in asthmatic bronchial mucosa. *Am J Respir Cell Mol Biol* 2005, 33(6):531–540.

16. Kariywasam HH, Aizen M, Barkans J, Robinson DS, Kay AB. Remodeling and airway hyperresponsiveness but not cellular inflammation persist after allergen challenge in asthma. *Am J Respir Crit Care Med* 2007, 175:896–904.

17. Laitinen LA, Laitinen A, Haahtela T. Airway mucosal inflammation even in patients with newly diagnosed asthma. *Am Rev Respir Dis* 1993, 147(3):697–704.

18. Bourdin A, Neveu D, Vachier I, Paganin F, Godard P, Chanez P. Specificity of basement membrane thickening in severe asthma. *J Allergy Clin Immunol* 2007, 119:1367–1374.

19. Brightling CE, Bradding P, Symon FA, Holgate ST, Wardlaw AJ, Pavord ID. Mast-cell infiltration of airway smooth muscle in asthma. *N Engl J Med* 2002, 346(22):1699–1705.

20. Okayama Y, Ra C, Saito H. Role of mast cells in airway remodeling. Curr Opin Immunol 2007, 57:197–203.

21. Holgate ST, Holloway J, Wilson S, Howarth PH, Haitchi HM, Babu S, Davies DE. *J Allergy Clin Immunol* 2006, 117:496–506.

22. Togias A. Rhinitis and asthma: evidence for respiratory system integration. *J Allergy Clin Immunol* 2003, 111(6):1171–1183; quiz 1184.

23. Gaga M, Lambrou P, Papageorgiou N, Koulouris NG, Kosmas E, Fragakis S, Sofios C, Rasidakis A, Jordanoglou J. Eosinophils are a feature of upper and lower airway pathology in non-atopic asthma, irrespective of the presence of rhinitis. *Clin Exp Allergy* 2000, 30(5):663–669.

24. Jeffery PK, Haahtela T. Allergic rhinitis and asthma: inflammation in one-airway condition. BMC Pulm Med 2006, 6(Suppl 1):S5.

25. Bousquet J, Jacot W, Vignola AM, Bachert C, Van Cauwenberge P. Allergic rhinitis: a disease remodeling the upper airways? *J Allergy Clin Immunol* 2004, 113(1):43–49.

26. Braunstahl GJ, Fokkens WJ, Overbeek SE, KleinJan A, Hoogsteden HC, Prins JB. Mucosal and systemic inflammatory changes in allergic rhinitis and asthma: a comparison between upper and lower airways. *Clin Exp Allergy* 2003, 33(5):579–587.

27. Bonay M, Neukirch C, Grandsaigne M, Lecon-Malas V, Ravaud P, Dehoux M, Aubier M. Changes in airway inflammation following nasal allergic challenge in patients with seasonal rhinitis. *Allergy* 2006, 61(1):111–118.

28. Braunstahl GJ, Kleinjan A, Overbeek SE, Prins JB, Hoogsteden HC, Fokkens WJ. Segmental bronchial provocation induces nasal inflammation in allergic rhinitis patients. *Am J Respir Crit Care Med* 2000, 161(6):2051–2057.

29. Braunstahl GJ, Overbeek SE, Fokkens WJ, Kleinjan A, McEuen AR, Walls AF, Hoogsteden HC, Prins JB. Segmental bronchoprovocation in allergic rhinitis patients affects mast cell and basophil numbers in nasal and bronchial mucosa. *Am J Respir Crit Care Med* 2001, 164(5):858–865.

30. Melen E, Bruce S, Doekes G, Kabesch M, Laitinen T, Lauener R, Lindgren CM, Riedler J, Scheynius A, van Hage-Hamsten M et al. Haplotypes of G protein-coupled receptor 154 are associated with childhood allergy and asthma. *Am J Respir Crit Care Med* 2005, 171(10):1089–1095.

31. Togias A. Systemic effects of local allergic disease. *J Allergy Clin Immunol* 2004, 113 (1 Suppl):S8–14.

32. Pin I, Gibson PG, Kolendowicz R, Girgis-Gabardo A, Denburg JA, Hargreave FE, Dolovich J. Use of induced sputum cell counts to investigate airway inflammation in asthma 1992, 47:25–29.

33. Spallarossa D, Battistini E, Silvestri M, Sabatini F, Fregonese L, Brazzola G, Rossi GA. Steroid-naive adolescents with mild intermittent allergic asthma have airway hyperresponsiveness and elevated exhaled nitric oxide levels. *J Asthma* 2003, 40(3):301–310.

34. Bisgaard H, Loland L, Oj JA. NO in exhaled air of asthmatic children is reduced by the leukotriene receptor antagonist montelukast. *Am J Respir Crit Care Med* 1999, 160(4):1227–1231.

35. Buchvald F, Baraldi E, Carraro S, Gaston B, De Jongste J, Pijnenburg MW, Silkoff PE, Bisgaard H. Measurements of exhaled nitric oxide in healthy subjects aged 4 to 17 years. *J Allergy Clin Immunol* 2005, 115(6):1130–1136.

36. Buchvald F, Eiberg H, Bisgaard H. Heterogeneity of FeNO response to inhaled steroid in asthmatic children. *Clin Exp Allergy* 2003, 33(12):1735–1740.

37. Malmberg LP, Petäys T, Haahtela T, Laatikainen T, Jousilahti P, Vartiainen E, Mäkelä MJ. Exhaled nitric oxide in healthy nonatopic school-age children: determinants and height-adjusted reference values. *Pediatr Pulmonol* 2006, 41:635–642.

38. Busse WW, Wanner A, Adams K, Reynolds HY, Castro M, Chowdhury B, Kraft M, Levine RJ, Peters SP, Sullivan EJ. Investigative bronchoprovocation and bronchoscopy in airway diseases. *Am J Respir Crit Care Med* 2005, 172(7):807–816.

39. Jeffery P, Holgate S, Wenzel S. Methods for the assessment of endobronchial biopsies in clinical research: application to studies of pathogenesis and the effects of treatment. *Am J Respir Crit Care Med* 2003, 168(6 Pt 2):S1–17.

40. Sont JK, Willems LN, Bel EH, vanKrieken JH, Vandenbroucke JP, Sterk PJ. Clinical control and histopathologic outcome of asthma when using airway hyperresponsiveness as an additional guide to long-term treatment. The AMPUL Study Group. *Am J Respir Crit Care Med* 1999, 159:1043–1051.

41. Ward C, Pais M, Bish R, Reid D, Feltis B, Johns D, Walters EH. Airway inflammation, basement membrane thickening and bronchial hyperresponsiveness in asthma. *Thorax* 2002, 57(4):309–316.

42. Lee SY, Kim JS, Lee JM, Kwon SS, Kim KH, Moon HS, Song JS, Park SH, Kim YK. Inhaled corticosteroid prevents the thickening of airway smooth muscle in murine model of chronic asthma. Pulm Pharmacol Ther 2008, 21:17–9.

43. Goleva E, Hauk PJ, Boguniewicz J, Martin RJ, Leung DY. Airway remodeling and lack of bronchodilator response in steroid-resistant asthma. *J Allergy Clin Immunol* 2007, 120:1065–72.

44. Pizzichini E, Leff JA, Reiss TF, Hendeles L, Boulet LP, Wei LX, Efthimiadis AE, Zhang J, Hargreave FE. Montelukast reduces airway eosinophilic inflammation in asthma: a randomized, controlled trial. *Eur Respir J* 1999, 14(1):12–18.

45. Nakamura Y, Hoshino M, Sim JJ, Ishii K, Hosaka K, Sakamoto T. Effect of the leukotriene receptor antagonist pranlukast on cellular infiltration in the bronchial mucosa of patients with asthma. *Thorax* 1998, 53(10):835–841.

46. Jeffery PK. The roles of leukotrienes and the effects of leukotriene receptor antagonists in the inflammatory response and remodelling of allergic asthma. *Clin Exp Allergy Rev* 2001, 1(2):148–153.

47. Panettieri RA, Tan EM, Ciocca V, Luttmann MA, Leonard TB, Hay DW. Effects of LTD4 on human airway smooth muscle cell proliferation, matrix expression, and contraction in vitro: differential sensitivity to cysteinyl leukotriene receptor antagonists. *Am J Respir Cell Mol Biol* 1998, 19(3):453–461.

48. Parameswaran K, Cox G, Radford K, Janssen LJ, Sehmi R, O'Byrne PM. Cysteinyl leukotrienes promote human airway smooth muscle migration. *Am J Respir Crit Care Med* 2002, 166(5):738–742.
49. Gueders MM, Bertholet P, Perin F, Rocks N, Maree R, Botta V, Louis R, Foidart JM, Noel A, Evrard B, Cataldo DD. A novel formulation of inhaled doxycycline reduces allergen-induced inflammation, hyperresponsiveness and remodeling by matrix metalloproteinases and cytokines modulation in a mouse model of asthma. Biochem Pharmacol 2008, 75:514–26.
50. Jain VV, Kitagaki K, Businga T, Hussain I, George C, O'Shaughnessy P, Kline JN. CpG-oligodeoxynucleotides inhibit airway remodeling in a murine model of chronic asthma. *J Allergy Clin Immunol* 2002, 110:867–872.
51. Camateros P, Tamaoka M, Hassan M, Marino R, Moisan J, Marion D, Guiot MC, Martin JG, Radzioch D. Chronic asthma-induced airway remodeling is prevented by toll-like receptor-7/8 ligand S28463. *Am J Respir Crit Care Med* 2007, 175:1241–1249.
52. Busse WW, Massanari M, Kianifard F, Geba GP. Effect of omalizumab on the need for rescue systemic corticosteroid treatment in patients with moderate-to-severe persistent IgE-mediated allergic asthma: a pooled analysis. *Curr Med Res Opin* 2007, 23:2379–2386.
53. Howarth PH, Babu KS, Arshad HS, Lau L, Buckley M, McConnell W, Beckett P, Al Ali M, Chauhan A, Wilson SJ, Reynolds A, Davies DE, Holgate ST. Tumour necrosis factor (TNFalpha) as a novel therapeutic target in symptomatic corticosteroid dependent asthma. *Thorax* 2005, 60:1012–1018.
54. Cox G, Thomson NC, Rubin AS, Niven RM, Corris PA, Siersted HC, Olivenstein R, Pavord ID, McCormack D, Chaudhuri R, Miller JD, Laviolette M. AIR Trial Study Group. Asthma control during the year after bronchial thermoplasty. *N Engl J Med* 2007, 356:1327–1337.
55. Lange P, Scharling H, Ulrik CS, Vestbo J. Inhaled corticosteroids and decline of lung function in community residents with asthma. *Thorax* 2006, 61:100–104.
56. Haahtela T, Jarvinen M, Kava T, Kiviranta K, Koskinen S, Lehtonen K, Nikander K, Persson T, Reinikainen K, Selroos O et al. Comparison of a beta 2-agonist, terbutaline, with an inhaled corticosteroid, budesonide, in newly detected asthma. *N Engl J Med* 1991, 325(6):388–392.
57. Haahtela T, Jarvinen M, Kava T, Kiviranta K, Koskinen S, Lehtonen K, Nikander K, Persson T, Selroos O, Sovijarvi A et al. Effects of reducing or discontinuing inhaled budesonide in patients with mild asthma. *N Engl J Med* 1994, 331(11):700–705.
58. Agertoft L, Pedersen S. Effects of long-term treatment with an inhaled corticosteroid on growth and pulmonary function in children. *Respir Med* 1994, 88:373–381.
59. Selroos O, Pietinalho A, Löfroos AB, Riska H. Effect of early vs. late intervention with inhaled corticosteroid in asthma. *Chest* 1995, 108:1228–1234.
60. Long-term effects of budesonide or nedocromil in children with asthma. The Childhood Asthma Management Program Research Group. *N Engl J Med* 2000, 343:1054–1063.
61. O'Byrne P, Pedersen S, Busse WW, Tan WC, Chen Y-Z, Ohlsson SV, Ullman A, Lamm CJ, Pauwels RA. Effects of early intervention with inhaled budesonide on lung function in newly diagnosed asthma. *Chest* 2006, 129:1478–1485.
62. Smith AD, Cowan JO, Brasset KP, Herbison GP, Taylor DR. Use of exhaled nitric oxide measurements to guide treatment in chronic asthma. *N Engl J Med* 2005, 352:2163–2173.
63. Haahtela T, Tuomisto LE, Pietinalho A, Klaukka T, Erhola M, Kaila M, Nieminen MM, Kontula E, Laitinen LA. A ten-year asthma programme in Finland: a major change for the better. *Thorax* 2006, 61:663–670.
64. Pavord ID, Ward R, Woltmann G, Wardlaw AJ, Sheller JR, Dworski R. Induced sputum eicosanoid concentrations in asthma. *Am J Respir Crit Care Med* 1999, 160(6):1905–1909.
65. Vaquerizo MJ, Casan P, Castillo J, Perpina M, Sanchis J, Sobradillo V, Valencia A, Verea H, Viejo JL, Villasante C et al. Effect of montelukast added to inhaled budesonide on control of mild to moderate asthma. *Thorax* 2003, 58(3):204–210.
66. Bjermer L, Bisgaard H, Bousquet J, Fabbri LM, Greening AP, Haahtela T, Holgate ST, Picado C, Menten J, Dass SB et al. Montelukast and fluticasone compared with salmeterol and fluticasone in protecting against asthma exacerbation in adults: one year, double blind, randomised, comparative trial. *BMJ* 2003, 327(7420):891.

67. Bousquet J, Van Cauwenberge P, Khaltaev N. Allergic rhinitis and its impact on asthma. *J Allergy Clin Immunol* 2001, 108(5 Suppl):S147–334.
68. Johansson SG, Haahtela T. World Allergy Organization Guidelines for Prevention of Allergy and Allergic Asthma. Condensed Version. *Int Arch Allergy Immunol* 2004, 135(1):83–92.
69. Haahtela T, Tamminen K, Malmberg LP, Zetterström O, Karjalainen J, Ylä-Outinen H, Svahn T, Ekström T, Selroos O. Formoterol as needed with or without budesonide in patients with intermittent asthma and raised NO levels in exhaled air: a SOMA study. *Eur Respir J* 2006, 28:748–755.
70. Holgate S, Bisgaard H, Bjermer L, Haahtela T, Haughney J, Horne R. McIvor A, Palkonen S, Price DB, Thomas M, Valovirta E, Wahn U. The Brussels Declaration: the need for change in asthma management. *Eur Respir J* 2008, 32:1433–42.

Occupational Asthma and Its Relationship to Occupational Rhinitis

Gianna Moscato and Eugenia Galdi

Introduction

Workplace exposure can induce or trigger asthma and cause the onset of different types of "work-related asthma" (WRA). This occurs in about 10–15% of adult asthma [1, 2]. WRA comprises two major entities, i.e. occupational asthma (OA), defined as a type of asthma "caused" by the workplace, and work-aggravated asthma (WAA), which is personal asthma that worsens at work due to other causes, and asthma variants, such eosinophilic bronchitis, potroom asthma and grain dust fever (Fig. 1) [3, 4]. OA has received the greatest attention, thanks to the pioneering work of Jack Pepys [5]. It is currently one of the most common forms of occupational lung disease in many industrialized countries [6, 7].

Occupational rhinitis (OR) is a disease of emerging relevance whose burden is considered to be largely underestimated in comparison with OA [8, 9]. Similarly to nonoccupational field [10], there is accumulating evidence of a strict relationship between OA and OR, supporting the concept that also in occupational field, asthma and rhinitis might be a unique disease with manifestations in different sites of the respiratory system (*'united airway disease'*). The evidence of this relationship comes from the observation of common epidemiologic [8], physiopathological, clinical and therapeutic features in both conditions, particularly when considering allergic mechanisms.

The purpose of the present chapter is to illustrate the different aspects of occupational asthma, including epidemiology, mechanisms, clinical aspects and diagnostic procedures, management, and preventive strategies, highlighting the common features shared by occupational rhinitis.

G. Moscato (✉) and E. Galdi
Allergy and Immunology Unit, Fondazione "Salvatore Maugeri", Institute of Research and Care, Scientific Institute of Pavia, Italy
e-mail: gmoscato@fsm.it

R. Pawankar et al. (eds.), *Allergy Frontiers: Clinical Manifestations,*
DOI: 10.1007/978-4-431-88317-3_19, © Springer 2009

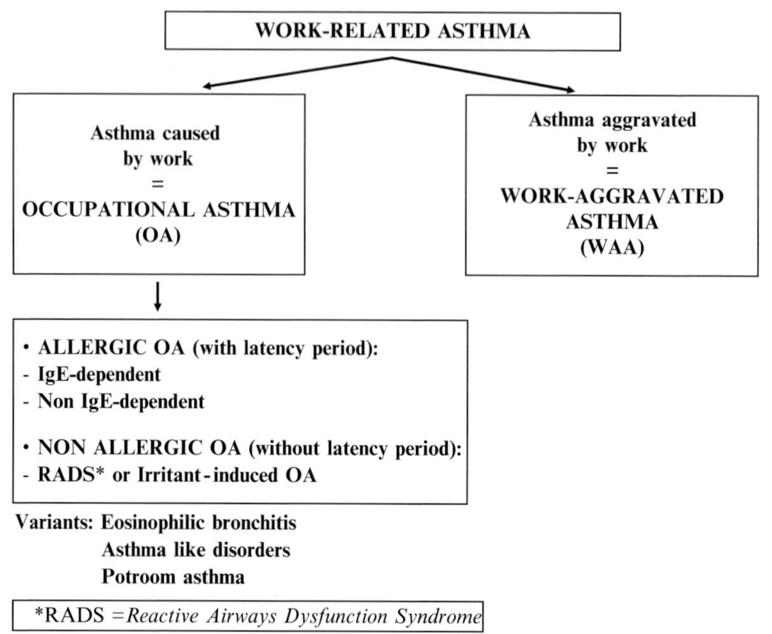

Fig. 1 Classification of work-related asthma

Definition and Classification

Occupational asthma is a disease characterized by variable airflow limitation and/or hyperresponsiveness and/or inflammation due to causes and conditions attributable to a particular occupational environment and not to stimuli encountered outside the workplace [11]. This type of work-related asthma should more appropriately be labelled "occupation-induced asthma" [3]. The key element is the presence of a causal relationship between workplace exposure and the development of asthma.

Two types of OA are distinguished by whether they appear after a latency period:

1. Allergic. OA appears after a latency period necessary for the worker to acquire sensitization to the causal agent. It encompasses OA caused by most high- (HMW) and certain low-molecular-weight (LMW) agents for which an IgE-mediated mechanism has been proven, and OA induced by some specific low-molecular-weight agents (such as isocyanates, western red cedar, acid anhydrides) in which the allergic mechanisms responsible have not yet been fully characterized.
2. Nonallergic. Characterized by the absence of a latency period. This clinical entity has been defined as irritant-induced asthma [12, 13]. The most

definitive form of irritant induced asthma is the "Reactive Airways Dysfunction Syndrome" (RADS), which occurs after single [14] or multiple [12] exposures to high concentrations of an irritating vapour, fume or smoke.

Allergic OA is the most common type of OA, accounting for more than 90% of cases [15].

Definition and classification of occupational rhinitis tailored on that of OA have recently been proposed by an *ad hoc* Task Force of the European Academy of Allergy and Clinical Immunology [9]. Among work-related rhinitis occupational rhinitis, i.e. rhinitis caused by work, and work-exacerbated rhinitis are distinguished. OR is defined as "an inflammatory disease of the nose, which is characterized by intermittent or persistent symptoms (i.e., nasal congestion, sneezing, rhinorrea, itching), and/or variable nasal airflow limitation and/or hypersecretion due to causes and conditions attributable to a particular work environment and not to stimuli encountered outside the workplace." OR may be allergic, appearing after a latency period, or non allergic, without latency period, occurring after a single (Reactive Upper Airway Dysfunction Syndrome, RUDS) or multiple exposure to irritants (irritant-induced OR).

Causal Agents and Mechanisms

Agents able to induce airway narrowing can be distinguished into "inducers" and "inciters" [16]. A "causal" agent is a substance able to act as an "inducer", i.e. to induce not only airway obstruction but also changes in airway inflammation and non specific bronchial hyperresponsiveness (NSBH). "Inciters" are agents able to trigger airway narrowing in subjects with pre-existing NSBH or asthma without inducing airway inflammation.

More than 300 substances have been identified as causal agents of OA. Lists are available in textbooks [17], and websites (www.asmanet.com, www.asthme.csst. qc.ca, www.eaaci.net). New causal agents are reported each year, and OA can be caused by agents not found on existing lists.

The causal agents of OA are classified into HMW- and LMW-agents. The prototypes of OA inducers are HMW proteins derived from animals or vegetables acting as complete antigens through an IgE-mediated mechanism. The same mechanism is strongly suggested, although not definitely demonstrated, for some LMW organic and inorganic compounds (i.e., platinum salts, trimellitic anhydrides, other acid anhydrides) which probably act as haptens, binding with body proteins to form functional antigens [15, 18]. The same HMW- and LMW- causal agents of OA may be involved in the aetiology of OR [8] (Table 1).

The mechanism of allergic IgE-mediated OA, and of allergic IgE-mediated OR, is similar to that of nonoccupational allergic asthma, or rhinitis: the inhaled sensitizer binds to specific IgE antibodies on the surface of mast-cells, basophils,

Table 1 Common aetiological agents of occupational asthma and rhinitis and examples of jobs in which they are used

Agents	Occupations
High molecular weight agents	
Animal-derived allergens	Laboratory workers
Food allergens (i.e. milk proteins, egg proteins)	Food processors
Fish and seafood protein	Trout, prawn, shrimp, crab and clam workers; acquarists and fish-food factory workers
Flour	Bakers
Latex	Health care workers, textile factory
Biological enzymes	Pharmaceutical and detergent industries
Low molecular weight agents	
Wood dusts	Carpenters, wood workers
Isocyanates	Painters, urethane mould workers
Anhydrides	Epoxy resin production, chemical workers
Colophony	Electronic workers
Persulphate salts	Hairdressers
Glutaraldehyde	Health care workers
Metals (platinum)	Platinum refinery
Drugs	Health care and pharmaceutical workers

and possibly macrophages and eosinophils, leading to a cascade of events that results in an influx and activation of inflammatory cells into the airway and in the release of inflammatory mediators [15, 18]. The asthmagenic mechanism of LMW-agents that currently represents at least half of the agents causing allergic OA is still lacking for most agents [4]. In this type of OA a mixed CD4/CD8 type 2/type 1 immunological response or induction of γ/δ-specific CD8 may play a role [15, 19]. Irrespective of the cause, either HMW- or LMW- agents, the pathology of allergic OA is the same, characterized by increased number of inflammatory cells (eosinophils, mast cells, macrophages, neutrophils, lymphocytes), extensive epithelial desquamation, epithelial cell ciliary abnormalities, smooth muscle hyperplasia, thickening of the reticular basement membrane. Airway inflammation contributes to the functional alterations of OA: NSBH and airflow obstruction [15, 18].

At high concentrations irritant materials are able to act as "inducers" leading to irritant, non-allergic OA or RADS. The mechanism of this type of OA is not well defined, but the damaged epithelium plays a central role, resulting in airway inflammation due to a loss of epithelial-derived relaxing factors, exposure of the nerve airway inflammation endings leading to neurogenic inflammation, and non specific activation of mast-cells with release of inflammatory mediators and cytokines [13]. An entity similar to RADS, the RUDS, has been proposed for OR as well [20], but the mechanisms are not known. At lower concentrations irritants generally act as "inciters" triggering airway narrowing in subjects with pre-existing or concurrent asthma. Multiple repeated exposure to low concentrations of irritants may lead to new-onset, irritant-induced OR whose mechanisms remain to be elucidated [21].

Epidemiology and Risk Factors

In 1999 in a comprehensive review of 43 epidemiological studies on occupationally associated asthma from 19 countries, Blanc and Toren [1] gave a median population attributable risk (PAR) estimate for occupationally associated asthma of 9% (range 5–19%). More recently, after a review of the published literature on the magnitude of the attributable risk of asthma due to occupation a median value of 15% (range 4–58%) has been proposed by Balmes et al. [2]. However these estimates are referred to occupationally associated asthma including both new onset disease caused by occupation (true occupational asthma, OA) and worsening of pre-existing asthma (work aggravated asthma, WAA), so that the real prevalence of OA remains uncertain. Moreover, most epidemiological studies regarding OA have been cross-sectional, which may underestimate the prevalence of OA due to the affected workers who left work [15].

The contribution of OR to the general burden of rhinitis in the general population is not known. From cross-sectional studies it is estimated that the prevalence of OR is 2–3 times that of OA [8].

Risk Factors for OA

Factors increasing the risk of developing OA have been identified for a number of occupational causal agents.

Exposure is the most important factor, and a positive dose–response relationship between the level of exposure and the development of OA has been shown for several agents (i.e. colophony, flour, western red cedar, isocyanates, crab, animal-derived allergens) in both prospective and retrospective studies [15, 18, 22–25]. Nevertheless, although the level of exposure is a critical factor for the development of OA, given the same level of exposure, only a small proportion of exposed subjects will develop OA, suggesting a role for host susceptibility [15, 18, 25]. Atopy, OR, NSBH, smoking and genetic factors have been variously associated with the development of OA. Atopy is a predisposing factor in workers exposed to HMW-agents, but the level of association is generally low. Having OR represents a risk factor for development of OA [26], although the positive predictive value appears low [27]. In cohort studies the presence of a measurable PC20FEV1 of histamine has also been shown to be associated with the development of OA [27, 28]. An association between smoking and development of OA has been shown for HMW- and for some LMW-agents causing asthma with an IgE-mediated mechanism, such as platinum salts and anhydride compounds [15], but the effect of cigarette smoking is still under debate [29]. Examples of HMW- and LMW-agents include platinum salts and anhydride compounds [14]. Genetic markers of OA have recently begun to be examined and available data suggest that HLA class II molecules, glutatione–transferase (GST) and N-aceyltransferase genotypes may play a role in the immune response to some occupational sensitizers, such as acid anhydrides, isocyanates, and platinum salts [15, 25, 30, 31].

To the same extent, asthma exposure and atopy have consistently emerged as the main potential determinants for the development of OR.

Natural History

Allergic OA

Natural history for the development of sensitization and OA has well been illustrated by Malo and Chan-Yeung [18, 32]: each step is associated with various modulating factors (Fig. 2). The rate of developing sensitization and OA may differ according to the nature of the agent and the intensity of exposure [18, 27, 32] and the latency period may vary from months to years. Most workers exposed to HMW-agents develop OA during the first 2 years of exposure, whereas in those exposed to LMW-agents symptoms develop more slowly [15]. Symptoms of rhinoconjunctivitis often precede the onset of asthma, particularly in the case of HMW-causal agents [33, 34]

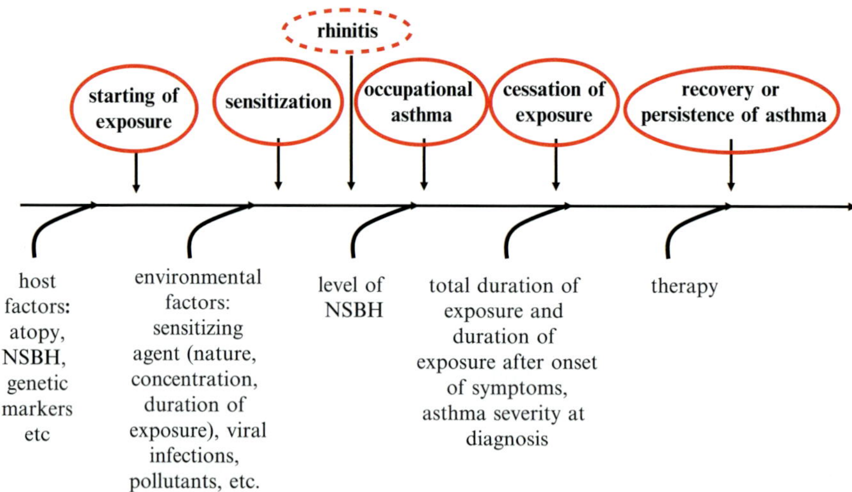

Fig. 2 Natural history of allergic occupational asthma

and rhinitis may be considered an early marker of OA. Once OA has developed, a crucial step for outcome is cessation of exposure to the causal agent, which is associated with improvement of both symptoms and functional variables [15, 35]. Nevertheless, even when exposure ceases, only a minority of subjects completely recover: about 70% of affected workers continue to experience symptoms even several years after avoidance of exposure [36, 37]. Prognosis is better in workers with shorter duration of symptoms before diagnosis and who are promptly removed from exposure [35, 38] whereas workers who continue to be exposed to the causal agent worsen with time [15, 35]. Once a worker is sensitized to an occupational agent, specific reactivity to the causal agent usually persists for 2 or more years after cessation of exposure [15] and may still be present even in patients who have become asymptomatic and with normalization of NSBH after cessation of exposure, so that in the case of re-exposure to the causal agent an asthmatic reaction may occur [15, 37]. Airway inflammation and remodeling of the airways are probably important contributors to the persistence of symptoms of OA and of NSBH, although their role is not yet completely clear [15, 37]. Treatment with inhaled corticosteroids has been shown to further improve clinical and functional parameters [37, 39].

Irritant-Induced OA

Outcome of irritant-induced asthma has been evaluated in few studies whose results show that NSBH can continue to improve in the 3 years following the accidental inhalation [13, 37, 40].

Clinical Aspects and Diagnosis

Symptoms

Symptoms of OA are the common symptoms of bronchial asthma, such as cough (more frequently dry), dyspnoea, wheezing, chest tightness; only their relationship to work induces the suspect to be of an occupational origin. Symptoms of upper airways, particularly rhinitis or rhinoconjunctivitis, are frequently associated (up to 92% of cases in the case of OA caused by HMW- agents) [33].

Diagnosis of OA

The diagnosis of OA has a two-sided objective: demonstrating the presence of asthma and confirming that it is caused by work. A detailed clinical history is a key step, since an occupational origin should be suspected for every new-onset asthma in an adult [18, 41, 42]. However, history alone has a low specificity for establishing a diagnosis of OA [43], and should be objectively confirmed. Objective testing encompasses a combination of tools which partially differ for allergic and for irritant-induced OA.

Allergic OA

The clinical investigation of allergic OA is a stepwise approach which includes clinical, physiological, immunological studies (Table 2) [44], and assessment of airway inflammation [15, 18, 45].

History should include a detailed occupational history aimed at collecting a thorough description of current worker's job duties, processes in adjacent work areas, recent changes in work processes or materials, and workplace hygiene conditions. Safety data sheets of the compounds to which the subject is directly and indirectly exposed should be gathered [18, 46]. Patient should also be questioned about previous jobs and exposure which may have contributed to sensitization and asthma. Medical history should investigate the type of symptoms (lower, upper airways) and their relationship to work exposure (immediate, late or dual onset after starting daily work). Symptoms may not be so obviously work-related, particularly when they first appear after the work shift has ended due to an isolated late airway response. In this case, diagnosis may be delayed since the relationship with work may not be recognized promptly by the patient or the physician [46].

Table 2 Diagnostic workup of allergic occupational asthma (Modified from [44])

History suggestive for OA and exposure documentation
Confirmation of bronchial asthma
    Variable airway limitation:
      Reversibility of bronchial obstruction
      Serial measurement of PEF
    Non specific bronchial challenges
Confirmation of work-relatedness of asthma
    Serial measurements of PEF, alone or associated to:
      Serial measurement of nonspecific bronchial responsiveness
      Serial assessment of airway inflammation
Confirmation of sensitization to occupational agents
    Skin tests (when available)
    In vitro tests (specific IgE or IgG) (when available)
Confirmation of causal role of occupational agents
    Specific inhalation challenges
OA, occupational asthma; PEF, peak expiratory flow

The relationship between symptoms and periods at and away from work must be assessed: at the onset of symptoms, improvement on weekends and holidays, and worsening on return to work is the rule (positive stop-resume test). By contrast, as exposure continues, symptoms may become persistent, thus a negative stop-resume test should not rule out the possibility of OA [46]. A history of pre-existing asthma does not exclude the possibility of developing OA after being exposed to sensitizing agents. Duration of employment at current job before onset of symptoms ("latency period"), duration of symptoms before diagnosis and information on individual risk factors such as atopy should be gathered [46].

The diagnosis of asthma is based on a compatible history and the presence of variable airflow limitation, or, in the absence of airflow limitation, the presence of NSBH [47]. The confirmation of the work-relatedness and causality of asthma is based on several methods (Table 2). Measurement of NSBH to pharmacological agents is an important step in the diagnostic workup. The absence of NSBH does not rule out the diagnosis of OA, unless the measurement is made after a person has worked for at least 2 weeks under his or her usual work conditions [18, 46]. The presence of NSBH requires further testing to confirm that asthma is related to work.

Serial measurements of peak expiratory flow (PEF) during periods at work and away from work is a useful method to objectively prove the relationship between symptoms and occupational exposure [48, 49]. PEF monitoring is a simple and reliable method, but it requires compliance and honesty of the subject. Combining PEF monitoring with serial measurements of NSBH at and away from work is helpful [48, 50], but does not change sensitivity or specificity of PEF monitoring alone [51, 52]. Since sputum eosinophils increased in subjects with OA when exposed and decreased after removal of exposure [53], the addition of induced sputum to PEF monitoring increases the specificity of this test [54].

Immunological tests in the diagnosis of OA are limited by the lack of commercially available or standardized reagents [18]. When feasible, immunological tests (prick tests and assessment of serum specific IgE) have shown good validity to document sensitization to an occupational allergen in the case of HMW sensitizers. They are of limited use for LMW sensitizers.

Specific inhalation challenge (SIC) is considered the gold standard for diagnosis of OA [46, 55]. During this test a subject is exposed to increasing doses of an occupational agent under controlled conditions with the aim of evaluating the inhalation-induced changes in respiratory function. SIC is simultaneously able to confirm the relationship between symptoms and occupational exposure, to relate symptoms to a specific agent, and to reproduce the temporal relationship between exposure and onset of symptoms. In the case of associated upper airway symptoms, the SIC can reproduce asthmatic and rhinitis symptoms at the same time. Several patterns of bronchial response have been described. Typical patterns include immediate, isolate late, and dual responses. False negative results may occur in the case of exposure to the wrong agent, exposure conditions not comparable with those in the workplace, or when the test is performed after a long time away from work (although complete desensitization is uncommon) [46, 55]. False positive results are uncommon if the test is properly conducted (control of baseline functional conditions, use of non irritant concentrations). SICs are time consuming, require proper facilities and should be carried out in specialized centres, also considering their potential danger of triggering severe asthmatic reactions. Thus, in general these tests remain available in relatively few centres [18]. This has led to a search for other tools that may be useful in the diagnosis of OA. The assessment of airway inflammation by means of non invasive methods such as induced sputum analysis [53, 56–58] and measurement of exhaled nitric oxide (eNO) [59, 60] has recently been proposed [45]. Exposure to occupational agents induces marked changes in sputum in subjects with OA sensitized to those agents [61–63]. When at work, subjects with OA both due to HMW- and to LMW-agents show a predominant eosinophilic airway inflammation which decreases or resolves after a period away from work [53]. A neutrophilic response may also be found, especially after exposure to isocyanates [57]. Increasing evidence supports the use of induced sputum as an additional tool in the investigation of OA in subjects still at work [58] particularly when SIC cannot be performed [45], or in addition to serial PEF monitoring at and away from work [54]. The role of eNO in the investigation of OA needs to be further investigated due to conflicting evidence reported in the literature [58, 60].

In the case of the presence of nasal symptoms in association with bronchial symptoms the confirmation of rhinitis and of its occupational origin should be made contemporarily to that of OA. The assessment of OR includes occupational and medical history, clinical examination of the nose, immunological test, and the specific challenge, which is considered the gold standard for diagnosis in OR as well [9].

Irritant-Induced OA

The diagnosis of OA is based on the clinical history and the demonstration of airway obstruction, NSBH or both [14]. History should show a single (or multiple) high exposure to an irritant agent, and appearance of symptoms shortly after the event in a subject without previous respiratory symptoms [18].

Management

The management of patients with OA depends on the type of OA, irritant-induced- or allergic-OA [15] (Table 3) and include environmental interventions aimed at avoiding or reducing exposure and pharmacologic treatment. The objectives are minimizing symptoms and their impact on the patients' life, and preventing the clinical, physiopathological and socioeconomic consequences of the disease. In the case of concomitant rhinitis symptoms, an integrated approach to the management of both rhinitis and asthma is strongly suggested [64].

Table 3 Management of occupational asthma

	Irritant-induced OA	Allergic OA
Exposure	Avoid exposure to high level of irritants	Avoid or substantially reduce exposure to the causal agent
Keeping the same job	Possible	Not advisable
Medicolegal measures	Notify national or regional authorities	Notify national or regional authorities
	Refer the patient to compensation boards	Refer the patient to compensation boards
Pharmacological therapy	Asthma therapy[a] (start soon after diagnosis)	Asthma therapy[a] (start soon after diagnosis)
Immunotherapy	No	Consider when available[b]

OA, occupational asthma

[a]Therapy based on asthma guidelines (see [47])

[b]At present scarcely evaluated, and only for a few HMW allergens (immunotherapy with latex extracts by subcutaneous or sublingual route seems to be useful)

In workers with irritant-induced OA further exposures to high concentrations of the irritant should be avoided [15], but the subject may continue his work if being exposed to low levels of the agent. In allergic OA complete cessation of exposure to the workplace sensitizer is the most desirable intervention, since a bulk of papers have shown that the likelihood of improvement or resolution of symptoms or preventing deterioration is greater in workers who have no further exposure to the causal agent [65]. However, a recent systematic review of studies on outcome of OA after cessation of exposure failed to show clear patterns of improvement relating to total duration of exposure, suggesting that further studies on the prognosis of OA and its determinants are needed [66]. As a matter of fact, since cessation of exposure has the worst socioeconomic consequences [36, 67] proper alternatives should be considered (see Section Prevention).

The management of OR has the same objectives of that of OA. Moreover, since rhinitis could be an early marker of OA, treatment strategies should aim to prevent the onset of OA. Environmental measures should focus on avoidance of exposure to the agent causing allergic OR. Nevertheless, having only few quantitative estimates both of the outcome of OR after environmental interventions and of the long-term risk of asthma among patients with OR [26, 27], and since complete avoidance of exposure may imply the same personal and socioeconomic consequences described for OA, in workplaces where the level of exposure can be significantly reduced, maintaining workers at their job may be considered a reasonable alternative [26, 27], provided that workers with OR are submitted to close medical surveillance [9].

Pharmacological treatment for patients with OA due to a respiratory sensitizer or to irritants should be the same as that for patients with nonoccupational asthma [47], although the effects on deterioration of lung function are controversial [36, 39]. The beneficial effects of inhaled corticosteroids are more evident when treatment starts soon after diagnosis [15, 39, 68]. The treatment of rhinitis does not differ from that of nonoccupational rhinitis [10]. The role of specific immunotherapy (SIT) with HMW allergens in OA has been scarcely evaluated, and only for a few allergens. From available data, SIT with latex extracts by subcutaneous or sublingual route seems to be useful in reducing cutaneous and respiratory symptoms, but systemic reactions have been reported [69]. At present SIT with latex is still under evaluation [69].

Medicolegal and Socio-economic Aspects

Once the diagnosis of OA is made the patient should be referred to compensation boards or similar agencies when appropriate. The national or regional authorities should be notified (Table 3). The physician should support the patient for obtaining adequate compensation. Proper and suitable re-adaptation programmes should be offered to the worker [18]. Affected workers often receive an inadequate protection [4] and several studies conducted in various countries have shown that OA is associated to considerable professional and financial consequences [36, 37, 40], 42–78% of subjects reporting a substantial loss of income [40]. More pronounced financial consequences result in workers who are removed from exposure [40], but even some subjects who don't change their job have negative financial consequences, due to sickness and lack of promotion [37]. The assessment for impairment-disability should be performed immediately after diagnosis, and 2 years after cessation of exposure since the maximum rate of improvement occurs at this time [15, 18]. Evaluation of physiological variables (airway caliber, degree of NSBH and/or airway reversibility), need for medication to control asthma, and quality of life [15, 18, 70] should be included in the assessment of impairment. Psychological evaluation has also been proposed [71].

Prevention

OA is a preventable disease. Clinicians and occupational health practitioners need to be actively involved with the primary, secondary and tertiary prevention of OA [35].

Primary prevention is designed to abate hazards before any damage has occurred, and it also takes into consideration environmental and host factors [15]. The most important measure is to reduce the level of exposure by elimination, substitution, or reduction of the agent/s causing OA [15, 18, 72]. An example is the use of powder-free and low-protein latex gloves in health care facilities which has led to a marked decrease in the incidence of latex-induced OA in recent years [73, 74]. Exposure limit values should be established for all high-risk agents of OA [15, 18]. An example is the bakeries, for which a permissible exposure limit of 0.5 mg/m^3

has been proposed [23, 75]. Even when complete avoidance is not possible, and reduction of levels to non-sensitizing concentrations cannot be achieved, maintaining low levels of sensitizers should reduce the risk of sensitization and OA, based on the knowledge that the risk of OA has a dose-response relationship [22, 24, 72]. Studies about usefulness of respiratory protective devices are few and small, and they offer protection when worn properly, removed safely, and either replaced or maintained regularly [66]. Although cigarette smoking has been demonstrated to increase the risk of sensitization to only a few agents, smoking should be discouraged in all workplaces [15, 18]. Due to the high prevalence of atopy in young adults and since atopy has a low predictive value for the development of OA, atopic subjects should not be excluded from high-risk workplaces [18], but a more strict environmental control of exposure and a more stringent medical surveillance are strongly recommended.

Secondary prevention aims to identify preclinical changes in the disease [15]. Workers exposed to known asthmagenic agents should undergo regular health surveillance [15, 35]. Medical surveillance programmes for OA are based on administration of a questionnaire before, and periodically after employment (the use of a validated questionnaire is recommended). Performing immunological and physiological tests may also be useful [76, 77]. Immunological sensitization generally precedes the development of OA, and it may be evaluated by skin tests: subjects with positive skin tests to HMW-agents should be monitored closely [15], although the positive predictive value of skin reactivity for the development of respiratory symptoms is low [27]. For subjects exposed to the same agents, the onset of rhinitis symptoms can be considered a predictor of the later development of OA, although some cohort-studies have shown a low positive predictive value [27]. However, the prevention of work-related rhinitis may provide an excellent opportunity to prevent OA. Bronchial responsiveness should also be evaluated: the onset of NSBH doesn't necessarily mean that a worker has OA [18], but a more frequent monitoring is necessary.

Tertiary prevention consists of early diagnosis and appropriate management of the disease in order to prevent permanent asthma [15, 35]. Early diagnosis allows early removal from exposure which makes more likely a positive outcome, but it is associated with the worst socioeconomic outcome [36, 67]. Alternative measures to reducing exposure to the causal agent, such as use of modified materials, improvement of workplace conditions, or relocation of the affected worker may be considered. Examples of successful alternative measures are reduction of exposure to latex [78] or substitution of non-isocyanate-containing paints. Keeping the worker at work with protective devices can help but still leads to deterioration of asthma [18]. The appropriate pharmacologic treatment (See Section Management) and a follow-up programme should be carried out, with periodic assessment of symptoms and lung function [4]. An additional component to enhance early diagnosis may be provision of effective education to workers and their primary care physicians in order to suspect the diagnosis of work related asthma early and have early investigation of this [72].

Conclusions

In conclusion, occupation accounts for 10–15% of adult asthma. Occupational asthma, i.e. asthma caused by work, has so far received the greatest attention. A wide spectrum of agents both HMW-proteins and LMW-compounds can induce OA, acting with allergic or non-allergic irritant mechanisms. The diagnosis needs to be made on firm grounds, as misdiagnosis may have substantial consequences. OA can lead to disability and to significant social and financial consequences, thus prevention is mandatory. A close relationship exists between OA and occupational rhinitis. OA and OR share the same etiological agents and mechanisms. In patients with OA, especially due to HMW-agents, symptoms of rhinitis are frequently found, and often the onset of these symptoms precedes that of asthma. In population studies the prevalence of OA and OR is similar and both population and cohort studies show that workers with OR have a greatest risk of developing asthma. The factors which facilitate this progression are not known, but prevention of OR may offer an excellent opportunity to prevent OA.

References

1. Blanc PD, Toren K (1999) How much adult asthma can be attributed to occupational factors? Am J Med 107: 580–587
2. Balmes J, Becklacke M, Blanc P, Henneberger P, Kreiss K, Mapp C, Milton D, Schwartz D, Toren K, Viegi G (2003) American Thoracic Society Statement. Occupational contribution to the burden of airway disease. Am J Respir Crit Care Med 167: 787–797
3. Vandenplas O, Malo J-L (2003) Definitions and types of work-related asthma: a nosological approach. Eur Respir J 21: 706–712
4. Malo J-L (2005) Future advances in work-related asthma and the impact on occupational health. Occup Med 55: 606–611
5. Pepys J (1980) Occupational asthma: review of present clinical and immunological status. J Allergy Clin Immunol 66: 179–185
6. Meredith S, Nordman H (1996) Occupational asthma: measures and frequency from four countries. Thorax 51: 435–440
7. Mannino DM (2000) How much asthma is occupationally related? Occup Med 15: 359–368
8. Siracusa A, Desrosiers M, Marabini A (2000) Epidemiology of occupational rhinitis: prevalence, aetiology and determinants. Clin Exp Allergy 30: 1519–1534
9. Moscato G, Vandenplas O, Gerth Van Wijk R, Malo J-L, Quirce S, Walusiak J, Castano R, De Groot H, Folletti I, Gautrin D, Yacoub MR, Perfetti L, Siracusa A. EAACI Task Force on Occupational Rhinitis (2008) Occupational rhinitis. Allergy 63: 969–980
10. Bousquet J, Khaltaev N, Cruz AA, Denburg J, Fokkens WJ, Togias A, Zuberbier T, Baena-Cagnani CE, Canonica GW, van Weel C, Agache I, Ait-Khaled N, Bachert C, Blaiss MS, Bonini S, Boulet MP, Bousquet PJ, Camargos P, Carlsen KH, Chen Y, Custovic A, Dahl R, Demoly P, Douagui H, Durham SR, van Wijk RG, Kalayci O, Kaliner MA, Kim YY, Kowalski ML, Kuna P, Le LT, Lemiere C, Li J, Lockey RF, Mavale-Manuel S, Meltzer EO, Mohammad Y, Mullol J, Naclerio R, O'Heir RE, Ohta K, Ouedraogo S, Palkonen S, Papadopoulos N, Passalacqua G, Pawankar R, Popov TA, Rabe KF, Rosado-Pinto J, Scadding GK, Simons FE, Toskala E, Valovirta E, van Cauwenberge P, Wang DY, Wickman M, Yawn BP, Yorgancioglu A, Yusuf OM, Zar H, Annesi-Maesano I, Bateman ED, Ben Kheder A,

Boakye DA, Bouchard J, Burney P, Busse WW, Chan-Yeung M, Chavannes NH, Chuchalin A, Dolen WK, Emuzyte R, Grouse L, Humbert M, Jackson C, Johnston SL, Keith PK, Kemp JP, Klossek JM, Larenas-Linnemann, Lipworth B, Malo JL, Marshall GD, Naspitz C, Nekam K, Niggemann B, Nizankowska-Mogilnicka E, Okamoto Y, Orru MP, Potter P, Price D, Stoloff SW, Vandenplas O, Viegi G, Williams D; World Health Organization; Ga(2)LEN; AllerGen (2008) Allegic Rhinits and its Impact on Asthma (ARIA) 2008 update (in collaboration with the World Health Organization, GA(2)LEN and AllerGen. Allergy 63 (86 suppl): 8–160

11. Bernstein IL, Bernstein DI, Chan-Yeung M, Malo J-L (2006) Definition and classification of asthma in the workplace. In: Bernstein IL, Chan-Yeung M, Malo J-L, Bernstein DI (eds) Asthma in the Workplace. Taylor & Francis, New York, pp 1–8

12. Tarlo SM, Broder I (1989) Irritant induced asthma. Chest 96: 297–300

13. Gautrin D, Bernstein IL, Brooks S (2006) Reactive airways dysfunction syndrome or irritant induced asthma. In: Bernstein IL, Chan-Yeung M, Malo J-L, Bernstein DI (eds) Asthma in the Workplace. Taylor & Francis, New York, pp 581–629

14. Brooks SM, Weiss MA, Bernstein IL (1985) Reactive airways dysfunction syndrome (RADS): persistent asthma syndrome after high level irritant exposures. Chest 88: 376–384

15. Mapp CE, Boschetto P, Maestrelli P, Fabbri LM (2005) Occupational asthma. Am J Respir Crit Care Med 172: 280–305

16. Newman-Taylor AJ (1995) Non-malignant diseases. Asthma. In: McDonald JC (ed) Epidemiology of Work-Related Diseases. BMJ, London, pp 117–143

17. Malo JL, Chan-Yeung M (2006) Appendix. Agents causing occupational asthma with key references. In: Bernstein IL, Chan-Yeung M, Malo J-L, Bernstein DI (eds) Asthma in the Workplace. Taylor & Francis , New York, pp 825–849

18. Malo JL, Chan-Yeung M (2001) Occupational asthma. J Allergy Clin Immunol 108: 317–328

19. Maestrelli P, Fabbri LM, Mapp CE (2006) Pathophysiology. In: Bernstein IL, Chan-Yeung M, Malo J-L, Bernstein DI (eds) Asthma in the Workplace. Taylor & Francis, New York, pp 109–140

20. Meggs WJ (1994) RADS and RUDS-the toxic induction of asthma and rhinitis. J Toxicol Clin Toxicol 32(5): 487–501

21. Castano R, Thériault G (2006) Defining and classifying occupational rhinitis. J Laryngol Otol 120: 812–817

22. Houba R, Heederik DJ, Doekes G, van Run PE (1996) Exposure-sensitization relationship for alpha-amylase allergens in the baking industry. Am J Respir Crit Care Med 154: 130–136

23. Heederik D, Venables KM, Malmberg P, Hollander A, Karlsson A-S, Renström A, Doekes G, Nieuwenhijsen M, Gordon S (1999) Exposure-response relationships for work-related sensitization in workers exposed to rat urinary allergens: results from a pooled study. J Allergy Clin Immunol 103: 678–684

24. Nieuwenhuijsen MJ, Putcha V, Gordon S, Heederik D, Venables KM, Cullinan P, Newman-Taylor AJ (2003) Exposure-response relations among laboratory animal workers exposed to rats. Occup Environ Med 60: 104–108

25. Mapp CE (2005) Genetics and the occupational environment. Curr Opin Allergy Clin Immunol 5: 113–118

26. Karjalainen A, Martikainen R, Klaukka T, Saarinen K, Uitti J (2003) Risk of asthma among Finnish patients with occupational rhinitis. Chest 123: 283–288

27. Gautrin D, Ghezzo H, Infante-Rivard C, Malo JL (2001) Natural history of sensitization, symptoms and diseases in apprentices exposed to laboratory animal. Eur Respir J 17: 904–908

28. Gautrin D, Infante-Rivard C, Ghezzo H, Malo J-L (2001) Incidence and host determinants of probable occupational asthma in apprentices exposed to laboratory animals. Am J Respir Crit Care Med 163: 899–904

29. Siracusa A, Marabini A, Folletti I, Moscato G (2006) Smoking and occupational asthma. Clin Exp Allergy 36: 577–584

30. Piirila P, Wikman H, Luukkonen R, Kaaria K, Rosenberg C, Nordman H, Norpaa H, Vainio H, Hirvonen A (2001) Glutathione S-transferase genotypes in allergic response to diisocyanate exposure. Pharmacogenetics 11: 437–445

31. Wikman J, Piirila R, Rosenberg C, Luukkonen R, Kaaria K, Nordman H, Norppa H, Vainio H, Hirvonen A (2002) N-acetyltransferase genotypes as modifiers of diisocyanate exposure-associated asthma risk. Pharmacogenetics 12: 227–233

32. Malo JL, Ghezzo H, D'Aquino C, L'Archeveque J, Cartier A, Chan-Yeung M (1992) Natural history of occupational asthma: relevance of type of agent and other factors in the rate of development of symptoms in affected subjects. J Allergy Clin Immunol 90: 937–944

33. Malo J-L, Lemière C, Desjardins A, Cartier A (1997) Prevalence and intensity of rhinoconjunctivitis in subjects with occupational asthma. Eur Respir J 10: 1513–1515

34. Storaas T, Steinvag SK, Florvaag E, Irgens A, Aasen TB (2005) Occupational rhinitis: diagnostic criteria, relation to lower airway symptoms and IgE sensitization in bakery workers. Acta Oto-Laryngoiatrica 125: 1211–1217

35. Abramson M, Sim MR (2006) Occupational asthma. Thorax 61: 741–742

36. Moscato G, Dellabianca A, Perfetti L, Bramé B, Galdi E, Niniano R, Paggiaro PL (1999) Occupational asthma: a longitudinal study on the clinical and socioeconomic outcome after diagnosis. Chest 115: 249–256

37. Ameille J, Descatha A (2005) Outcome of occupational asthma. Curr Opin Allergy Clin Immunol 5: 125–128

38. Chan-Yeung M (1995) Assessment of asthma in the workplace. ACCP consensus statement. American College of Chest Physicians. Chest 108: 1084–1117

39. Marabini A, Siracusa A, Stopponi R, Tacconi C, Abbritti G (2003) Outcome of occupational asthma in patients with continuous exposure: a 3-year longitudinal study during pharmacological treatment. Chest 124: 2372–2376

40. Vandenplas O, Toren K, Blanc PD (2003) Health and socioeconomic impact of work-related asthma. Eur Respir J 22: 689–697

41. Cockcroft DW (1990) Occupational asthma. Ann Allergy 65: 169–175

42. Quirce S, Sastre J (1998) Occupational asthma. Allergy 53: 633–641

43. Malo JL, Ghezzo H, L'Archeveque J, Lagier F, Perrin B, Cartier A (1991) Is the clinical history a satisfactory means of diagnosing occupational asthma? Am Rev Respir Dis 143: 528–532

44. Subcommittee on "Occupational Allergy" of the European Academy of Allerology and Clinical Immunology (1992) Guidelines for the diagnosis of occupational asthma. Clin Exp Allergy 22: 103–108

45. Moscato G, Malo J-L, Bernstein D (2003) Diagnosing occupational asthma: how. How much, how far? Eur Respir J 21: 879–885

46. Moscato G, Perfetti L, Galdi E (1997) Clinical evaluation of occupational asthma. Monaldi Arch Chest Dis 5: 469–473

47. Global Strategy for Asthma Management and Prevention, Global Initiative for Asthma (GINA) (2008) Available from: http://www.ginasthma.org

48. Moscato G, Godnic-Cvar J, Maestrelli P, Malo J-L, Burge PS, Coifman R (1995) Statement on self monitoring of peak expiratory flow in the investigation of occupational asthma. Official Statement. Eur Respir J 8: 1605–1610

49. Burge PS, Moscato G, Johnson A, Chan-Yeung M (2006) Physiological assessment: serial measurements of lung function and bronchial responsiveness. Bernstein IL, Chan-Yeung M, Malo J-L, Bernstein DI (eds) Asthma in the Workplace. Taylor & Francis, New York, pp 199–226

50. Cartier A, Pineau L, Malo J-L (1984) Monitoring of maximum expiratory peak flow rates and histamine inhalation tests in the investigation of occupational asthma. Clin Allergy 14: 193–196

51. Coté J, Kennedy S, Chan-Yeung M (1990) Sensitivity and specificity of PC20 and peak expiratory flow rate in cedar asthma. J Allergy Clin Immunol 85: 592–598

52. Perrin B, Lagier F, L'Archeveque J, Cartier A, Boulet LP, Coté J, Malo JL (1992) Occupational asthma: validity of monitoring of peak expiratory flow rates and non-allergic bronchial responsiveness as compared to specific inhalation challenge. Eur Respir J 51: 40–48

53. Lemiere C, Pizzichini MM, Balkissoon R, Clelland L, Efthimidias A, O'Shaughnessy D, Dolovich J, Hargreave FE (1999) Diagnosing occupational asthma: use of induced sputum. Eur Respir J 13: 482–488

54. Girard F, Chaboillez S, Cartier A, Coté J, Hargreave FE, Labrecque M, Malo JL, Tarlo SM, Lemiere C (2004) An effective strategy for diagnosing occupational asthma: use of induced sputum. Am J Respir Crit Care Med 170: 845–850

55. Vandenplas O, Malo JL (1997) Inhalation challenges with agents causing occupational asthma. Eur Respir J 10: 2612–2629

56. Djukanovic R, Sterk PJ, Fahy JV, Hargreave FE (2002) Standardised methodology of sputum induction and processing. Eur Respir J 20 (s37): 1s–55s

57. Anees W, Huggings V, Pavord ID, Robertson AS, Burge PS (2002) Occupational asthma due to low molecular weight agents: eosinophilic and non-eosinophilic variants. Thorax 57: 231–236

58. Lemiere C (2007) Induced sputum and exhaled nitric oxide as noninvasive markers of airway inflammation from work exposure. Curr Opin Allergy Clin Immunol 7: 133–137

59. Recommendations for standardized procedures for the on-line and off-line measurement of exhaled lower respiratory nitric oxide and nasal nitric oxide in adults and children (1999) Am J Respir Crit Care Med 160: 2104–2117

60. Babinova L, Baur X (2006) Increase in exhaled (eNO) after work-related isocyanate exposure. Int Arch Occup Environ Health 79: 387–395

61. Maestrelli P, Calcagni PG, Saetta M, Di Stefano A, Hosselet JJ, Santonastaso A, Fabbri LM, Mapp CE (1994) Sputum eosinophilia after asthmatic responses induced by isocyanates in sensitized subjects. Clin Exp Allergy 24: 29–34

62. Obata H, Cittrick M, Chan H, Chan-Yeung M (1999) Sputum eosinophils and exaled nitric oxide during late asthmatic reaction in patients with western red cedar asthma. Eur Respir J 13: 489–495

63. Moscato G, Pignatti P, Yacoub MR, Romano C, Spezia S, Perfetti L (2005) Occupational asthma and occupational rhinitis in hairdressers. Chest 128: 3590–3598

64. Castano R, Malo J-L (2007) Toward a 'united' management of 'united airways disease': the role of otorhinolaryngologists and pneumologists. Allergy 62: 708

65. Nicholson PJ, Cullinan P, Newman Taylor AJ, Burge PS, Boyle C (2005) Evidence based guidelines for the prevention, identification, and management of occupational asthma. Occup Environ Med 62: 290–299

66. Rachiotis G, Savani R, Brant A, MacNeill SJ, Newman Taylor A, Cullinan P (2007) Outcome of occupational asthma after cessation of exposure: a systematic review. Thorax 62: 147–152

67. Ameille J, Parion JC, Bayeux MC, Brochard P, Choudat D, Conso F, Devienne A, Garnier R, Iwatsubo Y (1997) Consequences of occupational asthma on employment and financial status: a follow-up study. Eur Respir J 10: 55–58

68. Malo JL, Cartier A, Coté J, Milot J, Lablanc C, Paquette L, Ghezzo H, Boulet LP (1996) Influence of inhaled steroids on the recovery of occupational asthma after cessation of exposure: an 18-month double-blind cross-over study. Am J Respir Crit Care Med 153: 953–960

69. Sastre J, Quirce S (2006) Immunotherapy: an option in the management of occupational asthma? Curr Opin Allergy Clin Immunol 6: 96–100

70. American Thoracic Society (1993) Guidelines for the evaluation of impairment/disability in patients with asthma. Am Rev Respir Dis 147: 1056–1061

71. Yacoub MR, Lavoie K, Lacoste G, Daigle S, L'Archevecque J, Ghezzo H, Lemiere C, Malo JL (2007) Assessment of impairment/disability due to occupational asthma through a multidimensional approach. Eur Respir J 29: 889–896

72. Tarlo SM, Liss GM (2005) Evidence based guidelines for the prevention, identification, and management of occupational asthma. Occup Environ Med 62: 288–289

73. Allmers H, Schmengler J, Skudlik C (2002) Primary prevention of natural rubber latex allergy in the German health care system through education and intervention. J Allergy Clin Immunol 110: 318–323

74. Liss GM, Tarlo SM (2001) Natural rubber latex-related occupational asthma: association with interventions and glove changes over time. Am J Ind Med 40(4): 347–353
75. Brant A (2007) Baker's asthma. Curr Opin Allergy Clin Immunol 7: 152–155
76. Tarlo SM, Malo J-L (2006) An ATS/ERS report: 100 key questions and needs in occupational asthma. Eur Respir J 27: 607–614
77. Liss GM, Nordman H, Tarlo SM, Bernstein DI (2006) Prevention and Surveillance. In: Bernstein IL, Chan-Yeung M, Malo J-L, Bernstein DI (eds) Asthma in the Workplace. Taylor & Francis, New York, pp 353–375
78. Vandenplas O, Jamart J, Delwiche JP, Evrard G, Larbanois A (2002) Occupational asthma caused by natural rubber latex: outcome according to cessation or reduction of exposure. J Allergy Clin Immunol 109: 125–130

Non-atopic Asthma: A Continuing Enigma

Chris Corrigan

Introduction

The terms "intrinsic" and "extrinsic" asthma derive from Rackeman's original recognition [1, 2] that, between individuals, external environmental factors may play a variable visible role in disease exacerbation. At this time, nothing was known about the cellular and molecular pathophysiology of asthma, and he considered the disease in non-atopic patients to be caused by an unknown, "intrinsic" process. Even at this early stage he noticed that patients with "intrinsic" asthma tend to have onset of symptoms later in life, were more commonly female, had disease that was more difficult to control and more frequently had rhinosinusitis. This distinction has become equated with the presence or absence of co-existing atopy, which is the tendency, inappropriately, to produce IgE antibodies against antigens encountered at mucosal surfaces ("allergens"). Atopy is conventionally defined by the presence of specific, circulating IgE to one or more of the panel of common aeroallergens as detected by skin prick or *in vitro* testing [3]. In non-atopic or "intrinsic" asthma, such antibodies are by definition not detectable by these tests. Strictly speaking, it is impossible to rule out the presence of atopy using these tests, since it is always possible to argue that a patient may have mounted a specific IgE response to obscure allergen that is not included even in an extensive panel of skin prick tests. One example of this is the recognition that many "non-atopic" patients may be sensitive to the fungus *Trichophyton* which causes tineal cutaneous infections, and which is not routinely included in panels of allergen solutions for skin prick testing [4]. In practice, however, 95% of atopic patients can be identified by positive skin prick tests to just a small range of aeroallergens such as grass pollen, cat dander and house and dust mite.

Rackeman's observations on the clinical distinctions between atopic and non-atopic asthma have been supported by more modern epidemiological studies such as

C. Corrigan (✉)
Professor of Asthma, Allergy and Respiratory Science, King's College London
School of Medicine, Department of Asthma, Allergy Respiratory Science and MRC
and Asthma UK Centre for Allergic Mechanisms of Asthma, 5th Floor, Tower Wing,
Guy's Hospital, London, SE1 9RT, UK
e-mail: chris.corrigan@kcl.ac.uk

R. Pawankar et al. (eds.), *Allergy Frontiers: Clinical Manifestations*,
DOI: 10.1007/978-4-431-88317-3_20, © Springer 2009

the Epidemiological Study on the Genetics and Environment of Asthma, Bronchial Hyperresponsiveness and Atopy [5]. Such studies [6] have shown that, in random samples of patients with asthma identified by validated questionnaires, increased age, female gender, chronic rhinosinusitis and more severe impairment of lung function are associated with an elevated chance of the patient being non-atopic. Conversely, the presence of other atopic diseases, such as hay fever, seasonal exacerbation of symptoms in line with the pollen season and earlier onset of disease increase the chance that the patient will be atopic. Even so, such studies have highlighted anomalies not easily explicable in terms of the presence or absence of IgE-mediated responses to allergens. For example, both atopic and non-atopic patients report symptoms of rhinitis with equal frequency [6], suggesting that non-atopic patients may have some pre-existing abnormality of the respiratory mucosa that allows these symptoms to develop even in the absence of mediator release from IgE-sensitized mast cells within the nasal mucosa. This same study showed that seasonal exacerbations of disease are features of both atopic and non-atopic asthma, in the former case during the summer months and in the latter case during the winter months. In non-atopic asthmatics, there is less likely to be a family history of asthma or allergy and development of symptoms is often preceded by an upper respiratory illness [7].

Do IgE-Dependent Mechanisms Play an Indispensable Role in Asthma Pathogenesis?

Asthma is characterized by bronchial hyperresponsiveness, or the propensity of the airways to constrict in response to a variety of stimuli that would not cause such constriction in patients without asthma. In atopic patients, the release of histamine and other mediators into the airways secondary to cross-linking of surface-bound, allergen-specific IgE on mast cells and basophils is one such stimulus. In fact, histamine hypersensitivity of the airways forms the basis of the "gold standard" histamine challenge diagnostic test for asthma. Consequently it is not surprising that allergen exposure of atopic individuals is associated with an increase in asthma symptoms, bronchial reactivity and deterioration in lung function [8, 9] (although interestingly it has proven difficult to demonstrate the converse, namely that allergen avoidance can improve asthma in atopic individuals [10], possibly because clinically effective avoidance is not possible in practice). Nevertheless, most clinicians would agree that atopic patients should avoid allergens to which they are sensitized and which clearly exacerbate symptoms of asthma and/or rhinitis, whereas in non-atopic patients such avoidance is irrelevant.

While allergen exposure exacerbates, or "triggers" asthma in atopic individuals, to go further and imply that this process *causes* asthma is more of a leap of faith: the simple observation that not all atopic subjects develop asthma, whereas some non-atopic subjects do, implies that IgE-mediated mast cell degranulation is neither necessary nor sufficient for the development of asthma. Nevertheless, the possibility of a role for IgE in both atopic and non-atopic asthma cannot be ignored. In addition to mast cell and basophil degranulation, IgE is also involved in allergen presentation through its binding to high- and low-affinity Fcε receptors on B cells and dendritic cells, where it captures allergen with high affinity and avidity, activating allergen-specific T and B cells, thereby perpetuating its own synthesis. It has long been known from epidemiological studies [11, 12] that, although total serum IgE concentrations in populations diminish with age, higher concentrations remain a predictor of poorer lung function at all ages, regardless of the presence or absence of asthma. A more recent study [13] showed that, in a large, unselected cohort of patients defined as atopic or non-atopic on the basis of skin prick testing, asthma was fivefold more prevalent and airways obstruction more severe in non-atopic subjects with serum IgE concentrations in excess of the "normal" upper limit of 150 IU/ml as compared with subjects with total serum IgE concentrations below this threshold. It is worth noting that these studies make no reference to the antigen specificity of the IgE, and indeed suggest that inappropriate IgE production is a risk factor for asthma independently of IgE-mediated responses to allergens. This might represent a causal relationship (IgE is involved in the causation of asthma by whatever mechanism) or it might reflect the fact that individuals inherit some abnormality of their respiratory mucosa which predisposes them both to asthma and inappropriate IgE synthesis (evidence is presented below that the respiratory mucosa is likely to be an important site of ongoing IgE synthesis), or both. It is to be hoped that, with the advent of new positional cloning techniques in genetics, which offers the possibility of identifying genes predisposing to particular phenotypes *a priori* and without bias as to preconceived ideas about mechanisms, genetic susceptibility to asthma and inappropriate IgE synthesis can be investigated independently, thus addressing the question whether or not there is any commonality between them. It is of interest in this regard that one of the first genes identified using this technique to be linked to an increased risk of asthma, ADAM33 [14], encodes a metalloproteinase expressed by a variety of normal lung cells, including bronchial smooth muscle and fibroblasts, but not by inflammatory leukocytes. This observation immediately suggests the hypothesis that alterations in the activity or expression of "normal" genes such as ADAM33 in the lung may underlie predisposition to asthma, rather than fundamental differences in immunological responses between individuals. The same principle might apply to inappropriate IgE synthesis. If inappropriate IgE synthesis is indeed involved in the causation of asthma even in non-atopic individuals, this begs questions as to whether IgE synthesis occurs on the respiratory mucosa of non-atopic asthmatics, what stimulates this synthesis and to what antigens the IgE might be directed. This is considered in more detail in the following section.

The Respiratory Mucosa as a Major Site of IgE Synthesis

The concentration of IgE in serum ($<1\,\mu g/ml$) is less than one ten thousandth that of IgG (10 mg/ml) making it the least abundant antibody class in the circulation. This should not be taken to imply, however, that small amounts of IgE are synthesized in the body, since most IgE is sequestered in mucosal tissues bound to high- and low-affinity IgE receptors, and IgE in the serum probably represents no more than the "spill over" from this process. This being the case, it is perfectly conceivable that IgE elaborated in the respiratory mucosa might not escape into the peripheral circulation in sufficient quantity to be detectable by skin prick or *in vitro* tests. There is now abundant evidence that B cells in the human respiratory mucosa undergo class switching to IgE synthesis and secrete mature IgE in both atopic and non-atopic asthmatics. Cells in the bronchial mucosa of non-atopic as well as atopic asthmatics show elevated expression of the high-affinity IgE receptor FcεRI [15]. Since IgE upregulates expression of its own receptor, this is indirect evidence of IgE synthesis. More compelling evidence for local IgE synthesis has come from the demonstration of elevated expression of IgE ε-heavy-chain germline gene transcripts and mature IgE mRNA in the bronchial mucosa of both non-atopic as well as atopic asthmatics compared with controls, in the absence of elevated numbers of B cells [16]. This observation has been further ratified by our recent demonstration of IgE circle transcripts in the bronchial mucosa of atopic and non-atopic asthmatics but not controls [17], confirming that the mucosal environment in asthmatics appears to be conducive to IgE switching. This most likely reflects elevated expression of the IgE class switching cytokines IL-4 and IL-13, as well as local T cell activation and CD40 ligand expression (see [18] and below). B-cell IgE class switching, as shown by the production of circle switch transcripts, has also been detected in the nasal mucosa of patients with allergic rhinitis [19]. This was increased in isolated nasal biopsies following culture with an allergen to which the patient was sensitized *ex vivo*, precluding the possibility that it could have occurred anywhere other than in the mucosa itself. Synthesis and secretion of mature, allergen-specific IgE have also been demonstrated in such biopsies cultured with allergen *ex vivo* [20]. Interestingly, the fraction of IgE expressed as a proportion of the total immunoglobulin secreted by these biopsies far exceeded that observed in the circulation, which is again consistent with the hypothesis that circulating IgE originates largely from the respiratory mucosa.

Despite these observations, and the high likelihood that the respiratory mucosa is a major site of IgE switching and synthesis in both atopic and non-atopic subjects, secretion of mature IgE within the bronchial mucosa of non-atopic asthmatics has yet to be demonstrated directly. Consequently, at present one can only speculate as to its antigen specificity. Some of it could conceivably be allergen-specific, despite the fact that allergen-specific IgE is by definition not detectable in the peripheral blood of these patients. IgE synthesis might also be induced by other environmental stimuli. Of topical interest in this regard are the "superantigens", so-called because they surpass the activity of conventional antigens, which activate single clones of antigen-specific T or B cells, in inducing polyclonal activation of entire subsets of T and B cells by interaction with conserved features of their antigen receptor structures [21]. The bacterium *Staphylococcus aureus* produces a range of enterotoxins which act as B and T cell superantigens. At least 20% of the population carries the commensal *S. aureus* in the nasal mucosa (the bronchial mucosa has not been similarly investigated). There is some evidence that *S. aureus* colonisation can enhance allergen-specific IgE responses in patients with allergic rhinitis [22]. Furthermore, IgE antibody specific for several of these toxins has been described in the serum of asthmatics more frequently than in controls and to a degree which can be correlated with disease severity [23]. These and other environmental influences may promote IgE synthesis in the respiratory mucosa of individuals regardless of their conventional atopic status. There are sources of superantigens in the respiratory mucosa other than from *S. aureus*.

In summary, these studies show that it is very likely that IgE is manufactured in the bronchial mucosa of non-atopic, as well as atopic asthmatics, raising the possibility that it may play a role in the causation and regulation of severity of asthma regardless of conventional atopic status. Firm proof of this might be obtained by investigating the effects of treatment of non-atopic asthmatics with humanized anti-IgE monoclonal antibody, which has so far been reserved for atopic asthmatics on the (unproven) assumption that it ameliorates disease by inhibiting allergen-specific IgE-mediated mast cell degranulation, a manoeuvre which has not so far been considered justified in non-atopic patients [24]. Clinical responses of "non-atopic" asthmatics to this therapy would provide direct evidence that IgE-mediated mechanisms play a causative role in asthma beyond the extent of simply releasing histamine from mast cells into hyperresponsive airways.

Finally, and at the risk of adding further confusion, it is pertinent to bear in mind that atopic status is not set in stone. It is typically assessed in scientific studies at a single point in time using skin prick or *in vitro* tests to a panel of "standard" aero-allergens. Few longitudinal studies of the epidemiology of atopic status have been performed on asthmatics, but a study of children with atopic dermatitis [25] showed that a number of them, originally defined as non-atopic on the basis of negative skin prick tests, developed one or more positive tests within the 10 year period of follow up. Analogously to asthma, such observations raise the questions whether inappropriate IgE responses and "atopic" dermatitis are inextricably linked or simply commonly occur together, and whether a change from skin test negativity to positivity represents a fundamental immunological upheaval or simply increased spill-over of allergen-specific IgE that was always there into the circulation. Direct application of aeroallergens to the skin of some patients with "atopic" dermatitis can induce a local delayed reaction, suggesting T cell-mediated hypersensitivity, even when skin prick tests to these allergens are negative [26]. Does this reflect an IgE-independent, T cell-mediated reaction to these allergens, or is IgE somehow involved?

Cellular and Molecular Pathology of Non-atopic Asthma

Analogously to the role of IgE, many studies over the past decade have revealed striking similarities in the cellular and molecular immunopathology of atopic and non-atopic asthma. The bronchial mucosal inflammatory cellular infiltrate is identical save for an excess of tissue macrophages in non-atopic patients [27, 28]. Furthermore, there appears to be equivalent, elevated expression not only of the key eosinophil-active cytokine IL-5 but also of the two B cell IgE-switching cytokines IL-4 and IL-13 in the bronchial mucosa of both atopic and non-atopic asthmatics as compared with atopy-matched controls [29–31], in the case of IL-5 and IL-4 at the mRNA and protein levels, and with a similar cellular distribution in T cells, mast cells and eosinophils. Furthermore, submucosal expression of mRNA encoding the α-subunits of the IL-4 [32] and IL-5 receptors [33] was elevated, compared with controls, in both patient groups. Mucosal expression of the eosinophil chemotactic chemokines eotaxin, eotaxin-2, RANTES, MCP-3 and MCP-4, as well as expression of the chemokine receptor CCR3, a ligand for these chemokines expressed on eosinophils and Th2-type T cells, was also similarly elevated, at least at the level of mRNA, compared with controls, in both atopic and non-atopic asthmatics [34, 35] and these molecules again showed a similar cellular distribution (predominantly epithelial cells, endothelial cells and macrophages in contrast to the cytokines).

The only described differences between the groups in terms of molecular pathology include the following: increased numbers of cells expressing the α-subunit of the GM-CSF receptor in the bronchial mucosa of non-atopic, as compared with atopic asthmatics, reflecting the increased numbers of tissue macrophages at this site in non-atopic patients [36, 37]; elevated numbers of induced sputum cells (mainly epithelial cells, eosinophils and macrophages) expressing mRNA and immunoreactivity for eotaxin in patients with non-atopic, but not atopic asthma as compared with controls [38]; and elevated concentrations of RANTES in bronchoalveolar lavage fluid (BALF) from non-atopic asthmatics [36, 39].

Expression of cytokines, even at the level of both mRNA and protein in the bronchial mucosa, may not however always equate with their release, and at least one group of researchers has produced data suggesting that T cells from the peripheral blood and BALF of non-atopic, as compared with atopic asthmatics are deficient in IL-4 release when stimulated *ex vivo* [40, 41]. There also exists evidence that STAT-6 mRNA expression may be deficient in the bronchial mucosa of non-atopic asthmatics [42], suggesting that IL-4 signalling may be deficient in these patients. Notwithstanding these reservations, however, the balance of evidence would seem to indicate that the cellular and molecular features of atopic and non-atopic asthma are strikingly similar, arguing that the immunopathogenesis of the disease is essentially the same despite the differences in the clinical phenotypic features. In particular, there is equivalent, elevated expression of IL-4 and IL-13, the key IgE switching cytokines in the bronchial mucosa of asthmatics regardless of whether or not they have positive skin prick tests, reinforcing the previous assertion that both groups of patients make IgE in the bronchial mucosa. Unfortunately this throws no further light on the question, reiterated repeatedly already, whether this IgE synthesis is causal to the disease or whether it serves merely to trigger disease in a subgroup of patients who have IgE which causes clinically significant responses to exogenous environmental agents.

Conclusion

Despite large inroads into understanding the comparative pathology of atopic and non-atopic asthma in the past decade, and appreciation that the airways mucosa is a key site of IgE synthesis, and that such synthesis may not always be detectable peripherally and not always directed against conventional "aeroallergens", non-atopic asthma remains an enigma. A working hypothesis of mechanisms of intrinsic asthma, built around the possible roles of IgE is presented in Fig. 1. In terms of the bronchial mucosal cellular infiltrate and local expression of cytokines and chemokines that are thought to be important in disease pathogenesis, atopic and non-atopic asthma are very similar diseases. Given this fact, one could conclude that atopy, and by implication IgE-mediated mechanisms are irrelevant to

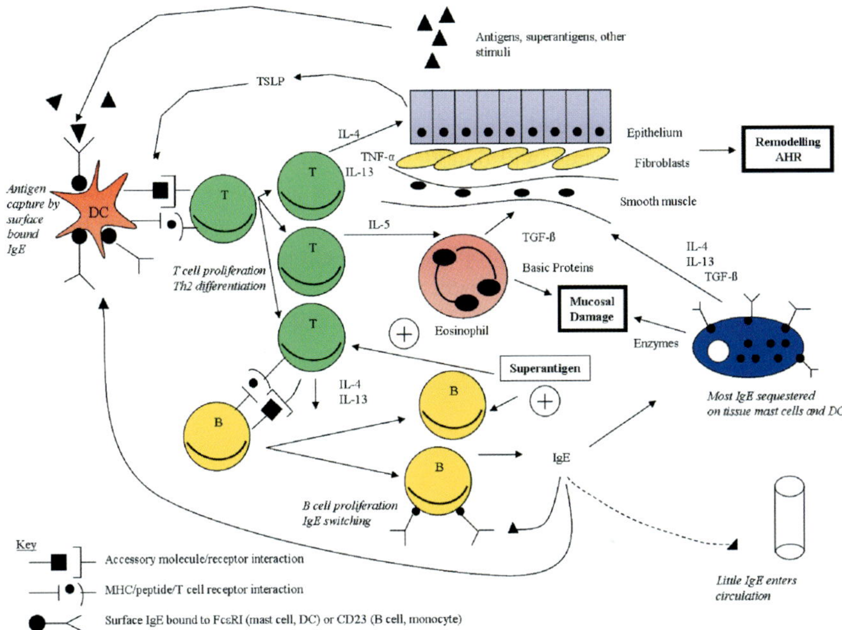

Fig. 1 Hypothetical overview of intrinsic asthma. Environmental stimuli, including allergens, viruses and pollutants act first on the airways epithelium producing mediators such as thymic stromal lymphopoietin (TSLP) which prime mucosal dendritic cells to interact with T cells and induce Th2 differentiation. An important accessory molecule in T cell/dendritic cell interaction induced by TSLP is OX40. Proliferating T cells produce remodelling cytokines such as IL-4, IL-13 and TNF-α which act on epithelial cells, fibroblasts and smooth muscle cells, and cytokines such as IL-5 which promote recruitment of eosinophils to the mucosal surface. Eosinophils also produce some remodelling cytokines, such as TGF-β, and, may cause local tissue damage through the release of basic proteins and other granule products. Antigen presentation by B cells to T cells in the mucosa causes immunoglobulin (Ig) production and, in the presence of IL-4 and IL-13 from T cells, IgE switching. IgE is sequestered largely in the mucosa bound to high- (FcεRI) and low-affinity receptors (CD23) on mast cells/basophils/dendritic cells (DC) and B cells/monocytes respectively. Environmental superantigens may cause oligoclonal T and B cell expansion. Epidemiologically, IgE production is associated with an increased risk of asthma regardless of whether or not allergen-specific IgE is detectable in the circulation. IgE may play a role in capture of antigens by dendritic cells, thus augmenting inflammation, and B cell differentiation by binding to CD23. Antigens other than allergens, such as viruses, may induce an IgE response. For these reasons IgE may play a role in asthma pathogenesis regardless of atopy, which is defined as detectable allergen-specific IgE in the periphery

asthma pathogenesis, and simply serve periodically to exacerbate disease in certain individuals. If this is so, then epidemiological and genetic studies directed at the genesis of atopy, rather than asthma, may be clouding, rather than clarifying our understanding of asthma pathogenesis. On the other hand, one could take the view that inappropriate IgE synthesis, and IgE-mediated mechanisms are an integral and indispensable part of asthma pathogenesis, regardless of clinical reactivity to allergens. The close epidemiological link between overall IgE synthesis and obstructive airways disease in atopic and non-atopic patients partially supports this view, although epidemiological associations do not prove causality and may simply reflect the fact that predisposition to both inappropriate IgE synthesis and asthma is commonly co-inherited. Further studies, particularly directed at whether IgE is in fact produced in the bronchial mucosa of non-atopic patients and what its allergen specificity might be, along with continued genetic studies unbiased by preconceptions of disease mechanisms, will doubtless serve to clarify these questions. At a time when anti-IgE therapy is readily available for asthma treatment [24], it has never been more important to clarify the role of IgE, since it may prove that such therapy is of therapeutic and even prophylactic benefit in both atopic and non-atopic patients alike. Conversely, abandonment of the shackles of an obligatory role for inappropriate IgE synthesis in asthma may open the door to a new appreciation of disease mechanisms and therapeutic avenues.

References

1. Rackeman FM (1947) A working classification of asthma. Am J Med 33:601–606
2. Rackeman FM, Burrage WS, Irwin JW (1950) Intrinsic asthma. Postgrad Med 8:134–140
3. Johansson SGO, Hourihane JO'B, Bousquet J (2001) A revised nomenclature for allergy: an EAACI position statement from the EAACI nomenclature task force [position paper]. Allergy 56:813–824
4. Mungan D, Bavbek S, Peksari V (2001) Trichophyton sensitivity in allergic and nonallergic asthma. Allergy 108:21–28
5. Kauffmann F, Dizier M-H (1995) EGEA (Epidemiological study on the Genetics and Environment of Asthma, bronchial hyperresponsiveness and atopy) – design issues. Clin Exp Allergy 25:19–22
6. Romanet-Manent S, Charpin D, Magnan A, Lanteaume A, Vervloet D (2002) Allergic vs. nonallergic asthma: what makes the difference? Allergy 57:607–613
7. Kroegel C, Jager L, Walker C (1997) Is there a place for intrinsic asthma as a distinct immuno-pathological entity? Eur Respir J 10:513–515
8. Sporik R, Holgate ST, Platts-Mills T (1990) Exposure to house dust mite allergen (*Der p1*) and the development of asthma in childhood. N Engl J Med 323:502–507
9. Peat JK, Salome CM, Woolcock AJ (1990) Longitudinal changes in atopy during a 4-year period: relation to bronchial hyperresponsiveness and respiratory symptoms in a population sample of Australian schoolchildren. J Allergy Clin Immunol 85:65–74
10. Gotzsche PC, Johansen HK, Hammarquist C (2001) House dust mite control measures for asthma [Cochrane review]. The Cochrane Library, issue 3. Oxford Update Software.
11. Barbee RA, Hallon M, Kaltenborn W (1987) A longitudinal study of serum IgE in a community cohort: correlations with age, sex, smoking and atopic status. J Allergy Clin Immunol 79:919–927

12. Burrows B, Martinez FD, Halonen M, Barbee RA, Cline MG (1989) Association of asthma with serum IgE levels and skin-test reactivity to allergens. N Engl J Med 320:271–277

13. Beeh KM, Ksoll M, Buhl R (2000) Elevation of total scrum immunoglobulin E is associated with asthma in nonallergic individuals. Eur Respir J 16:609–614

14. Van Eerdewegh P, Little RD, Dupuis J (2002) Association of the ADAM33 gene with asthma and bronchial hyperresponsiveness. Nature 418:426–430

15. Humbert M, Grant JA, Taborda-Barata L (1996) High-affinity IgE receptor (FcepsilonRI)-bearing cells in bronchial biopsies from atopic and nonatopic asthma. Am J Respir Crit Care Med 153:1931–1937

16. Ying S, Humbert M, Meng Q (2001) Local expression of epsilon germline gene transcripts and RNA for the epsilon heavy chain of IgE in the bronchial mucosa in atopic and nonatopic asthma. J Allergy Clin Immunol 107:686–692

17. Takhar P, Corrigan CJ, Smurthwaite L, O'Connor BJ, Durham SR, Lee TH, Gould HJ (2007) Class switch recombination to IgE in the bronchial mucosa of atopic and nonatopic patients with asthma. J Allergy Clin Immunol 119:213–218

18. Gould HJ, Takhar P, Harries HE, Durham SR, Corrigan CJ (2006) Germinal-centre reactions in allergic inflammation. Trends Immunol 27:446–445

19. Takhar P, Smurthwaite L, Coker CA, Fear DJ, Banfield GK, Carr VA, Durham SR, Gould HJ (2005) Allergen drives class switching to IgE in the nasal mucosa in allergic rhinitis. J Immunol 174:5024–5032

20. Smurthwaite L, Walker SN, Wilson DR, Birch DS, Merrett TG, Durham SR, Gould HJ (2001) Persistent IgE synthesis in the nasal mucosa of hay fever patients. Eur J Immunol 31:3422–3431

21. Gould HJ, Takhar P, Harries HE, Chevretton E, Sutton BJ (2007) The allergic march from *Staphylococcus aureus* superantigens to immunoglobulin E. Chem Immunol Allergy 93:106–136

22. Riechelmann H, Essig A, Duetschle T, Rau A, Rothermel B, Weschta M (2005) Nasal carriage of *Staphylococcus aureus* in house dust mite allergic patients and healthy controls. Allergy 60:1418–1423

23. Bachert C, Gevaert P, Howarth P, Holtappels G, van Cauwenberge P, Johansson SGO (2003) IgE to *Staphylococcus aureus* enterotoxins in serum is related to severity of asthma. J Allergy Clin Immunol 111:1131–1132

24. Berger WE (2002) Monoclonal anti-IgE antibody: a novel therapy for allergic airways disease. Ann Allergy Asthma Immunol 88:152–160

25. Novembre E, Cianferoni A, Lombardi E (2001) Natural history of "intrinsic" atopic dermatitis. Allergy 56:452–453

26. Kerschenlohr K, Decard S, Darsow U (2003) Clinical and immunologic reactivity to aeroallergens in "intrinsic" atopic dermatitis patients. J Allergy Clin Immunol 111:195–197

27. Bentley AM, Menz G, Storz C (1992) Identification of T lymphocytes, macrophages and activated eosinophils in the bronchial mucosa in intrinsic asthma: relationship to symptoms and bronchial responsiveness. Am Rev Respir Dis 146:500–506

28. Bentley AM, Durham SR, Kay AB (1994) Comparison of the immunopathology of extrinsic, intrinsic and occupational asthma. J Invest Allergol Clin Immunol 4:222–232

29. Humbert M, Durham SR, Ying S (1996) IL-4 and IL-5 mRNA and protein in bronchial biopsies from patients with atopic and nonatopic asthma: evidence against "intrinsic" asthma being a distinct immunopathologic entity. Am J Respir Crit Care Med 154:1497–1504

30. Ying S, Humbert M, Barkans J (1997) Expression of IL-4 and IL-5 mRNA and protein product by CD4 + and CD8 + T cells, eosinophils, and mast cells in bronchial biopsies obtained from atopic and nonatopic (intrinsic) asthmatics. J Immunol 158:3539–3544

31. Humbert M, Durham SR, Kimmitt P (1997) Elevated expression of messenger ribonucleic acid encoding interleukin-13 in the bronchial mucosa of atopic and non-atopic asthma. J Allergy Clin Immunol 99:657–665

32. Kotsimbos TC, Ghaffar O, Minshall EM (1998) Expression of the IL-4 receptor alpha-subunit is increased in bronchial biopsy specimens from atopic and nonatopic asthma subjects. J Allergy Clin Immunol 102:859–866

33. Yasruel Z, Humbert M, Kotsimbos TC (1996) Membrane-bound and soluble alpha IL-5 receptor mRNA in the bronchial mucosa of atopic and nonatopic asthmatics. Am J Respir Crit Care Med 154:1497–1504

34. Humbert M, Ying S, Corrigan C (1997) Bronchial mucosal expression of the genes encoding chemokines RANTES and MCP-3 in symptomatic atopic and nonatopic asthmatics: relationship to the eosinophil-active cytokines interleukin (IL)-5, granulocyte macrophage-colony-stimulating factor, and IL-3. Am J Respir Cell Mol Biol 16:1–8

35. Ying S, Meng Q, Zeibecoglou K (1999) Eosinophil chemotactic chemokines (eotaxin, eotaxin-2, RANTES, monocyte chemoattractant protein-3 (MCP-3), and MCP-4), and C-C chemokine receptor 3 expression in bronchial biopsies from atopic and nonatopic (intrinsic) asthmatics. J Immunol 163:6321–6329

36. Novak N, Bieber T (2003) Allergic and nonallergic forms of atopic diseases. J Allergy Clin Immunol 112:252–262

37. Kotsimbos AT, Humbert M, Minshall E (1997) Upregulation of alpha GM-CSF-receptor in nonatopic asthma but not in atopic asthma. J Allergy Clin Immunol 99:666–672

38. Zeibecoglou K, Ying S, Meng Q (2000) Expression of eotaxin in induced sputum of atopic and non-atopic asthmatics. Allergy 55:1042–1048

39. Folkard SG, Westwick J, Millar AB (1997) Production of interleukin-8, RANTES and MCP-1 in intrinsic and extrinsic asthmatics. Eur Respir J 10:2097–2104

40. Walker C, Bode E, Boer E, Hansel TT, Blaser K, Virchow JC (1992) Allergic and non-allergic asthmatics have distinct patterns of T-cell activation and cytokine production in peripheral blood and BAL. Am Rev Respir Dis 146:109–115

41. Virchow JC, Walker C, Hafner D (1995) T cells and cytokines in bronchoalveolar lavage fluid after segmental allergen challenge in atopic asthma. Am J Respir Crit Care Med 151:960–968

42. Christodoulopoulos P, Cameron L, Nakamura Y (2001) Th2 cytokine-associated transcription factors in atopic and nonatopic asthma: evidence for differential signal transducer and activator of transcription 6 expression. J Allergy Clin Immunol 107:586–591

Asthma in the Athlete

Kai-Håkon Carlsen

> *If from running, gymnastic exercises, or any other work, the breathing become difficult, it is called ASTHMA ($\alpha\sigma\theta\mu\alpha$); and the disease Orthopnœa ($o\rho\theta o\pi\nu o\iota\alpha$) is also called Asthma, for in the paroxysms the patients also pant for breath.[1].*
>
> Aereteus the Cappodocian

Introduction

With the citation above Aereteus already more than 2,000 years ago defined exercise-induced asthma (EIA), and this citation demonstrates the long-standing knowledge about the relationship between physical activity and asthma. Exercise induced asthma (EIA) is a general concern for asthmatic children and adolescents in growth as well as for top athletes in many different types of sports. EIA is an increasingly common occurrence among top athletes of several different types of sports. Traditionally this has been reported most often in athletes competing in endurance sports in cold climates, especially among cross-country skiers [2, 3], but also among swimmers [4, 5] and among endurance athletes active in summer sports [6]. The term EIA is used to describe symptoms and signs of asthma provoked by exercise, whereas exercise-induced bronchoconstriction (EIB) denotes the recorded reduction in lung function occurring after an exercise test or a natural occurring exercise.

Already in 1989, it was reported for the first time that high level endurance training increased non-specific bronchial hyperresponsiveness (BHR) to histamine depending on the intensity of the physical training [4]. Nine years later, the finding of inflammatory changes in bronchial biopsies from young skiers was reported [7]. The effect of the intensive physical activity repeatedly performed by the top-athletes may be enhanced by untoward environmental conditions during the activity, like cold ambient temperatures for winter sports and organic chlorine products from indoor swimming pools in swimmers [8].

K.-H. Carlsen (✉)
Voksentoppen, Ullveien 14, NO 0791 Oslo, Norway
e-mail: k.h.carlsen@medisin.uio.no

R. Pawankar et al. (eds.), *Allergy Frontiers: Clinical Manifestations*,
DOI: 10.1007/978-4-431-88317-3_21, © Springer 2009

Furthermore, the heavy exercise load during training with the resulting extremely high level of physical fitness and maximum oxygen uptake ($V'O_{2max}$) reached nowadays by elite athletes, may result in difficulties to discriminate between physiological and pathological limitations to maximum exercise. Thus it is important that our diagnosis of EIA and EIB is based upon good diagnostic criteria for EIB and BHR in athletes.

It is now recognised that the prevalence of EIA among top athletes has increased. In addition to the clinical expression of exercise-induced asthma among athletes, also other relationships create problems for the asthmatic athletes. Fear of a doping effect caused by asthmatic drugs as well as the frequent use of asthma drugs among athletes has caused the Medical Commission of the International Olympic Committee (IOC-MC) to set up strict rules and procedures for allowing the use of certain asthma drugs in sports. In the following a review will be given about the epidemiology of EIA among athletes, pathogenesis of EIA and the development of asthma and bronchial hyperrepsonsiveness (BHR) among athletes, diagnosis and treatment of exercise-induced asthma among athletes.

The Epidemiology of Asthma and Bronchial Hyperresponsiveness Among Athletes

From a screening programme organised by the US Olympic Committee, Voy reported that 67 out of 597 American Olympic Athletes for the Los Angeles 1984 Summer Olympic Games suffered from EIA or asthma. These 67 asthmatic athletes won 41 medals during the Olympic Games [9]. High prevalence of asthma was also reported from later Olympic Games [10], and in 1996 an asthma prevalence as high as 45% was reported in cyclists and mountain bikers compared to none in divers and weightlifters [11]. A questionnaire based survey on 2,060 competitive Swiss athletes of national and international standards reported lower respiratory symptoms in 7.1% and asthma attacks in 3.7% [12]. Langdeau et al. reported on the prevalence of BHR to metacholine (49%) in 100 competitive athletes of various sports compared to sedentary subjects (28%) and with varying prevalences among athletes performing their sports in cold air, dry air, humid air or a combination [13]. Lately, Anderson et al. as well as Fitch have reported on the use of inhaled drugs after applications for their use in the three latest Olympic Games [14–16]. Of all participating athletes 5.2% used inhaled ß$_2$-agonists in the Winter Olympic Games in 2002 [14] and 4.2% in the Summer Olympics in 2004 [15]. It appears that the usage of inhaled ß$_2$-agonists is largest in endurance sports.

Related to winter sports, Larsson et al. reported in 1993 that 23 of 42 elite cross country skiers had a combination of BHR and asthma symptoms compared to only one of 23 referents [3], whereas Heir and Oseid shortly thereafter showed in a questionnaire based report a prevalence of doctor diagnosed asthma of 14% in 155 actively competing skiers compared to 5% in twice matched controls, moreover the prevalence of asthma diagnosis increased with increasing age in the actively competing skiers [17]. Reports followed of high prevalences in Norwegian and Swedish skiers [18], in competitive figure skaters [19, 20], in elite cold-weather athletes [21] and among participants in the 1998 American Olympic National team for winter sports including gold medalists [22]. Figure 1 shows the distribution of bronchial responsiveness among the members of the Norwegian national cross-country skiing team in 2005, demonstrating that 43% of the skiers had a PD_{20} to meatcholine less than 8 µmol.

From summer sports, Feinstein et al. reported the presence of EIB in nine of 48 male football players [23], whereas BHR to methacholine ($PD_{20\text{-methacholine}}$ < 16.3 µmol) was found in 35.5% of the Norwegian national female soccer team [24].

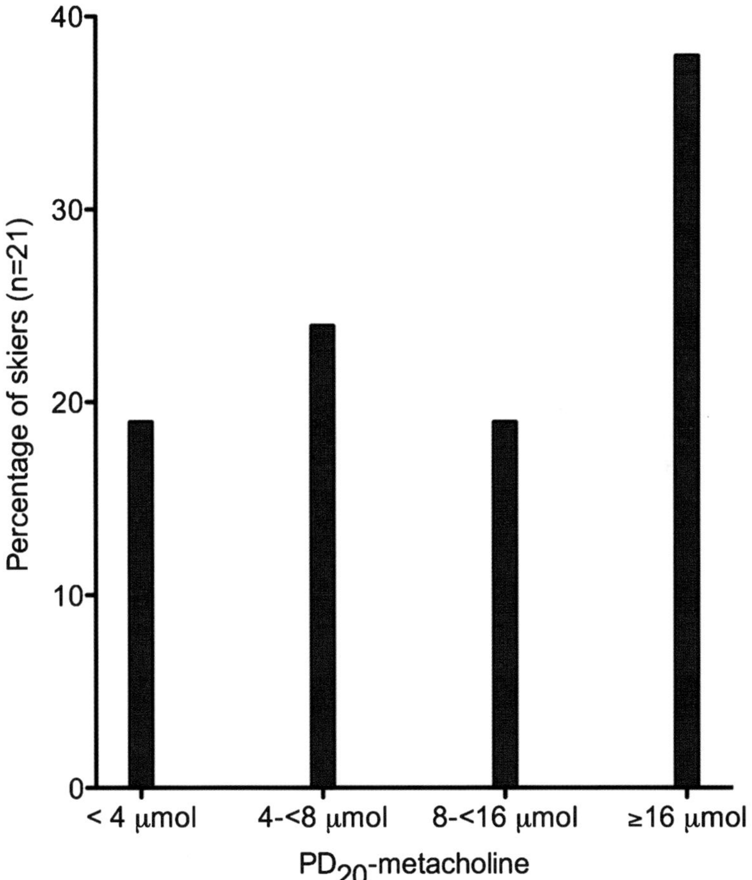

Fig. 1 Distribution of bronchial responsiveness to metacholine (PD_{20}) among the Norwegian national cross country skiing team before the competitive season in 2005. Levels are shown in percentage. There were 21 skiers on the team. The data shown are unpublished

Of Canadian professional football players 56% had positive bronchodilator test (increase in $FEV_1 \geq 12\%$) to inhaled salbutamol [25]. Among American track and field athletics, 10% of the men and 23% of the women suffered from EIB after a national competitive event with higher incidences after long-distance events [26].

Helenius and Haahtela have published a number of studies on Finnish elite track and field athletes. Physician diagnosed asthma was reported in 17% of long-distance runners, 8% of speed and power athletes and 3% of controls [27] whereas in another study total asthma (current asthma, physician diagnosed asthma or BHR) was found in 23% of the athletes compared to 4% of the controls, current asthma in 14% compared to 2% among controls and positive skin prick test (SPT) in 48% of the athletes compared to 36% among controls [28]. BHR to histamine was found in 48% of swimmers [5]. In 1,060 competing Italian summer athletes Maiolo et al. reported the prevalence of asthma to be 15% and atopy to be 18% [29]. A Norwegian report confirmed the finding of higher prevalence of asthma among endurance athletes as compared to speed and power athletes [30]. Employing the objective criteria for diagnosing asthma and/or BHR as given by the IOC-MC, Dickinson reported the prevalence among the British participants in the Olympic Games in 2000 and 2004 to be 21.2% and 20.7%, respectively, with a positive bronchoprovocation or bronchodilator test [31].

Pathogenesis of Exercise Induced Asthma

Presently, two main hypotheses are discussed to explain the relationship between physical activity and EIA. One relates to cooling of the airways in relationship to the increased ventilation during exercise, the other hypothesis relates to increased loss of water from the respiratory tract also caused by increased ventilation during exercise.

Firstly, McFadden and co-workers suggested that airway cooling due to respiratory heat loss leading to pulmonary vasoconstriction, and then followed by rewarming caused by secondary hyperaemia and pulmonary vasodilatation, is the probable cause of EIA [32].

Secondly, there are substantial evidence to indicate that EIA is effected through the release of mediators from mast cells and other inflammatory cells of the airways [33]. The lower respiratory tract is lined by ciliary epithelium coated by periciliary fluid. During breathing, respiratory vapour loss increases rapidly with increasing ventilatory rate [34] and increasingly so when inhaling cold air. Air of 37°C fully saturated with vapour contains 47 mg H_2O/L. Air of room temperature (22°C) with 50% relative humidity contains 22 mg H_2O/L, and air of −10°C with 50% relative humidity contains only 1 mg H_2O/L air. Thus with the high ventilation rates of top athletes (up to > 280 L/min) during exercise, the loss of water is considerable. The main factor causing the mediator release is now thought to be the change in osmolarity of the periciliary fluid lining the surface of the respiratory mucosal membranes, whether it is caused by respiratory heat loss or respiratory water loss [35]. The mediator release provoked by exercise is the main reason for considering EIA an indirect measure of bronchial reactivity [36].

Endurance Training and the Development of Asthma and Bronchial Hyperresponsiveness: Relationship to Environmental Factors

An increase in bronchial responsiveness was demonstrated in Norwegian competitive swimmers after a heavy swimming exercise [4] and then in young ski athletes during the competitive season [37]. Inflammatory changes with lymphoid aggregates in bronchial biopsies were demonstrated frequently in heavily trained young skiers without asthma, but with increased airways responsiveness to cold air compared to control subjects [7]. It seems that heavy and repeated physical endurance training over prolonged time periods in combination with non-optimal environmental conditions may contribute to the development of asthma among top athletes. This was first described among cross country skiers in Norway [2] and Sweden [3, 18], and later among endurance athletes in summer sports [38] and other types of sports [10, 11]. The risk for developing asthma increases markedly when intense and frequent endurance training is combined with untoward environmental factors. Heir et al. found that bronchial responsiveness to metacholine increased for up to 6 weeks after an upper respiratory tract infection [39], and also increased after training in a cold environment [40], as confirmed by other studies [41]. Increased occurrence of EIB and bronchial responsiveness among elite competitive swimmers has been connected to increased exposition to organic chloride products in indoor swimming pools [8, 42]. Also studies from school children with reports of increased prevalence of doctor-diagnosed asthma related to the time spent in swimming pools support this view [43–45]. Also other forms of pollution have impact upon physical performance in athletes [46].

Diagnosis of Exercise Induced Asthma and Bronchial Hyperresponsiveness in Athletes

A diagnosis of asthma or EIA/EIB ought to be made before starting treatment of asthma. An exact clinical history, examination with lung function measurements before and after inhalation of a ß_2-agonist, before and after a standardised exercise-test such as tread-mill run and/or a cold-air inhalation test and measurement of BHR by metacholine inhalation are parts of the diagnostic process. One important part of the diagnostic process is to follow up the patient to evaluate the treatment effect.

Assessment of Exercise Induced Bronchoconstriction

EIA may be diagnosed in different ways, running provokes EIB in children more easily than cycling [47]. Running for 6–8 min provokes greater decrease in post-exercise FEV_1 than running for shorter or longer time periods [48], and running on a motor-driven treadmill is particularly useful and easy to standardise. One way of standardisation useful to diagnose EIB in athletes is to employ a motor driven treadmill with an inclination of 5.5%, rapidly increasing speed until a steady heart rate of approximately 95% of calculated maximum is reached, maintaining this for 4–6 min. The widespread use of inhaled steroids necessitates this level of exercise [49]. Maximum heart rate is approximately calculated by taking 220 – the age of the patient. The heart rate can be measured electronically by devices such as the Sport-Tester PE 3000®. The running is performed with a room temperature of approximately 20°C and a relative humidity of approximately 40%. Lung function is measured before running, immediately after cessation of running, after 3, 6, 10, 15 and 20 min after running. FEV_1 is usually the lung function parameter employed, and a fall of 10% is usually taken as a sign of EIA.

In addition to diagnosing EIA, the reduction in FEV_1 after standardised exercise may be considered as a measure of non-specific bronchial reactivity [36] and used to evaluate the severity of asthma, as well as the effects of therapy [50]. When adding an extra stimulus to the exercise test, by combining running on a treadmill with the inhalation of dry cold air of −20°C, the sensitivity of the test is markedly increased while simultaneously maintaining a high degree of specificity [51].

Both ERS and ATS recommendations set a 10% reduction in FEV_1 as criterion for EIB [52, 53]. Also eucapnic voluntary hyperpnoea has been recommended and used successfully in a wide range of summer and winter athletes [54]. Eucapnic voluntary hyperpnoea has been found by some to have a higher sensitivity than exercise by itself [55].

The IOC-MC and the World Anti-Doping Association (WADA) have set up specific requirements for approving the use of inhaled steroids and inhaled β_2-agonists. This includes also the use of bronchodilator tests and other measures of bronchial responsiveness. For the asthmatic athlete, a thorough assessment including other laboratory measures such as bronchodilator reversibility and other ways of assessing bronchial responsiveness may become necessary, especially as EIB may represent a specific measure of asthma and EIB, but with a low sensitivity for the diagnosis.

Bronchodilator Response

Airways response to inhaled bronchodilators may detect airways obstruction, but has limited value as a basis for diagnosis of asthma [56]. The criterion for a positive bronchodilator response as recommended by European Respiratory Society is 12%

increase in FEV$_1$ expressed as percentage predicted after inhaled bronchodilator or a 200 mL increase [57]. Because of its simplicity, however, it is more common to record the increase in reversibility in per cent of baseline.

Measurement of Bronchial Hyperresponsiveness by Other Indirect Stimuli

EIB may be seen as a measure of indirect bronchial responsiveness by causing bronchoconstriction indirectly by release of mediators [36, 58]. Other indirect stimuli have also been used to assess bronchial responsiveness including inhalation of cold, dry air [59], of dry air [60], of hyperosmolar aerosols like hypertonic saline [61] and inhaled mannitol [60, 62, 63], and inhalation of adenosine monophosphate (AMP) [64]. On a general level it may be stated that indirect tests are more specific for asthma, whereas the direct tests are more sensitive, but do not to the same extent discriminate between asthma and other chronic lung disorders [51, 64, 65]. When combining two indirect stimuli such as cold air inhalation and exercise, the sensitivity may increase while maintaining a high level of specificity [51]. The method of inhalation of adenosine monophosphate has also demonstrated a higher degree of sensitivity while maintaining specificity [64]. It has been suggested by an independent panel of the Medical Commission of the International Olympic Committee to use eucapnic hyperventilation with dry air (with the addition of 5% CO$_2$) as a screening test for exercise- induced asthma in athletes [60]. Eucapnic hyperventilation of dry air of temperature 20–25°C has been demonstrated to correlate well with EIB. However, when performed for 4 min with dry cold air it has been shown to have a low sensitivity in adults to detect asthma and bronchial responsiveness [66]. On the other hand, one report showed higher sensitivity of eucapnic hyperventilation in young athletes to detect bronchial hyperresponsiveness than that of methacholine [67]. It has been demonstrated in several studies that the sensitivity of inhaling cold dry air is greater than the response to dry air only [68–71] including one recent study in pre-school children [72]. The eucapnic voluntary hyperpnoea protocol recommended by the IOC-MC independent panel uses 6 min of ventilation at 85% of maximum voluntary ventilation [60]. It was maintained that field tests consisting of the specific exercise type in the athlete's type of sport is optimal for diagnosing EIB. Rundell et al. demonstrated that 71% of athletes with EIB after a specific field test had a negative response to a laboratory treadmill test. However, the environmental conditions in their laboratory included a relative humidity of 60% which protects against EIB [73]. The same group reported a higher sensitivity of eucapnic hyperventilation than of exercise field test [74], as also was reported by Dickinson et al. [54]. On the other hand, with reference to the requirements set by IOC-MC, Stensrud et al. recently reported metacholine bronchial provocation to be much more sensitive to identify top athletes with direct/indirect bronchial hyperresponsiveness as compared to a competitive exercise field test (cross-country skiing competitive event) (75).

Measurement of Direct Bronchial Responsiveness Using a Pharmacological Agent

Different stimuli may cause different responses in the same persons. It has been found that thermal stimuli to the airways involve narrowing of bronchi at a segmental level, whereas inhaled methacholine has its effect more distally in the bronchi [76]. Hargreave [77] and Cockcroft [78] reported in the late 1970 ties the use of inhaled histamine or methacholine as a tool to measure bronchial responsiveness quantitatively. They demonstrated that the test differed between asthmatic patients and healthy individuals, and Cockroft reported that a histamine $PC_{20} \leq 8\,mg/mL$ had a sensitivity of 100% to diagnose asthma in a random sample of 500 college students, whereas the specificity was low. With a cut off of $1\,mg/mL$ the positive predictive value was 100, but the sensitivity low. Cockcroft concluded that a $PC_{20\text{-Histamine}} > 8$ or $16\,mg/mL$ ruled out current asthma in most instances in the absence of treatment with inhaled corticosteroids [79]. Later Yan et al. simplified the test measuring the totally cumulative inhaled dose instead of using concentrations at tidal breathing [80]. Later inspiration-triggered nebulisers have been combined with computer programs to calculate PD_{20} of the provocative agent (APS Jäger).

The use of different methods may mean that results from different laboratories are not always comparable [81]. Certain laboratories have developed their own methods with their own reference values.

In epidemiological general population studies, a defined level of PC_{20} or PD_{20} to histamine or methacholine does not always compare well to the diagnosis of asthma obtained by questionnaires [82]. When exercise challenge was compared with direct bronchial challenges, some children reacted to exercise and some to methacholine or histamine, probably demonstrating that the two methods describe different properties of the airways. Only 36% of athletes having a fall of 10% or more after eucapnic voluntary hyperpnoea had response to $7.8\,\mu mol$ of methacholine using the Yan technique. Some of these discrepancies may be accounted for by the deep breath technique used in the Yan technique [67]. When children with asthma and other chronic lung diseases were compared, it was found that exercise test had a very high specificity for asthma, but a low sensitivity, whereas methacholine challenge has a higher sensitivity but a low specificity [51, 65].

Anderson et al. chose cut off points on the basis of specificity rather than sensitivity for methacholine challenges to identify people with asthma, using cut off levels of methacholine challenges ($PC_{20} \leq 2\,mg/mL$) in athletes not treated by inhaled corticosteroids and PC_{20} of $13.2\,mg/mL$ for those treated with inhaled corticosteroids for more than 3 months, in order to obtain approval to use inhaled β_2-agonists in sports. These points were used for the applications received at the Olympic Games in 2002 [14]. Others felt that these cut off point rules were too strict [83].

The diagnosis of asthma in athletes sets the ground for permission to use inhaled β_2-agonists as reliever agents and inhaled corticosteroids as controller therapy in relationship to sports. There is overwhelming evidence that inhaled β_2-agonists and inhaled corticosteroids do not improve performance in healthy athletes.

A possible beneficial effect is thus limited to the asthmatic athlete through treatment of the disease. This favors an approach which should give priority to sensitivity over specificity in the use of laboratory methods as a tool in documenting the diagnosis of asthma in order to allow asthmatic athletes to be treated according to present guidelines, also when participating in sports. IOC-MC have changed their limits for metacholine provocation between each Olympic Games. It is therefore very important for the physician treating athletes to follow the latest regulations set up.

Differential Diagnoses to EIA in Athletes

There are several differential diagnoses to EIA, including exercise-induced vocal cord dysfunction [84, 85] and hyperventilation during exercise (Table 1). These conditions should be borne in mind, as many such patients have been given unnecessary drugs for treatment of asthma, including both inhaled steroids and ß₂-agonists, which will have no effect upon the exercise induced vocal cord dysfunction. Exercise-induced vocal cord dysfunction is more common among top trained female athletes during adolescence. Marked inspiratory stridor during maximal exercise with a flattening of the maximal inspiratory flow volume curve [86], is typical, in contrast to EIB in which case the dyspnoea occurs after exercise, and is expiratory due to the lower airways obstruction. Already taking a careful case

Table 1 Differential diagnoses to exercise-induced asthma

- **Exercise-induced asthma (EIA)**

  Symptoms occur shortly after physical exercise or sometimes during low grade exercise following hard.

  If observed: Expiratory dyspnoea, expiratory rhonchi and other signs of bronchial obstruction. Gradual improvement either spontaneously or after inhaled bronchodilator
- **Vocal cord dysfunction (VCD); exercise induced**

  Symptoms occur during maximum exertion. Symptoms disappear after stopping exercise (unless hyperventilating)

  If observed: Inspiratory stridor, audible inspiratory sounds from laryngeal area. No signs of bronchial obstruction. No effect of pre-treatment with inhaled bronchodilator
- **Poor physical fitness**

  Related to expectations

  High heart rate after low-grade exercise load
- **Other Chronic Lung disorders**
- **Other general diseases**

  Heart disease and others
- **Exercise induced arterial hypoxemia (EIAH)**

  Occurs in well-trained athletes with high maximum oxygen uptake ($V'O_{2max}$).

  Primarily due to diffusion limitations and ventilation-perfusion inequality. Incomplete diffusion in the healthy lung may be due to a rapid red blood cell transit time through the pulmonary capillary
- **Swimming-induced pulmonary edema (SIPE)**

history, asking if the dyspnoea occurs during maximal exercise or after completing the exercise; and if the dyspnoea is inspiratory or expiratory, may give useful information as to the probable diagnosis. Confirmation of the diagnosis may be obtained by direct laryngoscopia by use of a fibre laryngoscope during an intense exercise test [87].

Swimming-induced pulmonary oedema (SIPE) is another possible differential diagnosis to EIA. SIPE occur in well-trained swimmers after a heavy swimming session. This condition was recently reported in 70 previously healthy swimmers, who developed typical symptoms of pulmonary edema together with a restrictive pattern in pulmonary function, which remained for up to 1 week after the swimming incident [88].

Also other chronic disorders including heart diseases and other respiratory disorders may have effect upon physical performance and thus represent a possible differential diagnosis to EIA. Also poor physical fitness or overtraining may sometimes be misinterpreted as possible EIA, especially when physical fitness or exercise performance are not up to the expectations of the athletes, parents or trainers. Lack of success in sports may be explained by often minor respiratory complaints which may be mistaken for asthma.

Reports have been made concerning exercise-induced arterial hypoxemia [89]. This occurs especially in well-trained athletes and is thought to be due to diffusion limitations and ventilation-perfusion inequality. It is postulated that incomplete diffusion in the healthy lung may be due to a rapid red blood cell transit time through the pulmonary capillary. Physical training improves muscle strength and endurance, and increases ionotrophic and chronotrophic capacities of the cardiovascular system. No such effects of training occur in the respiratory tract. Ventilatory requirement may increase with no alteration in the capability of the airways and the lungs to produce higher flow rates or higher tidal volumes, and little or no change in the pressure-generating capability of inspiratory muscles [90]. The result is exercise induced arterial hypoxemia which may occur in up to 50% of highly trained athletes [91–93]. This reduction in arterial oxygen saturation may be confused with EIA.

Thus, there are several differential diagnoses to EIA. It is important to make a thorough examination and rule out possible differential diagnoses in order to be able to give optimal treatment and advice for the athlete.

Treatment of EIA in Athletes

In principle, EIA is treated by pre-medication shortly before physical activity and/ or by regular prophylactic anti-inflammatory treatment.

However, as relates to sports, the athletes must presently satisfy the regulations set up for the use of asthma drugs in sports by IOC-MC and WADA.

In order to be allowed to use the most common asthma drugs in relationship to international competitive sports, it is necessary to obtain permission to do so from World Anti Doping Association (WADA) or IOC-MC. IOC-MC gives the necessary permission in relationship to Olympic Games; WADA is responsible for other international competitive sports. IOC-MC set up restrictions for the use of inhaled ß$_2$-agonists already in 1993. These have later been modified repeatedly. It is necessary to apply before the competitions, and for some drugs the regulations also apply to the use out of competition. For the last Winter Olympic Games in Torino 2006, the following rules were applied by IOC:

One of the following objective tests must be satisfied:

(a) Positive bronchodilator test: ≥12% increase in FEV_1% predicted after inhalation of permitted beta-2-agonist.
(b) Exercise challenge or eucapnic voluntary hyperpnoea with a ≥10% fall in FEV_1.
(c) Metacholine: PC20 < 4 mg/mL or PD$_{20}$ ≤ 2 μmol in steroid naive subjects. If inhaled steroids > 3 months: PC20FEV1 ≤ 6.6 mg/ml or PD$_{20}$ ≤13.6 μmol. It is mandatory for accept of metacholine bronchial provocation tests to submit laboratory worksheets.
(d) WADA has used the following rules:

Topical steroids: There are presently no restrictions for topical use on skin, nose, eye. However, for the use of inhaled corticosteroids there are restrictions. Application (Therapeutic use exemption, TUE) is needed both for inhaled corticosteroids and inhaled ß$_2$-agonists. Inhaled ß2-agonists are also not permitted out-of competition. For the use of inhaled ß$_2$-agonists WADA has now declared: "It is preferred to leave to the professional judgement of the physician the medical conditions under which these drugs are to be prescribed" (Explanatory notes 2006). The team manager and team doctor are also responsible when an athlete is caught doping. A concentration of urinary salbutamol ≥ 1,000 ng/L is considered an adverse analytical finding regardless of the granting of any form of TUE.

Anti-Inflammatory Treatment

Anti-inflammatory treatment, especially inhaled steroids, is the most important treatment for asthma and for EIA. Most studies related to the effect upon EIA or EIB are performed on asthmatic patients with diagnosed EIB and not upon asthmatic athletes. However, both groups, patients with asthma and top athletes with asthma, probably benefit by the same type of treatment, and until specific studies in athletes are available, it is necessary to rely on studies performed in asthmatic patients.

Asthmatic well-trained athletes obtained a marked reduction in EIA after 1 week's treatment with inhaled steroids, as measured by the fall in FEV_1 after a standardised tread-mill run [94]. However, improvement in peripheral bronchial obstruction (MEF_{25-75}) required further treatment for 3–4 weeks [95]. Several other studies confirm these findings, and it is presently recognised that inhaled steroids represent the optimal treatment for controlling EIA.

Another treatment principle is the use of leukotriene-antagonists, taken orally. There are two main groups, leukotriene synthesis antagonists and leukotriene receptor antagonists. Two days treatment with a leukotriene synthesis inhibitor (zileuton) caused a protection of 40% against EIA [96]. Also in children the use of montelukast, a leukotriene receptor antagonist, led to a significant reduction in EIA after only 2 days treatment both in children and adults [97, 98]. These drugs reduce EIA, and a continuous effect has been observed without development of tolerance to the drug as has been observed in regular use of other types of treatment [99]. De Benedictis studied the prolonged effect upon EIB in asthmatic children by montelucast. He found that the protection obtained persisted over 4 weeks without tolerance development. However, when assessing the individual responses to the leukotriene anatagonist, there was a large number of non-responders to the drug [100]. This underlines the necessity to follow the athletes after starting treatment to evaluate the effect. It should be emphasized that no restrictions are put upon the use of leukotriene-antagonists in relationship to sports.

Also disodium cromoglycate (DSCG) and nedocromile sodium have been shown to improve EIA when taken before exercise. Some studies report an improvement of BHR after the use of DSCG, whereas other studies cannot confirm this finding [101, 102]. The most often reported effect of DSCG and nedocromile sodium upon EIA, is when taking the drugs before exercise [103].

Treatment Before Exercise

Several drugs taken before exercise protect against EIA. The effect should be evaluated by performing an exercise test or by observing the real life effect during training and competition. With a lack of effect, treatment should be adjusted, and, especially if the diagnosis of EIA is based upon history alone, the diagnosis should be reconsidered. The most usual therapeutic drugs employed before exercise by athletes, are inhaled β_2-agonists. Also DSCG and nedocromile sodium are useful in the pre-treatment of EIA, but inhaled β_2-agonists are more often employed. Taken within 15 min before physical activity, both groups of drugs reduce the exercise-induced fall in lung function, and to protect against EIA for up to 2 h after inhalation, whereas the combination DSCG and terbutaline protected for 4 h. Thus, combining the two drugs prolonged the protection [104]. Inhaled β_2-agonists are often preferred as protective treatment prior to physical activity. The protective effect against EIA is usually very good, both when bronchial constriction is present before exercise and not [105]. The short acting inhaled β_2-agonists; salbutamol and terbutaline are usually preferred.

Also inhaled long-acting β_2-agonists, salmeterol and formoterol, protects effectively against EIA [106]. Children with EIA will benefit from a long-acting protective drug, as they do not plan their activity beforehand. In athletes performing within endurance sports, a long-acting β_2-agonist may be of benefit as the usual β_2-agonists may last too short [107]. However, formoterol with its rapid onset of action may be used also as a protective agent immediately before exercise, and with the long-acting action effect of 12 h also as a prolonged protection. This may be preferable in long-distance endurance sports.

Recently, the oral leukotriene antagonists have been shown to protect against EIA and experience shows them to be effective also in relationship to sports. Montelukast protects for its entire therapeutic duration of 24 h [98]. In severe EIA, practical experience shows that a beneficial additive effect may be obtained by combining several protecting drugs such as inhaled β_2-agonists and leukotriene antagonists.

Ipratropium bromide may be effective in protecting against EIA in singular patients, though less useful than inhaled β_2-agonists, it may give an additional protective effect [108]. The optimal and individually adjusted use of asthma drugs enables asthmatic athletes to participate in competitive sports on an equal level with healthy competitors.

Relationship to Doping

Frequent use of any type of drug in relationship to competitive sports may cause suspicion that the drugs are used to improve physical performance, and not to treat medical illness. The frequent occurrence of EIA/EIB in participants in competitive sports has led to a high consumption of asthma drugs among athletes [2]. It has been debated if inhaled β_2-agonist in particular could improve performance, especially endurance performance. In animals it has been demonstrated that oral β_2-agonists (clenbuterol) in high doses may cause an increase in muscle mass and performance by striated muscle both by clenbuterol [109–114] and salbutamol [115, 116]. The use of systemic β_2-agonists in humans has been shown in some studies to enhance peak torque and muscle power [117, 118], whereas most studies do not demonstrate benefits for performance [119–122]. For inhaled β_2-agonists the findings are almost uniform in demonstrating a lack of improvement both on performance as regards peak torque and strength in all [123–127] except for one study [128] as well as endurance performance, both as regards short-acting [129–134] and long-acting β_2-agonists [135–140]. However, there are still restrictions in the international doping regulations as detailed above. Both inhaled steroids and inhaled β_2-agonists are allowed for use in sports in asthmatic athletes. Systemic β_2-agonists and systemic steroids are not allowed. From 1993 only the inhaled β_2-agonists salbutamol and terbutaline were allowed, but after studies demonstrating that salbutamol, terbutaline, salmeterol and formoterol do not improve performance in sports [137], salmeterol and formoterol have also been allowed for use in sports. The recently introduced oral leukotriene antagonists representing a new principle in asthma treatment, are presently allowed for use in sports, and no effect has been found upon performance during cold air conditions in well-trained athletes [141].

It is the responsibility of the athlete to know the doping rules. However, the physician treating athletes should know these rules, thereby avoiding prescribing drugs not permitted for the use in sports. According to the latest regulation from the World Antidoping Agency (WADA), both inhaled steroids and inhaled β_2-agonists are prohibited substances, and inhaled β_2-agonists are also prohibited out of competition without approval. If used in athletes participating in international events, an application to WADA should be made prior to the participation in the sports event. Information about asthma in relationship to sports is found on the WADA website at the following location: http://www.wada-ama.org/rtecontent/document/asthma_TUEC.pdf

References

1. Adams F. The extant works of Aretaeus, the Cappodician. London: The Sydenham Society; 1856.
2. Heir T, Oseid S. Self-reported asthma and exercise-induced asthma symptoms in high-level competitive cross-country skiers. Scand J Med Sci Sports 1994;4:128–33.
3. Larsson K, Ohlsen P, Larsson L, Malmberg P, Rydstrom PO, Ulriksen H. High prevalence of asthma in cross country skiers. BMJ 1993;307(6915):1326–9.
4. Carlsen KH, Oseid S, Odden H, Mellbye E. The response to heavy swimming exercise in children with and without bronchial asthma. In: Oseid S, Carlsen KH (eds) Children and Exercise XIII. Champaign, IL: Human Kinetics Publishers; 1989, pp. 351–60.
5. Helenius IJ, Rytila P, Metso T, Haahtela T, Venge P, Tikkanen HO. Respiratory symptoms, bronchial responsiveness, and cellular characteristics of induced sputum in elite swimmers. Allergy 1998 Apr;53(4):346–52.
6. Helenius IJ, Tikkanen HO, Haahtela T. Association between type of training and risk of asthma in elithe athletes. Thorax 1997;52:157–60.
7. Sue-Chue M, Karjalainen EM, Altraja A, Laitinen A, Laitinen LA, Naess AB, et al. Lymphoid aggregates in endobronchial biopsies from young elite cross-country skiers. Am J Respir Crit Care Med 1998;158(2):597–601.
8. Drobnic F, Freixa A, Casan P, Sanchis J, Guardino X. Assessment of chlorine exposure in swimmers during training. Med Sci Sports Exerc 1996;28(2):271–4.
9. Voy RO. The US Olympic Committee experience with exercise-induced bronchospasm, 1984. Med Sci Sports Exerc 1986 June;18(3):328–30.
10. Weiler JM, Metzger J, Donnelly AL, Crowley ET, Sharath MD. Prevalence of bronchial responsiveness in highly trained athletes. Chest 1986;90:23–8.
11. Weiler JM, Layton T, Hunt M. Asthma in United States Olympic athletes who participated in the 1996 Summer Games. J Allergy Clin Immunol 1998 Nov;102(5):722–6.
12. Helbling A, Jenoure P, Muller U. The incidence of hay fever in leading Swiss athletes. Schweiz Med Wochenschr 1990 Feb 17;120(7):231–6.
13. Langdeau JB, Turcotte H, Bowie DM, Jobin J, Desgagne P, Boulet LP. Airway hyperresponsiveness in elite athletes. Am J Respir Crit Care Med 2000 May;161(5):1479–84.
14. Anderson SD, Fitch K, Perry CP, Sue-Chu M, Crapo R, McKenzie D, et al. Responses to bronchial challenge submitted for approval to use inhaled beta2-agonists before an event at the 2002 Winter Olympics. J Allergy Clin Immunol 2003 Jan;111(1):45–50.
15. Anderson SD, Sue-Chu M, Perry CP, Gratziou C, Kippelen P, McKenzie DC, et al. Bronchial challenges in athletes applying to inhale a beta2-agonist at the 2004 Summer Olympics. J Allergy Clin Immunol 2006 Apr;117(4):767–73.
16. Fitch KD. beta2-Agonists at the Olympic Games. Clin Rev Allergy Immunol 2006 Oct;31(2–3):259–68.
17. Heir T, Oseid S. Self-reported asthma and exercise-induced asthma symptoms in high-level competitive cross-country skiers. Scand J Med Sci Sports 1994;4:128–33.
18. Sue-Chu M, Larsson L, Bjermer L. Prevalence of asthma in young cross-country skiers in central Scandinavia: differences between Norway and Sweden. Respir Med 1996 Feb;90(2):99–105.
19. Provost-Craig MA, Arbour KS, Sestili DC, Chabalko JJ, Ekinci E. The incidence of exercise-induced bronchospasm in competitive figure skaters. J Asthma 1996;33(1):67–71.

20. Mannix ET, Farber MO, Palange P, Galassetti P, Manfredi F. Exercise-induced asthma in figure skaters. Chest 1996;109(2):312–5.

21. Rundell KW, Im J, Mayers LB, Wilber RL, Szmedra L, Schmitz HR. Self-reported symptoms and exercise-induced asthma in the elite athlete. Med Sci Sports Exerc 2001 Feb;33(2):208–13.

22. Wilber RL, Rundell KW, Szmedra L, Jenkinson DM, Im J, Drake SD. Incidence of exercise-induced bronchospasm in Olympic winter sport athletes. Med Sci Sports Exerc 2000 Apr;32(4):732–7.

23. Feinstein RA, LaRussa J, Wang Dohlman A, Bartolucci AA. Screening adolescent athletes for exercise-induced asthma. Clin J Sport Med 1996;6(2):119–23.

24. Sødal A. Bronchial hyperreactivity, exercise induced asthma and allergy. A study of female national team athletes in soccer. Norwegian University of Sport and Physical Education; 1997.

25. Ross RG. The prevalence of reversible airway obstruction in professional football players. Med Sci Sports Exerc 2000 Dec;32(12):1985–9.

26. Schoene RB, Giboney K, Schimmel C, Hagen J, Robinson J, Sato W, et al. Spirometry and airway reactivity in elite track and field athletes. Clin J Sport Med 1997 Oct;7(4):257–61.

27. Helenius IJ, Tikkanen HO, Haahtela T. Association between type of training and risk of asthma in elite athletes. Thorax 1997;52:157–60.

28. Helenius IJ, Tikkanen HO, Sarna S, Haahtela T. Asthma and increased bronchial responsiveness in elite athletes: atopy and sport event as risk factors. J Allergy Clin Immunol 1998 May;101(5):646–52.

29. Maiolo C, Fuso L, Todaro A, Anatra F, Boniello V, Basso S, et al. Prevalence of asthma and atopy in Italian Olympic athletes. Int J Sports Med 2004 Feb;25(2):139–44.

30. Nystad W, Harris J, Borgen JS. Asthma and wheezing among Norwegian elite athletes. Med Sci Sports Exerc 2000 Feb;32(2):266–70.

31. Dickinson JW, Whyte GP, McConnell AK, Harries MG. Impact of changes in the IOC-MC asthma criteria: a British perspective. Thorax 2005 Aug;60(8):629–32.

32. Gilbert IA, McFadden ER, Jr. Airway cooling and rewarming. The second reaction sequence in exercise-induced asthma. J Clin Invest 1992;90:699–704.

33. Lee TH, Anderson SD. Heterogeneity of mechanisms in exercise-induced asthma. Thorax 1985;40:481–7.

34. Anderson SD. Exercise-induced asthma: Stimulus, mechanism and management. In: Barnes PJ, Roger IW, Thomson NC (eds) Asthma. Basic Mechanisms and Clinical Management. London: Academic; 1988, pp. 503–22.

35. Anderson SD, Daviskas E. The airway microvasculature and exercise induced asthma. Thorax 1992;47:748–52.

36. Pauwels R, Joos G, Van der Straten M. Bronchial responsiveness is not bronchial responsiveness is not asthma. Clin Allergy 1988;18:317–21.

37. Heir T. Longitudinal variations in bronchial responsiveness in cross-country skiers and control subjects. Scand J Med Sci Sports 1994;4:134–9.

38. Helenius IJ, Tikkanen HO, Haahtela T. Occurrence of exercise induced bronchospasm in elite runners: dependence on atopy and exposure to cold air and pollen. Br J Sports Med 1998 June;32(2):125–9.

39. Heir T, Aanestad G, Carlsen KH, Larsen S. Respiratory tract infection and bronchial responsiveness in elite athletes and sedentary control subjects. Scand J Med Sci Sports 1995;5:94–9.

40. Heir T, Larsen S. The influence of training intensity, airway infections and environmental conditions on seasonal variations in bronchial responsiveness in cross-country skiers. Scand J Med Sci Sports 1995;5:152–9.

41. Sandsund M, Faerevik H, Reinertsen RE, Bjermer L. Effects of breathing cold and warm air on lung function and physical performance in asthmatic and nonasthmatic athletes during exercise in the cold. Ann N Y Acad Sci 1997 Mar 15;813:751–6.

42. Drobnic F, Haahtela T. The role of the environment and climate in relation to outdoor and indoor sports. In: Carlsen KH, Delgado L, Del Giacco S (eds) Diagnosis, prevention and

treatment of exercise-related asthma, respiratory and allergic disorders in sports. Sheffield, UK: European Respiratory Society Journals Ltd; 2005, pp. 35–47.

43. Bernard A, Carbonnelle S, Michel O, Higuet S, De Burbure C, Buchet JP, et al. Lung hyperpermeability and asthma prevalence in schoolchildren: unexpected associations with the attendance at indoor chlorinated swimming pools. Occup Environ Med 2003 June;60(6):385–94.

44. Lagerkvist BJ, Bernard A, Blomberg A, Bergstrom E, Forsberg B, Holmstrom K, et al. Pulmonary epithelial integrity in children: relationship to ambient ozone exposure and swimming pool attendance. Environ Health Perspect 2004 Dec;112(17):1768–71.

45. Nickmilder M, Bernard A. Ecological association between childhood asthma and availability of indoor chlorinated swimming pools in Europe. Occup Environ Med 2007 Jan;64(1):37–46.

46. Pierson WE, Covert DS, Koenig JQ, Namekata T, Kim YS. Implications of air pollution effects on athletic performance. Med Sci Sports Exerc 1986 June;18(3):322–7.

47. Anderson SD, Silverman M, Tai E, Godfrey S. Specificity of exercise in exercise-induced asthma. Br Med J 1971 Dec 25;4(5790):814–5.

48. Silverman M, Anderson SD. Standardization of exercise tests in asthmatic children. Arch Dis Child 1972 Dec;47(256):882–9.

49. Carlsen KH, Engh G, Mørk M. Exercise induced bronchoconstriction depends on exercise load. Respir Med 2000 Aug 2;94:750–5.

50. Jonasson G, Carlsen KH, Hultquist C. Low-dose budesonide improves exercise-induced bronchospasm in schoolchildren. Pediatr Allergy Immunol 2000 May;11(2):120–5.

51. Carlsen KH, Engh G, Mørk M, Schrøder E. Cold air inhalation and exercise-induced bronchoconstriction in relationship to metacholine bronchial responsiveness. Different patterns in asthmatic children and children with other chronic lung diseases. Respir Med 1998;92(2):308–15.

52. Sterk PJ, Fabbri LM, Quanjer PH, Cockcroft DW, O'Byrne PM, Anderson SD, et al. Airway responsiveness. Standardized challenge testing with pharmacological, physical and sensitizing stimuli in adults. Report Working Party Standardization of Lung Function Tests, European Community for Steel and Coal. Official Statement of the European Respiratory Society. Eur Respir J Suppl 1993 Mar;16:53–83.

53. Crapo RO, Casaburi R, Coates AL, Enright PL, Hankinson JL, Irvin CG, et al. Guidelines for methacholine and exercise challenge testing-1999. This official statement of the American Thoracic Society was adopted by the ATS Board of Directors, July 1999. Am J Respir Crit Care Med 2000 Jan;161(1):309–29.

54. Dickinson JW, Whyte GP, McConnell AK, Harries MG. Screening elite winter athletes for exercise induced asthma: a comparison of three challenge methods. Br J Sports Med 2006 Feb;40(2):179–82.

55. Mannix ET, Manfredi F, Farber MO. A comparison of two challenge tests for identifying exercise-induced bronchospasm in figure skaters. Chest 1999 Mar;115(3):649–53.

56. Slieker MG, van der Ent CK. The diagnostic and screening capacities of peak expiratory flow measurements in the assessment of airway obstruction and bronchodilator response in children with asthma. Monaldi Arch Chest Dis 2003 Apr;59(2):155–9.

57. Quanjer PH, Tammeling GJ, Cotes JE, Pedersen OF, Peslin R, Yernault JC. Lung volumes and forced ventilatory flows. Report Working Party Standardization of Lung Function Tests, European Community for Steel and Coal. Official Statement of the European Respiratory Society. Eur Respir J Suppl 1993 Mar;16:5–40.

58. Anderson SD, Daviskas E. The mechanism of exercise-induced asthma is.... J Allergy Clin Immunol 2000 Sept;106(3):453–9.

59. Zach MS, Polgar G. Cold air challenge of airway hyperreactivity in children: dose-response interrelation with a reaction plateau. J Allergy Clin Immunol 1987;80:9–17.

60. Anderson SD, Argyros GJ, Magnussen H, Holzer K. Provocation by eucapnic voluntary hyperpnoea to identify exercise induced bronchoconstriction. Br J Sports Med 2001 Oct;35(5):344–7.

61. Boulet LP, Legris C, Thibault L, Turcotte H. Comparative bronchial responses to hyperosmolar saline and methacholine in asthma. Thorax 1987 Dec;42(12):953–8.

62. Brannan JD, Koskela H, Anderson SD, Chew N. Responsiveness to mannitol in asthmatic subjects with exercise- and hyperventilation-induced asthma. Am J Respir Crit Care Med 1998 Oct;158(4):1120–6.

63. Holzer K, Anderson SD, Chan HK, Douglass J. Mannitol as a challenge test to identify exercise-induced bronchoconstriction in elite athletes. Am J Respir Crit Care Med 2003 Feb 15;167(4):534–7.

64. Avital A, Springer C, Bar Yishay E, Godfrey S. Adenosine, methacholine, and exercise challenges in children with asthma or paediatric chronic obstructive pulmonary disease. Thorax 1995;50(5):511–6.

65. Godfrey S, Springer C, Noviski N, Maayan Ch, Avital A. Exercise but not metacholine differentiates asthma from chronic lung disease in children. Thorax 1991;46:488–92.

66. Koskela HO, Hyvarinen L, Brannan JD, Chan HK, Anderson SD. Sensitivity and validity of three bronchial provocation tests to demonstrate the effect of inhaled corticosteroids in asthma. Chest 2003 Oct;124(4):1341–9.

67. Holzer K, Anderson SD, Douglass J. Exercise in elite summer athletes: challenges for diagnosis. J Allergy Clin Immunol 2002 Sept;110(3):374–80.

68. Deal ECJ, McFadden ERJ, Ingram RHJ, Jaeger JJ. Hyperpnea and heat flux: initial reaction sequence in exercise-induced asthma. J Appl Physiol 1979 Mar;46(3):476–83.

69. Deal ECJ, McFadden ERJ, Ingram RHJ, Strauss RH, Jaeger JJ. Role of respiratory heat exchange in production of exercise-induced asthma. J Appl Physiol 1979 Mar;46(3):467–75.

70. McFadden ER, Jr., Nelson JA, Skowronski ME, Lenner KA. Thermally induced asthma and airway drying. Am J Respir Crit Care Med 1999 Jul;160(1):221–6.

71. Farley RD, Albazzaz MK, Patel KR. Role of cooling and drying in hyperventilation induced asthma. Thorax 1988 Apr;43(4):289–94.

72. Nielsen KG, Bisgaard H. Hyperventilation with cold versus dry air in 2- to 5-year-old children with asthma. Am J Respir Crit Care Med 2005 Feb 1;171(3):238–41.

73. Rundell KW, Wilber RL, Szmedra L, Jenkinson DM, Mayers LB, Im J. Exercise-induced asthma screening of elite athletes: field versus laboratory exercise challenge. Med Sci Sports Exerc 2000 Feb;32(2):309–16.

74. Rundell KW, Anderson SD, Spiering BA, Judelson DA. Field exercise vs laboratory eucapnic voluntary hyperventilation to identify airway hyperresponsiveness in elite cold weather athletes. Chest 2004 Mar;125(3):909–15.

75. Stensrud T, Mykland KV, Gabrielsen K, Carlsen KH. Bronchial hyperresponsiveness in skiers: field test versus methacholine provocation? Med Sci Sports Exerc 2007 Oct;39(10): 1681–6.

76. Kotaru C, Coreno A, Skowronski M, Muswick G, Gilkeson RC, McFadden ER, Jr. Morphometric changes after thermal and methacholine bronchoprovocations. J Appl Physiol 2005 Mar;98(3):1028–36.

77. Hargreave FE, Ryan G, Thomsom NC, O'Byrne PM, Latimer K, Juniper EF, et al. Bronchial responsiveness to histamine or metacholine in asthma: measurement and clinical significance. J Allergy Clin Immunol 1981;68:347–55.

78. Cockcroft DW, Ruffin RE, Dolovich J, Hargreave FE. Allergen-induced increase in non-allergic bronchial reactivity. Clin Allergy 1977;7:503–13.

79. Cockcroft DW, Murdock KY, Berscheid BA, Gore BP. Sensitivity and specificity of histamine PC20 determination in a random selection of young college students. J Allergy Clin Immunol 1992 Jan;89(1 Pt 1):23–30.

80. Yan K, Salome C, Woolcock AJ. Rapid method for measurement of bronchial responsiveness. Thorax 1983 Oct;38(10):760–5.

81. Chinn S, Burney P, Jarvis D, Luczynska C. Variation in bronchial responsiveness in the European Community Respiratory Health Survey (ECRHS). Eur Respir J 1997 Nov;10(11):2495–501.

82. Salome CM, Peat JK, Britton J, Woolcock AJ. Bronchial responsiveness in two populations of Australian schoolchildren. I. Relation to respiratory symptoms and diagnosed asthma. Clin Allergy 1987;17:271–81.

83. Bonini S, Brusasco V, Carlsen KH, Delgado L, Del Giacco SR, Haahtela T, et al. Diagnosis of asthma and permitted use of inhaled beta2-agonists in athletes. Allergy 2004 Jan;59(1):33–6.

84. Landwehr LP, Wood RP, Blager FB, Milgrom H. Vocal cord dysfunction mimicking exercise-induced bronchospasm in adolescents. Pediatrics 1996;98(5):971–4.

85. McFadden ERJ, Zawadski DK. Vocal cord dysfunction masquerading as exercise-induced asthma. a physiologic cause for "choking" during athletic activities. Am J Respir Crit Care Med 1996 Mar;153(3):942–7.

86. Refsum HE, Fønstelien E. Exercise-associated ventilatory insufficiency in adolescent athletes. In: Oseid S, Edwards AM (eds) The asthmatic child in play and sports. London: Pitmann; 1983, pp. 128–39.

87. Heimdal JH, Roksund OD, Halvorsen T, Skadberg BT, Olofsson J. Continuous laryngoscopy exercise test: a method for visualizing laryngeal dysfunction during exercise. Laryngoscope 2006 Jan;116(1):52–7.

88. Adir Y, Shupak A, Gil A, Peled N, Keynan Y, Domachevsky L, et al. Swimming-induced pulmonary edema: clinical presentation and serial lung function. Chest 2004 Aug;126(2):394–9.

89. Powers SK, Williams J. Exercise-induced hypoxaemia in highly trained athletes. Sports Med 1987 Jan;4(1):46–53.

90. Dempsey JA, Johnson BD, Saupe KW. Adaptations and limitations in the pulmonary system during exercise. Chest 1990 Mar;97(3 Suppl):81S–7S.

91. Powers SK, Martin D, Cicale M, Collop N, Huang D, Criswell D. Exercise-induced hypoxemia in athletes: role of inadequate hyperventilation. Eur J Appl Physiol Occup Physiol 1992;65(1):37–42.

92. Williams JH, Powers SK, Stuart MK. Hemoglobin desaturation in highly trained athletes during heavy exercise. Med Sci Sports Exerc 1986 Apr;18(2):168–73.

93. Durand F, Mucci P, Prefaut C. Evidence for an inadequate hyperventilation inducing arterial hypoxemia at submaximal exercise in all highly trained endurance athletes. Med Sci Sports Exerc 2000 May;32(5):926–32.

94. Papalia SM. Aspects of inhaled budesonide use in asthma and exercise Department of Human Movement, University of Western Australia. Thesis; 1996.

95. Henriksen JM, Dahl R. Effects of inhaled budesonide alone and in combination with low-dose terbutaline in children with exercise-induced asthma. Am Rev Respir Dis 1983;128(6):993–7.

96. Meltzer SS, Hasday JD, Cohn J, Bleecker ER. Inhibition of exercise-induced bronchospasm by zileuton: a 5- lipoxygenase inhibitor. Am J Respir Crit Care Med 1996;153(3):931–5.

97. Kemp JP, Dockhorn RJ, Shapiro GG, Nguyen HH, Reiss TF, Seidenberg BC, et al. Montelukast once daily inhibits exercise-induced bronchoconstriction in 6- to 14-year-old children with asthma. J Pediatr 1998 Sep;133(3):424–8.

98. Leff JA, Busse WW, Pearlman D, Bronsky E, Kemp J, Hendeles L, et al. Montelukast, a leukotriene-receptor antagonist, for the treatment of mild asthma and exercise-induced bronchoconstriction. N Engl J Med 1998;339:147–52.

99. Villaran C, O'Neill SJ, Helbling A, Van Noord JA, Lee TH, Chuchalin AG, et al. Montelukast versus salmeterol in patients with asthma and exercise- induced bronchoconstriction. J Allergy Clin Immunol 1999 Sept;104(3 Pt 1):547–53.

100. de Benedictis FM, del Giudice MM, Forenza N, Decimo F, de BD, Capristo A. Lack of tolerance to the protective effect of montelukast in exercise-induced bronchoconstriction in children. Eur Respir J 2006 Aug;28(2):291–5.

101. Freeman W, Williams C, Nute MG. Endurance running performance in athletes with asthma. J Sports Sci 1990;8(2):103–17.

102. Carlsen KH, Larsson K. The efficacy of inhaled disodium cromoglycate and glucocorticoids. Clin Exp Allergy 1996;26(Suppl 4):8–17.

103. Benedictis FM, Tuteri G, Bertotto A, Bruni L, Vaccaro R. Comparison of the protective effects of cromolyn sodium and nedocromil sodium in the treatment of exercise-induced asthma in children. J Allergy Clin Immunol 1994;94:684–8.

104. Woolley M, Anderson SD, Quigley BM. Duration of protective effect of terbutaline sulfate and cromolyn sodium alone and in combination on exercise-induced asthma. Chest 1990;97:39–45.

105. Anderson SD. Drugs and the control of exercise-induced asthma [editorial; comment]. Eur Respir J 1993;6:1090–2.

106. Green CP, Price JF. Prevention of exercise induced asthma by inhaled salmeterol xinafoate. Arch Dis Child 1992;67:1014–7.

107. Steffensen I, Faurschou P, Riska H, Rostrup J, Wegener T. Inhaled formoterol dry powder in the treatment of patients with reversible obstructive airway disease. A 3-month, placebo-controlled comparison of the efficacy and safety of formoterol and salbutamol, followed by a 12-month trial with formoterol. Allergy 1995;50(8):657–63.

108. De Lepeleire I, Reiss TF, Rochette F, Botto A, Zhang J, Kundu S, et al. Montelukast causes prolonged, potent leukotriene D4-receptor antagonism in the airways of patients with asthma. Clin Pharmacol Ther 1997 Jan;61(1):83–92.

109. Lynch GS, Hayes A, Campbell SP, Williams DA. Effects of beta 2-agonist administration and exercise on contractile activation of skeletal muscle fibers. J Appl Physiol 1996 Oct;81(4):1610–8.

110. Dodd SL, Powers SK, Vrabas IS, Criswell D, Stetson S, Hussain R. Effects of clenbuterol on contractile and biochemical properties of skeletal muscle. Med Sci Sports Exerc 1996 June;28(6):669–76.

111. Suzuki J, Gao M, Xie Z, Koyama T. Effects of the beta(2)-adrenergic agonist clenbuterol on capillary geometry in cardiac and skeletal muscles in young and middle-aged rats. Acta Physiologica Scandinavica 1997 Nov;161(3):317–26.

112. Hayes A, Williams DA. Contractile properties of clenbuterol-treated mdx muscle are enhanced by low-intensity swimming. J Appl Physiol 1997 Feb;82(2):435–9.

113. Lynch GS, Hayes A, Campbell SP, Williams DA. Effects of beta 2-agonist administration and exercise on contractile activation of skeletal muscle fibers. J Appl Physiol 1996 Oct;81(4):1610–8.

114. Duncan ND, Williams DA, Lynch GS. Deleterious effects of chronic clenbuterol treatment on endurance and sprint exercise performance in rats. Clin Sci (Lond) 2000 Mar;98(3):339–47.

115. Van Der Heijden HF, Zhan WZ, Prakash YS, Dekhuijzen PN, Sieck GC. Salbutamol enhances isotonic contractile properties of rat diaphragm muscle. J Appl Physiol 1998 Aug;85(2):525–9.

116. Buchanan R, Nielsen OB, Clausen T. Excitation- and beta(2)-agonist-induced activation of the Na(+)-K(+) pump in rat soleus muscle. J Physiol 2002 Nov 15;545(Pt 1):229–40.

117. Caruso JF, Signorile JF, Perry AC, Leblanc B, Williams R, Clark M, et al. The effects of albuterol and isokinetic exercise on the quadriceps muscle group. Med Sci Sports Exerc 1995 Nov;27(11):1471–6.

118. van Baak MA, Mayer LH, Kempinski RE, Hartgens F. Effect of salbutamol on muscle strength and endurance performance in nonasthmatic men. Med Sci Sports Exerc 2000 Jul;32(7):1300–6.

119. Violante B, Pellegrino R, Vinay C, Selleri R, Ghinamo G. Failure of aminophylline and salbutamol to improve respiratory muscle function and exercise tolerance in healthy humans. Respiration 1989;55(4):227–36.

120. Javaheri S, Smith JT, Thomas JP, Guilfoile TD, Donovan EF. Albuterol has no effect on diaphragmatic fatigue in humans. Am Rev Respir Dis 1988 Jan;137(1):197–201.

121. Lanigan C, Howes TQ, Borzone G, Vianna LG, Moxham J. The effects of beta 2-agonists and caffeine on respiratory and limb muscle performance. Eur Respir J 1993 Sep;6(8):1192–6.

122. Collomp K, Candau R, Collomp R, Carra J, Lasne F, Prefaut C, et al. Effects of acute ingestion of salbutamol during submaximal exercise. Int J Sports Med 2000 Oct;21(7):480–4.

123. Meeuwisse WH, McKenzie DC, Hopkins S, Road JD, Hopkins SR. The effect of salbutamol on performance in nonasthmatic athletes. Med Sci Sports Exerc 1992;24:1161–6.

124. Morton AR, Papalia SM, Fitch KD. Changes in anaerobic power and strength performance after inhalation of salbutamol in nonasthmatic athletes. Clin J Sport Med 1993;3:14–9.

125. Lemmer JT, Fleck SJ, Wallach JM, Fox S, Burke ER, Kearney JT, et al. The effects of albuterol on power output in non-asthmatic athletes. Int J Sports Med 1995 May;16(4):243–9.
126. Morton AR, Joyce K, Papalia SM, Carroll NG, Fitch KD. Is salmeterol ergogenic? Clin J Sport Med 1996;6(4):220–5.
127. McDowell SL, Fleck SJ, Storms WW. The effects of salmeterol on power output in nonasthmatic athletes. J Allergy Clin Immunol 1997 Apr;99(4):443–9.
128. Signorile JF, Kaplan TA, Applegate B, Perry AC. Effects of acute inhalation of the bronchodilator, albuterol, on power output. Med Sci Sports Exerc 1992;24:638–42.
129. Morton AR, Papalia SM, Fitch KD. Is salbutamol ergogenic?: the effects of salbutamol on physical performance in the high-performance nonasthmatic athletes. Clin J Sport Med 1992;2:93–7.
130. Meeuwisse WH, McKenzie DC, Hopkins SR, Road JD. The effect of salbutamol on performance in elite nonasthmatic athletes. Med Sci Sports Exerc 1992 Oct;24(10):1161–6.
131. Fleck SJ, Lucia A, Storms WW, Wallach JM, Vint PF, Zimmerman SD. Effects of acute inhalation of albuterol on submaximal and maximal VO2 and blood lactate. Int J Sports Med 1993 July;14(5):239–43.
132. Heir T, Stemshaug H. Sabutamol and high-intensity treadmill running in nonasthmatic highly conditioned athletes. Scand J Med Sci Sports 1995;5:231–6.
133. Unnithan VB, Thomson KJ, Aitchison TC, Paton JY. β2-Agonists and Running Economy in Prepubertal Boys. Pediatr Pulmonol 1994;17:378–82.
134. Goubault C, Perault MC, Leleu E, Bouquet S, Legros P, Vandel B, et al. Effects of inhaled salbutamol in exercising non-asthmatic athletes. Thorax 2001 Sept;56(9):675–9.
135. Carlsen KH, Ingjer F, Thyness B, Kirkegaard H. The effect of inhaled salbutamol and salmeterol on lung function and endurance performance in healthy well-trained athletes. Scand J Med Sci Sports 1997;7:160–5.
136. Sue-Chu M, Sandsund M, Helgerud J, Reinertsen RE, Bjermer L. Salmeterol and physical performance at −15 degrees C in highly trained nonasthmatic cross-country skiers. Scand J Med Sci Sports 1999 Feb;9(1):48–52.
137. Carlsen KH, Hem E, Stensrud T, Held T, Herland K, Mowinckel P. Can asthma treatment in sports be doping? The effect of the rapid onset, long-acting inhaled ß$_2$-agonist formoterol upon endurance performance in healthy well-trained athletes. Respir Med 2001 July;95(7):571–6.
138. Stewart IB, Labreche JM, McKenzie DC. Acute formoterol administration has no ergogenic effect in nonasthmatic athletes. Med Sci Sports Exerc 2002 Feb;34(2):213–7.
139. Riiser A, Tjorhom A, Carlsen KH. The effect of formoterol inhalation on endurance performance in hypobaric conditions. Med Sci Sports Exerc 2006 Dec;38(12):2132–7.
140. Tjorhom A, Riiser A, Carlsen KH. Effects of formoterol on endurance performance in athletes at an ambient temperature of −20 degrees C. Scand J Med Sci Sports 2007 Feb 19.
141. Sue-Chu M, Sandsund M, Holand B, Bjermer L. Montelukast does not affect exercise performance at subfreezing temperature in highly trained non-asthmatic endurance athletes [In Process Citation]. Int J Sports Med 2000 Aug;21(6):424–8.

Allergic Bronchopulmonary Aspergillosis

Viswanath P. Kurup and Alan P. Knutsen

Introduction

Allergic bronchopulmonary aspergillosis (ABPA) is a hypersensitivity lung disease caused by sensitization with *Aspergillus fumigatus* (Af) antigens [1, 2]. Af is a major component of the microflora of both indoor and outdoor environments. On exposure to the spores, hyphal fragments, and antigens of Af, susceptible individuals develop ABPA. ABPA occurs as a complication in 1–2% of all asthmatics and up to 7% or more among patients with cystic fibrosis (CF) [3–5].

Af and rarely other related fungi colonize the respiratory tract and release the antigens causing sensitization leading to the development of ABPA. This disease is characterized by a number of clinical and immunological features [5, 6]. These include, peripheral blood eosinophilia, immediate skin test reactivity to Af antigens, elevated total serum IgE, presence of precipitating antibodies to Af antigens, and elevated IgE, IgG, IgM, and IgA antibodies to Af antigens. Most ABPA patients demonstrate pulmonary infiltrates or a history of radiographically defined "pneumonias." Proximal bronchiectasis is present in most ABPA patients who have asthma. However, patients with milder form of ABPA may not have bronchiectasis, but may develop bronchiectasis if pulmonary infiltrates are not controlled. Without early recognition and treatment, ABPA may progress to end-stage pulmonary fibrosis [7, 8]. Prognosis depends on early diagnosis and effective anti-inflammatory therapy.

V.P. Kurup (✉)
Department of Pediatrics, Medical College of Wisconsin, Asthma and Allergy Center, 9000 West Wisconsin Avenue, Suite 408, Milwaukee, WI 53226, USA
e-mail: vkurup@mcw.edu, vkurup@yahoo.com

A.P. Knutsen
Pediatrics Research Institute, St. Louis University Health Sciences, 3662 Park Avenue, St. Louis, MO 63110, USA

R. Pawankar et al. (eds.), *Allergy Frontiers: Clinical Manifestations,*
DOI: 10.1007/978-4-431-88317-3_22, © Springer 2009

History

Hinson, Moon, and Plummer [2] presented eight cases of bronchopulmonary aspergillosis, which include pulmonary mycetoma as well as ABPA. The ABPA patients presented with chest pain, cough, and hemoptysis. Radiographic examination showed consolidation and fibrosis in the right upper lobe of the lungs. Peripheral blood eosinophilia and a history of persistent asthma were detected in all patients. Sputum plugs consisting of hyphal fragments were detected and Af grew from sputum cultures.

The first ABPA case from the US was reported by Patterson and Golbert [9], while the first pediatric case of ABPA was reported by Slavin et al. [10]. Although considered to be a rarity at that time, this disease has been recognized more frequently since then [1, 6]. Patterson and associates demonstrated elevated total serum IgE and elevated peripheral blood eosinophilia in a number of patients studied [3, 4, 6–8]. ABPA in CF was first reported in 1967 and since then the review of literature indicates a high prevalence of this disease [5, 11, 12]. Although only 25% of the asthmatics demonstrated skin test reactivity to Af, up to 60% of CF patients demonstrated skin test reactivity to Af. The radiological findings in CF without ABPA include proximal and distal bronchiectasis. Although, upper lobe bronchiectasis is characteristic of CF and ABPA, in some patients with mild CF, proximal without distal bronchiectasis is detected. Large mucoid impactions can be present on chest X-rays of both CF-ABPA and CF [5, 6]. The pulmonary infiltrate is usually transient and can be cleared by oral corticosteroid treatment.

Clinical Features and Diagnosis

Physical Examination

Physical examination results may be normal or may show features ranging from pneumonia, asthma with wheezing, or bronchiectasis with dry or moist rales [5, 6]. There may be mild cough when transient infiltrates are present. Temperature may be elevated or normal. There may be clubbing, cyanosis, tachypnea, and corpulmonale in the end stage ABPA. The diagnosis of ABPA should be considered in asthmatics of all ages. It has been described in young children, adolescents, and adults with symptoms of atopic diseases, especially asthma with episodic cough, purulent sputum, dyspnea, wheezing, fever, chills, malaise, and hemoptysis. As the disease progresses, features of fibrotic lung disease such as dyspnea and cough predominates. Not all clinical features may be present in every patient with ABPA.

The treatment with prednisone or other corticosteroids may suppress the eosinophilia, elevated total serum and specific IgE levels and the precipitating antibodies. Early in the disease, bronchiectasis may not be evident in ABPA, but may develop if not treated. In CF, all these features may be present even in the absence of ABPA [5, 6]. Because of these variables, ABPA should be considered in asthmatics even if all criteria are not present.

Diagnosis Criteria

The major clinical features of ABPA have been characterized by various authors [5, 6]. These criteria are listed in Table 1. The patients typically have persistent asthma that can be mild, moderate, or severe. Pulmonary infiltrates do not have to be present at all times, but when present, it may be in the posterior segment of the upper lobes or in the middle lobe. Peripheral blood eosinophilia may be present. Additional features include the presence of a late skin test response, following the immediate wheal and flare reaction. Although, rare presence of sputum plugs and demonstration of fungal elements by stain or culture may be significant.

Because of the overlapping features in CF and CF with ABPA, the CF Foundation Consensus Conference arrived at a minimum criteria for diagnosis of ABPA among CF patients (Table 2). The classical cases of ABPA show additional features [6].

Table 1 Diagnostic criteria for allergic bronchopulmonary aspergillosis in patients with asthma[a]

1. Asthma	Mild–severe persistent, also intermittent mild or seemingly no previous asthma
2. Elevated total IgE concentration	>1,000 ng/ml (417 U/ml)
3. Immediate skin reactivity to *A. fumigatus*	Nearly all patients are prick (epicutaneous) positive
4. Proximal bronchiectasis	Either present on chest roentgenograms or high resolution CT examination
5. Elevated serum anti-*A. fumigatus* IgE and or IgG antibodies	When compared to sera from patients with asthma and immediate skin reactivity to *A. fumigatus* but without sufficient criteria for ABPA
6. Precipitating antibodies to *A. fumigatus*	With appropriate antigens precipitins detected in a majority of ABPA
7. Pulmonary infiltrates	May be absent at the time of diagnosis but present in the upper lobes or middle lobe in classic cases, associated with peripheral blood eosinophilia

[a]Minimal essential criteria can include 1, 2, 3, 4 and 5 or 1, 2, 3, 4, and 7 [6]

Table 2 Minimal diagnostic criteria for allergic bronchopulmonary aspergillosis in patients with cystic fibrosis

1. Unexplained clinical deterioration such as worsening cough, wheezing, exercise intolerance, reduction of pulmonary function tests, or increased sputum
2. Elevated total serum IgE concentration >500 U/ml (may be suppressed by prednisone use)
3. Immediate skin reactivity to *Aspergillus* antigens or demonstration of anti-*A. fumigatus* IgE antibody in sera
4. Either (a) precipitating antibodies to *A. fumigatus* or demonstration of anti-*A. fumigatus* IgG or (b) new findings on chest roentgenograms (infiltrates or mucus plugs) or bronchiectasis on chest CT examination that have not cleared with standard physiotherapy and antibiotics

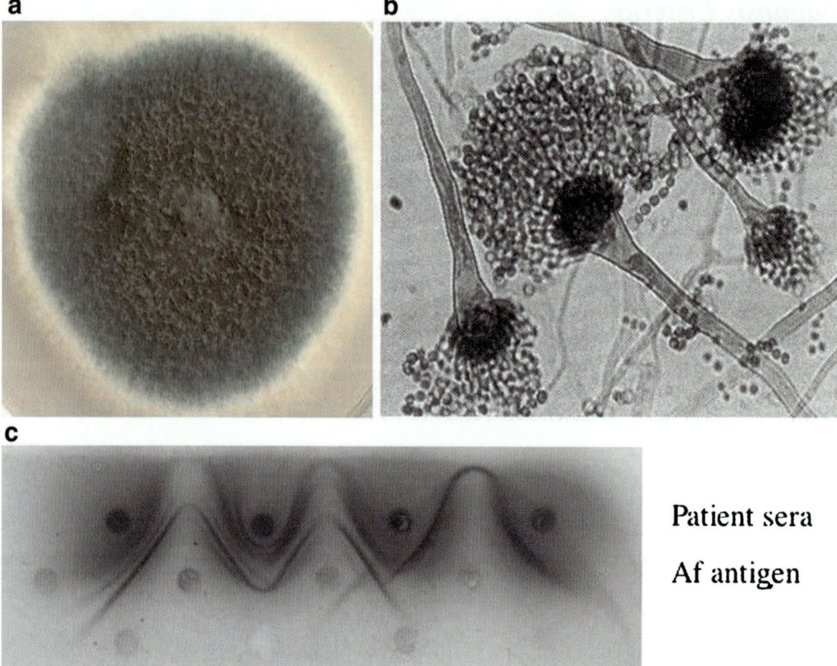

Fig. 1 (**a**) A colony of *A. fumigatus*, (**b**) conidial head and spores (**c**) reaction of ABPA serum with *Aspergillus* antigen showing precipitins by agar gel diffusion; outer wells – ABPA patient sera; Central wells – *Aspergillus fumigatus* antigen

Laboratory Diagnosis

Among the laboratory findings, the presence of immediate skin test reactivity to Af antigen [13] is a consistent finding. In one-third of the patients, the immediate wheal and flare skin test reaction is usually followed by a late-phase reaction (4–6 h Arthus reaction) of erythema and induration. False negative responses mostly are a result of the lack of potent reproducible and standardized antigens. Although several relevant recombinant antigens are currently available, they have not been extensively evaluated for their skin test reactivity.

The sputum, if present, may contain eosinophils, Charcot-Leyden crystals, and fungal hyphae. Sputum plugs may also be present and in most instances will grow *Aspergillus* in fungus cultures (Fig. 1). About 60% of the cases will show the presence of *Aspergillus* in the sputum. The peripheral blood eosinophils vary from 1,000 to 3,000 cells/ml of blood.

Serology may be helpful in the diagnosis of ABPA. Total serum IgE levels are elevated as in asthma and frequently may exceed very high levels. In untreated ABPA the total serum IgE levels may exceed over 60,000 ng/ml [5, 6]. Elevation of

Aspergillus specific IgE, IgG, and IgA have been detected in all ABPA patients, and the levels of these antibodies will be several fold greater than what is detected in *Aspergillus* skin test positive asthmatics. This parameter is important in delineating CF patients without ABPA, CF with asthma and allergy, and CF with ABPA.

Occasionally, the total serum IgE is elevated but not in the range fitting the diagnostic criteria for ABPA. Colonization with *Aspergillus* is especially common in CF patients, and pulmonary flares consisting of increased pulmonary symptoms, new pulmonary infiltrates, and decreased FEV_1, is most often due to a CF flare but may be an ABPA flare. Further studies examining the pulmonary inflammation of BAL or induced sputum identifying eosinophilia, inflammatory response and *Aspergillus* may help identify an ABPA flare [14]. Recently, Hartl et al. reported that thymus and activation regulation chemokine (TARC, CCL17) is increased in CF ABPA patients during flares of ABPA [15]. Chemokine receptor 4 (CCR4) is the receptor for TARC and is present on Th2 cells. Thus, increased TARC levels in ABPA may play a role in the Th2 skewing in ABPA. Interestingly, Knutsen did not observe increased CCR4 T cells in ABPA patients compared to non-ABPA atopic patients (unpublished observation). The role of using exhaled nitric oxide (eNO) has not been studied, but may be helpful. Additionally, genetic risk factors, especially HLA-DR restriction and IL-4Rα single nucleotide polymorphisms (see below) provide additional information of risk for development of ABPA.

Precipitating antibodies can be demonstrated by agar gel double diffusion (Fig. 1c) in up to 90% of patients with ABPA [7, 16]. Antibody responses differ considerably in patients with different *Aspergillus* induced diseases. Patients with ABPA demonstrate elevated levels of antigen specific IgE, IgG, and IgA in their sera [17]. The predominant isotypes represented are IgG_1 and IgG_2 antibodies in ABPA patients. The levels of Af specific IgE and IgG vary in allergic asthma and ABPA, and this feature has been used in differentiating these two groups. The reliability of laboratory results depends on the availability of reproducible antigens. Antigen extracts currently available lack purity and show frequent cross-reactivity with other fungal extracts. They also show considerable variations in their protein and carbohydrate contents, presence of toxins and C-reactive substance. Using conventional purification methods such as size exclusion chromatography, affinity chromatography, electrophoresis, isoelectric focusing, and chromatofocusing, reliable antigen preparations have been obtained from Af [18, 19].

Recombinant *A. fumigatus* Allergens

Search for purified relevant antigens for reliable diagnosis of ABPA has been continued using analytical methods. Most of these methods were time consuming and provided only very small quantities of antigens. With the advent of molecular methods, renewed attempts proved successful in isolating a number of relevant recombinant proteins. About 29 individual proteins have been expressed from

Table 3 Recombinant allergens from *Aspergillus fumigatus* approved by the Nomenclature Committee of the International Union of Immunological Societies (IUIS)*

Allergen	Name	Mol Size	Gene Reference
Asp f 1	Mitogillin	18	AAB07779
Asp f 2		37	AAC69357
Asp f 3	Peroxisomal Protein	19	AAB95638
Asp f 4		30	CAA04959
Asp f 5	Metalloprotease	40	CAA83015
Asp f 6	Manganese Superoxide Dismutase	26.5	AAB60779
Asp f 7		12	CAA11255
Asp f 8	Ribosomal Protein P2	11	CAB64688
Asp f 9		34	CAA11266
Asp f 10	Aspartic Protease	34	CAA59419
Asp f 11	Peptidyl prolyl isomerase	24	CAB44442
Asp f 12	Heat Shock Protein P90	90	AAB51544
Asp f 13	Alkaline Serine Protease	34	CAA77666
Asp f 15		16	CAA05149
Asp f 16		43	AAC61261
Asp f 17			CAA12162
Asp f 18	Vacuolar Serine Protease	34	CAA73782
asp f 22	Enolase	46	AAK49451
Asp f 23	Ribosomal Protein L3	44	AAM43909
Asp f 27	Cyclophilin	18*	
Asp f 28	Thioredoxin	12*	
Asp f 29	Thioredoxin	12*	
Asp f 34	Phi A Cellwall Protein		

*As of 2008

cloned genes of Af. Some of these proteins showed significant reactivity with sera from patients (Table 3). Although not extensively evaluated, these allergens show consistent reactivity comparable to native antigens of Af [20–24]. Among the recombinant allergens, only a few have been evaluated so far [20, 22, 25]. Since the allergenicity is usually directed against the peptide part of the molecule, prokaryotic expression systems were found to be satisfactory in most instances. However, glycosylated proteins have been successfully expressed in yeast and insect expression systems [26]. Molecular cloning and genetic engineering also provide the expression of significant proteins with predictable antibody binding. Similarly, sequences responsible for non-specific reactivity or cross-reactivity can be preferentially deleted by molecular engineering.

Cell-Mediated Immunity

Cell-mediated immunity studied using crude antigen extracts of Af failed to produce consistent results [27, 28]. Antigen induced peripheral blood mononuclear cell stimulation and cytokine production in ABPA patients, and in those with ABPA and CF, was highly variable. This diversity in response was thought to be due to the toxic and suppressive effects of certain components present in the crude antigen preparations. Purified native or recombinant allergens consistently produced more reproducible response. It was found that Asp f 2, a major allergen of ABPA, is capable of stimulating peripheral blood mononuclear cells (PBMC) from patients with ABPA [27]. T-cell clones generated from ABPA patients using Asp f 2 demonstrated epitopes capable of inducing specific cytokines [28]. Based on stimulation of T-cell clones by overlapping peptides, several specific epitopes have been identified of which two, 54–68 aa and 60–67 aa induced IL-4 and IL-5, but not IFN-γ. These regions of the molecule also bound to serum IgE antibodies of ABPA patients [28]. In the experimental mouse model of ABPA, peptide epitopes having specific T-cell response capable of inducing IFN-γ and IL-4 have been identified [29, 30].

Roentgenologic Manifestations

Chest Radiographs

The radiological features may be extremely helpful in the diagnosis of ABPA, and all suspected patients should be evaluated. In most patients with ABPA, central bronchiectasis can be demonstrated [31] (Fig. 2a). Central bronchiectasis is seen either as parallel-line opacities representing widening of the bronchi or as ring opacities. Parallel line opacities have been reported in 65–70% of ABPA patients, while ring shadows in 45–68% [6, 31]. The chest roentgenography showed a spectrum of changes which include both transient and permanent changes. The fleeting shadows appear and disappear in different parts of the lung. This represents acute or different exacerbation stages of the disease and reflects disease activity. Although no areas of the lung are excluded, the upper lobes are involved frequently. Permanent opacities reflect the irreversible fibrotic changes in the bronchial walls and parenchyma. Unlike transient changes these permanent opacities persists even during remission.

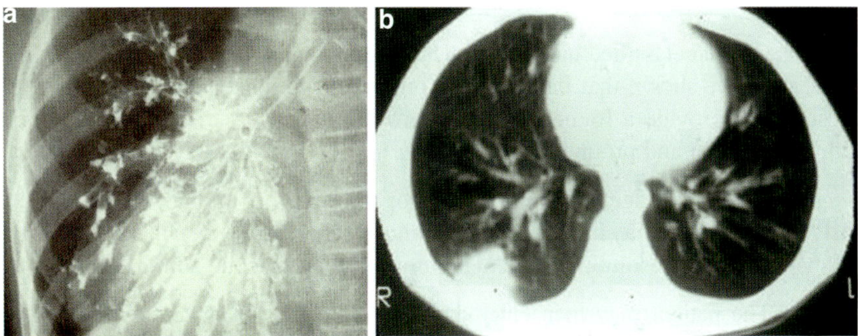

Fig. 2 (**a**) Chest bronchograph of an ABPA patient, (**b**) CT scan of the same patient

Computerized Tomography

Thin section on computerized tomography (CT) of the hilar and perihilar areas has considerable significance in the diagnosis of ABPA [6, 31]. In most patients with ABPA, bronchiectasis can be demonstrated safely by CT compared to bronchography (Fig. 2b). The CT chest scan allows determination of baseline evaluation of the bronchial tree and can be used to gauge response during treatment. It is however important to consider that some patients with strong evidence of ABPA do not have detectable bronchial changes [4]. Early treatment in these patients may prevent further progression of the disease. CT scans are also helpful in rapid, safe, and reliable diagnosis of ABPA in children with severe asthma and CF.

Histopathology

Patients presenting inconsistent radiologic and clinical picture may provide information from lung biopsy studies. However, due to the availability of other information, thoracotomy and lung biopsy are not commonly recommended for making an ABPA diagnosis. The pulmonary pathology of the disease is variable, non-specific, and may be different in the same biopsy specimen. Most specimens contained inspissated mucus and firm mucus plugs [32]. The histological findings included areas of eosinophilic pneumonia peripherally. The lesions may show pulmonary fibrosis, eosinophilic pneumonia, granulomas, and obliterative bronchiolitis. Fungi may be detected within bronchi, which are surrounded by eosinophil infiltrations. Invasion of pulmonary parenchyma by the fungus is rare. Pathologic findings of CF patients with ABPA also demonstrate either proximal or bronchocentric lesions. The infiltrations of inflammatory cells include lymphocytes, plasma cells, eosinophils, and monocytes [32].

Staging of ABPA

ABPA have been classified into five clinical stages ranging from acute to the fibrotic stage, and have shown that patients may progress from one stage to the other [6]. These stages provide a framework for improved diagnostic criteria that may help both in treatment and prognosis.

Stage 1: The acute stage is the early phase of the disease with classical features of ABPA. The patients may have all seven diagnostic characters given in Table 1. There will be a clear-cut resolution of all symptoms with prednisone administration.

Stage 2: The patient may then enter the stage of remission, where symptoms are absent and the underlying asthma is stable. Prednisone may be discontinued and there is an absence of new pulmonary infiltrates. The total serum IgE levels remain low and treatment may be discontinued, although inhaled corticosteroid may be needed for asthma management. This stage lasts a variable period and may remain permanent.

Stage 3: The third stage consists of recurrent exacerbation of the acute phase represented in Stage 1. Many of these patients have been treated as community acquired pneumonias in the past. During exacerbation, these patients may present all classical findings of ABPA, and they respond rapidly to corticosteroids therapy.

Stage 4: The patients with ABPA may develop corticosteroid dependent asthma despite the use of avoidance measures and pharmacotherapy. The asthma will be severe without corticosteroid therapy and other medications. Most patients will have elevated total serum IgE, anti-*Aspergillus* IgE and IgG, and precipitating antibodies. Some patients will convert from mild persistent asthma to severe persistent asthma when ABPA is present. Appropriate therapy of patients in this stage has resulted in stabilization of their conditions without further progression [8].

Stage 5: The final stage is fibrocavitary ABPA; an irreversible condition with widespread bronchiectasis, pulmonary fibrosis and resulting complications [6]. The prognosis in spite of oral prednisone, inhaled corticosteroids, leukotriene antagonists, and long-acting bronchodialators is poor. Some patients may have chronic sputum production and colonization of a respiratory tree with *A. fumigatus*, *pseudomonas aeruginosa*, *Bacillus cepacia*, *Hemophilus influenzae* or atypical mycobacteria. Pulmonary fibrosis results in fatalities in spite of pharmacotherapy in some patients.

Genetic Susceptibility

Genetic factors play a significant role in the pathogenesis of ABPA. Earlier studies have demonstrated that human leukocyte antigens (HLA) are involved in the disease. HLA Class II genes are prime candidates for eliciting immune responses leading to T cell receptor activation, culminating in IgE production (Fig. 3). The major histocompatibility complex (MHC) region contains numerous immune related genes that act specifically in various disease conditions. Genetic studies conducted on ABPA patients demonstrate a major role for HLA-DR alleles in susceptibility and HLA-DQ in protection. Three HLA-DR2 alleles (subtype DRB1 1501, 1503, and 1601) and three HLA-DR5 alleles (subtypes DRB1 1101, 1104, and 1202) facilitated T-cell activation [33–35]. ABPA patients are more than twice as likely to be positive for the crucial HLA-DR2 alleles than non-ABPA patients. These alleles have been shown to be associated with CF, general atopy, and ABPA, and may represent contributing factors in the development of ABPA. Several Af antigens, such as Asp f 1, Asp f 2, Asp f 4, and Asp f 6, may be HLA-DR2/DR5 restricted in ABPA. Interestingly, the presence of HLA-DQ2 even in the presence of HLA-DR2/DR5 contributed to resistance of the development of ABPA.

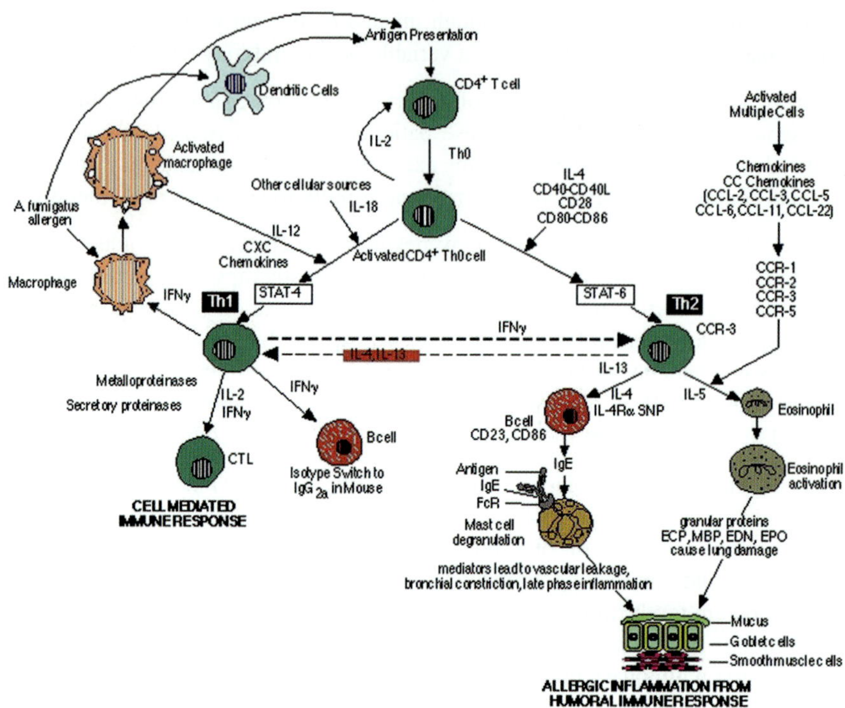

Fig. 3 Schematic presentation of the immunopathogenesis of ABPA

The deciphering of the human genome furthered our understanding of a number of diseases and the genes regulating susceptibility and protection. In recent years, a number of genes have been identified with verified association with allergy and asthma. These include ADAM33, PH-11, ESE-3, GPRA, SPINKS, DPP-10, etc. [36]. In addition, several single nucleotide polymorphisms have also been identified as having direct involvement in IgE synthesis, eosinophil generation, recruitment, and stimulation. Significant genes associated with asthma such as IL-4, IL-5, arginase, ornithine decarboxylase, mucine, metalloproteinase, etc. have been identified in mouse models of ABPA [36–38]. Further elucidation of the interactions among environment, gene, and immunity is essential for both in understanding ABPA and its management.

In asthmatic and CF–ABPA, polymorphisms of IL-4 alpha chain receptor (IL-4Rα), IL-13, and IL-10 have been examined [39]. IL-4Rα single nucleotide polymorphisms (SNPs), principally the ile75val SNP in the extracellular IL-4 receptor binding region has been identified in ABPA patients [40]. These IL-4Rα SNPs are associated with up-regulation of IL-4 stimulation. The IL-13 arg110gln SNP is associated with increased IL-13 stimulation and was observed in 38% of ABPA patients. Brouard et al. [41] were the first to report that the IL-10-1082G genotypes (GG and GA) were associated with increased risk of *Aspergillus* colonization and development of ABPA in CF patients. The IL-10-1082G genotype has been shown to be associated with increased IL-10 synthesis. Knutsen et al. [42] reported that the IL-10-1082G genotype was present in 90% of ABPA patients. Combining HLA-DR restriction (HLA-DR2, DR3, DR4, DR7) plus IL-4Rα SNP and IL-10-1082G genotype, the odds ratio was 8.6 (CI 3.2–22.5) for the development of ABPA.

Pathogenesis of ABPA

A diagrammatic presentation of our current knowledge of the pathogenesis of ABPA is depicted in Fig. 3. Fungi belonging to the genus *Aspergillus*, particularly Af, are distributed widely in nature, hence, exposure to the antigens leading to sensitization occurs in almost all individuals. Low levels of antibodies to Af have been reported in almost all individuals. Normal defense mechanism of the host usually protects the individual from further adverse responses. However, some individuals with pre-existing atopy may develop ABPA on exposure to Af.

In the pathogenesis of ABPA, the various allergens released by germinating spores play a major role [5, 43]. Af spores trapped in the bronchus on germination release catalases, proteases, phospholipases, superoxide dismutases, hemolysins, gliotoxins, and other molecules. These secreted antigens have a direct effect on bronchial epithelium in inducing a proinflammatory response [43]. The fungal spores and antigens are processed by antigen presenting cells, and the resulting response leads to the induction of a Th1 or Th2 response. The genetic role of this polarization is not fully understood although it has been shown that HLA-DR restrictions and IL-4Rα-single nucleotide polymorphism are involved in the pathogenesis of ABPA [40, 44].

Activated T-cells, particularly T-cells of the Th1 and Th2 types, may be responsible for the cumulative effect of the lung pathology in ABPA [44]. In addition to the eosinophils, T-, B-, and NK-cells are also involved in the immune response of ABPA. There was a 2:1 ratio of CD4$^+$ and CD8$^+$ T-cells in the lung lymphoid areas. ABPA patients also showed enhanced CD23 and particularly CD23$^+$, CD86$^+$ B-cells, and CD23$^+$ and CD4$^+$ T-cells.

In recent years, it has been shown that Af specific T-cell lines enhanced the B-cell IgE synthesis. CD4$^+$, CD25$^+$ T-cell phenotypes with a Th2 cytokine profile have been produced with Asp f 1 antigen. In recent studies with Asp f 2, f 3, and f 4 T-cell lines, a predominant Th2 response was detectable [44, 45].

The significant characteristics of ABPA are the enhanced IgE synthesis and increased eosinophil infiltration in the lung, both are induced and regulated by CD4$^+$ Th2 lymphocytes. T-lymphocytes regulate B-cell IgE secretion through cytokines such as IL-4 and IL-13. Similarly, eosinophil activation and differentiation are regulated by a number of cytokines and chemokines of which IL-5, RANTES, and eotaxins are more significant [45].

Mast cells and basophils also play a major role in releasing the mediators of anaphylaxis. The high affinity IgE receptor on mast cells (IgE FcRI) reacts with allergens resulting in degranulation of these cells releasing histamine and other vasoactive amines. Activated basophils also may secrete Th2 cytokines and lead to further activation and expansion of Th2 pathway, resulting in more IgE and eosinophil production [45].

In addition, *Aspergillus* allergens have biologic activity on the respiratory epithelia in addition to inducing allergic inflammatory responses. Kauffman et al. reported that Af proteases had a direct effect on the bronchial epithelia causing pro-inflammatory cytokine synthesis and desquamation [46]. Asp f 3 stimulated bronchial epithelia to secrete IL-6, IL-8, RANTES, and TGF-β, but not eotaxin (Knutsen, unpublished studies). Another mechanism that may be operative in mold-induced asthma and ABPA involves chitin, a major structural protein of the outer coating of fungi [47]. Chitin polarizes immune Th1 responses by suppressing Th2 responses. In humans, acidic mammalian chitinase degrades chitin shifting the responses toward a Th2 inflammatory response. Elevated chitinase has been associated with asthma and elevated IgE levels perhaps through an IL-13 pathway.

Immunotherapy and Vaccination

Specific immunotherapy and vaccination are the probable measures for controlling allergies. Due to the enhanced understanding of the immunopathogenesis and the availability of purified and well-characterized allergens, immunotherapy and vaccination have been looked upon with more optimism. The attention has been focused to reverse the Th2 type of immune response to a Th0 or a Th1 type of response [48]. These new directions include peptide immunotherapy, genetically engineered molecules with specificity, immunostimulatory sequences (CpG), and naked DNA vaccination [49]. Antigen specific immunotherapy constitutes synthetic peptides representing T-cell and B-cell specificity and genetically mutated allergens.

Pharmacotherapy

The goals of ABPA therapy are to control and prevent exacerbations of ABPA in order to stabilize the patients [50]. The treatment of patients with ABPA in asthma or ABPA in CF involves avoidance measures [6]. Concomitant gastroesophagal reflex disease (GERD), rhinitis, and sinusitis should be identified and treated. Those patients who produce sputum may be treated by chest percussion and physiotherapy. For acute exacerbation of bronchiectasis hospitalization may be needed [50].

Pharmacological treatment has consisted of oral corticosteroids, and has a dramatic effect on the recovery with marked reduction in the serum total IgE [7, 50] and clearance of pulmonary infiltrations and chest roentgenograms. For patients with pulmonary infiltrates, those are in Stages 1, 3, and 4, prednisone at a dose of 0.5 mg/kg/day given as a single dose for 2 week results in improvement of chest infiltrates and symptoms. This can be followed with an alternate week regimen, and based on the clearance of mucus, plugging, and infiltrates in CT scan, after 4–8 weeks, the prednisone can be tapered or discontinued. Treatment for asthma should be continued with inhaled corticosteroids and other medications. If the patients can be managed without prednisone for 6 months, and have no new pulmonary infiltrates, then they are considered to be in remission (Stage 2). Recurrence in these patients results from high exposure to fungal contamination or due to poor management of asthma. In the latter situation, the disease transforms to Stage 4 type (corticosteroid dependent ABPA). The Stage 4 patient often needs from 10 to 40 mg of prednisone on alternate days and inhaled corticosteroids and long-acting adrenergic agonists and leukotriene antagonists.

Although prednisone administration reduced the frequency of sputum expectoration, patients may continue to produce sputum plugs of Af. In those instances, itraconazole may have added significance in controlling the fungi and even in reducing or preventing the pulmonary infiltrates and airway inflammation, including sputum eosinophils and sputum ECP concentrations. The role of omalizumab in ABPA is unclear and information on safety and efficacy are lacking.

Summary and Future Directions

ABPA is a hypersensitivity lung disease resulting from exposure to Af spores, hyphal fragments, and antigens. Patients with ABPA show highly elevated serum IgE and *Aspergillus* specific IgE, IgG, and other isotypes. Peripheral blood eosinophilia, airway hyperresponse, and inflammatory responses are the major characteristic of ABPA. In recent years, a number of significant antigens have been cloned and purified from Af. The immune responses have been studied using these allergens. The genes and their expression in ABPA have not been understood well and need more studies. So also more information on immunotherapy and vaccination needs to be understood and should form a major initiative in the future research to control the disease.

Acknowledgment The editorial assistance of Donna Schrubbe is gratefully acknowledged.

References

1. Kurup VP, Apter AJ (1998) Immunology and Allergy Clinics of North America. W.B. Saunders, Philadelphia, PA, pp. 471–710
2. Hinson KFW, Moon AJ, Plummer NS (1952) Bronchopulmonary aspergillosis: a review and report of eight new cases. Thorax 7:317–333
3. Greenberger PA (1988) Allergic bronchopulmonary aspergillosis. In: Middleton E, Reed CE, Ellis EF, Adkinson NF, Yunginer JW (eds) Allergy Principle and Practice. Mosby, St. Louis, MO, pp. 1219–1236

4. Patterson R, Greenberger PA, Halwig JM, Liotta JL, Roberts M (1986) Allergic bronchopulmonary aspergillosis. Natural history and classification of early disease by serologic and roentgenographic studies. Arch Intern Med 146:916–918

5. Stevens DA, Moss RB, Kurup VP, Knutsen AP, Greenberger P, Judson MA, Denning DW, Crameri R, Brody AS, Light M, Skov M, Maish W, Mastella G, and the participants in the Cystic Fibrosis Foundation Consensus Conference (2003) Allergic bronchopulmonary aspergillosis in cystic fibrosis – state of the art: Cystic fibrosis foundation consensus conference. Clin Infect Dis 37:S225–S264

6. Greenberger PA (2005) Allergic bronchopulmonary aspergillosis: clinical aspects. In: Kurup VP (ed) Mold Allergy, Biology and Pathogenesis. Research Signpost, India, pp. 17–32

7. Greenberger PA, Patterson R (1986) Diagnosis and management of allergic bronchopulmonary aspergillosis. Ann Allergy 56:444–453

8. Patterson R, Roberts W (1995) Classification and staging of allergic bronchopulmonary aspergillosis. In: Patterson R, Greenberger PA, Roberts ML (eds) Allergic Bronchopulmonary Aspergillosis. Oceanside, Providence, RI, pp. 5–10

9. Patterson R, Golbert TM (1968) Hypersensitivity pneumonitis of the lung. Univ Mich Med Ctr Journal 34:8–11

10. Slavin RG, Stanczyk DJ, Lonigro AJ, Broun GO (1969) Allergic bronchopulmonary aspergillosis – a North American rarity. Clinical and immunologic characteristics. Am J Med 47:306–313

11. Nelson L, Collerame ML, Schwartz RM (1979) Aspergillosis and atopy in cystic fibrosis. Am Rev Respir Dis 120:863–873

12. Moss RB (2005) Fungal allergy in cystic fibrosis. In: Kurup VP (ed) Mold Allergy, Biology and Pathogenesis. Research Signpost, India, pp. 93–114

13. McCarthy DS, Pepys J (1971) Allergic bronchopulmonary aspergillosis: clinical immunology 2. Skin, nasal and bronchial tests. Clin Allergy 1:415–432

14. Knutsen AP, Warrier MR, Noyes B, Consolino J (2005) Allergic bronchopulmonary aspergillosis in a patient with cystic fibrosis: diagnostic criteria when the IgE level is < 500 IU/ml. Ann Allergy Asthma Immunol 95:488–493

15. Hartl D, Latzin P, Zissel G, Krane M, Krause-Etschmann S, Griese M.(2006) Chemokines indicate allergic bronchopulmonary aspergillosis in patients with cystic fibrosis. Am J Resp Crit care Med 173:1370–1376

16. Kurup VP, Kumar A (1991) Immunodiagnosis of aspergillosis. Clin Microbiol Rev 4:439–456

17. Kurup VP, Resnick A, Kalbfleish J, Fink JN (1990) Antibody isotype response responses in Aspergillus-induced diseases. J Lab Clin Med 115:298–303

18. Kurup VP, Madan T, Sarma UP (2004) Allergic bronchopulmonary aspergillosis: recent concepts and considerations. In: Domer JE, Kobayashi G (eds) The Mycota XII Human Fungal Pathogens. Springer, Berlin/Heidelberg, Germany, pp. 225–241

19. Kurup VP (2005) Aspergillus antigens: which are important? Med Mycol Suppl 43:S189–S196

20. Kurup VP, Banerjee B, Hemmann S, Greenberger PA, Blaser K, Crameri R (2000) Selected recombinant Aspergillus fumigatus allergens bind specifically to IgE in ABPA. Clin Exp Allergy 30:988–993

21. Crameri R, Jaussi R, Menz G, Blaser K (1994) Display of expression products of cDNA libraries on phage surfaces. A versatile system for selective isolation of genes by specific gene-product/ligand interaction. Eur J Biochem 226:53–58

22. Crameri R (1998) Recombinant Aspergillus fumigatus allergens: from the nucleotide sequences to clinical applications. Int Arch Allergy Immunol 115:99–114

23. Banerjee B, Kurup VP, Greenberger PA, Hoffman DR, Nair DS, Fink JN (1997) Purification of a major allergen, Asp f 2 binding to IgE in allergic bronchopulmonary aspergillosis, from culture filtrate of Aspergillus fumigatus. J Allergy Clin Immunol 99:821–827

24. Kumar A, Reddy LV, Sochanik A, Kurup VP (1993) Isolation and characterization of a recombinant heat shock protein of Aspergillus fumigatus. J Allergy Clin Immunol 91:1024–1030

25. Knutsen AP, Hutcheson PS, Slavin RG, Kurup VP (2004) IgE antibody to Aspergillus fumigatus recombinant allergens in cystic fibrosis patients with allergic bronchopulmonary aspergillosis. Allergy 59:198–203

26. Tang B, Banerjee B, Greenberger PA, Fink JN, Kelly KJ, Kurup VP (2000) Antibody binding of deletion mutants of Asp f 2, the major Aspergillus fumigatus allergen. Biochem Biophy Res Com 270:1128–1135

27. Knutsen AP, Chauhan B, Slavin RG (1998) Cell-mediated immunity in allergic bronchopulmonary aspergillosis. In: Kurup VP, Apter AJ (eds) Immunology and Allergy Clinics of North America. W.B. Saunders, Philadelphia, PA, pp. 575–599

28. Rathore VB, Johnson B, Fink JN, Kelly KJ, Greenberger PA, Kurup VP (2001) T cell proliferation and cytokine secretion to T cell epitopes of Asp f 2 in ABPA patients. Clin Immunol 100:228–235

29. Kurup VP, Hari V, Guo J, Murali PS, Resnick A, Krishnan M, Fink JN (1996) Aspergillus fumigatus peptides differentially express Th1 and Th2 cytokines. Peptides 17:183–190

30. Kurup VP, Banerjee B, Murali PS, Greenberger PA, Krishnan M, Hari V, Fink JN (1998) Immunodominant peptide epitopes of allergen, Asp f 1 from the fungus Aspergillus fumigatus. Peptides 19:1469–1477

31. Shah A (2005) Radiological aspects of allergic bronchopulmonary aspergillosis and allergic Aspergillus sinusitis. In: Kurup VP (ed) Mold Allergy, Biology and Pathogenesis. Research Signpost, India, pp. 147–162

32. Martin T, Chetty A (2005) Allergic fungal diseases of the lung: Pathology. In: Kurup VP (ed) Mold Allergy, Biology and Pathogenesis. Research Signpost, India, pp. 163–175

33. Chauhan B, Hutcheson PS, Slavin RG, Bellone CJ (2003) MHC restriction in allergic bronchopulmonary aspergillosis. Front Biosci 8:s140–s148

34. Chauhan B, Santiago L, Kirschmann DA, Hauptfeld V, Knutsen AP, Hutcheson PS, Woulfe SL, Slavin RG, Schwartz HJ, Bellone CJ (1997) The association of HLA-DR alleles and T cell activation with allergic bronchopulmonary aspergillosis. J Immunol 159:4072–4076

35. Chauhan B, Hutcheson PS, Slavin RG (2005) Genetics of fungal allergy. In: Kurup VP (ed) Mold Allergy, Biology and Pathogenesis. Research Signpost, India, pp. 309–322

36. Kurup VP, Raju RP (2005) Genes in asthma and allergy. In: Kurup VP (ed) Mold Allergy, Biology and Pathogenesis. Research Signpost, India, pp. 323–334

37. Zimmermann N, King NE, Laporte J, Yang M, Mishra A, Pope SM, Muntel EE, Witte DP, Pegg AA, Foster PS, Hanid Q, Rothenberg ME (2003) Dissection of experimental asthma with DNA microarray analysis identifies arginase in asthma pathogenesis. J Clin Invest 111:1863–1874

38. Kurup VP, Raju R, Manickam P (2005) Profile of gene expression in a murine model of allergic bronchopulmonary aspergillosis. Infect Immun 73:4381–4384

39. Knutsen AP (2006) Genetic and respiratory tract risk factors for aspergillosis: ABPA and asthma with fungal sensitization. Med Mycol 44:S61–S70

40. Knutsen AP, Kariuki B, Consolino JD, Warrier MR (2006) IL-4 alpha chain receptor (IL-4Rα) polymorphisms in allergic bronchopulmonary aspergillosis. Clin Mol Allergy 3:1–6

41. Brouard J, Knauer N, Boelle P-Y, Corvol H, Henrion-Caude A, Flamant C, Bremont F, Delaisi B, Duhamel J-F, Marguet C, Roussey M, Miesch M-C, Chadelat K, Boule M, Fauroux B, Ratjen F, Grasemann H, Clement A (2005) Influence of interleukin-10 on airways colonization by Aspergillus fumigatus in cystic fibrosis patients. J Infect Dis 191:1988–1991

42. Warrier MR, Chauhaqn B, Slavin RG, Knutsen AP (2006) IL-4 alpha chain receptor (IL-4Rα) polymorphism: Genetic risk factors in the development of allergic bronchopulmonary aspergillosis. Trends in Diphtheria research, Nova Science Publishers. Inc. pp 37–62.

43. Kauffman HF, Heijink IH (2005) Airway remodeling in fungal allergy. In: Kurup VP (ed) Mold Allergy, Biology and Pathogenesis. Research Signpost, India, pp. 237–255

44. Knutsen AP, Mueller KR, Levine AD, Chauhan B, Hutcheson PS, Slavin RG (1994) Asp f 1 CD4 + TH2-like T-cell lines in allergic bronchopulmonary aspergillosis. J Allergy Clin Immunol 94:215–221

45. Knutsen AP (2005) Immune responses in allergic bronchopulmonary aspergillosis and fungal allergy. In: Kurup VP (ed) Mold Allergy, Biology and Pathogenesis. Research Signpost, India, pp 209–235

46. Kauffman HF, Tomee JF, van de Riet MA, Timmerman AJ, Borger P (2000) Protease-dependent activation of epithelial cells by fungal allergens leads to morphologic changes and cytokine production. J Allergy Clin Immunol 105:1185–1193

47. Chatterjee R, Batra J, Das S, Sharma SK, Ghosh B (2008) Genetic association of acidic mammalian chitanse with atopic asthma and serum total IgE levels. J Allergy Clin Immunol 122:202–208
48. Banerjee B, Kelly KJ, Fink JN, Henderson JD Jr, Bansal NK, Kurup VP (2004) Modulation of airway inflammation by immunostimulatory CpG oligodeoxynucleotides in a murine model of allergic aspergillosis. Infect Immun 72:6087–6094
49. Svirshchevskaya EV, Frolova E, Alekseeva L, Kotzareva O, Kurup VP (2000) Intravenous injection of major and cryptic peptide epitopes of ribotoxins, Asp f 1 inhibit T-cell response induced by crude Aspergillus fumigatus antigen in mice. Peptides 21:1–8
50. Fink JN (1998) Therapy of allergic bronchopulmonary aspergillosis. In: Kurup VP, Apter AJ (eds) Immunology and Allergy Clinics of North America. W.B. Saunders, Philadelphia, PA, pp. 655–661

Mechanisms of Anaphylaxis

Stephen F. Kemp and Richard F. Lockey

Background

Anaphylaxis is an acute, potentially lethal multi-system syndrome resulting from the sudden release of mast cell- and basophil-derived mediators into the circulation, and it cannot completely be prevented [1]. It most often results from immunologic reactions to foods, medications, insect stings, and allergen immunotherapy injections, but it can be induced by any agent capable of producing a sudden, systemic degranulation of mast cells or basophils [2]. Anaphylaxis remains a clinical diagnosis based on probability and pattern recognition. Cause-and-effect often is confirmed historically in subjects who experience objective findings of anaphylaxis upon the inadvertent reexposure to the causative agent. Lifetime personal risk of anaphylaxis is thought to be 1–3%, with a mortality rate of 1% [2].

Anaphylaxis consists of some or all of the following signs and symptoms: diffuse erythema, pruritus, urticaria and/or angioedema; bronchospasm; laryngeal edema; hyperperistalsis; hypotension; and/or cardiac arrhythmias. Other symptoms can occur such as nausea, vomiting, lightheadedness, uterine cramps, a generalized flushing sensation, headache, feeling of impending doom, and unconsciousness. Cutaneous manifestations of anaphylaxis are the most common overall, but these may be delayed or absent in rapidly progressive anaphylaxis. Anaphylaxis often causes signs and symptoms within 5–30 min, but some reactions may not develop for several hours. Respiratory compromise and cardiovascular collapse are responsible for most fatalities [2, 3]. The more rapid the onset of the signs and symptoms of anaphylaxis following exposure to an offending stimulus, the more likely the reaction will be life-threatening. An analysis of 202 anaphylaxis fatalities over a 10-year period in the

S.F. Kemp (✉)
Division of Clinical Immunology and Allergy, Department of Medicine, The University of Mississippi Medical Center, 2500 North State Street, Jackson, MS 39216, USA

R.F. Lockey
Division of Allergy and Immunology, Department of Internal Medicine, University of South Florida College of Medicine and the James A. Haley Veterans Administration Hospital, 13000 Bruce B. Downs Blvd. (111D), Tampa, FL 33612, USA

R. Pawankar et al. (eds.), *Allergy Frontiers: Clinical Manifestations*, 367
DOI: 10.1007/978-4-431-88317-3_23, © Springer 2009

United Kingdom determined that the interval between eating a causative food and fatal cardiopulmonary arrest averaged 25–35 min, which was longer than for drugs (mean, 5 min in-hospital; 10–20 min pre-hospital) or insect stings (10–15 min) [3].

Some authors reserve the term *anaphylaxis* for IgE-dependent events and utilize the term *anaphylactoid* to describe IgE-independent reactions that otherwise are clinically indistinguishable. The World Allergy Organization has proposed replacing this traditional nomenclature with *immunologic* (IgE-mediated and non-IgE-mediated [e.g., IgG and immune complex complement-mediated]) and *non-immunologic* anaphylaxis [4]. A clinical, working definition of anaphylaxis has been proposed and is discussed elsewhere [1]. Reactions may be immediate and uniphasic or may be delayed in onset, biphasic, or protracted.

Proposed Immunopathologic Mechanisms

Gell and Coombs first classified immunopathologic (hypersensitivity) reactions into four types: I, immediate (IgE-dependent); II, cytotoxic (IgG, IgM-dependent); III, immune complexes (IgG, IgM-complex dependent); and IV, delayed (T-lymphocyte-dependent) [5]. Sell has proposed an alternate classification system based on seven immunopathologic mechanisms with both protective and destructive functions [6]. These are: (1) immune-mediated inactivation/activation reactions of biologically active molecules; (2) antibody-mediated cytotoxic or cytolytic reactions; (3) immune complex reactions; (4) allergic reactions; (5) T lymphocyte-mediated cytotoxicity; (6) delayed hypersensitivity; and (7) granulomatous reactions. Mechanism 4 in this classification includes IgE-dependent anaphylaxis, but several of these immunopathologic mechanisms may be responsible for anaphylaxis in a given individual. For example, transfusion-related anaphylaxis has cytotoxic features and aggregate anaphylaxis involves immune complex formation (e.g., complexes of immunoglobulin administered parenterally), both of which do not involve IgE and yet cause anaphylaxis. Table 1 classifies representative agents of anaphylaxis by pathophysiologic mechanism.

The pathogenesis of anaphylaxis arguably is fairly obscure and its complexity can adversely impact clinical management. Complex genetic factors and environmental exposure have important roles, but murine models demonstrate two distinct mechanisms of anaphylaxis that also probably apply to humans. The first, which is the mechanism classically associated with human allergic disease, is both IL-4 and IL-4 receptor dependent. It is characterized by an allergen/antigen cross-linking allergen-specific IgE bound to FcεRI receptors on mast cells and/or basophils. This results in the subsequent release of inflammatory mediators and cytokines that produce the smooth muscle contraction and increased vascular contractility associated with clinical anaphylaxis. The second mechanism is IgE-independent; requires proportionately more antigen and antibody than the first pathway; is mediated by IgG, FcγRIII receptors, and macrophages; and can block IgE-dependent anaphylaxis by mediating an interaction between mast cell FcεRI and FcγRIIb receptors. Both

Table 1 Representative agents that cause anaphylaxis

IgE-dependent
  Foods
  Medications
  Insect bites and stings
  Allergen vaccines
  Latex
  Exercise (possibly, in food- and medication-dependent events)
  Hormones
  Animal or human proteins
  Colorants (insect-derived, such as carmine)
  Polysaccharides
  Enzymes
IgE-independent
  Nonspecific degranulation of mast cells and basophils
    Opioids
    Muscle relaxants
    Idiopathic
    Physical factors
      Exercise
      Temperature
  Disturbance of arachidonic acid metabolism
    Aspirin and other nonsteroidal anti-inflammatory drugs (NSAIDs)[a]
  Immune aggregates
    Intravenous immunoglobulin
    Dextran (possibly)
    Possibly antihaptoglobin in anhaptoglobinemia (in Asians)
  Cytotoxic
    Transfusion reactions to cellular elements (IgM, IgG)
  Multimediator complement activation/activation of contact system
    Radiocontrast media
    Dialysis membranes
    Protamine (possibly)

[a]These reactions are almost always drug-specific (unlike the cross-reactivity observed in aspirin-exacerbating respiratory disease) they require two or more previous specific drug exposures, and the subject group characteristically has no underlying asthma or nasal polyps.

mechanisms release platelet activating factor (PAF), while only the IgE-dependent mechanism releases histamine [7, 8].

Antigen-specific IgG antibody blocks IgE-dependent anaphylaxis in immunized mice without precipitating IgE-independent anaphylaxis when anaphylaxis is induced by low-dose allergen, but not when induced by high-dose allergen [7]. No IgG-dependent anaphylaxis in humans has been reported, but some anaphylactic reactions have been described for which no specific IgE antibodies or mast cell degranulation (e.g., tryptase elevations) could be detected. Some of these cases might reflect immunoglobulin-independent activation of inflammatory cells. However, some investigators have speculated that the mechanism might be the well characterized IgG/FcγRIII/macrophage/PAF interaction observed in murine anaphylaxis. Human IgG receptors are capable of activating macrophages to secrete PAF, thus enabling potential FcγRIII-dependent anaphylaxis [7].

Chemical Mediators of Anaphylaxis

Biochemical mediators and chemotactic substances are released systemically during anaphylaxis by the degranulation of mast cells and basophils. These include preformed granule-associated substances such as histamine, tryptase, chymase, and heparin; histamine-releasing factor and other cytokines; and newly generated lipid-derived mediators such as prostaglandin D_2, leukotriene B_4, PAF, and the cysteinyl leukotrienes, LTC_4, LTD_4, and LTE_4 [2].

The development and severity of anaphylaxis also depend on the responsiveness of cells targeted by these mediators. IL-4 and IL-13 are cytokines important in the initial generation of antibody and inflammatory cell responses to anaphylaxis. No comparable studies have been conducted in humans, but anaphylactic effects in the mouse depend on IL-4Rα-dependent IL-4/IL-13 activation of the transcription factor, signal transducer and activator of transcription 6 (STAT-6). The most rapid, dramatic effect of IL-4 on murine anaphylaxis is a three- to sixfold increase in responsiveness of targeted cells to inflammatory and vasoactive mediators, including histamine, cysteinyl leukotrienes, serotonin, and PAF [7].

Eosinophils may be pro-inflammatory (e.g., release of cytotoxic granule-associated proteins) or anti-inflammatory (e.g., metabolism of vasoactive mediators) [9, 10]. A guinea-pig anaphylaxis model suggests that eosinophils already present in chronically inflamed airways may participate in the immediate phase response to allergen exposure, as well as the role traditionally expected in the late-phase allergic response [11]. Potential implications for anaphylaxis in humans have not been studied.

Histamine and Tryptase

Histamine activates H_1 and H_2 receptors. Pruritus, rhinorrhea, tachycardia, and bronchospasm are caused by activation of the H_1 receptors, whereas both H_1 and H_2 receptors mediate headache, flushing, and hypotension [12].

H_3 receptors have been implicated in the canine model of anaphylaxis [13]. These inhibitory presynaptic receptors modulate release of endogenous norepinephrine from sympathetic fibers that innervate the cardiovascular system. Pretreatment of study animals with the H_3 receptor antagonist, thioperamide maleate, is associated with a higher heart rate and greater left ventricular systolic function compared to the non-treatment group or the other treatment arms involving receptor blockade for H_1, H_2, cyclooxygenase, and leukotriene pathways [13]. Potential implications for human subjects and anaphylaxis have not been studied.

Tryptase is concentrated selectively in the secretory granules of human mast cells and is released when these cells degranulate. It can activate complement, coagulation pathways, and the kallikrein-kinin contact system with the potential clinical consequences of hypotension, angioedema, clotting, and clot lysis (disseminated intravascular coagulation) [10]. Release of β-tryptase (mature tryptase) stored in mast cell secretory granules is more specific for activation than α-protryptase, which is an inactive monomer. Levels of total tryptase peak 60–90 min after the onset of anaphylaxis and can persist as long as 5 h after the onset of symptoms [10]. Tryptase levels generally correlate with the clinical severity of anaphylaxis [14]. However, a dichotomy seems to exist in the magnitude of tryptase elevations for those individuals experiencing anaphylaxis after parenteral exposure (e.g., injection, insect sting) versus oral exposure (e.g., food ingestion). In an analysis of anaphylaxis fatalities, the parenterally exposed subjects had higher serum levels of tryptase and lower levels of antigen-specific IgE, whereas those who succumbed after oral challenge had low tryptase levels and comparatively high levels of antigen-specific IgE [15]. This difference may be related to the mast cell phenotype first encountered by the culprit antigen. Tryptase- and chymase-containing (MC_{TC}) mast cells have approximately threefold predominance in connective tissue over tryptase-containing (MC_T) mast cells, whereas the latter cells predominate in the mucosa of the lung and small intestine [15].

Elevations of histamine and tryptase may not correlate clinically. In an emergency department study evaluating subjects who presented with acute allergic reactions, elevated histamine was observed in 42 of 97 subjects but only 20 exhibited increased tryptase levels [16]. Serum histamine levels also correlate with the severity and persistence of cardiopulmonary manifestations but not with the formation of urticaria [16, 17].

Possibly because fatal anaphylaxis can occur quickly, many subjects have no distinguishing gross pathologic features at autopsy [18]. Post-mortem measurements of serum tryptase may be useful in establishing anaphylaxis as the cause of death in subjects experiencing sudden death of uncertain cause [15, 19, 20]. However, post-mortem tryptase levels have also been reported in non-anaphylactic fatalities, including those due to sudden infant death syndrome, trauma, and heroin injection, all of which can cause mast cell degranulation [10, 21–24]. Thus, the practical utility for post-mortem measurement of tryptase is likely limited to confirming anaphylaxis fatalities where clinically suspected.

Metabolites of arachidonic acid include products of the lipoxygenase and cyclooxygenase pathways. Of note, leukotriene B_4 is a chemotactic agent and thus theoretically may contribute to the late phase of anaphylaxis and to protracted reactions [10].

Nitric Oxide in Anaphylaxis

Nitric oxide (NO), a potent autacoid vasodilator, is apparently involved in the complex interaction of regulatory and counter-regulatory mediators in mast cell activation, including anaphylaxis [25, 26]. *L*-arginine is converted to NO as histamine binds to H_1-receptors during phospholipase-C-dependent calcium mobilization. Physiologically, NO participates in the homeostatic control of vascular tone and regional blood pressure. However, its net effects in anaphylaxis appear to be detrimental vascular smooth muscle relaxation and enhanced vascular permeability [27].

NO may be produced endogenously by inducible nitric oxide synthase (iNOS) or by the constitutively expressed isoforms, endothelial NOS (eNOS) and neuronal NOS (nNOS). eNOS and nNOS presumably produce low amounts of NO for physiologic and/or anti-inflammatory functions, whereas inflammation-associated expression of iNOS and subsequent overproduction of NO and activation of guanylate cyclase have been implicated in the cardiovascular morbidity and mortality associated with septic shock. It has widely been presumed that this mechanism also applies in anaphylaxis [28].

Cauwels and colleagues, however, suggest that eNOS, rather than iNOS, is a critical mediator of anaphylactic shock experimentally produced by injecting mice with PAF [29]. eNOS-knockout mice survived PAF injection and soluble guanylate cyclase inhibitors had no effect on the anaphylaxis. Induction of phosphoinositide 3-kinase (PI3K) and protein kinase Akt-mediated phosphorylation were absolutely protective. The authors conclude PAF anaphylaxis in mice depends on PI3K/Akt and eNOS-derived NO [29].

Other Inflammatory Pathways Are Probably Important

During severe episodes of anaphylaxis, activation of complement, coagulation pathways, and the kallikrein-kinin contact system also occurs. Much of the supporting evidence derives from data obtained during experimental insect sting challenges. Decreases in C4 and C3 and generation of C3a have been observed in anaphylaxis. The lectin pathway (innate immune response) of complement activation does not appear to be involved [30]. Demonstrable evidence for coagulation pathway activation during severe anaphylaxis includes decreases in factor V, factor VIII, and fibrinogen, and fatal disseminated intravascular coagulation in some instances [3, 17]. Decreased high molecular weight kininogen and the formation of kallikrein-C1 inhibitor and factor XIIa-C1 inhibitor complexes indicate contact system activation [17, 31]. Kallikrein activation not only generates bradykinin but also activates factor XII. Factor XII itself can cause clotting and clot lysis via plasmin formation, an action which itself can activate complement.

In contrast, some mediators may have anti-inflammatory, modulatory effects that limit anaphylaxis. For example, chymase may facilitate the conversion of angiotensin I to angiotensin II, theoretically helping to counteract hypotension during anaphylaxis. Heparin opposes complement activation, modulates tryptase activity, and inhibits clotting, plasmin, and kallikrein [10, 17, 32].

Shock Organs in Anaphylaxis

Organ system involvement, which varies from species to species, determines the clinical course of anaphylaxis of whatever etiology. Factors that determine a specific "shock organ" include variations in the immune response; the location of smooth muscle; and the distribution and rate of degradation and responsiveness to chemical mediators [33]. In the guinea pig there is bronchial smooth muscle constriction, which leads to bronchospasm, hypoxemia, and death [34, 35]. Anaphylaxis in rabbits produces fatal pulmonary artery vasoconstriction with right ventricular failure [35, 36]. The primary shock organ in the dog is the venous system of the liver which contracts and produces severe hepatic congestion [35]. In humans, the predominant shock organs are the lung and the heart, and fatalities are divided equally between respiratory arrest and circulatory collapse [3, 37].

The Heart as Shock Organ in Anaphylaxis

Chemical mediators of anaphylaxis appear to affect the myocardium directly [17, 38]. H_1 receptors mediate coronary artery vasoconstriction and increase vascular permeability, whereas H_2 receptors increase atrial and ventricular contractile forces, atrial rate, and coronary artery vasodilation. The interaction of H_1 and H_2 receptor stimulation appears to mediate decreased diastolic pressure and increased pulse pressure [39]. Animal studies suggest a possible modulatory role for H_3 receptors [13]. Platelet-activating factor (PAF) also decreases coronary blood flow, delays atrioventricular conduction, and has depressor effects on the heart [40].

Anaphylaxis has been associated clinically with myocardial ischemia and with conduction defects, atrial and ventricular arrhythmias, and T-wave abnormalities [40]. Whether such changes are related to direct mediator effects on the myocardium, or to exacerbation of pre-existing myocardial insufficiency by the hemodynamic stress of anaphylaxis, or to either exogenous (therapeutically administered) or endogenous epinephrine is unclear [17, 38, 40, 41]. Raper and Fisher describe two previously healthy subjects who developed profound myocardial depression during anaphylaxis [38]. Echocardiography, nuclear imaging, and hemodynamic measurements confirmed the presence of myocardial dysfunction. The anaphylaxis treatment was supplemented with intra-aortic balloon counter-pulsation to provide hemodynamic support. Balloon counter-pulsation was required for up to 72 h because of persistent myocardial depression, even though other clinical signs of anaphylaxis resolved. Both subjects recovered with no subsequent evidence of myocardial dysfunction. Thus, the heart can be the primary target of anaphylaxis, even in subjects with no prior cardiovascular disease.

In a retrospective review of pre-hospital anaphylactic fatalities in the United Kingdom, the postural history was known for ten individuals [42]. Four of the ten fatalities were associated with the assumption of an upright or sitting posture and postmortem findings were consistent with pulseless electrical activity and an "empty heart" attributed to reduced venous return from vasodilation and concomitant volume redistribution.

Increased vascular permeability during anaphylaxis can transfer up to 35% of the intravascular fluid into the extravascular space within 10 min [43]. This shift in effective blood volume causes compensatory catecholamine and endothelin release and activates the renin-angiotensin-aldosterone system [31, 44, 45], all of which have variable clinical effects. Some subjects experience abnormal elevations of peripheral vascular resistance (maximal vasoconstriction yet shock persists due to diminished intravascular volume) [46], while others have decreased systemic vascular resistance, despite elevated levels of catecholamines [47]. These differences have important clinical implications since the latter scenario may respond favorably to therapeutic doses of vasoconstrictor agents while the former is vasoconstrictor-unresponsive and requires large-volume fluid resuscitation.

Non-pharmacologic Myocardial Ischemia in Anaphylaxis

Since mast cells accumulate at sites of coronary atherosclerotic plaques, some investigators have suggested that anaphylaxis may promote plaque rupture, thus risking myocardial ischemia [48, 49]. Stimulation of the H_1 histamine receptor may also produce coronary artery vasospasm [49–51].

Calcitonin gene-related peptide (CGRP) released during anaphylaxis may help to counteract coronary artery vasoconstriction during anaphylaxis [52, 53]. CGRP, a sensory neurotransmitter widely distributed in cardiovascular tissues, relaxes vascular smooth muscle and has cardioprotective effects in animal models of anaphylaxis [54].

Bradycardia During Anaphylaxis

Tachycardia is the rule, but bradycardia may occur during anaphylaxis and thus may not be as useful to distinguish anaphylaxis from a vasodepressor reaction as previously presumed. Relative bradycardia (initial tachycardia followed by a reduction in heart rate despite worsening hypotension) has been reported previously in experimental settings such as insect sting anaphylaxis [17, 31, 55].

Two distinct phases of physiologic response occur in mammals subjected to hypovolemia. The initial phase is a baroreceptor-mediated sympatho-excitatory response comprised of increased cardiac sympathetic drive and simultaneous withdrawal of resting vagal drive, which together produce tachycardia and peripheral vasoconstriction [56]. When effective blood volume falls by 20–30%, a second phase follows which is characterized by withdrawal of vasoconstrictor drive, relative or absolute bradycardia, increased vasopressin, further catecholamine release as the adrenal axis becomes more active, and hypotension [56, 57]. Atropine administered therapeutically in this hypovolemic scenario reverses the bradycardia but not the hypotension.

Conduction defects and sympatholytic medications may also produce bradycardia [2]. Excessive venous pooling with decreased venous return (also seen in vasodepressor reactions) may activate tension-sensitive sensory receptors in the infero-posterior portions of the left ventricle, thus resulting in a cardio-inhibitory (Bezold-Jarisch) reflex that stimulates the vagus nerve and causes bradycardia [10].

Conclusion

Anaphylaxis is complex and involves numerous immunopathologic mechanisms and interactions. Well-characterized animal models clearly would facilitate a better understanding of the pathophysiologic mechanisms of anaphylaxis and might ultimately assist in diagnosis and treatment, particularly of anaphylactic shock.

References

1. Sampson HA, Muñoz-Furlong A, Campbell RL, et al. (2006) Second symposium on the definition and management of anaphylaxis: summary report. J Allergy Clin Immunol 117: 391–7.
2. Kemp SF, Lockey RF (2002) Anaphylaxis: a review of causes and mechanisms. J Allergy Clin Immunol 110:341–8.
3. Pumphrey R (2004) Anaphylaxis: can we tell who is at risk of a fatal reaction? Curr Opin Allergy Clin Immunol 4:285–90.
4. Johansson SGO, Bieber T, Dahl R, et al. (2004) Revised nomenclature for allergy for global use: report of the Nomenclature Review Committee of the World Allergy Organization, October 2003. J Allergy Clin Immunol 113:832–6.
5. Coombs RRA, Gell PGH (1975) Classification of allergic reactions responsible for clinical hypersensitivity and disease. In: Gell PGH, Coombs RRA, Lachmann PJ (eds) Clinical Aspects of Immunology, 3rd ed. Blackwell Scientific, Oxford, pp. 761–81.
6. Sell S (1996) Immunopathology. In: Rich RR, Fleisher TA, Schwartz BD, Shearer WT, Strober W (eds) Clinical Immunology: Principles and Practice. Mosby, St. Louis, MO, pp. 449–77.
7. Finkelman FD, Rothenberg ME, Brandt EB, et al. (2005) Molecular mechanisms of anaphylaxis: lessons from studies with murine models. J Allergy Clin Immunol 115:449–57.
8. Strait RT, Morris SC, Finkelman FD (2006) IgG blocking antibodies inhibit IgE-mediated anaphylaxis in vivo through both antigen interruption and FcγRIIb cross-linking. J Clin Invest 116:833–41.
9. Goetzl EJ, Wasserman SI, Austin KF (1975) Eosinophil polymorphonuclear leukocyte function in immediate hypersensitivity. Arch Pathol 99:1–4.
10. Lieberman P (2003) Anaphylaxis and anaphylactoid reactions. In: Adkinson NF Jr, Yunginger JW, Busse WW, et al. (eds) Middleton's Allergy: Principles and Practice, 6th ed. Mosby-Year Book, St. Louis, MO, pp. 1497–1522.
11. Erjefält JS, Korsgren M, Malm-Erjefält M, et al. (2003) Acute allergic responses induce a prompt luminal entry of airway tissue eosinophils. Am J Respir Cell Mol Biol 29:439–48.
12. Kaliner M, Sigler R, Summers R, Shelhamer JH (1981) Effects of infused histamine: analysis of the effects of H-1 and H-2 receptor antagonists on cardiovascular and pulmonary responses. J Allergy Clin Immunol 68:365–71.
13. Chrusch C, Sharma S, Unruh H, Bautista E, Duke E, Becker A, et al. (1999) Histamine H3 receptor blockade improves cardiac function in canine anaphylaxis. Am J Respir Crit Care Med 160:142–9.
14. Schwartz LB (2004) Effector cells of anaphylaxis: mast cells and basophils. Novartis Found Symp 257:65–74.

15. Yunginger JW, Nelson DR, Squillace DL, et al. (1991) Laboratory investigations of death due to anaphylaxis. J Forensic Sci 36:857–65.
16. Lin RY, Schwartz LB, Curry A, et al. (2000) Histamine and tryptase levels in patients with acute allergic reactions: an emergency department-based study. J Allergy Clin Immunol 106:65–71.
17. Smith PL, Kagey-Sobotka A, Bleecker ER, Traystman R, Kaplan AP, Gralnick H, et al. (1980) Physiologic manifestations of human anaphylaxis. J Clin Invest 66:1072–80.
18. Pumphrey RS, Roberts IS (2000) Postmortem findings after fatal anaphylactic reactions. J Clin Pathol 53:273–6.
19. Ansari MQ, Zamora JL, Lipscomb MF (1993) Postmortem diagnosis of acute anaphylaxis by serum tryptase analysis. A case report. Am J Clin Pathol 99:101–3.
20. Schwartz HJ, Yunginger JW, Schwartz LB (1995) Is unrecognized anaphylaxis a cause of sudden unexpected death? Clin Exp Allergy 25:866–70.
21. Platt MS, Yunginger JW, Sekula-Perlman A, Irani AM, et al. (1994) Involvement of mast cells in sudden infant death syndrome. J Allergy Clin Immunol 94:250–6.
22. Randall B, Butts J, Halsey JF (1995) Elevated postmortem tryptase in the absence of anaphylaxis. J Forensic Sci 40:208–11.
23. Edston E, van Hage-Hamsten M (1998) β-Tryptase measurements post-mortem in anaphylactic deaths and in controls. Forensic Sci Int 93:135–42.
24. Edston E, Gidlund E, Wickman M, Ribbing H, van Hage-Hamsten M (1999) Increased mast cell tryptase in sudden infant death – anaphylaxis, hypoxemia or artifact? Clin Exp Allergy 29:1648–54.
25. Palmer RMJ, Ferrige AG, Moncada S (1987) Nitric oxide release accounts for the biological activity of endothelium derived relaxing factor. Nature 327:524–6.
26. Coleman JW (2002) Nitric oxide: a regulator of mast cell activation and mast cell-mediated inflammation. Clin Exp Immunol 129:4–10.
27. Mitsuhata H, Shimizu R, Yokoyama MM (1995) Role of nitric oxide in anaphylactic shock. J Clin Immunol 15:277–83.
28. Lowenstein CJ, Michel T (2006) What's in a name? eNOS and anaphylactic shock. J Clin Invest 116:2075–8.
29. Cauwels A, Janssen B, Buys E, et al. (2006) Anaphylactic shock depends on PI3K and eNOS-derived NO. J Clin Invest 116:2244–51.
30. Windbichler M, Echtenacher B, Takahashi K, et al. (2006) Investigations on the involvement of the lectin pathway of complement activation in anaphylaxis. Int Arch Allergy Immunol 141:11–23.
31. van der Linden P-WG, Struyvenberg A, Kraaijenhagen RJ, Hack CE, van der Zwan JK (1993) Anaphylactic shock after insect-sting challenge in 138 persons with a previous insect-sting reaction. Ann Intern Med 118:161–8.
32. Kaplan AP, Joseph K, Silverberg M (2002) Pathways for bradykinin formation and inflammatory disease. J Allergy Clin Immunol 109:195–209.
33. James LP Jr, Austen KF (1964) Fatal and systemic anaphylaxis in man. N Engl J Med 270:597–603.
34. Warren S, Dixon FJ (1948) Antigen tracer studies and histologic observations in anaphylactic shock in the guinea pig. Part 1. Am J Med Sci 216:136–45.
35. Lockey RF, Bukantz SC (1974) Allergic emergencies. Med Clin North Am 58:147–56.
36. Coca AF (1919) The mechanism of the anaphylaxis reaction in the rabbit. J Immunol 4:219–31.
37. Greenberger PA, Rotskoff BD, Lifschultz B (2007) Fatal anaphylaxis: postmortem findings and associated comorbid diseases. Ann Allergy Asthma Immunol 98:252–7.
38. Raper RF, Fisher MM (1988) Profound reversible myocardial depression after anaphylaxis. Lancet 1:386–8.
39. Bristow MR, Ginsburg R, Harrison DC (1982) Histamine and the human heart: the other receptor system. Am J Cardiol 49:249–51.

40. Marone G, Bova M, Detoraki A, et al. (2004) The human heart as a shock organ in anaphylaxis. Novartis Found Symp 257:133–49.
41. Wittstein IS, Thiemann DR, Lima JAC, et al. (2005) Neurohumoral features of myocardial stunning due to sudden emotional stress. N Engl J Med 352:539–48.
42. Pumphrey RS (2003) Fatal posture in anaphylactic shock. J Allergy Clin Immunol 112:451–2.
43. Fisher MM (1986) Clinical observations on the pathophysiology and treatment of anaphylactic cardiovascular collapse. Anaesth Intensive Care 14:17–21.
44. Hermann K, Rittweger R, Ring J (1992) Urinary excretion of angiotensin I, II, arginine vasopressin and oxytocin in patients with anaphylactoid reactions. Clin Exp Allergy 22:845–53.
45. von Tschirschnitz M, von Eschenbach CE, Hermann K, Ring J (1993) Plasma angiotensin II in patients with Hymenoptera venom allergy during hyposensitization [abstract]. J Allergy Clin Immunol 91:283.
46. Hanashiro PK, Weil MH (1967) Anaphylactic shock in man: report of two cases with detailed hemodynamics and metabolic studies. Arch Intern Med 119:129–40.
47. Fahmy NR (1981) Hemodynamics, plasma histamine and catecholamine concentrations during an anaphylactoid reaction to morphine. Anesthesiology 55:329–31.
48. Kovanen PT, Kaartinen M, Paavonen T (1995) Infiltrates of activated mast cells at the site of coronary atheromatous erosion or rupture in myocardial infarction. Circulation 92:1084–8.
49. Kounis NG (2006) Kounis syndrome (allergic angina and allergic myocardial infarction): a natural paradigm? Int J Cardiol 110:7–14.
50. Abela GS, Picon PD, Friedl SE, Gebara OC, Miyamoto A, Federman M, et al. (1995) Triggering of plaque disruption and arterial thrombosis in an atherosclerotic rabbit model. Circulation 91:776–84.
51. Steffel J, Akhmedov A, Greutert H, et al. (2005) Histamine induces tissue factor expression: implications for acute coronary syndromes. Circulation 112:341–9.
52. Rubin LE, Levi R (1995) Protective role of bradykinin in cardiac anaphylaxis: coronary-vasodilating and antiarrhythmic activities mediated by autocrine/paracrine mechanisms. Circulation Research 76:434–40.
53. Schuligoi R, Amann R, Donnerer J, Peskar BA (1997) Release of calcitonin gene-related peptide in cardiac anaphylaxis. Naunyn-Schmiedeberg's Arch Pharmacol 355:224–9.
54. Rang WQ, Du YH, Hu CP, et al. (2003) Protective effects of calcitonin gene-related peptide-mediated evodiamine on guinea-pig cardiac anaphylaxis. Naunyn-Schmiedeberg's Arch Pharmacol 367:306–11.
55. Brown SGA, Blackman KE, Stenlake V, Heddle RJ (2004) Insect sting anaphylaxis: prospective evaluation of treatment with intravenous adrenaline and volume resuscitation. Emerg Med J 21:149–54.
56. Schadt JC, Ludbrook J (1991) Hemodynamic and neurohumoral responses to acute hypovolemia in conscious mammals. Am J Physiol 260:H305–18.
57. Demetriades D, Chan LS, Bhasin P, et al. (1998) Relative bradycardia in patients with traumatic hypotension. J Trauma 45:534–9.

Drug Hypersensitivity: Clinical Manifestations and Diagnosis

Pascal Demoly and Antonino Romano

Introduction

Drug hypersensitivity reactions (DHRs) represent the adverse effects of certain drugs, which clinically resemble allergy and are provoked by a dose tolerated by normal subjects. The revised nomenclature for allergy classifies allergic reactions to drugs as IgE-mediated or non-IgE-mediated [1]. However, numerous reactions with symptoms suggestive of allergy are often erroneously considered to be real drug allergies. They occur in a small percentage of patients only and are generally not predictable. The aetiologies of these reactions include non-specific histamine release (e.g., by opiates, radiocontrast media, and vancomycin), bradykinin accumulation (induced by angiotensin-converting enzyme inhibitors), complement activation (by protamine), induction of leukotriene synthesis (by aspirin and other non steroidal anti-inflammatory agents) and bronchospasm (e.g., that induced by SO_2 released by drug preparations containing sulfites). In most cases, the underlying disease is the cause of the exanthema (e.g., in the case of an upper respiratory tract infection) or, since drugs are often taken during meals, a food allergy may be involved.

DHRs may represent up to one-third of adverse drug reactions. They can be life-threatening, require or prolong hospitalisation, and entail changes in the drug prescription [2]. They concern more than 7% of the general population and therefore represent an important public health problem [3]. Both under-diagnosis (due to under-reporting [4, 5]) and over-diagnosis (due to the over-use of the term "allergy" [6]) have to be considered. Misclassification based on the drug allergy history may have consequences on individual treatment choices, and can lead to the use of more expensive and less effective drugs. Clinical manifestations are heterogeneous and range from maculopapular exanthema to anaphylactic shock, which may be fatal (Table 1) [7].

P. Demoly (✉)
Professor and Head, Allergy Department, Meladies Respiratories-Hôpital Arnaud de Villeneuve, University Hospital of Montpellier-Inserm U657, 34295 Montpellier cedex 05-France
e-mail: demoly@montp.inserm.fr

A. Romano
Unità di Allergologia, Complesso Integrato Columbus, via G. Moscati, 31, I-00168 Rome, Italy; IRCCS Oasi Maria S.S., Troina, Italy

R. Pawankar et al. (eds.), *Allergy Frontiers: Clinical Manifestations,*
DOI: 10.1007/978-4-431-88317-3_24, © Springer 2009

Table 1 Classification of drug hypersensitivities (Adapted from [7])

Type	Type of immune response	Pathophysiology	Clinical symptoms	Chronology of the reaction
I	IgE	Mast cells and basophil degranulation	Anaphylactic shock	A few minutes to 1 h after the last intake of the drug
			Angio-oedema Urticaria Bronchospasm	
II	IgG and FcR	FcR-dependent cell death	Cytopenia	5–15 days after the start of treatment
III	IgM or IgG and complement or FcR	Deposition of immune complexes	Serum sickness	7–8 days for serum sickness
			Urticaria	
			Vasculitis	7–21 days after the start of treatment for vasculitis
IVa	Th1 (IFNγ)	Monocytic inflammation	Eczema	5–21 days after the start of treatment
IVb	Th2 (IL-5 and IL-4)	Eosinophilic inflammation	Maculo-papular exanthema, bullous exanthema	2–6 weeks after the start of treatment for DRESS
IVc	Cytotoxic T cells (perforin, granzyme B, FasL)	Keratinocyte death mediated by CD4 or CD8	Maculo-papular exanthema, bullous exanthema, pustular exanthema	2 days after the start of treatment for fixed drug eruption, 7–21 days after the start of treatment for Stevens-Johnson syndrome and TEN
IVd	T cells (IL-8/ CXCL8)	Neutrophilic inflammation	Acute generalised exanthematous pustulosis	Less than 2 days

Currently, to evaluate DHRs it is important to distinguish between immediate and non-immediate reactions. The former occur within the first hour after the last drug administration and are manifested clinically by urticaria, angioedema, rhinitis, bronchospasm, and anaphylactic shock. Non-immediate reactions occur more than 1 h after the last drug administration. The main non-immediate reactions are maculopapular eruptions and delayed-appearing urticaria/angioedema.

The diagnosis of hypersensitivity reactions to drugs requires knowledge of the scientific literature with, for the more recently introduced drugs, access to Medline searches and to the Committee on Safety of Medicine Reports. The lack of case studies involving a particular compound does not mean that it cannot induce allergic reactions. The diagnosis is actually based on the history, clinical manifestations, and, if possible, skin tests and biological tests. Few available clinical and biological tools are available and not all of them have been fully evaluated. Moreover, a definite diagnosis of DHRs is required in order to take the proper preventive measures.

Under the aegis of the *European Academy of Allergology and Clinical Immunology* (www.eaaci.net), the *European Network of Drug Allergy* (ENDA) is working towards the establishment of diagnostic tools in daily practice.

Clinical History

Clinical history should be extremely thorough and should take into account the symptomatology, any previous exposure, the time elapsed between the last dose and the onset of symptoms, the effect of stopping treatment, any other medication involved (both at the time of the reaction and since), and the general medical background of the patient. Data should be recorded in a uniform format, such as the questionnaire developed by the ENDA [8], which is available in many different languages (Annex 1). Diagnosis is more difficult when patients are not seen during the acute phase, in which case photographs are helpful. When patients are seen during the reaction, the suspected drugs should be stopped, particularly if danger signs such as widespread bullous or hemorrhagic lesions or mucosal affections are present (Table 2) [9].

The main limits of the history are incompleteness, the lack of accuracy and the erroneous attribution of responsibility to a certain drug. Moreover, the clinical picture of drug allergy is very heterogeneous, mirroring many distinct pathophysiological events. Thus, for drug allergy diagnosis, many doctors rely on the history and various reference manuals. They do not attempt to prove the relationship between the drug intake and the symptoms or to clarify the underlying pathomechanism of the reaction. Such an attitude leads to a misunderstanding of the epidemiology and the pathophysiology of this highly important field. In cases where a hypersensitivity reaction is suspected, if the drug is essential and/or frequently prescribed (e.g., β-lactams and non-steroidal anti-inflammatory drugs (NSAIDs)), a certified

Table 2 Clinical and biological danger signs suggesting severe cutaneous and/or systemic reactions (Adapted from [9])

Centrofacial oedema
Dysphonia, hypersialorrhea (laryngeal angioedema)
Drop in blood pressure
Involvement of extended body surface (>60%)
Painful skin
Atypical target lesions
Positive Nikolsky's sign
Epidermolysis, vesicles, bulla
Hemorrhagic or necrotic lesions
Mucosal erosions or aphtous lesions
Systemic signs (high fever, malaise)
Blood cytopenia
Eosinophilia
Affection of internal organs: hepatic cytolysis, proteinuria

Table 3 Allergy tests according to clinical symptoms (Adapted from [9])

Clinical symptoms	Potential pathogenesis	Diagnostic tests
Urticaria Angioedema	Type I allergy, non-allergic hypersensitivity, rarely: type III allergy	Prick and intradermal tests, specific IgE assays, and mediator release/cellular tests (BAT)
Anaphylaxis	Type I allergy, non-allergic hypersensitivity	Prick and intradermal tests, specific IgE assays, and mediator release/cellular tests (BAT)
Maculopapular exanthem	Type IV allergy	Patch and late-reading intradermal tests, LTT, and LTA
Vesicular-bullous exanthem	Type IV allergy	Patch tests, LTT, and LTA
Pustular exanthem	Type IV allergy	Patch and late-reading intradermal tests, LTT, and LTA
Fixed drug eruption	Type IV allergy	Patch tests in the affected area

BAT, flow cytometry basophil activation test; LTT, lymphocyte transformation test; LTA, lymphocyte activation test

diagnosis should be performed and tests should be carried out in a specialised centre. Only a formal diagnosis of drug hypersensitivity reactions allows the measures required for prevention and treatment to be brought into play. For these drugs, the prudent principle of avoidance of the suspect drug may be insufficient. This procedure could lead to the exclusion of drugs that do not necessarily give rise to reactions and are widely used. However, such exclusion is a valid option until a specialist consultation can be scheduled.

The specific allergy diagnosis should be carried out 4 weeks after the complete clearing of all clinical symptoms and signs. On the other hand, after a time interval longer than 6–12 months, some drug tests may have turned negative, resulting in false negative results. According to the clinical manifestations, a hypothesis on pathogenesis should be generated (Table 3) to select appropriate testing procedures [9, 10].

Skin and Patch Tests

Skin tests are the most common form of allergy testing. Because of their greater sensitivity, skin tests cannot yet be replaced by *in vitro* tests. However, the diagnostic value of skin tests has not been fully assessed for all drugs, and the different centres have rarely shared their experiences over the past decades. Skin tests have to be performed according to the suspected pathomechanism. Both immediate-reading prick and intradermal tests are particularly important in the diagnosis of an IgE-dependent mechanism. They should be performed 4–6 weeks after the reaction. The prick test is recommended for initial screening due to its simplicity, safety, and high specificity. Intradermal tests are accomplished by injecting 0.02–0.03 ml of an allergen intradermally, raising a small bleb measuring 3 mm in diameter. Readings should be taken after 15–20 min, if immediate reactions are analysed, and after 24 and 72 h for evaluation of non-immediate (late) reactions. In selected cases, additional readings (e.g., after 96 h) are sometimes recommended, as time intervals between testing and positive test reactions may vary [10].

Patch, or epicutaneous, testing is useful in diagnosing cases of eczematous contact forms of allergy like those observed in pharmaceutical workers. Patch-test positivity can also occur in non-immediate cutaneous reactions to systemically administered drugs like penicillins and anticonvulsants [10–12].

In a patch, test the allergen is usually applied on the back of the patient for 2 days by using Finn Chambers or an equivalent fixed with "hypoallergic" tape. Readings should be done when the patch test is removed, and 1 day later. Additional readings after 96 h or more might also be needed in some cases. Sometimes reactions occur earlier or much later (as in the case of corticosteroids and phenylephrine). Patients should be instructed to report any reactions occurring earlier or later to the doctor. Scoring is done according to international standards [10].

Skin-test sensitivity and predictive values vary, depending on the culprit drug; in any case, it is high for penicillins, muscle relaxants, heterologous sera, and enzymes.

With regard to β-lactams, a recent article by Blanca et al. [13] reviewed the results of skin tests in the hypersensitivity to these antibiotics and provided evidence for their continued need. In both the ENDA position paper [14] and the American practice parameters [15], skin testing with penicilloyl-polylysine (PPL) and minor determinant mixture (MDM) represents the first-line method for diagnosing immediate hypersensitivity reactions to β-lactams. In most countries, however, these classic penicillin reagents are not available because Allergopharma and Hollister-Stier ceased their production in 2004. Nevertheless, two recent studies [16, 17] proved that the penicillin reagents (PPL and MDM) produced in Spain by Diater (DAP, Madrid, Spain) are a reliable and safe alternative to the Allergopharma ones, with a very similar specificity and sensitivity.

In evaluating subjects with immediate reactions to β-lactams, the aforesaid protocols [14, 15] recommend the use of benzyl-penicillin, amoxicillin, ampicillin, and any other suspect β-lactam, in addition to PPL and MDM.

With regard to cephalosporins, recent studies have contributed to the standardisation of skin testing with these β-lactams and to proving its usefulness in evaluating subjects with immediate reactions to cephalosporins [18–20].

Skin testing with cephalosporins, as well as with carbapenems, is also useful in discovering safe alternatives in penicillin-allergic subjects. In a study regarding 128 patients with a well-established IgE-mediated hypersensitivity to penicillins [21], all 101 patients who displayed negative skin tests for cefuroxime, ceftazidime, ceftriaxone, and cefotaxime and accepted challenges with cefuroxime axetil and ceftriaxone tolerated them. In two of our recent studies [22, 23], we found a 0.9% rate of positive responses to skin tests with imipenem/cilastatin and meropenem among 112 and 104 adults, respectively, with a well-demonstrated IgE-mediated hypersensitivity to penicillins. In these two studies [22, 23], all negative subjects who agreed to imipenem/cilastatin and/or meropenem challenges tolerated them.

Skin tests continue to be regularly used in order to assess patients with immediate reactions during general anaesthesia, as well as to decrease the risk of such reactions by identifying patients sensitised to anaesthetic drugs and/or other compounds to be administered during the procedure and providing safe alternatives to them.

In this regard, the guidelines devised by the Société Française d'Anesthésie et de Réanimation and endorsed by the ENDA are available [24].

With regard to compounds other than muscle relaxants and β-lactams, the literature data suggest that immediate- and delayed-reading skin tests with iodinated contrast media (ICM) are appropriate in patients with severe immediate hypersensitivity reactions and in those with non-immediate skin reactions following administration of ICM, respectively [25, 26]. Kanny et al. [27] diagnosed a cell-mediated hypersensitivity in 12 patients with non-immediate reactions to ICM, mainly maculopapular eruptions, on the basis of positive responses to delayed-reading skin tests and/or patch tests, as well as to *in vitro* tests. In a study by Kvedariene et al. [28], which evaluated 44 consecutive patients with histories of ICM hypersensitivity by skin tests, 10 patients (23%) displayed positive responses: 8 had immediate positive responses, and 2 had delayed ones. Skin tests were more often positive in patients with immediate reactions (9 of 32) as compared with those with non-immediate ones (1 of 11). However, the sensitivity, specificity, and predictive value of ICM skin testing are not yet fully established, and are being addressed in a multi-centre ENDA study.

In a review by Bircher et al. regarding hypersensitivity reactions to anticoagulant drugs [29], skin tests with immediate and delayed readings are indicated as reliable diagnostic tools for evaluating subjects with heparin- or hirudins-induced urticaria/anaphylaxis or heparin-induced delayed plaques. However, skin testing is contraindicated if necrosis from heparins or coumarins is suspected.

A recent study by Leguy-Seguin et al. [30] proved that intradermal tests are a useful tool in evaluating subjects with immediate hypersensitivity reactions to platinum salts. Moreover, their high negative predictive value allows safe re-treatments by detecting alternatives to the positive compounds.

When the responsible allergen is not the parent drug, but a metabolite, it is crucial to test the latter, if available. A study by Popescu et al. [31] assessed five patients with delayed-onset, IgE-mediated hypersensitivity reactions to cyclophosphamide, by performing skin tests with the parent drug and its metabolites. All patients displayed positive responses to one or more metabolites, whereas none of them was positive to the parent drug.

With regard to the involvement of drug metabolites in cell-mediated reactions, Lee et al. [32] evaluated 13 patients who had suffered cutaneous reactions to carbamazepine by performing patch tests with the parent drug and its main metabolite, carbamazepine epoxide; 10 of the 13 patients were positive to patch tests, 2 of them only to the metabolite.

Provocation Tests

These remain the gold standard for the identification of a responsible drug when allergologic tests are negative, not available, or not validated. Provocation tests have the finest sensitivity, but can only be performed under the most rigorous surveillance conditions, and are therefore restricted to certain specialised centres with on-site intensive care facilities [33]. These tests are especially required for NSAIDs, local anaesthetics, antibiotics other than β-lactams, or β-lactams when skin tests and serum specific IgE assays are negative. They should be performed after a certain time interval following the hypersensitivity reaction (at least 1 month) using the same drug as in the initial case. The route of administration depends on the suspected drug. The precise challenge procedure varies a great deal from one team to another and guidelines for the performance of provocation tests in drug allergies have been proposed by the ENDA [33]. Recent studies, which performed drug provocation tests [34, 35], have confirmed the data of Messaad et al. [6], not only allowing drug hypersensitivity to be diagnosed, but also excluding it in more than 80% of reactions suffered by patients with negative results in skin tests and/ or *in vitro* tests. Provocation tests should not be performed if the responsible drug is infrequently used, or several alternatives exist. They are contraindicated in case of severe hypersensitivity reactions, such as the Stevens-Johnson syndrome, toxic epidermal necrolysis (TEN), acute generalised exanthematous pustolosis (AGEP), and drug reactions with eosinophilia and systemic symptoms (DRESS).

Biological Tests

Serum specific IgE assays (radioallergosorbent tests, or RAST, and immunoenzymatic assays, or ELISA) are still the most common *in vitro* methods for evaluating immediate reactions. These tests are available only for a few drugs, such as some β-lactams, muscle relaxants, and insulin. It should also be remembered that the results should be interpreted with caution. A negative test does not exclude the responsibility of the drug; in fact, the absence of specific circulating IgE does not rule out a diagnosis of allergy. The demonstration of isolated drug-specific IgE (to penicillins [36], muscle relaxants [37], chymopapain or tetanus toxoid, for example) by itself does not constitute a diagnosis of a drug allergy. However, in conjunction with clinical findings (e.g., typical symptoms of rapid onset), the IgE-dependent mechanism can be pinpointed [36].

Studies comparing skin tests and specific IgE assays indicate that the two methods are not totally equivalent. Although these *in vitro* tests appear to be less sensitive than skin testing, the aforesaid ENDA position paper [14] recommends them, because there are patients with immediate reactions displaying skin-test negativity and specific-IgE-assay positivity. Therefore, serum specific IgE assays can reduce the need for drug provocation tests. In an aforementioned study of ours [18], we performed sepharose-radioimmunoassays (sepharose-RIAs) with cefaclor and the responsible cephalosporins in 70 of 76 patients who had suffered immediate reactions, mostly anaphylactic shocks. Considering the positivity of at least one of the two sepharose-RIAs, specific IgE were detected in 47 (67.1%) of these 70 patients; 5 of them were skin-test negative and were not challenged.

Serum specific IgE assays are extremely useful when skin tests are not reliable, such as those performed with quinolones. Manfredi et al. [38] carried out a sepharose-RIA in 55 patients with immediate reactions to quinolones, detecting serum specific IgE in 54.5% of cases.

Cross-reactivity among several drugs may also be explored by using quantitative inhibition.

The release of histamine from whole blood in the presence of the drug correlates well with skin tests and specific IgE for muscle relaxants but is not reliable for many other drugs [39]. Moreover, it is costly and requires a high level of technical expertise. The usefulness of measuring sulfidopeptide leukotrienes still requires further validation in both IgE-dependent allergies and non-IgE-dependent hypersensitivity reactions [40]. In cases of acute clinical reactions, measurements of plasma histamine or serum tryptase could confirm the role played by basophils and mast cells, whatever the cause of the degranulation [41].

In patients with immediate reactions, a flow cytometric basophil activation test (BAT) to detect specific surface markers with monoclonal antibodies can also be carried out. At present, the most commonly used antigens in BATs are CD63, CD203c and CRTH2 (chemoattractant receptor-homologous molecule expressed on T-helper 2 cells) [42]. There is evidence that the BAT can contribute to the diagnosis of anaphylactic reactions to several drugs, particularly muscle relaxants, β-lactams, and NSAIDs [42–46].

As far as β-lactams are concerned, in two studies [44, 45] evaluating 58 and 70 patients, respectively, with immediate reactions to these antibiotics, BAT sensitivity was about 50% and specificity over 90%. However, additional comprehensive studies in large samples are needed in order to further validate the technique and provide a definitive evaluation of its sensitivity.

The measure of drug-specific IgM or IgG is of interest only in cases of drug-induced cytopenia or hypersensitivity reactions to dextrans. For drug-induced type II and III allergic reactions, the following tests can be performed: Coombs' test, the *in vitro* hemolysis test, the determination of complement factors and circulating immune complexes.

The lymphocyte transformation test (LTT) is a useful tool for evaluating cell-mediated hypersensitivity reactions, such as maculopapular exanthems, bullous disorders, AGEP, and DRESS induced by drugs like aminopenicillins, anticonvulsants, ICM, and quinolones [25, 47–49]. However, the LTT is frequently negative in patients with TEN, fixed drug eruptions, and vasculitis [48].

In the aforementioned study by Kanny et al. [27], patients with non-immediate hypersensitivity reactions to ICM were assessed not only by the LTT (three of four were positive), but also by a new *in vitro* method, the lymphocyte activation test (LAT). The LAT measured by means of cell-cycle analysis through DNA content was positive to the responsible ICM in one patient; the LAT measured by means of upregulation of the activation marker CD69 was positive to the culprit ICM in another one, and negative in a third patient. These results require confirmation in a larger sample of subjects.

Conclusion

The diagnosis of drug hypersensitivity often relies on clinical histories, skin tests, and a few validated *in vitro* tests, such as serum specific IgE assays, which are available only for a few drugs. The sensitivity of these tests is not absolute; in selected cases, therefore, provocation tests – which are the gold standard, but are also cumbersome and possibly harmful – are necessary. However, new diagnostic tools, such as the BAT and the LAT, have been developed and are under validation. Their routine use could increase the sensitivity of diagnostic work-ups, thus reducing the need for drug provocation tests.

A definite diagnosis of hypersensitivity reactions to drugs is required in order to take the proper preventive measures. Such measures include a declaration to the Committee on Safety of Medicine Reports, the issue of an "Allergy Card" specifying the culprit agent(s), and the delivery of both a list of drugs to avoid and a list of possible alternatives. The patient is also asked to make his or her allergies known prior to all prescriptions and surgical operations and to read the leaflet included with any drugs to be taken. The lists can never be exhaustive and should be frequently updated. Similarly, the questioning (to elicit any history of allergy) of each patient by each clinician prior to prescribing a drug is essential from both a medical and a legal point of view. Preventive measures by pre-medication (e.g., slow injection and preparations with glucocorticosteroids and anti-histamines) mainly concern non-allergic hypersensitivity reactions (for example, to vancomycin, certain anaesthetics, and chemotherapy drugs).

The possibility of desensitisation should always be considered when the offending drug is essential and no alternatives exist, as in the following cases: sulfonamides in HIV-infected patients [50], quinolone hypersensitivity in some cystic fibrosis patients, serious infections in patients allergic to penicillins, allergy to tetanus vaccine, hemochromatosis with allergy to desferoxamine, hypersensitivity to aspirin and other NSAIDs in patients for whom the necessity for these drugs to treat either a cardiac or rheumatoid illness is clear [51]. Rapid desensitisation protocols have also been performed for cancer patients with DHRs to chemotherapy agents, such as taxanes, platinum salts, doxorubicin, and monoclonal antibodies, when alternative regimens were limited by the tumor sensitivity and the need to provide first-line therapy [52].

References

1. Johansson S, Bieber T, Dahl R, et al. (2004) Revised nomenclature for allergy for global use: Report of the Nomenclature Review Committee of the World Allergy Organization, October 2003. J Allergy Clin Immunol 113:832–836
2. Gomes ER, Demoly P (2005) Epidemiology of hypersensitivity drug reactions. Curr Opin Allergy Clin Immunol 5:309–316

3. Gomes E, Cardoso MF, Praça F, et al. (2004) Self reported drug allergy in a general adult Portuguese population. Clin Exp Allergy 34:1597–1601

4. Backstrom M, Mjorndal, Dahlqvist R (2004) Under-reporting of serious adverse drug reactions in Sweden. Pharmacoepidemiol Drug Saf 13:483–487

5. Mittmann N, Knowles SR, Gomez M, et al. (2004) Evaluation of the extent of under-reporting of serious adverse drug reactions: the case of toxic epidermal necrolysis. Drug Saf 27:477–487

6. Messaad D, Sahla H, Benahmed S, et al. (2004) Drug provocation tests in patients with a history suggesting an immediate drug hypersensitivity reaction. Ann Intern Med 140:1001–1006

7. Pichler WJ (2003) Delayed drug hypersensitivity reactions. Ann Intern Med 139:683–693

8. Demoly P, Kropf R, Bircher A, Pichler WJ (1999) Drug hypersensitivity questionnaire. Allergy 54:999–1003

9. Bircher AJ (2005) Symptoms and danger signs in acute drug hypersensitivity. Toxicology 209:201–207

10. Brockow K, Romano A, Blanca M, et al. (2002) General considerations for skin test procedures in the diagnosis of drug hypersensitivity. Allergy 57:45–51

11. Barbaud A, Reichert-Penetrat S, Trechot P, et al. (1998) The use of skin testing in the investigation of cutaneous adverse drug reactions. Br J Dermatol 139:49–58

12. Romano A, Blanca M, Torres MJ, et al. (2004) Diagnosis of nonimmediate reactions to beta-lactam antibiotics. Allergy 59:1153–1160

13. Blanca M, Romano A, Torres MJ, et al. (2007) Continued need of appropriate betalactam-derived skin test reagents for the management of allergy to betalactams. Clin Exp Allergy 37:166–173

14. Torres MJ, Blanca M, Fernandez J, et al. (2003) Diagnosis of immediate allergic reactions to beta-lactam antibiotics. Allergy 58:961–972

15. Joint Task Force on Practice Parameters, the American Academy of Allergy, Asthma and Immunology, the American Academy of Allergy, Asthma and Immunology, and the Joint Council of Allergy, Asthma and Immunology (1999) Executive summary of disease management of drug hypersensitivity: a practice parameter. Ann Allergy Asthma Immunol 83:665–700

16. Rodríguez-Bada JL, Montañez MI, Torres MJ, et al. (2006) Skin testing for immediate hypersensitivity to betalactams: comparison between two commercial kits. Allergy 61:947–951

17. Romano A, Viola M, Bousquet JP, et al. (2007) A comparison of the performance of two penicillin reagent kits in the diagnosis of β-lactam hypersensitivity. Allergy 62:53–58

18. Romano A, Guéant-Rodriguez RM, Viola M, et al. (2005) Diagnosing immediate reactions to cephalosporins. Clin Exp Allergy 35:1234–1242

19. Antunez C, Blanca-Lopez N, Torres MJ, et al. (2006) Immediate allergic reactions to cephalosporins: evaluation of cross-reactivity with a panel of penicillins and cephalosporins. J Allergy Clin Immunol 117:404–410

20. Guéant JL, Guéant-Rodriguez RM, Viola, M et al. (2006) IgE-mediated hypersensitivity to cephalosporins. Curr Pharm Des 12:3335–3345

21. Romano A, Guéant-Rodriguez RM, Viola M, et al. (2004) Cross-reactivity and tolerability of cephalosporins in patients with immediate hypersensitivity to penicillins. Ann Intern Med 141:16–22

22. Romano A, Viola M, Guéant-Rodriguez RM, et al. (2006) Imipenem in patients with immediate hypersensitivity to penicillins [Letter]. N Engl J Med 354:2835–2837

23. Romano A, Viola M, Guéant-Rodriguez RM, et al. (2007) Brief communication: tolerability of meropenem in patients with IgE-mediated hypersensitivity to penicillins. Ann Intern Med 146:266–269

24. Mertes PM, Laxenaire MC, Lienhart A, et al. (2005) Reducing the risk of anaphylaxis during anaesthesia: guidelines for clinical practice. J Invest Allergy Clin Immunol 15:91–101

25. Brockow K, Christiansen C, Kanny G, et al. (2005) Management of hypersensitivity reactions to iodinated contrast media. Allergy 60:150–158

26. Guéant-Rodríguez RM, Romano A, Barbaud A, et al. (2006) Hypersensitivity reactions to iodinated contrast media. Curr Pharm Des 12:3359–3372
27. Kanny G, Pichler W, Morisset M, et al. (2005) T cell–mediated reactions to iodinated contrast media: evaluation by skin and lymphocyte activation tests. J Allergy Clin Immunol 115:179–185
28. Kvedariene V, Martins P, Ruanet L, Demoly P (2006) Diagnosis of iodinated contrast media hypersensitivity: results of a 6-year period. Clin Exp Allergy 36:1072–1077
29. Bircher AJ, Harr T, Hohenstein L, Tsakiris DA (2006) Hypersensitivity reactions to anticoagulant drugs: diagnosis and management options. Allergy 61:1432–1440
30. Leguy-Seguin V, Jolimoy G, Coudert B, et al. (2007) Diagnostic and predictive value of skin testing in platinum salt hypersensitivity. J Allergy Clin Immunol 119:726–730
31. Popescu NA, Sheehan MG, Kouides PA, et al. (1996) Allergic reactions to cyclophosphamide: delayed clinical expression associated with positive immediate skin tests to drug metabolites in five patients. J Allergy Clin Immunol 97:26–33
32. Lee AY, Chey WY (2003) Patch testing with carbamazepine and its main metabolite carbamazepine epoxide in cutaneous adverse drug reactions to carbamazepine. Contact Dermatitis 48:137–139
33. Aberer W, Bircher A, Romano A, et al. (2003) Drug provocation testing in the diagnosis of drug hypersensitivity reactions: general considerations. Allergy 58:854–863
34. Wong BB, Keith PK, Waserman S (2006) Clinical history as a predictor of penicillin skin test outcome. Ann Allergy Asthma Immunol 97:169–174
35. Wöhrl S, Vigl K, Stingl G (2006) Patients with drug reactions – it is worth testing? Allergy 61:828–934
36. Fontaine C, Mayorga L, Bousquet PJ, et al. (2007) Relevance of the determination of serum-specific IgE antibodies in the diagnosis of immediate beta-lactam allergy. Allergy 62:47–52
37. Guéant JL, Mata E, Monin B, et al. (1991) Evaluation of a new reactive solid phase for radio-immunoassay of serum specific IgE against muscle relaxant drugs. Allergy 46:452–458
38. Manfredi M, Severino M, Testi S, et al. (2004) Detection of specific IgE to quinolones. J Allergy Clin Immunol 113:155–160
39. Demoly P, Lebel B, Messaad D, et al. (1999) Predictive capacity of histamine release for the diagnosis of drug allergy. Allergy 54:500–506
40. Lebel B, Messaad D, Kvedariene V, et al. (2001) Cysteinyl-leukotriene release test (CAST) in the diagnosis of immediate drug reactions. Allergy 56:688–692
41. Watkins J, Wild G (1993) Improved diagnosis of anaphylactoid reactions by measurement of serum tryptase and urinary methylhistamine. Ann Fr Anesth Reanim 12:169–172
42. Ebo DG, Sainte-Laudy J, Bridts CH, et al. (2006) Flow-assisted allergy diagnosis: current applications and future perspectives. Allergy 61:1028–1039
43. Kvedariene V, Kamey S, Ryckwaert Y, et al. (2006) Diagnosis of neuromuscular blocking agent hypersensitivity reactions using cytofluorimetric analysis of basophils. Allergy 61:311–315
44. Sanz ML, Gamboa PM, Antépara I, et al. (2002) Flow cytometric basophil activation test by detection of CD63 expression in patients with immediate-type reactions to betalactam antibiotics. Clin Exp Allergy 32:277–286
45. Torres MJ, Padial A, Mayorga C, et al. (2004) The diagnostic interpretation of basophil activation test in immediate allergic reactions to betalactams. Clin Exp Allergy 34:1768–1775
46. Sanz ML, Gamboa P, de Weck AL (2005) A new combined test with flowcytometric basophil activation and determination of sulfidoleukotrienes is useful for in vitro diagnosis of hypersensitivity to aspirin and other nonsteroidal anti-inflammatory drugs. Int Arch Allergy Immunol 136:58–72
47. Nyfeler B, Pichler WJ (1997) The lymphocyte transformation test for the diagnosis of drug allergy: sensitivity and specificity. Clin Exp Allergy 27:175–181
48. Pichler WJ, Tilch J (2004) The lymphocyte transformation test in the diagnosis of drug hypersensitivity. Allergy 59:809–820

49. Schmid DA, Depta JP, Pichler WJ (2006) T cell-mediated hypersensitivity to quinolones. Clin Exp Allergy 36:59–69
50. Demoly P, Messaad D, Sahla H, et al. (1998) Six-hour trimethoprim-sulfamethoxazole graded challenge in HIV-infected patients. J Allergy Clin Immunol 102:1033–1036
51. Castells M (2006) Desensitization for drug allergy. Curr Opin Allergy Clin Immunol 6:476–481
52. Castells M (2006) Rapid desensitization for hypersensitivity reactions to chemotherapy agents. Curr Opin Allergy Clin Immunol 6:271–277

Annex 1 Questionnaire for drug hypersensitivities (Adapted from [8])

DRUG HYPERSENSITVITY QUESTIONNAIRE

INVESTIGATOR: Date of protocol: ....
Name:...Center:..

Address:...Tel/Fax/E-mail: ....

PATIENT:
Name:..Date of birth:..........................Age:..............years
Weight:..............kg   Height:.................cm
Profession:...Origin:...Sex: □ M   □ F
Riskgroups: □ Medical staff □ Pharmaceutical Industries □ Farmers □ others (specify)...............................

CURRENT COMPLAINTS:..
....
....
....

DRUG REACTION: **DATE OF REACTION:**...
(Multiple boxes can be ticked; underline the choice if necessary; chronology can be characterized with numbers)

♦ CUTANEOUS SYMPTOMS: ♦ DIFFERENTIAL DIAGNOSIS:
□ Maculopapular exanthema
□ Macular exanthema   □...
□ Urticarious exanthema
□ AGEP (Acute generalized exanthemous pustulosis)   □...
□ Eczematoid exanthema
□ Erythema exudativum multiforme   □...
□ Bullous exanthema
□ Stevens Johnson Syndrome / TEN (Lyell)
□ Fixed drug exanthema   ♦ CONTRIBUTING FACTORS:
□ Purpura -> Thrombocyte count :........................... □ Viral infections: □ Flu like infection □ Other:...................
      □ palpable   □ haemorrhagic-necrotizing   □ Fever
      □ Visceral organ involvement:........................... □ Suspicion of photosensitivity ? □ No □ Yes   □ Unknown
□ Contact dermatitis □Topic cause □Haematogenous cause □............. □ Stress
□ Urticaria vasculitis   □ Exercise
□ **ONLY** Pruritus   □ Other (specify): ....
□ Urticaria   ....
□ Angioedema/Location/s: ....
□ Conjunctivitis   ♦ EVOLUTION:
□ Other (specify):...   *Intensity*

□ Morphology/Location/s:...

♦ EFFLORESCENCES: Distribution / Dynamics (??)   **h / days**

□ generalized

♦ GASTROINTESTINAL AND RESPIRATORY SYMPTOMS: ♦ ASSOCIATED SYMPTOMS:
□ Nausea/Emesis   □ Involvement of: □ Liver □ Kidney □ Other (specify): ....
□ Diarrhea   □ Fever..........°C
□ Gastro intestinal cramps   □ Malaise
                                                         □ Pain/Burning □ Location/s:...
□ Cough   □ Edema   □ Location/s:...
□ Dysphonia   □ Arthralgia/Myalgia □ Location/s:...
□ Dyspnea   PEFR or FEV1:............................... □ Lymphadenopathy
□ Wheezing/Bronchospasm   □ Other (specify):...

□ Rhinitis   ♦ CARDIOVASCULAR SYMPTOMS:
□ Rhinorrhea   □ Tachykardia   Pulse rate: ..../min
□ Sneezing   □ Hypotension   Blood pressure: ....mmHg
□ Nasal obstruction   □ Collapse
□ Other (specify):... □ Arrhythmia
                                                         □ Other (specify): ....

♦ PSYCHIC SYMPTOMS:
□ Fear/Panic reaction   □ Vertigo   ♦ INVOLVEMENT OF OTHER ORGANS :
□ Fainting   *(eg. peripheral neuropathy, lung involvement, cytopenia....)*
□ Paraesthesia/Hyperventilation   □...
□ Sweating   □...
□ Other (specify):... □...

(continued)

Annex 1 (continued)

♦ SUSPICIOUS DRUGS:

Drug's generic name ± additives Indication:	Daily dose / Route of application / Duration of therapy:	Interval between dose and reaction	Previous therapy with this drug:
1.	...............mg/d; ....; ....d		☐ No ☐ Unknown ☐ Yes -> Symptoms:..
2.	...............mg/d; ....; ....d		☐ No ☐ Unknown ☐ Yes -> Symptoms:..
3.	...............mg/d; ....; ....d		☐ No ☐ Unknown ☐ Yes -> Symptoms:..
4.	...............mg/d; ....; ....d		☐ No ☐ Unknown ☐ Yes -> Symptoms:..
5.	...............mg/d; ....; ....d		☐ No ☐ Unknown ☐ Yes -> Symptoms:..
6.	...............mg/d; ....; ....d		☐ No ☐ Unknown ☐ Yes -> Symptoms:..

♦ MANAGEMENT FOLLOWING ACUTE DRUG REACTION: ☐ No therapy
☐ Stop of suspicious drugs No.# ....
☐ Antihistamines   ☐ local   ☐ systemic
☐ Corticosteroids   ☐ local   ☐ systemic
☐ Bronchodilatators ☐ local   ☐ systemic
☐ Shock treatment   ☐ Epinephrine ☐ Plasma expanders ☐ Other: ....
☐ Change to substitute/s:
　　　　☐ Type/Name: ....
　　　　☐ Tolerance: ....
　　　　☐ Other (specify):..
☐ Dosis reduction (Drug.............................)...
☐ Other (specify)...
　　　　..

♦ DRUG TAKEN SINCE WITHOUT ANY REACTION:
....
....
....
....

CURRENT DRUGS: .... ☐ Antihistamines ....
　　　　　　　　　　　　　　　　　　　　　　　　☐ β-Blockers ....
....
....

PERSONAL HISTORY:

1) HAVE SIMILIAR SYMPTOMS BEEN OBSERVED WITHOUT THE INTAKE OF THE SUSPICIOUS DRUGS ?☐ Yes ☐No ☐Unknown

2) MEDICAL HISTORY:
☐ Asthma   ☐ Autoimmune (Sjögren, Lupus, etc)   ☐ Urticaria pigmentosa / syst. mastocytosis
☐ Nasal polyposis   ☐ Lymphoprolific (ALL, CLL, Hodgkin, etc.)   ☐ Chronic urticaria
☐ Cystic fibrosis   ☐ Intervertebral disk surgery   ☐ HIV positivity
☐ Diabetes   ☐ Liver:..   ☐ Kidney: ....
☐ Other/Specification: ....

3) ALLERGIC DISEASES: ....
　　(eg. pollinosis, atopic dermatitis, food allergy, hymenoptera venom allergy, latex allergy, etc.)

4) DRUG REACTIONS DURING FORMER SURGERY: .... ☐ Dentist ☐ Local anaesthesia☐ General anaesthesia (No:.....)

5) REACTIONS DURING FORMER VACCINATIONS: .... ☐ Polio   ☐ Tetanus ☐ Rubella ☐ Measles ☐ Hepatitis B
　　　　　　　　　　　　　　　　　　　　　　.................................... ☐ Diphteria ☐ Other:.................................☐ Unknown

FAMILY HISTORY: Allergies / Drug allergies:
....
....
....

REMARKS:
....
....
....

Immunological Principles of Drug Hypersensitivity

Anna Zawodniak and Werner J. Pichler

Introduction

Adverse drug reactions (ADR) are a major public health problem. They are common, occasionally severe and have an impact on the use of medications and cause socioeconomic losses [1]. Most of the ADRs represent predictable side effects due to a known pharmacological action of the drug and do not involve immunological processes. These reactions are classified as type A and type B. Examples of type A reactions are sleepiness with some antihistamines, accumulation of drug derived compounds in the skin resulting in hyperpigmentation (amiodaron, antimalarials, minocycline, quinolones) or a pharmacologic inhibition of the proliferation and differentiation of epidermal cells, hair follicles or a sebaceous glands inducing alopecia (cytostatics), or severe dryness (isoretinoin). In such cases the prescribing physician can evaluate the benefit/risk ratio and often also provide advices for preventing or alleviating the adverse reactions.

Unlike type A reactions, type B reactions are not predictable and their development appears to be dependent on both genetic and environmental factors. Drug Hypersensitivity Reactions (DHRs) belong to type B reactions and account for about one sixth of all adverse drug reactions. They comprise drug allergic reactions, which according to the Nomenclature Review Committee of the World Allergy Organization, refer to DHRs where a definite immunological mechanism, either IgE- or T-cell-mediated, is demonstrated [2], and pseudoallergic reactions (non-immune mediated hypersensitivity). Pseudoallergic reactions clinically resemble a true allergy and involve effector-cells of the immune system (e.g. basophilic and eosinophilic leucocytes, mast cells) but no specific immune reaction to the drug can be proven in standardized tests.

In this chapter the concepts on how small molecular drugs can activate the immune system are discussed. The hapten, prohapten and p-i concept are presented,

A. Zawodniak and W.J. Pichler (✉)
Division of Allergology, Clinic for Rheumatology and Clinical Immunology/Allergology,
Inselspital, University of Bern, CH-3010, Bern, Switzerland
e-mail: werner.pichler@insel.ch

R. Pawankar et al. (eds.), *Allergy Frontiers: Clinical Manifestations*,
DOI: 10.1007/978-4-431-88317-3_25, © Springer 2009

and recent data about the involvement of the innate immune system are also presented. Immune reactions to larger proteins like biologicals are not discussed.

Immune Recognition of the Drug

People are constantly confronted with chemicals (xenobiotics), which constitute one of the important interventions in modern medicine. Their doubtless enormous success has, regretfully a darker side, namely unwanted side effects. A substantial amount of side effects of drugs is due to an interaction of small chemicals with the immune system. This will be discussed in detail in this chapter.

General Principles of Immune System Activation

An immune reaction starts with the involvement of the innate system. The antigen stimulates the innate immune system via e.g. Toll like receptors (TLR) on dendritic cells (DC), thereby setting an initial alarm signal. The activated dendritic cells function as antigen presenting cells (APC) as they take up and process complex antigens into short peptides, which subsequently are presented as peptide – MHC (major histocompatibility complex) complexes to T cells in a suitable environment, mainly in lymph nodes. Peptides that are derived from proteins synthesized and degraded in cytosol are presented by MHC class I molecules and activate CD8 T cells. The reactive CD8 T cells secrete cytokines and are able to kill cells displaying foreign peptides derived from cytosolic pathogens, such as viruses. In contrast, MHC class II molecules present peptides derived from extracellular proteins and degraded in endocytic vesicles. These structures interact with CD4 T cells, which produce cytokines and modulate the action of other immune cells like macrophages, B cells, and CD8 T cells [3, 4]. Due to the enormous number ($>10^{12}$) of different T cell receptors (TCRs), the ensuing immune response is variable and efficient to eliminate infectious agents.

Hapten Concept

Drugs, as a low-molecular weight compounds (MW < 1,000 D) are thought to be too small to elicit such an immune response per se. The understanding of the recognition of small molecules like drugs by B- and T-cells is based primarily on the hapten hypothesis [5, 6]. Haptens are chemically reactive molecules that are able to undergo stable covalent binding to the larger proteins or peptides. Covalently modified soluble autologous proteins (e.g. albumins) or cell bound proteins (e.g. integrins) can be taken up by antigen presenting cells and processed (broken down into small fragments). The derived hapten-modified peptides are transported to the cell surface for presentation to T-cells in MHC molecules. It is also possible that the hapten binds directly to the immunogenic peptide presented by the MHC molecule. In this case, no processing is required [7, 8]. Alteration of the MHC molecule directly has also been observed [9] (Fig. 1).

A predominant humoral immune response may occur, if the hapten-modification affects soluble and cell bound proteins, but exclusive T cell response can be seen if the hapten binds directly to the MHC-peptide complexes themselves.

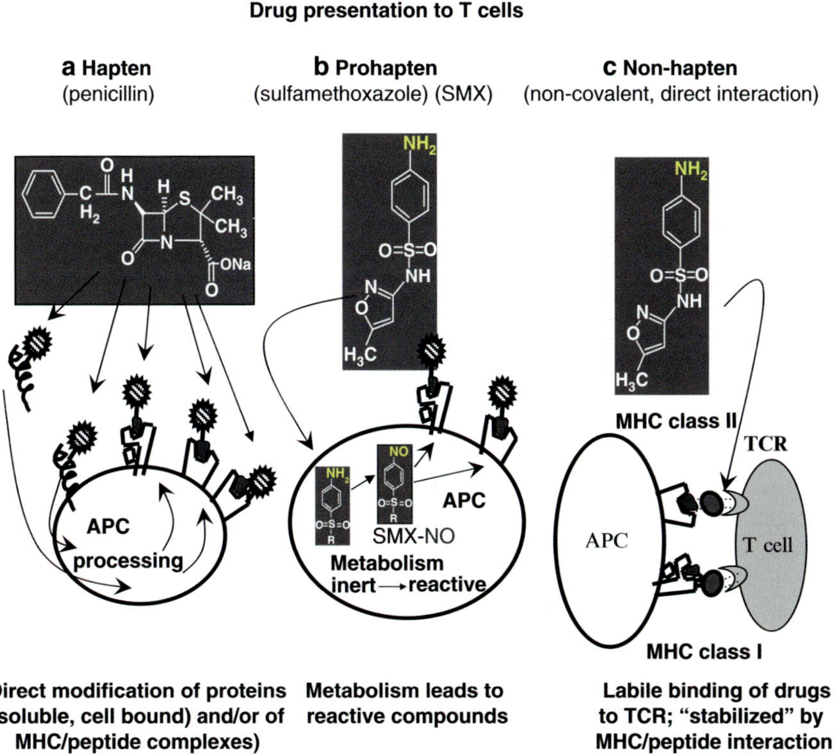

Fig. 1 Drug presentation to T cells. (**a**) Hapten-like drugs (like penicillin) can bind covalently and modify soluble or cell bound molecules. They can even bind directly to the major histocompatibiliy complex (*MHC*)/peptide complex on antigen presenting cells (*APC*), either to the embedded peptide or to the MHC molecule itself. (**b**) Pro-haptens, require metabolic activation to become haptens. The metabolism leads to the formation of a chemically reactive compound (e.g. from sulfamethoxazole [*SMX*] to the chemically reactive form *SMX-NO*). The metabolite may modify cell bound or soluble proteins, similar to a real hapten. (**c**) Non-hapten pathway (p-i-concept, *p*harmacological *i*nteraction with *i*mmune receptors) does not require covalent association of the drug with the MHC molecule. The chemically inert drug seems to bind directly to the T cell receptor (*TCR*). Full T cell stimulation requires an interaction with the MHC molecule. This type of drug stimulation is restricted to certain drugs that fit into TCRs and results in an exclusive T cell stimulation

The chemical haptens have often a tendency to bind covalently to a certain amino acid within a protein. The typical example is penicillin G. It tends to bind covalently to accessible lysine groups within soluble or cell bound proteins. The binding can occur via the beta-lactam ring, by binding as penicilloyl to the lysine. Alternatively, the binding can occur to cysteine residues via the SH group of the thiazolidine ring. The identification of the relevant protein modification and the nature of the binding are difficult since the number of potential target proteins is very high and many nucleophilic binding sites are available for chemical binding in any given protein. Consequently, formation of distinct antigenic epitopes can occur and lead to a great heterogeneity of immune responses and clinical pictures in drug hypersensitivity.

Pro-Hapten Concept

Many drugs are not chemically reactive per se and are not able to form a covalent binding with proteins and peptides, but can still elicit allergic side effects. An example of such a drug is sulfamethoxazole (SMX). It is an important and well characterized antimicrobial agent which unfortunately leads to hypersensitivity reactions in 1–3% of the general population, and in up to 50% of patients with HIV infection [10]. Sulfmethoxazole is metabolized by CYP2C9 in human liver to a metabolite that can be easily oxidized to nitroso-sulfamethoxazole (NO-SMX). Nitroso-sulfamethoxazole acts as a hapten and covalently binds to cellular proteins forming a potential immunogenic epitope [11, 12] (Fig. 1).

Metabolism occurs in the liver, where it may not necessarily induce an immune response, but actually can induce tolerance [13]. If reactive compounds escape the tolerogenic environment of the liver and reach the local lymph nodes, where an immune response may develop, an accompanying hepatitis may occur [14]. On the other hand, the metabolite produced in the liver may be of intermediate reactivity but can be further oxidized outside the liver causing a systemic syndrome like DRESS/DiHS (drug related eosinophilia with systemic symptoms or drug induced hypersensitivity syndrome). If such oxidation would happen in the skin, it might be presented on the membrane of the keratinocytes that, thereby, might become targets for cytotoxic T cells in drug eruptions.

Drugs and Innate System Activation

Both, pro-haptens and haptens need to somehow activate the innate immune system as they induce an activation of naïve T cells. The primary sensitization to a drug most likely happens in the lymph nodes. The key players of the sensitization phase are professional antigen presenting cells (APCs), namely activated dendritic cells (DCs). In order to get fully activated, DC must receive a threshold level of signaling, which probably derives from a number of sources. DC responds to such signaling by increased cell surface expression of costimulatory receptors, particularly CD40, CD80/86 and/or cytokine secretion, which in turn provide additional signals for activation and phenotypic differentiation of T cells (Fig. 2). It is possible that drugs themselves may induce a danger signal, e.g. by direct interaction with receptors found on the surface of DC. As an example, imidazoquinoline and imiquimod can directly interact with toll-like receptors (TLR7/8 and TLR7

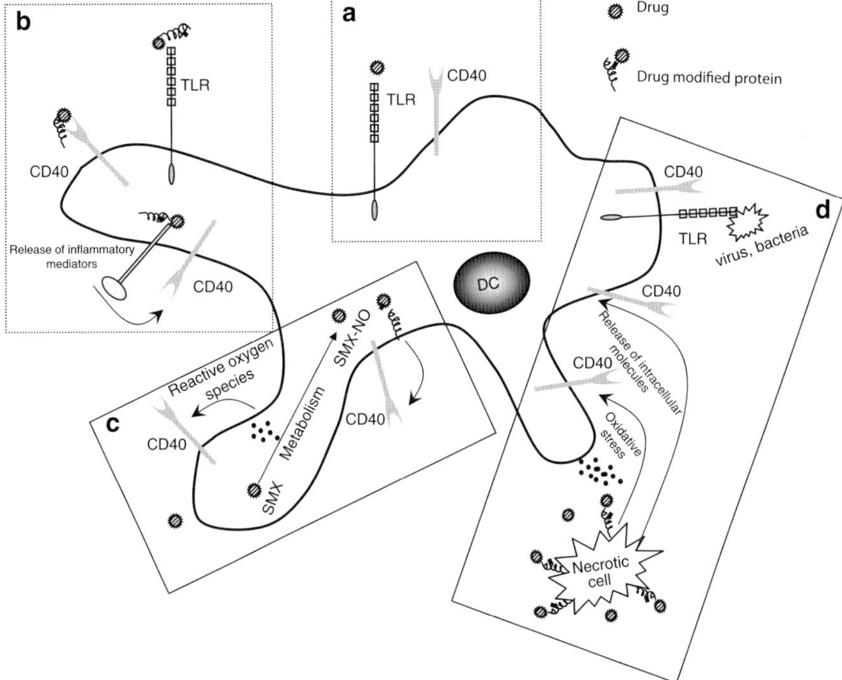

Fig. 2 Maturation signals for dendritic cells (*DC*) in drug hypersensitivity. (**a**) Some drugs like imidazoquinoline and imiquimod may directly interact with toll-like receptors (*TLR* 7/8) on the surface of dendritic cells, potentially causing danger signal for immature DCs. (**b**) Reactive drug metabolites may covalently bind to extra- or/and intracellular dendritic cell proteins. This binding can lead to stimulation of DC and e.g. upregulation of CD40 molecule on the surface of DC or to the release of inflammatory mediators inducing a mature state in DC. This has been demonstrated for some haptens causing contact dermatitis, as well as for the widely used drugs like amoxycil in and sulfamethoxazole (*SMX*). (**c**) DCs contain some of drug metabolizing enzymes which have a capacity to catalyze e.g. SMX metabolite formation. These reactive metabolites can covalently modify different intracellular proteins leading to DC activation, moreover auto-oxidative conversion of SMX-NHOH to *SMX-NO* can generate reactive oxygen species and oxidative stress, both known inducers of DC maturation. (**d**) A number of indirect signals, possibly caused by some toxic effect of the drugs, may induce the release of intracellular molecules from necrotic cells into extracellular matrix, cause apoptotic cell death, or may induce oxidative stress. Hormonal or environmental conditions (surgical trauma, other diseases) and virus or bacterial infections can also cause DC maturation, which may enhance reactions to drugs

respectively) [15–17]. Surprisingly these drugs are actually not inducing hypersensitivity, although they are used for topical skin treatment (normally the most sensitizing pathway). Reactive drug metabolites, acting as a haptens, may induce mature state in DC, e.g. by binding of electrophilic chemical allergens to thiol-rich dendritic cell proteins [18–20]. This has been demonstrated for some haptens causing contact dermatitis [21, 22] as well as for the widely used drugs like amoxycil in and sulfamethoxazole which upregulate CD40 expression on DC [23, 24]. I Surprisingly, one group actually postulated that the difference between amoxycil in allergic and not allergic individuals is due to differences in the DC as only patient's DC, but not DC from control subjects, upregulated CD40 on the surface after stimulation with amoxycil in [24]. On the other hand Sanderson et al. observed that SMX could induce maturation changes in DCs derived form both allergic and non-allergic individuals [23].

Moreover, it has been observed that DC contains some drug metabolizing enzymes and that they have a capacity to catalyze SMX metabolite formation [23]. These reactive metabolites can covalently modify different intracellular proteins leading to DC activation. However, the bioactivation and CD40 upregulation is not necessarily due to covalent binding. An auto-oxidative conversion of SMX-NHOH to SMX-NO can generate reactive oxygen species and oxidative stress, both known inducers of DC maturation.

There are also a number of indirect signals that can cause changes in dendritic cell activation. SMX-NO can bind covalently to cysteine residues in cellular proteins which could a cause direct toxicity [25] and necrotic cell death. Release of intracellular molecules from necrotic cells into extracellular matrix stimulates increased CD40 expression on DC [26–29]. Apoptotic cell death and induction of oxidative stress can also provide DC maturation signals. Other stimuli that lead to the activation of the DC include conserved microbial products which interact with TLRs (see Fig. 2). Some authors postulate also that hormonal or environmental conditions (surgical trauma, other diseases) [30, 31] can serve as factors increasing DC activation.

According to these data it is possible that, either the drug processing itself or the binding of the chemically reactive compound would stimulate the partial maturation and migration of DCs to the lymph nodes. In the lymph node, presentation of the hapten-carrier molecule by DC\LC may then lead to the local stimulation and expansion of the hapten specific T cells.

While this concept is well documented for contact dermatitis, it does not explain all features of systemic drug hypersensitivity, for instance metabolism in the skin is very moderate and restricted to some enzymes. Neither epidermal cells nor DC cells are "professional" metabolizers and the amount of reactive metabolites that they are capable of producing is very low [32] and it is not sure if such a in situ production of reactive metabolites is sufficient to induce an immune response. It is also controversial whether a complex metabolism, as required for some drugs, can occur in the skin. Moreover, if the metabolism occurs in the liver, why would the generated metabolites preferentially go to the skin, when they could form hapten-carrier complexes all over the body?

The p-i Concept

According to the hapten and pro-hapten concept, drugs and other substances that are not chemically active and therefore incapable of coupling to a macromolecular carrier, would not be antigens and could not induce hypersensitivity reactions. However this has been challenged recently by clinical, immunological and biochemical evidences that neither can be explained neither by hapten nor pro-hapten models. The p-i concept indicates that not only immunological but also pharmacological (direct interaction between T-cell receptor and the drug) activation of the immune system are possible by drugs (p-i concept) (see Fig. 1).

Clinical Data

1. Some of the drugs causing delayed hypersensitivity reactions are able to stimulate specific immune response to a drug at the first encounter, before an immune response has had time to evolve. Other reactions happen to occur in less than 3 days which seems to be too short to mount a specific immune response.
2. Delayed hypersensitivity reaction can be caused by drugs that are not known to be metabolized to the reactive compounds.
3. It has also been observed that many inert drugs, unable to form hapten–carrier complex in the skin, can nevertheless cause positive skin tests with lymphocyte infiltration.

Immunologic Data

1. Using T cell clones, mostly chemically inert drugs and only occasionally chemically reactive metabolites were found to stimulate T cells via the T-cell receptor (TCR) in an MHC-dependent way. It was shown in particularly for lamotragine [33], carbamazepine [34], sulfamethaxazol (SMX) [35, 36], mepivacaine [37] and lidocaine [38], p-phenylendiamine [39], ciproxin or moxifloxacin, and radio contrast media (RCM) [40, 41]. Moreover, some drugs such as RCM or lidocaine, have no known metabolism resulting in a reactive metabolite, and the p-i concept offers the only plausible explanation for their ability to induce delayed type T-cell mediated reactions.
2. Drug specific TCC could be activated even in the presence of glutaraldehyde fixed antigen presenting cells (APCs). These APCs were unable to take up, process or intracellulary metabolize the drugs [33–37].
3. Upon pulsing of APCs (incubation of APCs with the drug for 18 h followed by two washing steps), which obviously removes the drug, no T cell stimulation

was observed for lidocaine, lamotrigine, carbamazapine, ciproxin and SMX [33, 34, 36, 42]. The reactive metabolite of SMX, namely SMX-NO, which acts as a hapten and is able to covalently modify the MHC-peptide complex, was still able to stimulate hapten-reactive T-cells after the same procedures.

4. TCCs react quasi immediately after encountering the specific drug as revealed by a rapid and sustained intracellular Ca^{2+} increase. The kinetics of T cell activation is simply too fast for any involvement of antigen processing or metabolism, which might need >60 min to occur. Moreover, the kinetics of TCR-downregulation on drug reactive TCCs after encountering the inert drug are similar to the recognition of pre-processed, immunogenic peptides (occurring within the first 30 min), clearly differing from the recognition of proteins, which requires several hours.

All these observations lead to the conclusion that drugs could directly stimulate T-cell receptors. This metabolism-and processing-independent stimulation would depend primarily on the structural features of the inert drug, that enable it to fit into some of the $>10^{12}$ available T-cell receptors. The interaction of the drug with the TCR receptor is labile, since it can be easily reversed by simple washing, while the covalent hapten binding to MHC is not. In pharmacological terms, this means that the binding of the drug to the TCR has a low affinity, probably in the millimolar to micromolar range.

The p-i Concept Does Not Rely on Activation of the Innate Immune System

The stimulatory potential of the drug-TCR interaction may decisively depend on the readiness of the T cell to react to a minor signal like a drug. The p-i mechanism of T-cell stimulation does not require biotransformation of the inert drug to a chemically reactive compound. Actually, according to the p-i concept, no involvement/stimulation of the innate immune system is required [43]: the drug binding to TCR is probably only able to activate T cells which were previously primed and represent effector memory T cells, as such T-cells, in contrast to naïve T-cells, have a substantially lower threshold of activation and are less dependent on the costimulation by e.g. CD28. Thus, the signal provided by drug binding to the TCR activates T cells with an additional specificity. On the other hand, it cannot be ruled out that, if a costimulatory effect of the drug on the innate immune system is also provided, it may further enhance the response.

This concept explains also the important role of generalized virus infections as cofactors for drug hypersensitivity. The threshold of T cell activation might be further lowered by massive immune stimulation of T cells as it occurs during a generalized herpes [31, 44] or human immunodeficiency virus (HIV) infections [45], but also during exacerbations of autoimmune diseases. These generalized inflammations are accompanied by high cytokine levels and an increased expression of

MHC- and costimulatory molecules. Consequently T cells are pre-activated and more ready to react to a minor signal like binding of a drug to its TCR. This would explain the high occurrence of drug hypersensitivity in these diseases. Thus, the p-i concept does not imply the induction of own immune response but postulates that it is a consequence of a cross-reactivity of the TCR which reacts with a drug and an unknown peptide structure.

Relationship Between Viral Infections and Drug Hypersensitivity Reactions

A relationship between viral infection and the simultaneous or subsequent development of drug eruption has been often observed in the clinical situation. Ampicillin "rash" during infection mononucleosis and the highly increased risk of developing drug eruptions in AIDS are perhaps the best known examples.

A peculiar syndrome is the so called Drug-induced Hypersensitivity Syndrome (DiHS), also called Drug Rash with Eosinophilia and Systemic Symptoms (DRESS): It is very often associated with the reactivation of herpes viruses (HHV6, CMV, EBV) [31, 46], and this reactivation has been incorporated in the diagnostic algorithm proposed by Japanese researchers [47].

In this syndrome antibodies to herpes viruses and herpes-viral genome and viruses can be observed in the 2–4 week after allergy symptoms started. It often leads to a clinical deterioration long after cessation of the drug treatment. What is the explanation? Japanese researchers have proposed a hypothesis involving the concept of immunoreconstitution [46]. We would propose that DiHS/DRESS is a disease where the antigen, recognized by the T cells triggered by the p-i concept, is ubiquitously present and that the drug-stimulated T cells are directed to it:

(a) *"Virus and immune-reconstitution hypothesis"*: some very peculiar clinical features of DiHS/DRESS, like delayed onset (usually 2–4 weeks, often even 10–12 weeks after start of treatment), multiorgan involvement (dermatitis, hepatitis, nephritis, pneumonitis, myocarditis, thrombosis, thyroiditis, rhabdomyolysis [48–50]), lymphadenopathy and lymphocytosis resemble a generalized virus infection. Japanese researchers therefore postulated that DiHS is actually *a viral disease, modified by drug intake*: The viral activation of the immune system may facilitate the reactivity to the drug, thus explaining the immune response to the drug found in patch and in vitro tests. The drugs causing DiHS/DRESS like carbamazepine, are also immunosuppressive, and therefore the detectable immune response to the virus is delayed. This explains, why the viral antibody tests are initially negative, but become positive after a while, namely when the drug treatment is stopped (similar to the immune reconstitution syndrome). This is an interesting hypothesis, but it is doubtful whether it can explain the great number of elicitors of DiHS/DRESS, many of which are not known to be immunosuppressive.

(b) We would like to propose a different, *"drug-virus cross-reactivity hypothesis"*: Herpes virus infections are constantly controlled by T cells, and this control involves a high proportion of circulating T cells, as 2–>4% of circulating T cells react to CMV, EBV and other virally derived peptides. Moreover, these viruses infect often immune cells like T cells and monocytes.

Carbamazepine, lamotrigine, sulfapyrin, etc. are drugs able to induce a strong drug specific, polyclonal immune response. These drugs seem to stimulate via the p-i mechanism and activate preferentially preactivated T cells which includes the activation of herpes-virus peptide specific T cells – as these cells represent a substantial proportion of circulating T cells and as they are specific for endogeneous herpes viruses and have a lower threshold of activation due to the constant presence of the viral peptides. Thus a drug-induced but virus-peptide specific T cell response develops. These drug activated T cells may home to different organs and react with the viral peptides presented in multiple organs. This may be one factor explaining the damage to multiple organs as it is typical for DiHS/DRESS. It can also explain the persistence of symptoms after cessation of drug therapy as the activated T cells might be reactivated by virus-peptide presenting cells. But why can one find even herpes viruses, if it is only reactivation of virus-specific T cells by drugs?

Herpes viruses are harboured in T cells themselves, some of which are stimulated by the drug. Their activation may lead to the production of more herpes viruses and induction of an immune response to it. This explains the appearance of viruses 2–4 weeks after stopping the drug treatment, and the aggravation of symptoms at that time period. This cross-reactivity hypothesis would make DiHS/DRESS an example for an immune reaction elicited by the p-i concept, where the real antigen for the stimulated T cells would be available in the body.

Immunogenetic and Pharmacogenetic Risk Factors of Drug Allergy

Any drug is assumed to be able to elicit hypersensitivity reactions, but clearly antibiotics, non steroidal anti-inflammatory drugs (NSAID) and antiepileptics are those drugs most frequently causing them. There is evidence that various factors can increase the risk of sensitization and the severity of clinical symptoms in drug hypersensitivity reactions. A summary of these risk factors is shown in Table 1.

The unpredictable nature of drug hypersensitivity reactions prompted an intensive search for genetic factors with the major emphasis on pharmacogenetic factors [51]. An altered metabolism was thought to be a good explanation for the appearance of drug hypersensitivity in a small subset of treated persons. Impaired acetylation of SMX may lead to elevated production of reactive metabolites (SMX-NHOH and SMX-NO) that behaved as haptens [52] and slow acetylation phenotype or genotype was proposed as a risk factor for allergy to sulfonamides [53] especially in patients with AIDS [54]. On the other hand some large prospective cohorts in HIV positive patients treated with sulfonamides [55, 56] did not confirm suspected metabolic risk

Table 1 List of factors increasing the risk of sensitization and the severity of clinical symptoms in drug hypersensitivity

State of immune activation – infections may stimulate the immune system and thus lower the threshold to react to drugs

The dose – important in all DH, both for the sensitization and elicitation

The duration of treatment – some DH appear only if treatment is given for days to weeks

Female sex – can increase the frequency of DH

Immunogenetic predisposition – in particular HLA-B alleles for severe forms of DH; also dependent on race (e.g. Han Chinese)

Pharmacogenetic predisposition – has been detected quite rarely

Epicutaneous application of a drug – clearly increases the probability of a sensitization compared to oral or parenteral treatments

Atopy – normally not associated with a higher risk of drug hypersensitivity, but an atopic predisposition may prolong the detectability of drug specific IgE in the serum

DH, drug hypersensitivity; Ig, immunoglobulin

factors for sulfonamide induced cutaneous reactions. Recent study excluded most of the polymorphisms in drug metabolism as a predisposing factor, however suggests further in vitro and in vivo studies on the role of glutathione S-transferase P1 variants [57]. The polymorphism in the tumor necrosis factor promoter region may have a role in the severity of the carbamazepine hypersensitivity [58].

Thus, extensive research did not reveal any clear and convincing pharmacogenetic predispositions. This is quite in contrast to recent data on a striking HLA-association of certain, mostly severe drug hypersensitivity reactions with HLA-class I alleles. HLA-B alleles, which are the most polymorphic HLA-alleles are involved in carbamazepine (HLA-B*1502) induced SJS/TEN in Han Chinese [59] but not in Caucasians [60] and in abacavir induced DRESS syndrome (HLA-B*5701 together with hsp70) in Caucasians [61]. It seems that in these reactions a certain HLA-B allele favors the presentation of certain peptides able to optimally present the drug as a hapten. However, preliminary data could not prove this hapten-peptide concept. Alternatively, many of the drugs involved can stimulate the T cells via the p-i mechanism. In this case, only certain MHC-class B alleles might be able to supplement the T cell stimulation by the drug (p-i mechanism), while others do not. Absence of the supplementing MHC-allele may thus render the T cell insufficiently responsive to the drugs.

Classification of Drug Hypersensitivity Reactions

Drug hypersensitivity reactions are notorious for their great variability. This can, to a certain extent, be traced back to the peculiar nature of drugs as allergens: A drug, which is a hapten (also derived from a prohapten), may bind to many different structures and thus elicit different types of immune reactions (see Fig. 3). To account for this heterogeneity and to better explain the various clinical pictures, Gell and Coombs have classified drug hypersensitivity as well as other immune reactions into four categories termed type I–IV reactions [62]. It relies on IgE, on complement fixing antibodies and on T cell reactions, which orchestrate different

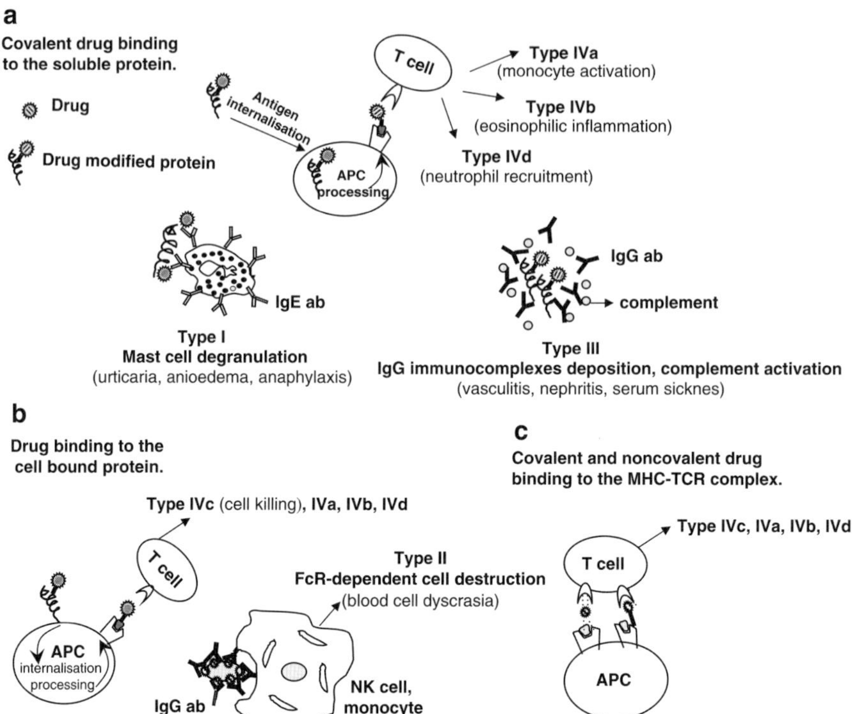

Fig. 3 Covalent and non-covalent interactions of drugs with various soluble and cell bound proteins account for the diversity of drug hypersensitivity reactions. (**a**) Soluble protein, modified by the covalent drug binding, may be internalized, processed and presented by the antigen presenting cells (*APC*) to drug specific T cells. Once activated, these T cells orchestrate further immune reaction by release of various cytokines. In type IVa interferon (INF) gamma, in type IVb interleukin 5 (IL-5) and IL-4 and in type IVd IL-8 are produced. Drug modified soluble protein can also cross-link IgE antibodies (*IgE ab*) on the surface of mast cell, causing mast cell degranulation (Type I response) or induce IgG antibodies (*IgG ab*) production, activation of complement and immunocomplexes deposition (Type III response). (**b**) If the drug binds to cell bound protein, drug/protein complex can be internalized, processed and presented by the APC to drug specific T cells. As discussed above, T cells produce different cytokines and can further modulate immune response. Cell associated antigens are often presented in the context of major histocompatibility complex (MHC) class I molecule to cytotoxic T lymphocytes (CTL) (Type IVc response). Drug modified cell bound proteins can also activate complement and induce specific IgG ab. production. Cells coated by IgG antibodies and complement are phagocytosed by Fc receptor positive (*FcR*) cells, like natural killer (*NK*) cells and monocytes (Type II response). (**c**) Drugs may bind directly to the (MHC)/peptide complex on APC, either to the embedded peptide or to the MHC molecule itself. Direct interaction of the drug with the T cell receptor (TCR) is also possible (see p-i concept). In this case the drug can initiate all kinds of T cell responses (IVa–IVc)

forms of inflammations. These reactions are tightly connected, as e.g. the maturation of B cells to IgE- or IgG-producing plasma cells depends on the help of T cells. Thus, e.g. type I and type IVb as well as type II or III with type IVa reactions occur often together, and the clinical picture is probably dominated by the prevalent immune reaction (see Fig. 3).

Type 1 represents immediate reactions. It is based on formation and binding of drug/antigen-specific IgE antibodies to the high-affinity Fc-IgE receptors on mast cells and basophiles. Cross-linking of these receptors leads to the liberation of various mediators, eliciting symptoms such as urticaria, angioedema, rhinitis, bronchoconstriction and the most severe form, anaphylaxis. Type II and type III reactions rely on the formation of complement fixing IgG antibodies (IgG1, IgG3). Occasionally, IgM is involved. These reactions are similar, as both depend on the formation of immune complexes and interaction with complement and Fc-IgG receptors (Fc-IgGI, IIa and IIIa) bearing cells (macrophages, NK cells, granulocytes, platelets) but the target structures and physiological consequences are different. In Type II reactions IgG mediated cytotoxic mechanisms, account mainly for blood cell dyscrasias such as hemolytic anemia and trombocytopenia. The clinical symptoms of Type III reactions may be immuno-complexes mediated small vessel vasculitis and/or serum sickness. Type IV reactions are mediated by T cells, causing the so-called "delayed type hypersensitivity reactions," with the most typical example being contact dermatitis or delayed skin test to tuberculin. This classification reflects distinct immune mechanisms and explains the heterogeneous presentation of drug hypersensitivity and has been helpful in clinical practice. However, recent findings and detailed analysis of T-cell subsets and function showed some limitation of this classification. For example, the Coombs and Gell classification did not account for bullous or pustular skin eruption or hepatitis, because cytotoxic T-cells mechanism was not included, and the regulation of neutrophils by T cells was not yet investigated. Immunologic research has revealed that all four types of reactions require an involvement of T cells, which provide help by generating cytokines acting as switch factors for immunoglobulin isotype switch. Moreover, T cells have been found to differ in cytokines produced, which results in distinct pathologies [63]. Therefore T cell meditated type IV reactions have recently been revised and further sub-classified into IVa–IVd [6].

Type IVa corresponds to Th1-type immune reactions: Th1 type T cells activate macrophages by secreting large amounts of interferon-γ, drive the production of complement fixing antibody isotypes involved in type II and III reactions (IgG1, IgG3), and are co-stimulatory for proinflammatory responses (tumor necrosis factor, IL-12) and CD8+ T cell responses.

Type IVb corresponds to the Th2 type immune response. Th2 T cells secrete the cytokines IL-4, IL13 and IL-5, which promote B cell production of IgE and IgG4, macrophage deactivation and mast cell and eosinophil responses: The high production of the Th2 cytokine IL-5 leads to an eosinophilic inflammation, which is the characteristic inflammatory cell type in many drug hypersensitivity reactions [6]. In addition, there is a link to type I reactions, as Th2 cells boost IgE production by IL-4/IL-13 secretion.

Type IVc T cells themselves can also act as effector cells: They emigrate to the tissue and can kill tissue cells like hepatocytes or keratinocytes in a perforin/granzymeB and FasL dependent manner [64, 65]. Such reactions are occurring in most drug induced delayed hypersensitivity reactions, mostly together with other type IV reactions (monocyte, eosinophil or polymorphonuclear leucocyte's recruitment and activation). Cytotoxic T cells thus play an important role in maculopapular or bullous skin diseases as well as in neutrophilic inflammations (acute generalized exanthematous pustulosis, AGEP), and in contact dermatitis. Type IVc reactions appear to be dominant in bullous skin reactions like Stevens-Johnson syndrome (SJS) and toxic epidermal necrolysis (TEN), where activated CD8+ T cells kill keratinocytes, but may also be the dominant cell type in hepatitis or nephritis.

Type IVd Recently it was shown that CXCL8 and GM-CSF producing T cells recruit neutrophilic leukocytes via CXCL8 release and prevent their apoptosis via GM-CSF release [66]. Thus T cells could coordinate (sterile) neutrophilic inflammations of the skin, in particular AGEP. Besides AGEP, such T cell reactions are also found in Behçet disease and pustular psoriasis [67]. The relationship of these T cells to the recently described IL-17 producing T cells which can also activate and recruit PMN (polymorphonuclear) leucocytes, needs to be clarified.

Taken together, the number and proportion of activated CD4 and CD8 T cells, intrinsic specificity and most importantly cytokine environment appear to be a key factors for the nature and severity of drug allergic reactions. T-cell cytokines IL-4 and IL-5 and the cutaneous migration of eosinophils have been associated with maculopapular reactions [68], IL-8 and neutrophil recruitment are associated with pustular reactions [66, 69], while the cytokine INF-gamma is connected to bullous reactions [34, 64]. Until recently, less serious cutaneous hypersensitivity reactions were thought to involve predominantly CD4+ T cells exhibiting lower levels of cytotoxicity [33, 34, 70–72]. However, drug specific CD4+ and CD8+ cytotoxic T cells, have recently been isolated from the same hypersensitivity patients and were found to express perforin- and/or Fas-mediated cytotoxic capacity following stimulation with the drug [73]. Moreover it remains difficult to believe that drug specific cytotoxic T lymphocytes (CTLs), which were shown to be main effector cells in the most severe formation of a drug hypersensitivity reaction, toxic epidermal necrolysis (TEN) [64, 74], are solely responsible for the massive apoptosis, since similar CTLs were found in the epidermis of patients with mild maculopapular drug eruption, in the absence of necrolysis [70]. Indeed, recently the secretory molecule granulsin was shown to be a key cytotoxic mediator responsible for disseminated keratinocyte death in SJS-TEN [75]. The drug hypersensitivity reactions are therefore fascinating and complex diseases where a small chemical compound can elicit a strong systemic immune reaction. A lot of effort is needed to explore and better understand the pathomechanisms of these immune-mediated side effects.

Conclusions

Drug hypersensitivity reactions represent a major clinical problem. Their clinical characteristics are very heterogeneous as drugs can actually elicit all types of immune reactions. The antigenicity of drugs relies on the fact that small molecules can bind covalently to carrier proteins, which become modified and then behave like a foreign antigenic protein. Such modification of soluble or cell bound proteins can induce humoral and T cell mediated immune reactions, particularly, if the drug or the metabolite is stimulating the innate immune system as well or is given into an already activated immune system. In addition, drugs can directly interact with immune receptors like the highly polymorphic αβ T cell receptors and thereby stimulate some cells of the specific immune system via their surface receptors for antigen. This new concept is named **p**harmacological interaction with **i**mmune receptors (p-i-concept). The p-i concept supplements the hapten concept and explains many of the peculiar findings in drug hypersensitivity. Improving our understanding of drug allergies not only allows us to better understand the general immunologic mechanisms but would also open new possibilities for immunopharmacology.

References

1. Lazarou J, Pomeranz BH, Corey PN (1998) Incidence of adverse drug reactions in hospitalized patients: a meta-analysis of prospective studies. JAMA 279:1200–1205
2. Johansson S, Bieber T, Dahl R, et al. (2004) Revised nomenclature for allergy for global use: report of the Nomenclature Review Committee of the World Allergy Organization, October 2003. J Allergy Clin Immunology 113:832–836
3. Romagnani S (1997) The Th1/Th2 paradigm. Immunol Today 18:263–266
4. Janeway CA, Travers P, Walport M, Sholmchik MJ (2001) Immunobiology: The Immune System in Health and Disease. New York: Garland Science
5. Naisbitt DJ, Gordon SF, Pirmohamed M, Park BK (2000) Immunological principles of adverse drug reactions: the initiation and propagation of immune responses elicited by drug treatment. Drug Saf 23:483–507
6. Pichler WJ (2003) Delayed drug hypersensitivity reactions. Ann Intern Med 139:683–693
7. Padovan E, Bauer T, Tongio MM, Kalbacher H, Weltzien HU (1997) Penicilloyl peptides are recognized as T cell antigenic determinants in penicillin allergy. Eur J Immunol 27:1303–1307
8. Mauri-Hellweg D, Zanni M, Frei E, Bettens F, Brander C, Mauri D, Padovan E, Weltzien HU, Pichler WJ (1996) Cross-reactivity of T cell lines and clones to beta-lactam antibiotics. J Immunol 157:1071–1109
9. Morel E, Bellon T (2007) Amoxicillin conjugates to HLA class I molecules and interferes with signalling through the ILT2/LIR-1/CD85j inhibitory receptor. Allergy 62:190–196
10. van der Ven AJ, Koopmans PP, Vree TB, van der Meer JW (1991) Adverse reactions to co-trimoxazol in HIV infection. Lancet 338:431–433
11. Naisbitt DJ, Hough SJ, Gill HJ, Pirmohamed M, Kitteringham NR, Park BK (1999) Cellular disposition of sulphamethoxazole and its metabolites: implications for hypersensitivity. Br J Pharmacol 126:1393–1407
12. Manchanda T, Hess D, Dale L, Ferguson SG, Rieder MJ (2002) Haptenation of sulfonamide reactive metabolites to cellular proteins. Mol Pharmacol 62:1011–1026
13. Crispe IN (2003) Hepatic T cells and liver tolerance. Nat Rev Immunol 3:51–62
14. Bowen DG, Zen M, Holz L, Davis T, McCaughan GW (2004) The site of primary T cell activation is a determinant of the balance between intrahepatic tolerance and immunity. J Clin Invest 114:701–712
15. Jurk M, Kritzler A, Schulte B, Tluk S, Schetter C, Krieg AM, Vollmer J (2006) Modulating responsiveness of human TLR7 and 8 to small molecule ligands with T-rich phosphorothiate oligodeoxynucleotides. Eur J Immunol 36:1815–1826
16. Prins R, Craft N, Bruhn KW, Khan-Farooqi H, Koya RC, Stripecke R, Miller JF, Liau LM (2006) The TLR-7 agonist, imiquimod, enhances dendritic cell survival and promotes tumor antigen-specific T cell priming: relation to central nervous system antitumor immunity. J Immunol 176:157–164

17. Rifkin IR, Leadbetter EA, Busconi L, Viglianti G, Marshak-Rothstein A (2005) Toll-like receptors, endogenous ligands, and systemic autoimmune disease. Immunol Rev 204:27–42
18. Aiba S, Terunuma A, Manome H, Tagami H (1997) Dendritic cells differently respond to haptens and irritants by their production of cytokines and expression of co-stimulatory molecules. Eur J Immunology 27:3031–3038
19. Bruchhausen S, Zahn S, Valk E, Knop J, Becker D (2003) Thiol antioxidants block the activation of antigen-presenting cells by contact sensitizers. J Invest Dermatol 121:1039–1044
20. Becker D, Valk E, Zahn S, Brand P, Knop J (2003) Coupling of contact sensitizers to thiol groups is a key event for the activation of monocytes and monocyte-derived dendritic cells. J Invest Dermatol 120:233–238
21. Aiba S, Manome H, Nakagawa S, Mollah ZU, Ohtani T, Yoshino Y, Tagami H (2003) p 38 Mitogen-activated protein kinase and extracellular signal-regulated kinases play distinct roles in the activation of dendritic cells by two representative haptens, NiCl2 and 2,4-dinitrochlorobenzene. J Invest Dermatol 120:390–399
22. Arrighi JF, Rebsamen M, Rousset F, Kindler V, Hauser C (2001) A critical role for p38 mitogen-activated protein kinase in the maturation of human blood-derived dendritic cells induced by lipopolysaccharide, TNF-alpha, and contact sensitizers. J Immunol 166:3837–3845
23. Sanderson JP, Naisbitt DJ, Farrell J, Ashby CA, Tucker MJ, Rieder MJ, Pirmohamed M, Clarke SE, Park BK (2007) Sulfamethoxazole and its metabolite nitroso sulfamethoxazole stimulate dendritic cell costimulatory signaling. J Immunol 178:5533–5542
24. Rodriquez PR, Lopez S, Mayorga C, Antunez C, Fernandez TD, Torres MJ, Blanca M (2006) Potential involvement of dendritic cells in delayed-type hypersensitivity reactions to beta-lactams. J Allergy Clin Immunol 118:949–956
25. Naisbitt DJ, Farrell J, Gordon SF, Maggs JL, Burkhart C, Pichler WJ, Pirmohamed M, Park BK (2002) Covalent binding of the nitroso metabolite of sulfamethoxazole leads to toxicity and major histocompatibility complex-restricted antigen presentation. Mol Pharmacol 62:628–637
26. Scheibner KA, Lutz MA, Boodoo S, Fenton MJ, Powell JD, Horton MR (2006) Hyaluronan fragments act as an endogenous danger signal by engaging TLR2. J Immunol 177:1272–1281
27. Beere HM (2005) Death versus survival: functional interaction between the apoptotic and stress-inducible heat shock protein pathways. J Clin Invest 115:2633–2639
28. Shi Y, Evans JE, Rock KL (2003) Molecular identification of a danger signal that alerts the immune system to dying cells. Nature 425:516–521
29. Shi Y, Zheng W, Rock KL (2000) Cell injury releases endogenous adjuvants that stimulate cytotoxic T cell responses. Proc Natl Acad Sci USA 97:14590–14595
30. Uetrecht JP (1999) New concepts in immunology relevant to idiosyncratic drug reactions: the "danger hypothesis" and innate immune system. Chem Res Toxicology 12:387–395
31. Descamps V, Valance A, Edlinger C (2001) Association of human herpesvirus 6 infection with drug reaction with eosinophilia and systemic symptoms. Arch Dermatol 137:301–304
32. Reilly TP, Lash LH, Doll MA, Hein DW, Woster PM, Svensson CG (2000) A role for bioactivation and covalent binding within epidermal keratinocytes in sulfonamide-induced cutaneous drug reactions. J Invest Dermatol 114:1164–1173
33. Naisbitt DJ, Farrell J, Wong G, Depta JP, Dodd CC, Hopkins JE, Gibney CA, Chadwick DW, Pichler WJ, Pirmohamed M, Park BK (2003) Characterization of drug-specific T cells in lamotrigine hypersensitivity. J Allergy Clin Immunol 111:1393–1403
34. Naisbitt DJ, Britschgi M, Wong G, Farrell J, Depta JP, Chadwick DW, Pichler WJ, Pirmohamed M, Park BK (2003) Hypersensitivity reactions to carbamazepine: characterization of the specificity, phenotype, and cytokine profile of drug-specific T cell clones. Mol Pharmacol 63:732–741
35. Schnyder B, Mauri-Hellweg D, Zanni M, Bettens F, Pichler WJ (1997) Direct, MHC-dependent presentation of the drug sulfamethoxazole to human alphabeta T cell clones. J Clin Invest 100:136–141
36. Zanni MP, von Greyerz S, Schnyder B, Brander KA, Frutig K, Hari Y, Valitutti S, Pichler WJ (1998) HLA-restricted, processing- and metabolism-independent pathway of drug recognition by human alpha beta T lymphocytes. J Clin Invest 102:p1591–p1598

37. Zanni MP, von Greyerz S, Hari Y, Schnyder B, Pichler WJ (1999) Recognition of local anesthetics by alphabeta+ T cells. J Invest Dermatol 112:197–204
38. Zanni MP, Mauri-Hellweg D, Brander C, Wendland T, Schnyder B, Frei E, von Greyerz S, Bircher A, Pichler WJ (1997) Characterization of lidocaine-specific T cells. J Immunol 158: 1139–1148
39. Sieben S, Kawakubo Y, Al Masaoudi T, Merk HF, Blomeke B (2002) Delayed-type hypersensitivity reaction to paraphenylenediamine is mediated by 2 different pathways of antigen recognition by specific alphabeta human T-cell clones. J Allergy Clin Immunology 109:1005–1011
40. Christiansen C (2002) Late-onset allergy-like reactions to X-ray contrast media. Curr Opin Allergy Clin Immunol 2:333–339
41. Christiansen C, Pichler WJ, Skotland T (2000) Delayed allergy-like reactions to X-ray contrast media: mechanistic considerations. Eur Radiol 10:1965–1975
42. Schmid DA, Pichler W (2006) T cell-mediated hypersensitivity to quinolones: mechanisms and cross-reactivity. Clin Exp Allergy 36:59–69
43. Pichler WJ (2005) Direct T-cell stimulations by drugs, bypassing the innate immune system. Toxicology 209:95–100
44. Suzuki Y, Inagi R, Aono T, Yamanishi K, Shiohara T (1998) Human herpesvirus 6 infection as a risk factor for the development of severe drug-induced hypersensitivity syndrome. Arch Dermatol 134:1108–1112
45. Coopman SA, Johnson RA, Platt R, Stern R (1993) Cutaneous disease and drug reactions in HIV infection. N Engl J Med 328:1670–1674
46. Shiohara T, Inaoka M, Kano Y (2006) Drug-induced hypersensitivity syndrome (DIHS): a reaction induced by a complex interplay among herpesviruses and antiviral and antidrug immune responses. Allergol Int 55:1–8
47. Shiohara T, Iijima M, Ikezawa Z, Hashimoto K (2007) The diagnosis of a DRESS syndrome has been sufficiently established on the basis of typical clinical features and viral reactivations. Br J Dermatol 156:1083–1084
48. Taliercio CP, Olney BA, Lie JT (1985) Myocarditis related to drug hypersensitivity. Mayo Clin Proc 60:463–468
49. Engel JN, Mellul VG, Goodman DB (1986) Phenytoin hypersensitivity: a case of severe acute rhabdomyolisis. Am J Med 81:938–930
50. Descamps V, Collot S, Houhou N, Ranger-Rogez S (2003) Human herpesvirus-6 encephalitis associated with hypersensitivity syndrome. Ann Neurol 53:280
51. Pirmohamed M, Park BK (2001) Genetics susceptibility to adverse drug reactions. Trends Pharmacol Sci 22:298–305
52. Shear NH, Spielberg SP, Grant DM, Tanq BK, Kalow W (1986) Differences in metabolism of sulfonamides predisposing to idiosyncratic toxicity. Ann Intern Med 105:179–184
53. Wolkenstein P, Charue D, Laurent P, Revuz J, Roujeau JC, Bagot M (1995) Metabolic predisposition to cutaneous adverse drug reactions: role in toxic epidermal necrolysis caused by sulfonamides and anticonvulsants. Arch Dermatol 131:544–551
54. Carr A, Gross AS, Hoskins JM, Penny R, Cooper DA (1994) Acetylation phenotype and cutaneous hypersensitivity to trimethoprim-sulphamethoxazole in HIV-infected patients. AIDS 8:333–337
55. Pirmohamed M, Alfirevic A, Vilar J, Stalford A, Wilkins EG, Sim E, Park BK (2000) Association analysis of drug metabolizing enzyme gene polymorphisms in HIV-positive patients with co-trimoxazole hypersensitivity. Pharmacogenetics 10:705–713
56. Wolkenstein P, Loriot MA, Aractinqi S, Cabelquenne A, Beaune P, Chosidow O (2000) Prospective evaluation of detoxification pathways as markers of cutaneous adverse reactions to sulphonamides in AIDS. Pharmacogenetics 10:821–828
57. Wolkenstein P, Loriot MA, Flahault A, Cadilhac M, Caumes E, Eliaszewicz M, Beaune P, Roujeau JC, Chosidow O, The EG (2005) Association analysis of drug metabolizing enzyme gene polymorphisms in AIDS patients with cutaneous reactions to sulfonamides. J Invest Dermatol 125:1080–1082

58. Pirmohamed M, Lin K, Chadwick D, Park BK (2001) TNFalpha promoter region gene polymorphisms in carbamazepine-hypersensitive patients. Neurology 56:890–896
59. Chung WH, Hunq SI, Honq HS, Hsih MS, Yang LC, Ho HC, Wu JY, Chen YT (2004) Medical genetics: a marker for Stevens-Johnson syndrome. Nature 428:486
60. Alfirevic A, Jorgensen AL, Williamson PR, Chadwick DW, Park BK, Pirmohamed M (2006) HLA-B locus in Caucasian patients with carbamazepine hypersensitivity. Pharmacogenetics 7:813–818
61. Mallal S, Nolan D, Witt C, Masel G, Martin AM, Moore C, Sayer D, Castley A, Mamotte C, Maxwell D, James I, Christiansen FT (2002) Association between presence of HLA-B*5701, HLA-DR7, and HLA-DQ3 and hypersensitivity to HIV-1 reverse-transcriptase inhibitor abacavir. Lancet 359:727–732
62. Gell PGH, Coombs RRA (1963) Classification of allergic reactions responsible for clinical hypersensitivity and disease. In: Gell PBH, Coombs RRA (eds) Clinical Aspects of Immunology. Oxford, England: Blackwell, pp 317–337
63. Romagnani S (2004) Immunologic influences on allergy and the TH1/TH2 balance. J Allergy Clin Immunol 113:395–400
64. Nassif A, Bensussan A, Dorothee G, Mami-Chouaib F, Bachot N, Bagot M, Boumsell L, Roujeau JC (2002) Drug specific cytotoxic T-cells in the skin lesions of a patient with toxic epidermal necrolysis. J Invest Dermatol 118:728–733
65. Schnyder B, Frutig K, Mauri-Hellweg D, Limat A, Yawalkar N, Pichler WJ (1998) T-cell-mediated cytotoxicity against keratinocytes in sulfamethoxazol-induced skin reaction. Clin Exp Allergy 28:1412–1417
66. Britschgi M, Steiner UC, Schmid S, Depta JP, Senti G, Bircher A, Burkhart C, Yawalkar N, Pichler WJ (2001) T-cell involvement in drug-induced acute generalized exanthematous pustulosis. J Clin Invest 107:1433–1441
67. Keller M, Spanou Z, Schaerli P, Britschgi M, Yawalkar N, Seitz M, Villiger PM, Pichler WJ (2005) T cell-regulated neutrophilic inflammation in autoinflammatory diseases. J Immunol 175:7678–7686
68. Yawalkar N, Shrikhande M, Hari Y, Nievergelt H, Braathen LR, Pichler WJ (2000) Evidence for a role for IL-5 and eotaxin in activating and recruiting eosinophils in drug-induced cutaneous eruptions. J Allergy Clin Immunol 106:1171–1176
69. Schaerli P, Britschgi M, Keller M, Steiner UC, Steinmann LS, Moser B, Pichler WJ (2004) Characterization of human T cells that regulate neutrophilic skin inflammation. J Immunol 173:2151–2158
70. Yawalkar N, Hari Y, Frutig K, Egli F, Wendland T, Braathen LR, Pichler WJ (2000) T cells isolated from positive epicutaneous test reactions to amoxicillin and ceftriaxone are drug specific and cytotoxic. J Invest Dermatol 115:647–652
71. Schnyder B, Burkhart C, Schnyder-Frutig K, von Greyerz S, Naisbitt DJ, Pirmohamed M, Park BK, Pichler WJ (2000) Recognition of sulfamethoxazole and its reactive metabolites by drug-specific CD4+ T cells from allergic individuals. J Immunol 164:6647–6654
72. Pichler WJ (2003) Lessons from drug allergy: against dogmata. Curr Allergy Asthma Rep 3:1–3
73. Kuechler PC, Britschgi M, Schmid S, Hari Y, Grabscheid B, Pichler WJ (2004) Cytotoxic mechanisms in different forms of T-cell-mediated drug allergies. Allergy 59:613–622
74. Le Cleach L, Delaire S, Boumsell L, Bagot M, Bourgault-Villada I, Bensussan A, Roujeau JC (2000) Blister fluid T lymphocytes during toxic epidermal necrolysis are functional cytotoxic cells which express human natural killer (NK) inhibitory receptors. Clin Exp Immunol 119:225–230
75. Chung WH, Hung SI, Yang JY, Su SC, Huang SP, Wei CY, Chin SW, Chiou CC, Chu SC, Ho HC, Yang CH, Lu CF, Wu JY, Liao YD, Chen YT. (2008) Granulysin is a key mediator for disseminated keratinocyte death in Stevens-Johnson syndrome and toxic epidermal necrolysis. Nat Med 14:1343–1350

Food Allergy: Mechanisms and Clinical Manifestations

Stephan C. Bischoff

Introduction

Food allergy (FA) is defined as an adverse reaction to food (ARF) caused by an individually occurring immunologic hypersensitivity against food antigen. This definition clearly separates FA from other forms of ARF not mediated by immunologic mechanisms such as intolerance reactions caused by enzyme deficiencies or toxic reactions caused by contaminating microbes or chemicals. Since ARF is common in the general population – about 20–30% seems to be afflicted – the rather small subgroup of patients suffering from true food allergy needs to be identified by validated diagnostic means. According to recent epidemiologic data, 1/4 of children and 1/10 of adults with ARF have true FA based on immunologic mechanisms, either IgE-mediated or other forms (Table 1). Accordingly, the prevalence of food allergy is 3–8% in small children, and 1–3% in teenagers and adults [1–4]. The fact that food allergy is preferentially a disease of the early years of life is related to our current understanding of the mechanisms of food allergy closely related to the integrity of the gastrointestinal (GI) barrier. The GI mucosa is the site of sensitization and challenge, but not necessarily the shock organ. Actually, any organ can be involved, but in most cases, symptoms manifest at the level of the skin, the GI or respiratory mucosa, or a combination thereof [4]. In the present chapter, our current understanding of the mechanisms, the clinical presentation, comprehensive diagnostic means, and therapeutic strategies are reviewed. Apart from the children aspects, particular emphasis will be on adults suffering from FA manifesting in the GI tract, because this form of FA has been often neglected in the past.

S.C. Bischoff (✉)
Professor of Medicine, Department of Nutritional Medicine and Immunology,
University of Hohenheim, Stuttgart, Germany
e-mail: bischoff.stephan@uni-hohenheim.de

R. Pawankar et al. (eds.), *Allergy Frontiers: Clinical Manifestations*,
DOI: 10.1007/978-4-431-88317-3_26, © Springer 2009

Table 1 Epidemiology of adverse reactions to food (ARF) and food allergy (FA)

ARF (20–30%)			
Children		Adults	
FA (3–8%)	Other (10–20%)	FA (1–3%)	Other (20–25%)
IgE-mediated	Infections	IgE-mediated	Food intolerances
IgE-independent	Unclear	IgE-independent	Irritable bowel syndrome
			Other diseases ($\rightarrow$ Table 4)

Mechanisms

Basis of any allergic reaction is an adequate antigen exposure, an abnormal immune response, a genetic predisposition, and an "acquired" predisposition, e.g., an impaired mucosal barrier, which might be of particular relevance for food allergy, but possible also for other forms of allergic diseases [4, 5].

Food allergens (mostly proteins) are to a large extent, but by far not totally degraded during passage through the stomach and the intestine. Studies showed that about 2% of the food proteins ingested daily (about 50–100 g/day) reach the intestinal mucosa in intact form. This is necessary to establish a mucosal immune response, which normally leads to the generation of immunologic tolerance provided that the mucosal barrier is intact. This normal immune response is observed in all individuals and can be estimated by the generation of food-antigen-specific T cells (memory cells) and food-antigen-specific IgA and IgG production. The characteristics of the most relevant food allergens, and the key elements involved in allergic inflammation will be discussed in more detail.

Triggering Food Allergens

The most relevant food allergens triggering disease are dependent on age of the patient, and on eating habits of a population, therefore on the geographic region. In small children chicken eggs, cow's milk, soy, and wheat are common food allergens. In some countries (US, UK, France, less in Germany, and other countries) peanuts also play a significant role as triggers for FA, which is of particular importance because peanut allergy requires only tiny amounts of peanut allergen, which causes particularly often life-threatening events. Apart from peanuts, other food allergens such as nuts (hazelnuts, walnuts, etc.), fish, shellfish, milk, and egg are frequent triggers of fatal allergic reactions, which are more often induced by food, drugs and venoms compared to pollens and other inhalative allergens [6, 7]. With increasing age, the spectrum of relevant food allergens changes. Egg, milk, soy and wheat become less important, while food allergens cross-reactive with pollen allergens increase in relevance instead. This change is most prominent in adults, in whom most food allergies are related to pollen-associated or other airborne allergen-associated food allergens. Some of the relevant cross-reactive food allergens are listed in Table 2. The importance of different cross-reactive groups is very much dependent on the geographic region, the local pollen exposure and eating habits. On the other hand, the fact that food allergens cross-reactive with airborne allergens are the dominant ones in adults seems to be a world-wide phenomenon [8, 9].

IgE-Mediated and IgE-Independent Abnormal Immune Responses

The best characterized hypersensitivity reaction to food is the IgE-mediated type I-reaction according to Coombs and Gell, who distinguished four types of hypersensitivity reactions according to the antigen-recognizing molecules (type I, IgE; type II, red blood cells surface molecules; type III, IgG complexes; type IV, allergen-specific T cells) [10]. Type I reactions, which are also taken as a basis for many cases of bronchial asthma, seasonal rhinitis, and atopic skin diseases, are divided into an immediate phase and a late phase occurring facultatively a few hours after the immediate phase.

The immediate phase is characterized by the IgE-dependent activation of mast cells and basophils and the release of pro-inflammatory mediators from these cells such as histamine, proteases, leukotrienes, and cytokines. This reaction requires a preceding sensitization phase in which the specific immune system is challenged with allergen in a way that leads to the production of sufficient amounts of specific IgE. This IgE is bound to the surface of mast cells and basophils because they express the high-affinity IgE receptor. Once the cell is "loaded" with specific IgE, a second challenge can lead to crosslinking of surface-bound IgE. This is an activation signal for the cells which in response start to degranulate and release mediators like histamine and protease from their granules within a few seconds. At the same time, the cells start to synthesize mediators leading to a more sustained release of mediators such as eicosanoids and cytokines.

The late phase is characterized by the infiltration of the tissue with further inflammatory cells such as neutrophils, eosinophils, and lymphocytes. These cells are attracted by mediators such as TNFα, IL-5, IL-4 and IL-3 release by mast cells and basophils upon IgE-dependent immediate-type activation. The role of mast cells in this clinically more important late phase reaction, as well as in hypersensitivity reactions other than type I reactions, such as type IV hypersensitivity reactions also occurring during allergic reactions, has been clearly documented [4]. Such mechanisms play a role in milk and soy protein-induced enteropathy, as well as in celiac disease. Immunological reactions to food can also be caused by a combination of IgE-dependent and IgE-independent reactions. Especially type IV

Table 2 Examples of food allergens cross-reacting with inhalative allergens (See also www. allergome.org)

1. Birch pollen (frequent in Northern Europe)

Cross-reacting with

- Hazelnuts
- Pome fruits and Stone fruit
- Carrots and Celery (Spices)

Common allergen epitopes

- Bet v 1 (pathogenesis-related protein 10): Major allergen
- Bet v 2 (birch profiling): Minor allergen
- Bet v 6 (isoflavon reductase-like protein, cross-reactive with exotic fruits): Minor allergen

2. Mugwort (frequent in Middle and Southern Europe)

Cross-reacting with

- Carrots and Celery, Spices
- Fruits (mango, grapes, litschi)
- Seeds of sunflowers, pistachios and cabbage

Common allergen epitopes

3. Gras pollens (only Southern Europe)

Cross-reacting with

- Tomato
- Melon
- Peanuts and Soy

Common allergen epitopes

4. Ragweed (frequent in the USA)

Cross-reacting with

- Melon
- Zucchini
- Cucumber
- Banana

Common allergen epitopes

5. Lipid transfer protein (LTP) allergy (in Northern Europe, severe reactions!)

Cross-reacting with

- Peach
- Apricot, Plum, Apple

Common allergen epitopes

- LTP

6. House dust mites (ubiquitous)

Cross-reacting with

- Crustaceae
- Seafruit

Common allergen epitopes

- Tropomyosine

7. Latex (*Ficus benjamini*)

Cross-reacting with

- Banana
- Kiwi
- Avocado etc.

Common allergen epitopes

See also www.allergome.org

hypersensitivity reactions to food proteins can be expected, due to the presence of food antigen-specific T helper cells and cytotoxic T-cells [4, 5]. Most importantly, human mast cells induce the recruitment and local activation of eosinophils by expressing factors such as IL-5 upon IgE-dependent activation, and induce the recruitment of neutrophils by releasing IL-8 and TNFα. The latter has been shown in vitro for both human and murine mast cells, as well as in murine disease models [11, 12]. In comparison to mouse mast cells, however, the amount of TNF produced by human mast cells on a per-cell-basis is small, compared with monocytes, and the portion that is preformed and stored in granules is even smaller, although it is consistently detectable [13]. Nevertheless, human mast cells, even by releasing small quantities of preformed TNF might be responsible for the discrete neutrophil infiltration typically seen at sites of allergic inflammation.

In vitro studies indicate that human mast cells also participate in regulating lymphocyte functions in the course of allergic inflammation. Upon IgE-crosslinking, mast cells produce IL-13, a cytokine that supports the production of allergen-specific IgE by B cells. The release of IL-13 can be further increased by the presence of IL-4, which is known to shift the cytokine profile produced by human mast cells away from pro-inflammatory cytokines such as TNF, IL-1 and IL-6, to TH2 cytokines including IL-13 [14]. Human mast cells can also regulate T-cell functions, for example through PGD2, which almost exclusively derives from activated mast cells and is released during allergic reactions [15]. Recently, exciting new functions of PGD2 have been identified that indicate a particular role for PGD2 at the onset and for the perpetuation of asthma in young adults. The lipid mediator evokes airway hypersensitivity and chemotaxis of T cells, basophils and eosinophils through interaction with two receptors, the prostanoid DP receptor (PTGDR) on granulocytes and smooth muscle cells, and CRTH2 (chemoattractant receptor-homologous molecule expressed on TH2 cells) on TH2 cells [16, 17]. Furthermore, gene-mutation analyses have identified PTGDR as an asthma-susceptibility gene [17]. Apart from PGD2, other human mast-cell mediators such as LTB4, CCL3 and CCL4, OX40 ligand and TNF are involved in recruiting T cells and triggering T-cell-mediated adaptive immune responses, including memory induction, which enhance and perpetuate allergic reactions [18].

However, mast cells, at least under normal conditions, are not a relevant source of IL-4. It has been repeatedly claimed that mast cells, in addition to TH2 cells, produce IL-4; however, well-performed in vitro studies using mature human mast cells from non-allergic individuals, as well as mouse in vivo studies, could not confirm such findings [14, 19, 20]. Instead, TH2 cells and basophils seem to be the relevant sources of IL-4 in humans, whereas mast cells, if at all, might contribute to local IL-4 production under allergic conditions [21]. This fits with the recent in vivo finding in mice that basophils are crucial for the induction of IgE-mediated chronic allergic inflammation, for which T cells, and even mast cells, were dispensable [22].

Inflammatory mediators derived from mast cells und eosinophils are primarily responsible for the clinical symptoms of patients with food allergies. These patients have an increased level of histamine (or methyl histamine), tryptase, eosinophilic cationic protein (ECP), IL-5 and TNFα in serum, urine, intestinal lavages, and stool samples [4, 23].

Histological examinations show that mast cells and eosinophils degranulate in the intestinal mucosa after localized provocation testing and that they release mediators such as cytokines [24]. These cells are no longer understood to be solely inflammatory cells, but also as immune modulatory cells, which contribute to homeostasis in the intestines and to the suppression of bacteria and parasites [4].

Not only is the specific immune system involved in immunological hypersensitivity reactions, but also the innate immune system. The characterization of key molecules belonging to the innate immune defense mechanism, such as defensins, mucin or synactin and their possible mutation in people with allergies, is therefore of the utmost importance for the understanding of the mechanisms and the development of new therapy concepts [25]. Disorders of the innate immune system can also be responsible for deviations of the specific immune system, which lead, for example, to an over-production of specific IgE.

During an allergic reaction, naive lymphocytes of the GALT give rise to the production of Th2-cytokines such as IL-4 and IL-13, which encourage the development of IgE-producing plasma cells. Allergen-specific T-cells, which apart from IL-4 und IL-13 also produce IL-5, can actually be isolated in the blood, skin and mucosa of patients with FA. These cytokines do not only regulate the IgE-synthesis (IL-4, IL-13), but also the colonization and activation of inflammatory cells such as mast cells (IL-4) and eosinophilic granulocytes (IL-5) [4, 5].

Clinical studies have shown that IgE is produced locally in the respiratory and gastrointestinal mucosa. This might explain why serum IgE evaluations and skin tests do not closely correlate with mucosal allergic reactions in the intestines. In atopic patients, the increased IgE levels are closely related to IL-13, whose gene is attributed to a polymorphism, which is associated with atopy. The IgE-induced, allergic immune response can therefore be divided into three phases: the clinically silent sensitization phase, usually during infancy or childhood; the symptomatic effector phase, which is composed of an acute and a facultatively delayed reaction; and the chronic, organ-destroying phase, which can be the outcome of reoccurring delayed reactions [4].

In intestinal allergic reactions, activated mast cells have been proposed to induce the inflammation, tissue transformation and fibrosis observed in both allergic and non-allergic processes, such as Crohn's disease [4, 26]. More recently, it became evident that mast cells stimulated by IgE crosslinking also trigger local nerve responses resulting in pain and diarrhea [27, 28]. It has become apparent in recent years that the enteric nervous system (ENS) plays a role in regulating allergic inflammatory cells such as lymphocytes, mast cells and eosinophils. The morphologic-functional association between immune cells and nerve cells has mainly been described for mast cells and in some cases has been extended to include eosinophils [29]. It should be emphasized, that not only is the GALT innervated, but conversely, the ENS is also regulated in a crucial manner by mediators derived from mucosal immune cells [4, 30]. Such neuro-immune interactions may explain the frequent psychological and functional accompanying symptoms, which characterize many patients with allergic and other chronic bowel disorders.

A delayed development of the protective IgA system within the gut-associated lymphoid tissue (GALT) in the postnatal phase, or a particularly pronounced switch to IgE-producing B lymphocytes is associated with an enhanced risk for the development of allergic diseases. IgA-synthesis is induced mainly by TGF-ß from Th3 cells and external triggers, whilst IgE-synthesis is dependent on CD40 ligands, as well as the cytokines IL-4 and IL-13, which are produced by the Th2 cells and inflammatory cells (mast cells, basophils) [5]. In contrast, Th1 cytokines such as IFNg inhibit the activity of Th2 cells, which explains how a controlled Th1-dominant immune response, triggered, for example, by certain bacterial products, can contribute to restricting a primary pre-existingTH2 response in the bowels and thus prevent an over-production of IgE. Such procedures support the "hygiene theory" claiming that high hygiene standard in particular during the early years of life may support not only the development of immunologic diseases such as allergy including food allergy, but also other immunological diseases such as rheumatic arthritis, type 1 diabetes mellitus and chronic inflammatory intestinal disorders [31, 32].

Loss of Oral Tolerance – the Role of the Mucosal Barrier

The GI barrier forms the largest barrier of the body to the environment (estimated 400 qm, compared to the respiratory mucosa 100–200 qm or the skin 2 qm). The GI barrier consists of a complex interaction of different elements such as a mucus layer, secretory products like sIgA and defensins protecting the host against infection, and the commensal flora, the epithelial barrier, an extensive mucosal immune system comprising innate immune cells (mast cells, eosinophils, macrophages) and adaptive immune cells (lymphocytes, GALT), and, most importantly, an enteric nervous system (ENS) acting, to a large extent, independently of the central nervous system (CNS) and controlling all major functions of the GI tract (secretion, absorption, motility, immune defense).

Any impairment of the GI barrier, either because of immaturity in early life or acquired during later life, promotes the development of food allergy, and, possibly, other forms of allergy, because oral tolerance cannot be established or maintained. Common causes for an acquired impairment of the GI muosa are infections (bacterial, viral), toxins (e.g. bacterial toxins such as Clostridium difficile), or disturbances of the GI flora (e.g. caused by treatment with antibiotics). Interestingly, such conditions are known to be associated with the onset of food allergy suggesting a causal link between such events. For example, FA is most common in newborns and small children in whom the GI barrier is not yet fully maturate. Once these children become elder, most of them lose spontaneously their allergy, most likely because of maturation of the GI barrier, and this establishment of host defense and tolerance induction. The situation is more complex in adults, but possibly similar mechanisms could play a role. The hygiene hypothesis, which has been well established by multiple epidemiologic studies and became partly confirmed by experimental studies, suggests that particular conditions such as life style, reduced bacterial exposure because of high hygiene standard or frequent use of antibiotics might promote an impairment of the GI barrier and thus the development of intestinal hypersensitivity against food proteins and other antigens such as bacterial antigens derived from the gut lumen. Interestingly, not only allergy, but also other chronic inflammatory diseases such as IBD and RA increase under such conditions. Therefore, it is tempting to speculate that an impaired GI barrier caused by particular environmental conditions and life style factors may lead to the increased occurrence of immune-mediated chronic diseases including food allergy [4, 5].

Clinical Presentation

Food allergy is not associated with specific clinical presentation, but with typical symptoms that vary depending on the organs involved (Table 3). In children, the classical manifestations are the skin and the GI mucosa, therefore symptoms such as diarrhea and skin disease (atopic dermatitis, which is facultatively caused by an allergic mechanism, or other forms such as pruritus without other efflorescences, or

Table 3 Immune-mediated food allergy

I.	Mucosal manifestation	
	GI mucosa:	Oral allergy syndrome (mostly IgE-mediated)
		Nausea and vomiting (mostly IgE-mediated)
		Diarrhea, flatulence and pain
		Eosinophilic inflammation (possibly allergy-based)
		"Irritable bowel syndrome" (mast cell-related)
		Celiac disease (IgA-mediated)
	Respiratory	allergic rhinitis and conjunctivitis (mostly IgE-mediated)
	Mucosa	Asthma bronchiale (mostly IgE-mediated)
		Otitis serosa (children)
II.	Skin manifestion	
		Urticaria and quincke-edema
		Flush, pruritus (mostly IgE-mediated)
		Atopic dermatitis (possibly allergy-based)
III.	Systemic manifestation	
		Systemic anaphylaxis (mostly IgE-mediated)
		Generalized edema
		Vasculitis (?)
IV.	Other manifestations (mostly not IgE-mediated)	
	Joints	Arthritis, fibromyalgia
	Nervous system	Migraine headaches
		Chronic fatigue
		Psychic disturbances
		Hyperactivity syndrome (children)

urticaria) are most frequent in children suffering from food allergy [33]. Whereas skin symptoms can be more easily related to atopic disease, GI symptoms are either related to allergy or to infections which needs to be distinguished. In adults, food allergy triggers most often the oral allergy syndrome (OAS), which occurs almost exclusively as an immediate, IgE-mediated reaction. The short time interval between allergen exposure and onset of symptoms such as itching of the buccal mucosa, and the classical set of food like apples and other pome fruits that triggers the OAS make diagnosis usually easy. More complicated are cases presenting delayed reactions occurring hours or even days after food challenge. These reactions are difficult to diagnose, because the history is often unclear and inconsistent, the patients are frequently altered on the psychological level, and the mechanisms do not typically involve IgE. Therefore, they cannot be confirmed by classical diagnostic means such as skin tests or measurement of specific IgE in serum. In most cases, such forms need the confirmation by a kind of double-blind placebo-controlled food challenge (DBPCFC) [4].

Allergy symptoms range from minor impairments to life-threatening shock reactions. Approximately one third of the patients with real food allergies suffer from gastrointestinal (GI) symptoms such as nausea, vomiting, cramps, flatulence and diarrhea. Others complain of skin problems (urticaria, Quincke edema, atopic dermatitis), respiratory symptoms (rhinitis, bronchial asthma), shock symptoms or less clearly defined systemic ailments (migraine, fatigue syndrome, edema, hypotension, arthritis etc.) [34–36]. While dermatological, respiratory and systemic signs of allergies are sufficiently well-known and established, this is not so for GI manifestations, which are frequently caused by food antigens and are difficult to diagnose and treat [4].

In case of GI-related FA, a long list of other diseases have to be considered that might also be responsible for the common combination of GI symptoms and adverse reactions to food, which afflicts 20–30% of the general population in industrialized countries (Table 4). The number of diseases that must be excluded is

Table 4 Differential diagnosis of ARF associated with GI symptoms

ARF	20–30%
ARF with GI symptoms	~20%
Lactose intolerance	~5%
Irritable bowel syndrome	~5%
Other carbohydrate intolerances	~2%
Histamine intolerance:	~1%?
Impairment of GI flora	~1%?
Food allery with GI symptoms	~0.5%
Celiac disease	~0.4%
Inflammatory bowel disease	~0.3%
Other organic causes	~0.2%
Unclear (projection?)	~5%?

Data derived from pooled epidemiologic data (? indicates estimations because of lacking comprehensive epidemiologic studies)

much longer in adults, especially in older adults, compared to children. In children, basically other inflammatory diseases, either of infectious origin (bacterial and viral diarrhea), or immune mediated diseases such as IBD or celiac disease, need to be excluded. In adults, not only additional common diseases such as lactose intolerance, other carbohydrate intolerances, histamine intolerance, have to be ruled out but also ulcers, tumor diseases, and the irritable bowl syndrome. This requires specific diagnostic means, because the clinical symptoms are too much overlapping among these diseases making it almost impossible to differentiate based just on clinical presentation [4].

IgE-Independent FA

Food-induced enteropathy is a childhood illness and is characterized by protracted diarrhea and vomiting, which leads to a clinical picture of malassimilation. Protein-losing enteropathy can lead to edema, abdominal distension, nausea, vomiting, diarrhea and anemia. Infectious and metabolic diseases, lymphangioectasy and celiac disease are to be diagnostically differentiated. Underlying mechanisms include the formation of immune complexes and abnormal T-cell reactions after the consumption of milk, soy and other foods, such as egg, fish, cereals, rice, vegetables and meat [33]. Normally, there is no detectable specific IgE against these foods. The diagnosis is based on endoscopic and histological findings (increased intraepithelial lymphocytes and eosinophilic granulocytes, villous atrophy), as well as on elimination diets and re-exposure.

Eosinophilic GI Disorders and Allergy

Eosinophilic esophagitis and gastro-esophageal reflux disease (GERD): Investigations involving milk elimination in children with reflux symptoms showed that approximately one third of the reflux conditions are caused by cow's milk [37]. In such cases, classical medicinal anti-reflux treatment does not lead to any improvement and histological investigation shows a marked infiltration with eosinophilic granulocytes, which gives the illness its name. Typical symptoms include vomiting, retrosternal pains and dysphagia due to strictures, sometimes also signs of asthma. Recent studies have demonstrated that this illness is by no means limited to children, but can also affect adults to a still largely undefined extent [38, 39].

Eosinophilic gastroenteritis: It is characterized by eosinophilic infiltration of the gastric/enteric mucosa, muscularis, or serosa. Abdominal pains, vomiting, diarrhea occur simultaneously in over 50% of the patients. Ascites is seen in patients with serosa infiltrations. More than two thirds of the cases show eosinophilia also in the peripheral blood. The differential diagnosis of the eosinophilic gastroenteritis in children includes parasites, IBD, connective tissue diseases, tumors and drug allergies. The eosinophilic gastroenteritis itself is closely associated, in 50–70% of the cases, with food allergies and other atopic diseases [4, 38, 39].

It should be emphasized that FA, contrary to FI, can lead to a life-threatening anaphylaxis. Indeed, FA is considered to be the main cause of anaphylaxis in industrial countries such as the USA and Europe [40]. The prevalence of the peanut allergy (0.5–7% of adults in the USA and UK) and its potential fatal consequences has already had an impact on regulations in institutions ranging from school canteens to airlines. Occasionally, the anaphylaxis only appears under simultaneous physical effort, for example, in an anaphylaxis triggered by a cereal and induced by exercise. Acetylsalicylate and other NSAID can likewise contribute to an increase in the allergic symptoms.

Diagnostic Means

The diagnosis of food allergy is primarily based on a carefully performed patient's history with detailed informations about the type of symptoms, the suspected food triggers, and the time interval between food challenge and start of symptoms. Moreover, information on allergies other than FA, on the family history, and on efforts to exclude other possible diseases causing similar symptoms is mandatory. If patient history and exclusion diagnosis support the suspect of allergy, specific allergy tests like skin tests (Prick and others) as well as laboratory tests (measurement of total and specific IgE against allergens selected individually according to the patient's history, formally called RAST) need to be performed [41].

Specific indications for the measurement of specific IgE are the suspected sensitization against food antigens that cannot be easily tested in skin tests (for example: histamine or protease-rich food such as tomato), suspected fatal reactions against food, substantial skin diseases including urticaria factitia, drug treatment that might impair skin test results, and babies and small children who would possibly not tolerate skin testing. Interestingly, cut-off levels of specific IgE have been published for some allergens (egg 7 kU/l, milk15 kU/l, fish 20 kU/l, peanut 14 kU/l) that must be exceeded to confirm food allergy per se without the need for further confirmation by other means [42]. However, this interesting result could be confirmed only partially by a more recent study from Germany [43], possibly because the definition of confirmed food allergy symptoms was more detailed. In individual cases, other laboratory tests such as histological examinations of mucosal samples e.g. for eosinophilia, or special laboratory parameters such as measurement of basophils activation markers (CD63, CD203c), or mast cell and eosinophil mediators like ECP, EDN (Methyl-)Histamine, or tryptase can be helpful. If the results are not consistent, a PBPCFC procedure might be reasonable.

Because of the possibility that food allergen-specific IgE can be produced only locally, both skin test and measurement of specific IgE (formerly called RAST) might yield false negative results. On the other hand, since those tests indicate allergen sensitization, and not necessarily allergic disease, both tests might also yield false positive results. Indeed, both are true and occur more often than anticipated (about 30% of cases depending on the allergen and the organs involved). Therefore, the diagnosis of FA should never be based just on such allergy tests, at least not if the history does not fit clearly with the laboratory results. In case of any doubts, a DBPCFC should be performed.

In case of suspected GI allergy, additional tests such as screening tests like measurement of calprotecin in feces, eosinophil-related tests such as histology and measurement of eosinophil markers like EDN in feces and other body fluids, hemoccult tests, microbiological examinations as well as endoscopy and sonography are helpful [4, 44, 45]. Lactose intolerance and other carbohydrate intolerances should be excluded by H2 breath tests, facultatively combined with an appropriate genetic test for the detection of lactose gene mutations [46]. Usually, the right consortium of physicians should be involved (allergologist, pediatrician, dermatologist, pneumologist, and/or gastroenterologist).

A supervised provocation test, in the form of a DBPCFC, is necessary in ambiguous cases, whereby food antigens are taken either orally, in the form of a gelatin capsule, or fed directly into the intestines by means of a tube. The DBPCFC method is viewed as the gold standard for confirmation of the diagnosis of FA and should constitute an obligatory component of the diagnosis in all uncertain cases [4, 41]. On the other hand, even this procedure has weaknesses, especially in regard to the clarification of a FA with GI manifestations. The readout of these tests is, as far as GI symptoms are concerned, hardly standardized and validated, i.e. this is a subjective rather than an objective test. Secondly, no immunological reaction is verified, that means, the test checks for intolerance to food, but not for an allergy [4]. Several attempts have been made to develop a gastrointestinal equivalent of the allergy skin tests, in which food allergens are administered to the stomach or bowel mucosa and reactions such as reddening or swelling of the mucous membrane are detailed. This approach was conceived back in the 1930s and later further developed in the form of gastric, duodenal and, most recently, colonic provocations. Particularly the coloscopic allergen provocation (COLAP) has been validated as a localized test procedure in clinical studies, and offers an alternative to oral provocation tests for gastroenterological patients [24]. Despite the obvious advantages of localized testing, these are not routinely employed in clinics, due to the expense and the necessity of endoscopic expertise. On the other hand, the endoscopic examination and histology represent the basis for the diagnosis of other immunological reactions of the GI tract to food, such as celiac disease, food-protein induced gastroenteropathies in children, or eosinophilic gastroenteritis.

Further informations can be obtained from guidelines published by the American Gastroenterological Association (AGA) on the diagnosis and treatment of food allergies [41, 47].

The complex diagnostic procedure recommended in patients with GI manifestations of food allergy is summarized in Fig. 1.

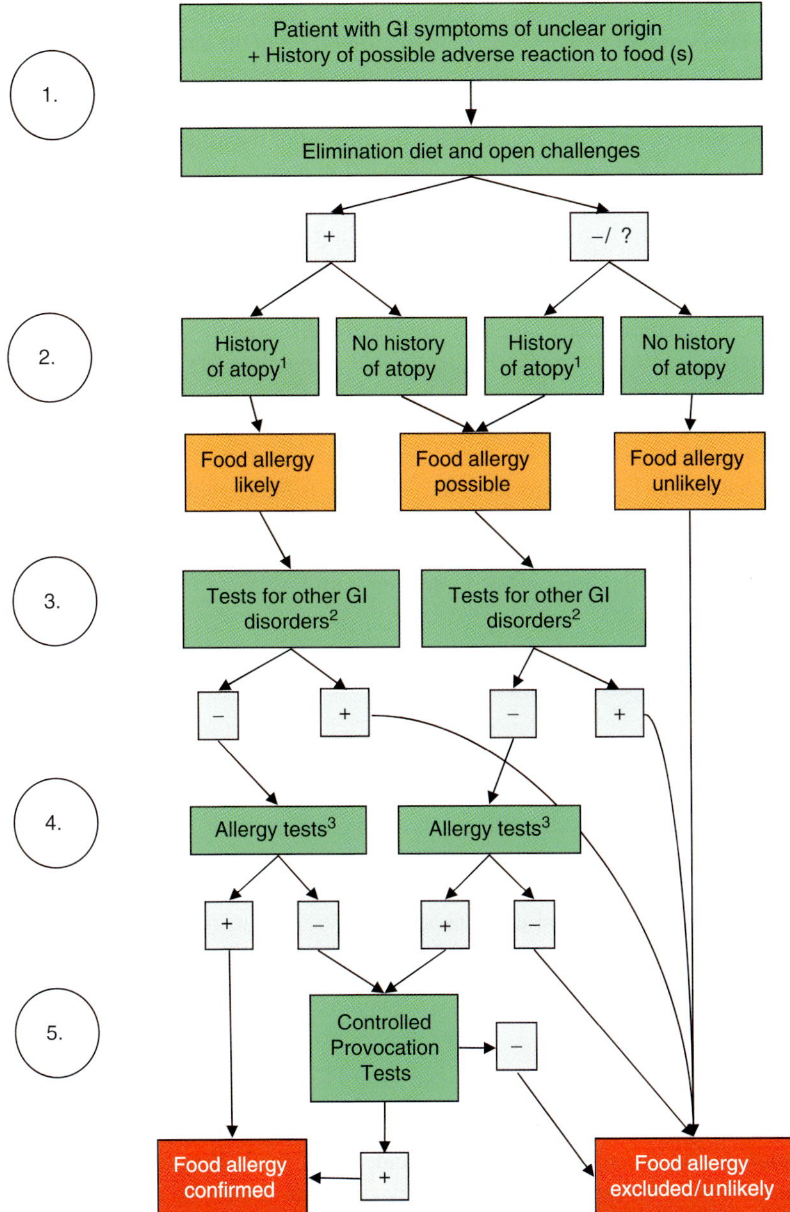

Fig. 1 Flowchart for the diagnosis of food allergies (Modified according to Bischoff and Crowe [4])

Therapy

Basis Therapy

The basis for treating food allergy is the avoidance of exposure to the allergen(s) that cause(s) the symptoms. This is particularly important in the case of a peanut allergy, in which even tiny traces of allergens can initiate substantial reactions. However, the practicability of such elimination diets is limited. They necessitate well-trained counselors, time, and a lot of motivation on the part of the affected persons. Dietetic counseling should comprise not only information on what must be avoided but also on what is allowed or at least allowed in limited quantities. Moreover, the patients should be educated in reading and understanding the labeling of food. Finally, the dietician should preview a follow-up counseling to avoid continuation of unsuccessful diets and iatrogenic induction of malnutrition [41, 47].

If an elimination diet cannot be implemented thoroughly or, if not all of the provocative foodstuffs are clearly identifiable, supplementary medicinal treatment becomes necessary. In such cases, a bowel-friendly compound of chromoglycate is obtainable [48]. In more complicated cases (short-term) treatment with corticosteroids may be unavoidable. So far it has not been researched in controlled studies, as to what extent locally effective steroids such as budesonide are suitable for the treatment of gastrointestinal food allergies [4]. To date, no evident data exist neither for the application of oral or systemic desensitization, nor for prophylactic medicinal treatment, nor similar approaches in dealing with FA.

Medical Emergency Treatment

Since an undesired exposure to food antigens cannot always be avoided, patients with an anaphylactic history must be equipped with a so-called emergency kit. The chief component of this kit is adrenaline, whose application must be carefully learnt by affected persons for emergency situations. The kit should also include a corticosteroid (2×100 mg prednisolone equivalent), as well as an antihistamine (e.g. 2×2 mg Tavergil®). People with food allergies should also learn to read and understand the labels on foodstuffs, in respect to hidden or cross-reactive allergens [49, 50].

FA Prevention

A hypo-allergenic diet is recommended for atopic mothers during pregnancy and the lactation period, in order to reduce the incidence of food allergies in their children. Foodstuffs with an especially high allergy potential should be introduced into an endangered baby's diet at a later date, in order to minimize the likelihood of a food allergy arising. In general, total breast feeding over 6 months is recommended, followed by a period of another 6 months of partial breast feeding [51, 52].

Studies have been recently published, according to which, probiotics, e.g. lactobacillus rhamnose GG, are capable of reducing the incidence of allergies in children from high-risk families. For example, the prevalence of food-induced atopic dermatitis can be reduced by approximately 50% through treatment with lactobacillus GG, during and immediately after pregnancy, as surveys 2 and/or 4 years after birth of the children have shown [53]. However, these exciting data could not be fully confirmed in recent follow-up studies from other research groups [54–56].

Future Therapeutic Directions

Immunotherapy – an Approach to a Causal Therapy of FA?

Subcutaneous immunotherapy (SCIT) has been used not only in pollen-allergic individuals, but also in individuals with pollen-associated food allergy with some success. For example, according to Asaro et al. apple-induced OAS could be reduced by 50–100% after SCIT with birch pollen extract in 83% of patients [57]. Similar findings were made more recently by Bolhaar et al. [58]. However, other publications did not confirm these positive results [59, 60], and even the group of Asero et al. reported that the initial benefits of SCIT disappeared within time in 50% of cases [61]. For patients with confirmed peanut allergy, a SCIT with peanut extract revealed a reduction of symptoms following DBPCFC of 67–100% in three patients who completed the trial (out of 11 patients who were included). The rate of adverse reactions was 13.3% of all injections, and included one case of death [62]. More recently, first data were published on sublingual immunotherapy (SLIT) using hazelnut extract in patients with hazelnut allergy. The trial showed a significant improvement of hazelnut tolerance after verum SLIT compared to control SLIT suggesting a potential of SLIT therapy in FA [63, 64]. However, more studies are needed to confirm these promising results. Alternatively, oral tolerance induction was examined by oral administration of steadily increasing doses of food allergen up to 3–5 g food protein (40–60 steps in 2–3 months). Several reports suggested effectiveness [65–67], but not a single RCT is available to confirm the results [68]. Therefore, the value of this approach cannot be estimated finally at the moment, and in particular, the long-term effectiveness needs to be confirmed [69]. In summary, immunotherapy could become a valuable additional tool to treat FA by a causal approach; however, more clinical data and data on how to perform it are required. At present, the SLIT approach seems to be most promising.

Anti-IgE Therapy

In selected cases (e.g. severe peanut allergy) anti-IgE therapy using humanized antibodies directed against the Fc part of IgE can be considered. Leung et al. could show that the threshold dose inducing symptoms could be enhanced in patients with serious peanut allergy. Thus, the amount of allergen that might induce a fatal reaction will be somewhat higher for some time following anti-IgE therapy [70].

Other New Approaches

Instead of immunotherapy using classical allergen extracts, the development of new treatments tools such as tolerogenic peptides, recombinant epitopes for desensitization, and DNA-vaccination with allergen-DNA might help to improve the effectiveness of future immunotherapy. In addition, methods have been developed for the genetic or chemical modification of antigen-structures of food allergens, with the aim of reducing the allergen potential [71]. Finally, anti-cytokine-antibodies or cytokine-receptor antagonists against Th2-cytokines, such as IL-4 and anti-c-kit-antibodies functioning as new anti-mast cell medicaments [72, 73] are currently examined for their potential in FA treatment.

Summary

Adverse reactions to food affect more than 20% of the general population in industrialized countries. In about one fourth of the affected children and one tenth of affected adults, such incompatibilities are based on an allergy defined as an immune-mediated disease. Gastrointestinal symptoms occur in 1/2–1/3 of the cases. Food allergies are caused by IgE-dependent or IgE-independent immunological reactions. The diagnosis is founded on meticulous self and family history, a symptom-orientated eliminatory diagnosis, specific allergy tests, and in problematic cases, a controlled provocation procedure. Although none of these methods can lead to confirmation or exclusion of a "food allergy" in their own right, the combination of the various testing processes offers a reliable instrument when submitting a diagnosis. Currently, the basis of any successful treatment of food allergy is a carefully conducted elimination diet, which can be accompanied by medical treatment with anti-histamines or cromoglycate. In case of unclear history or history of systemic anaphylaxis, equipment with an emergency set of drugs including an epinephrine syringe is mandatory. The role of specific immunotherapy, either with food allergens or with cross-reactive pollen allergens, as alternative treatment option in patients with food allergy is currently under investigation.

References

1. Bjorksten B (2001) The epidemiology of food allergy. Curr Opin Allergy Clin Immunol 1:225–227
2. Grundy J, Matthews S, Bateman B, Dean T, Arshad SH (2002) Rising prevalence of allergy to peanut in children: data from 2 sequential cohorts. J Allergy Clin Immunol 110:784–789

3. Zuberbier T, Edenharter G, Worm M, Ehlers I, Reimann S, Hantke T, Roehr CC, Bergmann KE, Niggemann B (2004) Prevalence of adverse reactions to food in Germany – a population study. Allergy 59:338–345

4. Bischoff S, Crowe SE (2005) Gastrointestinal food allergy: new insights into pathophysiology and clinical perspectives. Gastroenterology 128:1089–1113

5. Brandtzaeg PE (2002) Current understanding of gastrointestinal immunoregulation and its relation to food allergy. Ann N Y Acad Sci 964:13–45

6. Sampson HA, Mendelson L, Rosen JP (1992) Fatal and near-fatal anaphylactic reactions to food in children and adolescents. N Engl J Med 327:380–384

7. Pumphrey RS, Gowland MH (2007) Further fatal allergic reactions to food in the United Kingdom, 1999–2006. Allergy Clin Immunol 119:1018–1019

8. Rodriguez J, Crespo JF (2002) Clinical features of cross-reactivity of food allergy caused by fruits. Curr Opin Allergy Clin Immunol 2:233–238

9. Vieths S, Scheurer S, Ballmer-Weber B (2002) Current understanding of cross-reactivity of food allergens and pollen. Ann N Y Acad Sci 964:47–68

10. Coombs RR (1992) The Jack Pepys lecture. The hypersensitivity reactions – some personal reflections. Clin Exp Allergy 22:673–680

11. Furuta GT, Schmidt-Choudhury A, Wang MY, Wang ZS, Lu L, Furlano RI, Wershil BK (1997) Mast cell-dependent tumor necrosis factor alpha production participates in allergic gastric inflammation in mice. Gastroenterology 113:1560–1569

12. Malaviya R, Navara C, Uckun FM (2001) Role of Janus kinase 3 in mast cell-mediated innate immunity against gram-negative bacteria. Immunity 15:313–321

13. Galli SJ, Nakae S, Tsai M (2005) Mast cells in the development of adaptive immune responses. Nat Immunol 6:135–142

14. Lorentz A, Schwengberg S, Sellge G, Manns MP, Bischoff SC (2000) Human intestinal mast cells are capable of producing different cytokine profiles: role of IgE receptor cross-linking and IL-4. J Immunol 164:43–48

15. Dahlen SE, Kumlin M (2004) Monitoring mast cell activation by prostaglandin D2 in vivo. Thorax 59:453–455

16. Brightling CE, Bradding P, Symon FA, Holgate ST, Wardlaw AJ, Pavrod ID (2002) Mast cell infiltration of airway smooth muscle in asthma. N Engl J Med 346:1699–1705

17. Oguma T, Palmer LJ, Birben E, Sonna LA, Asano K, Lilly CM (2004) Role of prostanoid DP receptor variants in susceptibility to asthma. N Engl J Med 351:1752–1763

18. Bischoff SC (2007) Role of mast cells in allergic and non-allergic immune responses: comparison of human and murine data. Nat Rev Immunol 7:93–104

19. Bischoff SC, Sellge G, Lorentz A, Sebald W, Raab R, Manns MP (1999) IL-4 enhances proliferation and mediator release in mature human mast cells. Proc Natl Acad Sci USA 96:8080–8085

20. Min B, Prout M, Hu-Li J, Zhu J, Jankovic D, Morgan ES, Urban JF Jr, Dvorak AM, Finkelmann FD, LeGros G, Paul WE (2004) Basophils produce IL-4 and accumulate in tissues after infection with a Th2-inducing parasite. J Exp Med 200:507–517

21. Bradding, P, Feather IH, Wilson S, Barding PG, Heusser CH, Holgate ST, Howarth PH (1993) Immunolocalization of cytokines in the nasal mucosa of normal and perennial rhinitic subjects. The mast cell as a source of IL-4, IL-5, and IL-6 in human allergic mucosal inflammation. J Immunol 151:3853–3865

22. Mukai K, Matsuoka K, Taya C, Suzuki H, Yokozeki H, Nishioka K, Hirokawa K, Etori M, Yamashita M, Kubota T, Minegishi Y, Yonekawa H, Karasuyama H (2005) Basophils play a critical role in the development of IgE-mediated chronic allergic inflammation independently of T cells and mast cells. Immunity 23:191–202

23. Majamaa H, Laine S, Miettinen A (1999) Eosinophil protein X and eosinophil cationic protein as indicators of intestinal inflammation in infants with atopic eczema and food allergy. Clin Exp Allergy 29:1502–1506

24. Bischoff SC, Mayer J, Wedemeyer J, Meier PN, Zeck-Kapp G, Wedi B, Kapp A, Cetin Y, Gebel M, Manns MP (1997) Colonoscopic allergen provocation (COLAP): a new diagnostic approach for gastrointestinal food allergy. Gut 40:745–753

25. Wehkamp J, Fellermann K, Herrlinger KR, Bevins CL, Stange EF (2005) Mechanisms of disease: defensins in gastrointestinal diseases. Nat Clin Pract Gastroenterol Hepatol. Sept 2:406–415
26. Macdonald TT, Monteleone G (2005) Immunity, inflammation, and allergy in the gut. Science 307:1920–1925
27. Barbara G, Stanghellini V, De Giorgio R, Cremon C, Cottrell GS, Santini D, Pasquinelli G, Morselli-Labate AM, Grady EF, Bunnett NW, Collins SM, Corinaldesi R (2004) Activated mast cells in proximity to colonic nerves correlate with abdominal pain in irritable bowel syndrome. Gastroenterology 126:693–702
28. Wood JD (2004) Enteric neuroimmunophysiology and pathophysiology. Gastroenterology 127:635–657
29. Jansen SC, van Dusseldorp M, Bottema KC, Dubois AE (2003) Intolerance to dietary biogenic amines: a review. Ann Allergy Asthma Immunol 91:233–240
30. Wood JD, Alpers DH, Andrews PL (1999) Fundamentals of neurogastroenterology. Gut 45:II6–II16
31. Blumer N, Herz U, Wegmann M, Renz H (2005) Prenatal lipopolysaccharide-exposure prevents allergic sensitization and airway inflammation, but not airway responsiveness in a murine model of experimental asthma. Clin Exp Allergy 35:397–402
32. Rook GA, Brunet LR (2005) Microbes, immunoregulation, and the gut. Gut 54:317–320
33. Sicherer SH (2003) Clinical aspects of gastrointestinal food allergy in childhood. Pediatrics 111:1609–1616
34. Leung DY, Bieber T (2003) Atopic dermatitis. Lancet 361:151–160
35. Chong SU, Worm M, Zuberbier T (2002) Role of adverse reactions to food in urticaria and exercise-induced anaphylaxis. Int Arch Allergy Immunol 129:19–26
36. Roberts G, Patel N, Levi-Schaffer F, Habibi P, Lack G (2003) Food allergy as a risk factor for life-threatening asthma in childhood: a case-controlled study. J Allergy Clin Immunol 112:168–174
37. Bhat K, Harper A, Gorard DA (2002) Perceived food and drug allergies in functional and organic gastrointestinal disorders. Aliment Pharmacol Ther 16:969–973
38. Rothenberg ME (2004) Eosinophilic gastrointestinal disorders (EGID). J Allergy Clin Immunol 113:11–28
39. Furuta GT, Liacouras CA, Collins MH, Gupta SK, Justinich C, Putnam PE, Bonis P, Hassall E, Straumann A, Rothenberg ME (2007) First International Gastrointestinal Eosinophil Research Symposium (FIGERS) Subcommittees. Eosinophilic esophagitis in children and adults: a systematic review and consensus recommendations for diagnosis and treatment. Gastroenterology 133:1342–1363
40. Bock SA, Munoz-Furlong A, Sampson HA (2001) Fatalities due to anaphylactic reactions to foods. J Allergy Clin Immunol 107:191–193
41. American Gastroenterological Association position statement: guidelines for the evaluation of food allergies (2001) Gastroenterology 120:1023–1025
42. Sampson HA (2001) Utility of food-specific IgE concentrations in predicting symptomatic food allergy. J Allergy Clin Immunol 107:891–896
43. Celik-Bilgili S, Mehl A, Verstege A, Staden U, Nocon M, Beyer K, Niggemann B (2005) The predictive value of specific immunoglobulin E levels in serum for the outcome of oral food challenges. Clin Exp Allergy 35:268–273
44. Bischoff SC, Grabowsky J, Manns MP (1997) Quantification of inflammatory mediators in stool samples of patients with inflammatory bowel disorders and controls. Dig Dis Sci 42:394–403
45. Schröder O, Naumann M, Shastri Y, Povse N, Stein J (2007) Prospective evaluation of faecal neutrophil-derived proteins in identifying intestinal inflammation: combination of parameters does not improve diagnostic accuracy of calprotectin. Aliment Pharmacol Ther 1.26:1035–1042
46. Simren M, Stotzer PO (2006) Use and abuse of hydrogen breath tests. Gut 55:297–303

47. Mukoyama T, Nishima S, Arita M, Ito S, Urisu A, Ebisawa M, Ogura H, Kohno Y, Kondo N, Shibata R, Hurusho M, Mayumi M, Morikawa A (2007) Guidelines for diagnosis and management of pediatric food allergy in Japan. Allergol Int 56:349–361
48. Edwards AM (1995) Oral sodium cromoglycate: its use in the management of food allergy. Clin Exp Allergy 25(Suppl 1):31–33
49. Muraro A, Roberts G, Clark A, Eigenmann PA, Halken S, Lack G, Moneret-Vautrin A, Niggemann B, Rance F (2007) EAACI task force on anaphylaxis in children. The management of anaphylaxis in childhood: position paper of the European academy of allergology and clinical immunology. Allergy 62:857–871
50. Joint Task Force on Practice Parameters, American Academy of Allergy, Asthma and Immunology, American College of Allergy, Asthma and Immunology, Joint Council of Allergy, Asthma and Immunology (2005) The diagnosis and management of anaphylaxis: an updated practice parameter. J Allergy Clin Immunol 115(Suppl 3):483–523
51. Matheson MC, Erbas B, Balasuriya A, Jenkins MA, Wharton CL, Tang ML, Abramson MJ, Walters EH, Hopper JL, Dharmage SC (2007) Breast-feeding and atopic disease: a cohort study from childhood to middle age. J Allergy Clin Immunol 120:1051–1057
52. Friedman NJ, Zeiger RS (2005) The role of breast-feeding in the development of allergies and asthma. J Allergy Clin Immunol 115:1238–1248
53. Kalliomaki M, Salminen S, Poussa T, Arvilommi H, Isolauri E (2003) Probiotics and prevention of atopic disease: 4-year follow-up of a randomised placebo-controlled trial. Lancet 361:1869–1871
54. Taylor AL, Dunstan JA, Prescott SL (2007) Probiotic supplementation for the first 6 months of life fails to reduce the risk of atopic dermatitis and increases the risk of allergen sensitization in high-risk children: a randomized controlled trial. J Allergy Clin Immunol 119:184–191
55. Brouwer ML, Wolt-Plompen SA, Dubois AE, van der Heide S, Jansen DF, Hoijer MA, Kauffman HF, Duiverman EJ (2006) No effects of probiotics on atopic dermatitis in infancy: a randomized placebo-controlled trial. Clin Exp Allergy 36:899–906
56. Folster-Holst R, Muller F, Schnopp N, Abeck D, Kreiselmaier I, Lenz T, von Ruden U, Schrezenmeir J, Christophers E, Weichenthal M (2006) Prospective, randomized controlled trial on Lactobacillus rhamnosus in infants with moderate to severe atopic dermatitis. Br J Dermatol 155:1256–1261
57. Asero R (1998) Effects of birch pollen-specific immunotherapy on apple allergy in birch pollen-hypersensitive patients. Clin Exp Allergy 28:1368–1373
58. Bolhaar ST, Tiemessen MM, Zuidmeer L, van Leeuwen A, Hoffmann-Sommergruber K, Bruijnzeel-Koomen CA, Taams LS, Knol EF, van Hoffen E, van Ree R, Knulst AC (2004) Efficacy of birch-pollen immunotherapy on cross-reactive food allergy confirmed by skin tests and double-blind food challenges. Clin Exp Allergy 34:761–769
59. Möller C (1989) Effect of pollen immunotherapy on food hypersensitivity in children with birch pollinosis. Ann Allergy 62:343–345
60. Hansen KS, Khinchi MS, Skov PS, Bindslev-Jensen C, Poulsen LK, Malling HJ (2004) Food allergy to apple and specific immunotherapy with birch pollen. Mol Nutr Food Res 48:441–448
61. Asero R (2003) How long does the effect of birch pollen injection SIT on apple allergy last? Allergy 58:435–438
62. Oppenheimer JJ, Nelson HS, Bock SA, Christensen F, Leung DY (1992) Treatment of peanut allergy with rush immunotherapy. J Allergy Clin Immunol 90:256–262
63. Enrique E, Pineda F, Malek T, Bartra J, Basagaña M, Tella R, Castelló JV, Alonso R, de Mateo JA, Cerdá-Trias T, San Miguel-Moncín Mdel M, Monzón S, García M, Palacios R, Cisteró-Bahíma A (2005) Sublingual immunotherapy for hazelnut food allergy: a randomized, double-blind, placebo-controlled study with a standardized hazelnut extract. J Allergy Clin Immunol 116:1073–1079
64. Pajno GB (2007) Sublingual immunotherapy: the optimism and the issues. J Allergy Clin Immunol 119:796–801

65. Buchanan AD, Green TD, Jones SM, Scurlock AM, Christie L, Althage KA, Steele PH, Pons L, Helm RM, Lee LA, Burks AW (2007) Egg oral immunotherapy in nonanaphylactic children with egg allergy. J Allergy Clin Immunol 119:199–205
66. Patriarca G, Nucera E, Roncallo C, Pollastrini E, Bartolozzi F, De Pasquale T, Buonomo A, Gasbarrini G, Di Campli C, Schiavino D (2003) Oral desensitizing treatment in food allergy: clinical and immunological results. Aliment Pharmacol Ther 17:459–465 Erratum in: Aliment Pharmacol Ther 17:1205
67. Patriarca G, Nucera E, Pollastrini E, Roncallo C, De Pasquale T, Lombardo C, Pedone C, Gasbarrini G, Buonomo A, Schiavino D (2007) Oral specific desensitization in food-allergic children. Dig Dis Sci 52:1662–1672
68. Niggemann B, Staden U, Rolinck-Werninghaus C, Beyer K (2006) Specific oral tolerance induction in food allergy. Allergy 61:808–811
69. Rolinck-Werninghaus C, Staden U, Mehl A, Hamelmann E, Beyer K, Niggemann B (2005) Specific oral tolerance induction with food in children: transient or persistent effect on food allergy? Allergy 60:1320–1322
70. Leung DY, Sampson HA, Yunginger JW, Burks AW Jr, Schneider LC, Wortel CH, Davis FM, Hyun JD, Shanahan WR Jr (2003) Avon longitudinal study of parents and children study team. Effect of anti-IgE therapy in patients with peanut allergy. N Engl J Med 13(348):986–993
71. Valenta R (2002) The future of antigen-specific immunotherapy of allergy. Nat Rev Immunol 2:446–453
72. Wenzel S, Wilbraham D, Fuller R, Getz EB, Longphre M (2007) Effect of an interleukin-4 variant on late phase asthmatic response to allergen challenge in asthmatic patients: results of two phase 2a studies. Lancet 370:1422–1431
73. Jensen BM, Metcalfe DD, Gilfillan AM (2007) Targeting kit activation: a potential therapeutic approach in the treatment of allergic inflammation. Inflamm Allergy Drug Targets 6:57–62

Lactose and Fructose Intolerance

Eitan Amir and Peter J. Whorwell

Lactose and Fructose Intolerance

Lactose and fructose are important carbohydrates, which are included in the human diet throughout the world. Maldigestion or malabsorption of these carbohydrates is very common in both normal patients and those with bowel symptoms [1]. Studies show that the frequency of maldigestion of lactose may be as high as 98% [2] while the prevalence of fructose malabsorption has been shown to be as high as 60% [3–6]. Not all patients with such carbohydrate malabsorption develop symptoms. However, in selected subjects, carbohydrate malabsorption is associated with symptomatology such as bloating, flatulence, abdominal pain and diarrhoea. When these manifestations are present, the subject is considered to have "carbohydrate intolerance" [7].

This chapter will present the latest evidence regarding the intolerance to both lactose and fructose and explore how these disorders impact clinical practice in the field of functional bowel disease.

Lactose Intolerance

Introduction

Lactose is a disaccharide, which is present in milk and many processed foods. It is, therefore, found in significant quantities in the diets of people across the whole world. Since only monosaccharides are absorbed across the intestinal epithelium, disaccharides such as lactose must be enzymatically cleaved into their monosaccharide

E. Amir
Department of Medical Oncology, Christie Hospital NHS Trust, Wilmslow Road, Manchester M20 4BX, UK

P.J. Whorwell (✉)
University Hospitals of South Manchester, Education and Research Centre, Wythenshawe Hospital, Southmoor Road, Wythenshawe, Manchester, M23 9LT, UK

R. Pawankar et al. (eds.), *Allergy Frontiers: Clinical Manifestations,*
DOI: 10.1007/978-4-431-88317-3_27, © Springer 2009

components prior to absorption. Abnormalities of lactose hydrolysis lead to the build up of lactose within the gut and this is thought to contribute to symptomatology.

Epidemiology

Lactose maldigestion is a prevalent disorder with marked geographic variability. Evidence [8, 9] shows that at least 50% of people in South America, Africa and Asia suffer from this disorder. Certain areas in Asia in particular show prevalence rates approaching 100%. In North America it is estimated that 15% of Caucasians, 53% of Mexican-Americans and 80% of African-Americans are affected, while in Europe prevalence rates vary from 2% in Scandinavia to approximately 70% in Southern Europe.

This geographic variability is also seen in the age of manifestation of symptoms, with subjects of African or Asian origin developing symptoms in early childhood compared with Caucasians who are affected predominantly in adolescence [8].

Males and females tend to be affected equally [10]; however, several studies [11–13] have shown that women who are lactose intolerant regain the ability to digest lactose during pregnancy.

Clinical Features

Symptoms of lactose intolerance include diarrhoea, abdominal bloating and pain, flatulence, nausea and borborygmi. The mechanism of loose stools induced by unabsorbed carbohydrate is well documented: the osmotic load of the carbohydrate causes secretion of fluid and electrolytes until osmotic equilibrium is reached [14, 15]. Dilatation of the intestine, caused by the osmosis, induces an acceleration of small intestinal transit, which increases with the degree of maldigestion [16].

Pathophysiology

Lactose maldigestion occurs due to inability to break down lactose to its components galactose and glucose [17]. The effects of the processing of this maldigested lactose within the colon is thought to be the cause of intolerance symptoms.

Recent evidence shows that lactose maldigestion has two predominant causative factors: a deficiency of the enzyme lactase and abnormal oro-caecal transit time [18]. The latter of these incorporates both gastric emptying time and small bowel transit time.

Lactase Deficiency

Lactase, which is normally produced by the intestinal brush borders exists in high concentrations in neonates, but during weaning, its activity begins to decline. This process, which has been shown to occur in the majority of the world's population, is thought to be genetically programmed and irreversible [19].

Following the neonatal period, all humans show a reduction of lactase activity with consequential reduction in lactose digestion. The level of this reduction in activity is highly variable. In the 1960s this variability was thought to be an acquired trait [20], but more recent evidence shows that it is, in fact, genetically determined. Enattah and colleagues [21] showed that lactose maldigestion is associated with a non-coding variation in the MCM6 gene (present on chromosome 2q21). This variation consists of a C/T(-13910) polymorphism located in an intron of the MCM6 gene. This locus is present 14 kb upstream from the lactase gene itself. The role of the variation in lactase may be unrelated to the MCM6 gene itself. This study showed that the presence of the C allele in place of the T allele was mostly associated with hypolactasia with all individuals with lactase deficiency being found to be homozygous with respect to the C allele. This polymorphism has now been developed into a screening test for lactose intolerance [22]. A further variation consisting of a G/A(-22018) polymorphism has also been described upstream of the lactase gene [23]; however, its significance in isolation is unclear.

Mucosal Damage

The concept of enteric infection causing lactose intolerance is well recognised. Intolerance can develop in people who had hitherto been tolerant to lactose. This phenomenon is likely to be secondary to mucosal injury, including infectious gastroenteritis, particularly if it affects the small bowel [24].

This theory is based on data from several observational studies. Langman and colleagues investigated endoscopic duodenal biopsies of symptomatic subjects. They found that the presence of moderate to severe duodenal lesions was associated with a significant decrease in all disaccharidase activity. However, in mild lesions, only lactase activity was reduced [25]. This may be explained by the fact that lactase activity is maximal at the distal part of the villus and hence is more susceptible to damage. Investigators also found that treatment of the underlying disorder leads to improvement in lactase activity, although this did lag behind the return of other intestinal function. In fact, it showed that symptoms of lactose intolerance persisted for months after resolution of other intestinal symptoms.

The transient nature of this post-inflammatory disaccharide maldigestion has also been shown in a study of children, with acute gastroenteritis, in Poland [26]. In this study, the authors showed that carbohydrate intolerance was present in approximately one in seven of their cohort. However, evidence of maldigestion was shown to persist for only 5 days. In view of the age of the sample population, assessment of symptoms was not undertaken.

Other causes of mucosal injury causing lactose intolerance have also been described. Studies have shown that diseases of the small bowel such as Coeliac and Crohn's disease can cause both lactose maldigestion [27, 28] and delayed oro-caecal transit time [38, 39]. Furthermore, Tursi et al. [29] showed that most patients affected by symptomatic, uncomplicated diverticular disease developed transient lactose maldigestion. In this study, laboratory evidence of maldigestion continued for only a few days, but again data on duration of *symptoms* were not collected. Finally, further work has shown that reversible hypolactasia can result from administration of 5-Fluoro-uracil based chemotherapy [30].

Abnormal Oro-Caecal Transit Time

Studies have shown that non-absorbable sugars can accelerate small intestinal transit time [31–33]. This phenomenon is thought to be caused by an increased intestinal liquid volume resulting from the osmotic effect of the malabsorbed sugars. It is postulated that the increased volume causes intestinal distension and stimulation of motility [34]. However, work by Vonk and colleagues [18] showed that the increased rate of transit was likely to be a person-specific factor, independent of the lactase activity level. This is supported by various studies, which have shown large inter-individual differences in small intestinal transit time in lactose maldigestion [35–37].

Conversely, however, lactose maldigestion is often associated with disorders in which the oro-caecal transit time is prolonged. Small bowel diseases, such as Coeliac disease or Crohn's disease are associated with both lactose maldigestion [27, 28] and delayed oro-caecal transit time [38, 39]. It has been proposed that small bowel bacterial overgrowth is the mechanism by which delayed transit time causes intolerance symptoms [40].

A review by Tursi [41] therefore, concluded that lactose intolerance is most likely influenced by a variety of factors such as lactose maldigestion, abnormal oro-caecal transit time (which may be shortened or prolonged) and small bowel bacterial overgrowth.

Diagnosis

Lactose intolerance is often diagnosed on a clinical basis. The most commonly utilised process is that of an empirical trial of dietary lactose avoidance. Despite the ease of this method, a number of methods of diagnosing lactose maldigestion have been developed, specifically, lactose breath test, direct lactase enzyme activity and genetic testing for common polymorphisms.

Lactose Breath Test

The lactose breath test involves the intake of 50 g of lactose orally, followed by measurement of breath hydrogen every 30 min for 3 h. A breath hydrogen of 20 ppm above the nadir indicates lactose maldigestion [42]. This test, although highly specific has a relatively poor sensitivity of approximately 34% [43]. It is also weakened by the fact that symptoms are not routinely recorded during the test [44] and hence, includes those with asymptomatic lactose maldigestion as well as those with true intolerance.

Direct Lactase Enzyme Activity

Direct lactase enzyme activity can be performed on tissue obtained from a small intestinal biopsy. This test is invasive, as it usually requires an upper gastrointestinal endoscopy. Furthermore, its reliability is sometimes low because disaccharidase activity in a particular small biopsy specimen does not necessarily reflect the activity of this enzyme in the rest of the small bowel [45].

Genetic Testing

The presence of the two genetic polymorphisms described above have led to the development of specific genetic tests to help diagnose lactose maldigestion. These tests have only recently been developed and the literature has opposing data on their application. One study [46] has shown that genotyping for the C/T(-13910) polymorphism is a reliable test for adult-type hypolactasia with high sensitivity and specificity, while another [47] has suggested that its use should be restricted to patients of north European origin. The latter study based its advice on data showing that the presence of the alternative allele C at this site is not a good predictor of hypolactasia in many non-Northern Europeans [48, 49]. Furthermore, this method also, relies on a small bowel biopsy and is, therefore, associated with the risks that obtaining this entail.

In summary, despite the development of advanced methods, the ease of utilising dietary lactose avoidance makes this the most appropriate first line investigation. However, if this fails and lactose intolerance remains suspected, other investigations such as those detailed above may be helpful.

Management

Treatment of lactose maldigestion is only required in those with symptoms suggestive of lactose intolerance [50]. Unfortunately, there are no internationally accepted guidelines for the treatment of lactose intolerance and hence, the usual therapeutic approach is that of exclusion of dairy and dairy-related products from the diet of affected individuals. However, elimination of these from the diet has many nutritional disadvantages, especially relating to an associated fall in bone mineral density [51]. As a result, alternative approaches have been assessed, most of which have aimed to prolong contact time between enzyme and substrate, delay oro-caecal transit time and therefore, enhance colonic adaptation.

Beta-Galactosidase

Beta-Galactosidase is an exogenous lactase enzyme, which can be obtained from a variety of yeasts and fungi.

Initial studies of the use of Beta-Galactosidase were conducted by adding the soluble enzyme in liquid form to milk a number of hours prior to consumption [52–55]. These showed that this so called "pre-incubated milk" both reduced hydrogen breath excretion on lactose breath testing, as well as reduced symptoms after ingestion. However, these studies relied on data derived from very small populations and the methodology did not involve control arms. Furthermore, practicality aspects have meant that the addition of lactase to milk prior to ingestion has never been routinely utilised as a treatment modality.

Consequently, multiple studies have looked into whether the addition of lactase at the time of eating instead of using pre-incubated milk were of any benefit [56–59]. The most recent of these studies, by Montalto and colleagues [59], randomised 30 lactose intolerant subjects into a double blind, placebo controlled trial and showed that hydrogen excretion and symptom score were no different in the two arms. Further work on Beta-galactosidase has studied its safety in laboratory animals [60]. This study showed that there were no significant dose-related changes in body weights, feed consumption, organ weights, urinalysis, haematological profiles, biochemistry, or histopathological profiles.

Solid lactase preparations of exogenous lactase have also been made available in the form of capsules or tablets. They are an alternative to the soluble liquid form of lactase described above, and their efficacy also appears to be confirmed [61]. However, they are less effective than pre-hydrolysed milk, most likely due to the inactivation of the enzyme by gastric proteases [50].

On balance, therefore, it appears that the addition of exogenous lactase in the form of Beta-galactosidase is effective, practical and safe.

Yoghurt and Probiotics

The association between ingestion of *fermented* milk products and improvements in lactose digestion is well established [62, 63]. The fermentation of milk into yoghurt is usually carried out by incubating milk with two species of lactic acid bacteria, specifically, *L. bulgaricus* and *S. thermophilus* [64]. These bacteria hydrolyse lactose during the fermentation process and it is estimated that the lactose content is subsequently reduced by 25–50%. Unfortunately, this process leads to the formation of lactic acid, which contributes to the sour taste of yoghurt that some patients find unpalatable.

To overcome this problem, *L. acidophilus* can be substituted for lactic acid bacteria to produce unfermented "sweet milk". However, multiple studies [65–67] have shown the inadequate effectiveness of this milk in reducing symptoms. A proposed explanation for this is that the availability of bacterial Beta-galactosidase is the main factor in improving lactose digestion and this is reduced in the case of *L. acidophilus*. De Vrese and colleagues [68] showed that bacteria need an intact cell wall to protect their intracellular enzymes during exposure to gastric acid and against the actions of bile. It has been suggested that *L. bulgaricus*, despite having equivalent Beta-galactosidase activity and the same lactose active transport mechanism as *L. acidophilus*, has a softer cell wall membrane and hence is better adapted to release its enzymes than *L. acidophilus* [69].

A further study [70] has shown that yoghurt can delay gastric emptying and intestinal transit and, therefore, it optimises the effect of Beta-galactosidase in the small intestine.

Delaying Oro-Caecal Transit Time

Pharmacological approaches that delay both gastric emptying and intestinal transit time have been well studied. Peuhkuri and colleagues [71] undertook a double blind placebo controlled trial of propantheline and metoclopramide on lactose digestion. They found that propantheline induced a prolongation of gastric emptying and thus improved lactose tolerance compared with both metoclopramide and placebo. A similar study looking at intestinal transit showed improvement in symptoms after administration of loperamide [72].

The use of high calorie foods in place of pharmacological agents has also been studied with varying results. Leichter et al. [73] showed that full-fat milk improved carbohydrate absorption by slowing both gastric emptying and intestinal transit. However, work by Vesa and colleagues [74] disputed this by showing no improvement in lactose tolerance after ingestion of high energy milk.

It therefore appears that pharmacological approaches are more efficacious than dietary attempts to delay transit, although some would question the advisability of using a pharmacological approach to this long term problem.

Adaptation

As described above, lactase undergoes an irreversible reduction in its activity after the neonatal period. However, it has been reported that continuous dietary intake of lactose reduces the severity of gastrointestinal symptoms [75, 76]. It has been proposed that this "adaptation" is related to both changes in the gut microflora as well as to changes in colonic function.

Various studies have tried to explain this phenomenon in detail: Hertzler et al. [77] showed that after daily ingestion of milk for 10 days, levels of faecal Beta-galactosidase were elevated. It was hypothesized that the origin of this enzyme was from gut microbes, which increased their level of lactose fermentation activity. This was confirmed by Hill and colleagues [78] who showed that the presence of malabsorbed lactose enhanced the fermentation ability of various gut bacteria. These included bifidobacteria and lactic acid bacteria, which can metabolise lactose without producing hydrogen. Further work by Perman et al. [79] suggested that the acidic products of fermentation inhibit the production of hydrogen and hence reduce symptoms.

However, work by Briet and colleagues [80] suggested that this adaptation could be explained by the placebo effect. In their double-blind controlled trial, it was shown that following intake of lactose for 13 consecutive days, there was a measurable increase in faecal Beta-galactosidase, reduced hydrogen excretion and improved symptoms. However, after comparison with the control group, no evidence of metabolic adaptation was found.

Montalto and colleagues [81] reviewed the above evidence and together with their clinical experience suggested a therapeutic management plan. This included a temporary lactose free diet to obtain remission of symptoms followed by gradual re-introduction of lactose without overcoming the individual threshold dose. It was recommended that the threshold dose could then be increased with the aid of both pharmacological and non-pharmacological strategies as detailed above.

Lactose and Pharmaceutical Agents

Lactose is widely used by the pharmaceutical industry as a filler or diluent in oral capsule, powder and tablet formulations. It is also used as a carrier for drugs in dry powder inhalers as well as in combination with sucrose in the preparation of sugar-coating solutions [82].

The total quantity of lactose that may be ingested through the administration of pharmaceutical agents seldom exceeds 2 g a day. Therefore, the use of medications containing lactose is unlikely to result in gastrointestinal symptoms in the majority of people [82]. A review of the literature has uncovered a few case reports of intolerance to lactose in medication [83–86]; therefore, for a small number of patients, lactose-free medication may be required.

Complications

Lactose intolerance is considered to be a relatively benign condition with few complications. Historically, it has been assumed that patients with lactose intolerance have a reduced intake of calcium as a result of either low-dairy or dairy-free diets. It has therefore been proposed that lactose intolerance could be a potential cause of osteopenia or osteoporosis.

The current literature is rather conflicting on the link between lactose intolerance and loss of bone mineral density. A large population based study of perimenopausal women in Finland [87] did show that lactose intolerance slightly reduced perimenopausal bone mineral density, possibly through reduced calcium intake. However, a smaller study of adult women in the United States [88] showed no correlation between expired hydrogen content and bone mass at various sites. It therefore concluded that there was no association between lactose intolerance and loss of bone density. A possible explanation for the disparity of the above results is the different methodologies for determining the presence of lactose intolerance, which were used in these studies.

A more recent case control study from Austria [89] showed that individuals with lactose intolerance, verified by the hydrogen breath test, did not appear to be at risk for accelerated bone loss. Nevertheless, a relationship between vertebral fractures and lactose intolerance cannot be excluded, as a few individuals with severe lactose intolerance had a large number of vertebral fractures.

Fructose Intolerance

Introduction

Fructose is a hexose monosaccharide, which is consumed frequently in Western diets. It is found in three main forms: as free fructose (present in fruits and honey); as a constituent of the disaccharide sucrose; or as fructans, a polymer of fructose (present in some vegetables and wheat) [90]. Unlike glucose, fructose does not have an active transport mechanism, but is absorbed by facilitative diffusion, a method that has limited capacity [91]. Therefore, fructose is liable to be malabsorbed and its presence in large quantities in the gut may give rise to symptoms similar to those in lactose intolerance.

Fructose Intolerance should not to be confused with *Hereditary* Fructose Intolerance (HFI), which is an autosomal recessive condition in which there is an inborn error of fructose metabolism caused by deficiency of the liver enzyme aldolase B.

Epidemiology

As described above, lactose intolerance is a well recognised cause of non-specific gastrointestinal complaints. However, less is known about the significance of other carbohydrates such as fructose.

Mishkin and colleagues [92] reported that between 40–55% of their cohort of patients with functional dyspepsia had fructose malabsorption. A Danish study [6], also showed a high proportion of fructose malabsorption in a small cohort of patients with functional bowel disorders. Several other uncontrolled studies [3, 93, 94] have also corroborated these data, and therefore, investigators have suggested that fructose malabsorption was more prevalent in patients with functional bowel disease (36–75%) than in healthy subjects (0–50%).

However, these data have not been confirmed by the only controlled study on the subject [95], which showed that the frequency of incomplete fructose absorption was not significantly different in patients with gastrointestinal symptoms than in controls. A possible explanation for this could be that patients with functional bowel disorders and incomplete fructose absorption describe higher symptom scores than those with functional bowel disease who absorb fructose adequately [6]. This might be a result of a heightened visceral sensitivity which is described in such disorders [96].

Clinical Features

Symptoms of fructose intolerance are similar to the constellation of symptoms associated with lactose intolerance. They can therefore, include abdominal distension, bloating and discomfort, excessive flatus and diarrhoea.

As is the case with lactose intolerance, it is the presence of an osmotic load in the gut, which draws fluid into the lumen and consequently leads to pain and bloating. Similarly, the fermentation of fructose by colonic bacteria has been shown to be the mechanism by which excess flatus and diarrhoea are manifested [3].

Pathophysiology

As described above, only monosaccharides can be absorbed across the intestinal epithelium. Glucose has a dedicated transporter, which actively transports it across the epithelium even against a concentration gradient. Other monosaccharides such as fructose rely on passive diffusion through a carrier mediated facilitated diffusion process.

Studies have isolated GLUT5, one of the glucose transport family transporters, as having a high affinity to fructose [97]. This transporter, which is found on the luminal surface of small intestinal epithelial cells, is thought to be responsible for fructose absorption from the intestinal lumen into enterocytes. A further glucose transporter called GLUT2 is thought to be responsible for the transportation of fructose from the enterocyte into the portal circulation.

Initial work on the mechanism of fructose malabsorption suggested the possible presence of mutant forms of the GLUT5 transporter protein. However, evidence from sequence analyses has shown that isolated fructose malabsorption does not result from the expression of a mutant GLUT5 protein [97].

Molecular studies have shown that GLUT5 expression can be induced by the presence of fructose within the gut lumen [98, 99]. However, if the capacity of diffusion of GLUT5 is exceeded, GLUT2 can be employed to assist in absorption of any excess luminal fructose. Gouyon and colleagues [100] reported that GLUT2, which is normally located in the basolateral membrane, could be recruited to the apical brush-border membrane upon ingestion of a fructose-rich meal. They therefore proposed that suboptimal recruitment of GLUT2 or its defective intestinal membrane insertion might be the mechanism for fructose malabsorption.

The mouse GLUT5 transporter has recently been cloned and it is hoped that this may allow for improved future investigation of the mechanisms regulating fructose absorption [101].

Other physiological principles underlying potential malabsorption of fructose have been identified from the literature. It has been shown that fructose absorption can be enhanced by the presence of either glucose [91] or amino acids [102] within the intestinal lumen. Furthermore, it has been shown that ingestion of fructose together with the sugar alcohol sorbitol impedes fructose absorption [103].

The precise mechanism by which glucose enhances fructose absorption has not been definitively ascertained. However, it is postulated that glucose provides a stronger stimulus for increased expression of the GLUT family of transporters [91]. This phenomenon may explain why fructose, if given as sucrose, or in equimolar combination with glucose, can be well absorbed even in subjects with proven fructose malabsorption [6, 91, 104].

It is therefore proposed that the amount of fructose ingested in excess of glucose is likely to be an important determinant of fructose malabsorption. However, despite this, a high fructose load can still lead to malabsorption of fructose independently of the presence or absence of facilitators of its absorption [104].

Other hypotheses to explain the improved absorption of fructose in the presence of glucose and amino acids have been formed. Two studies have suggested that active transportation of amino acids and glucose into the enterocyte causes a "solvent drag" and hence enhances passive diffusion [105, 106]. A further study by Elias and colleagues [107] suggested that glucose caused a delay in gastric emptying and hence facilitated fructose absorption.

Sorbitol is one of several naturally occurring sugar alcohols and is used extensively as a "sugar-free" sweetener in many foods. It is incompletely absorbed [108] in the small intestine and appears to compete with fructose for absorption. Rumessen and colleagues [103] showed that sorbitol and fructose doses that are fully absorbed when ingested separately are incompletely absorbed when taken together. A further study [109] has suggested that the presence of both fructose and sorbitol in the gut accelerates transit by its synergistic osmotic effect and suggested this mechanism for the poor absorption of fructose in this context.

Diagnosis

Similar to other carbohydrates, incomplete absorption of fructose can be identified non-invasively by measuring breath hydrogen after a fructose load. Colonic fermentation of undigested carbohydrates produces a cocktail of short-chain fatty acids, hydrogen and carb higher doses on dioxide. Hydrogen cannot be metabolised by humans and hence must be excreted in breath or flatus or consumed by colonic bacteria to produce methane and sulphides. In general, a rise in breath hydrogen of more than 20 ppm peaking 2–3 h after ingestion of fructose is indicative of incomplete absorption [110]. Unfortunately, there is no international consensus over what constitutes an appropriate dose and concentration of fructose for such tests [111]. However, it is felt that lower fructose loads are more specific for recognition of fructose intolerance as higher doses are most likely to overwhelm the fructose absorptive capacity even of normal individuals [112].

Furthermore, the process of hydrogen breath testing is not without flaws. It relies on hydrogen-producing flora outnumbering hydrogen-consuming bacteria and is prone to false negative results. It has therefore been proposed that individuals should at first be subjected to a hydrogen breath test with lactulose (a non-absorbable, synthetic disaccharide) and if this does not induce a hydrogen breath response, it is likely they lack the necessary flora. In this group of patients, testing for methane may identify malabsorption [113].

Management

Despite the substantial data on the pathogenesis of fructose intolerance, there are few published guidelines on its management. Shepherd and colleagues [114] attempted to address this deficiency in the literature by undertaking a retrospective study to evaluate a potentially successful diet therapy in patients with fructose malabsorption.

This diet included what was described as three "novel" principles. Firstly, there was an attempt to balance free fructose with glucose-rich foods. Secondly, the total fructose load was limited irrespective of whether the glucose content was equivalent or in excess to the fructose content. Finally, the diet included a reduced intake of fructans. Wheat is a major source of fructans in the diet [115] and hence reduction of its consumption was central. This leaves an important unanswered question, specifically, whether it is the reduction of fructans, which contributed to symptom relief or whether it was due to other dietary factors such as a reduction in the intake of insoluble fibre.

This diet was not effective for all patients with the authors reporting that 74% of their studied population showed significant symptomatic benefit. Furthermore, their methodology was limited in that it was not controlled, was analysed retrospectively, and the follow up period was as short as 2 months in some subjects.

Complications

Fructose intolerance is a benign condition with no known complications described in the literature.

Summary

The management of non-specific abdominal symptoms can sometimes prove to be a complex conundrum. Among the multitude of differential diagnoses is carbohydrate malabsorption, the prevalence of which is often underestimated. Lactose and fructose are important dietary carbohydrates that are included in human diet all over the world. Furthermore, there is a large body of evidence to show that malabsorption of these sugars is both prevalent and clinically relevant.

References

1. Fernandez-Banares F, Esteve-Pardo M, de Leon R, Humbert P, Cabre E, Lovet JM, Gassullm A. Sugar malabsorption in functional bowel disease: clinical implications. Am J Gastroenterol 1993; 88: 2044–2050.
2. Scrimshaw NS, Murray EB. The acceptability of milk and milk products in populations with a high prevalence of lactose intolerance. Am J Clin Nutr 1988; 48: 1083–1159.
3. Ravich WJ, Bayless TM, Thomas M. Fructose: incomplete intestinal absorption in humans. Gastroenterology 1983; 84: 26–29.
4. Truswell AS, Seach JM, Thorburn AW. Incomplete absorption of pure fructose in healthy subjects and the facilitating effect of glucose. Am J Clin Nutr 1988; 48: 1424–1430.
5. Nelis GF, Vermeeren MAP, Jansen W. Role of fructose– sorbitol malabsorption in the irritable bowel syndrome. Gastroenterology 1990; 99: 1016–1020.
6. Rumessen JJ, Gudmand-Hoyer E. Functional bowel disease: malabsorption and abdominal distress after ingestion of fructose, sorbitol, and fructose-sorbitol mixtures. Gastroenterology 1988; 95: 694–700.
7. Shaw AD, Davies GJ. Lactose intolerance: problems in diagnosis and treatment. J Clin Gastroenterol 1999; 28: 208–216.
8. Scrimshaw NS, Murray EB. Prevalence of lactose maldigestion. Am J Clin Nutr 1988; 48: 1086–1098.
9. Sahi T. Genetics and epidemiology of adult-type hypolactasia. Scand J Gastroenterol 1994; 29: 7–20.
10. Rao DR, Bello H, Warren AP, Brown GE. Prevalence of lactose maldigestion: influence and interaction of age, race, and sex. Dig Dis Sci 1994; 39: 1519–1524.
11. Szilagyi A, Salomon R, Martin M, Fokeeff K, Seidman E. Lactose handling by women with lactose malabsorption is improved during pregnancy. Clin Invest Med 1996; 19: 416.
12. Villar J, Kestler E, Castillo P, Juarez A, Menendez R, Solomons NW. Improved lactose digestion during pregnancy: a case of physiologic adaptation? Obstet Gynecol 1988; 71: 697.
13. Paige DM, Witter FR, Bronner YL, Kessler LA, Perman JA, Paige TR. Lactose intolerance in pregnant African-American women. J Am Coll Nutr 1997; 16: 488.
14. Launiala K. The effect of unabsorbed sucrose and mannitol on the small intestinal flow rate and mean transit time. Scand J Gastroenterol 1968; 3: 665–671.
15. Christopher NL, Bayless TM. Role of the small bowel and colon in lactose-induced diarrhea. Gastroenterology 1971; 60: 845–852.
16. Ladas S, Papanikos J, Arapakis G. Lactose malabsorption in Greek adults: correlation of small bowel transit time with the severity of lactose intolerance. Gut 1982; 23: 968–973.
17. Gilat T, Russo S, Gelman-Malachi E, Aldor TA. Lactase in man: a nonadaptable enzyme. Gastroenterology 1972; 62: 1125–1127.
18. Vonk RJ, Priebe MG, Koetse HA. Lactose intolerance: analysis of underlying factors. Eur J Clin Invest 2003; 33: 70–75.
19. Wang Y, Harvey CB, Hollox EJ, Phillips AD, Poulter M, Clay P, Walker-Smith JA, Swallow DM. The genetically programmed down-regulation of lactase in children. Gastroenterology 1998; 114: 1230–1236.
20. Cuatrecasas P, Lockwood DH, Caldwell JR. Lactase deficiency in the adult: a common occurrence. Lancet I 1965: 14–18.
21. Enattah NS, Sahi T, Savilahti E, Terwilliger JD, Peltonen L, Jarvela I. Identification of a variant associated with adult-type hypolactasia. Nature Genet 2002; 30: 233–237.
22. Rasinpera H, Savilahti E, Enattah NS, Kuokkanen M, Totterman N, Lindahl H, Jarvela I, Kolho KL. A genetic test which can be used to diagnose adult-type hypolactasia in children. Gut 2004; 53: 1571–1576.
23. Olds LC, Sibley E. Lactase persistence DNA variant enhances lactase promoter activity in vitro: functional role as a cis regulatory element. Hum Mol Genet 2003; 12: 2333–2340.

24. Parry SD, Barton JR, Welfare MR. Is lactose intolerance implicated in the development of post-infectious irritable bowel syndrome or functional diarrhoea in previously asymptomatic people? Eur J Gastroenterol Hepatol 2002; 14: 1225–1230.
25. Langman JM, Rowland R. Activity of duodenal disaccharidases in relation to normal and abnormal mucosal morphology. J Clin Pathol 1990; 43: 537–540.
26. Szajewska H, Kantecki M, Albrecht P, Antoniewicz J. Carbohydrate intolerance after acute gastroenteritis – a disappearing problem in Polish children. Acta Paediatr 1997; 86: 347–350.
27. Bode S, Gudmand-Hoyer E. Incidence and clinical significance of lacose malabsorption in adult coeliac disease. Scand J Gastroenterol 1988; 32: 484–488.
28. Mishkin B, Yalovsky M, Mishkin S. Increased prevalence of lactose malabsorption in Crohn's disease patients at low risk for lactose malabsorption based on ethnic origin. Am J Gastroenterol 1997; 92: 148–153.
29. Tursi A, Brandimarte G, Giorgetti GM, Elisei W. Transient lactose malabsorption in patients affected by symptomatic uncomplicated diverticular disease of the colon. 1: Dig Dis Sci 2006; 51: 461–465.
30. Osterlund P, Ruotsalainen T, Peuhkuri K, Korpela R, Ollus A, Ikonen M, Joensuu H, Elomaa I. Lactose intolerance associated with adjuvant 5-fluorouracil-based chemotherapy for colorectal cancer. Clin Gastroenterol Hepatol 2004; 2: 696–703.
31. Launiala K. The effect of unabsorbed sucrose and mannitol on the small intestinal flow rate and mean transit time. Scand J Gastroenterol 1968; 3: 665–671.
32. La Brooy SJ, Male PJ, Beavis AK, Misiewicz JJ. Assessment of the reproducibility of the lactulose H2 breath test as a measure of mouth to caecum transit time. Gut 1983; 24: 893–896.
33. He T, Priebe MG, Welling GW, Vonk RJ. Effect of lactose on oro-cecal transit in lactose digesters and maldigesters. Eur J Clin Invest 2006; 36: 737–742.
34. Christopher NL, Bayless TM. Role of the small bowel and colon in lactose-induced diarrhoea. Gastroenterology 1971; 60: 845–852.
35. Argenyi EE, Soffer EE, Madsen MT, Berbaum KS, Walkner WO. Scintigraphic evaluation of small bowel transit in healthy subjects: inter- and intrasubject variability. Am J Gastroenterol 1995; 90: 938–942.
36. Degen LP, Phillips SF, Kost L, Thomforde G. Does the menstrual cycle really influence gastrointestinal transit? Gastroenterology 1994; 106: A484.
37. Read NW. Small bowel transit time of food in man: measurement, regulation and possible importance. Scand J Gastroenterol Suppl 1984; 96: 77–85.
38. Tursi A. Clinical implications of delayed orocecal transit time and bacterial overgrowth in adult patients with Crohn's disease. J Clin Gastroenterol 2001; 32: 274–275.
39. Tursi A, Brandimarte G, Giorgetti GM, Nasi G. Assessment of orocecal transit time in different localisation of Crohn's disease and its possible influence on clinical response to therapy. Eur J Gastroenterol Hepatol 2003; 15: 69–74.
40. Husebye E. Gastrointestinal motility disorders and bacterial overgrowth. J Intern Med 1995; 237: 419–427.
41. Tursi A. Factors influencing lactose intolerance. Eur J Clin Invest 2004; 34: 314–315.
42. Joseph F, Rosenberg AJ. Breath hydrogen testing: diseased versus normal patients. J Pediatr Gasterenterol Nutr 1988; 7: 787–791.
43. Matthews SB, Waud JP, Roberts AG, Campbell AK. Systemic lactose intolerance: a new perspective on an old problem. Postgrad Med J 2005; 81: 167–173.
44. Fauchi AS, Braunwald E, Isselbacher KJ. Disorders of the gastrointestinal system. In: Harrison's principles of internal medicine. 14th ed. New York: McGraw-Hill; 1998: 631 pp.
45. Shaw AD, Davies GJ. Lactose intolerance: problems in diagnosis and treatment. J Clin Gastroenterol 1999; 28: 208–216.
46. Büning C, Genschel J, Jurga J, Fiedler T, Voderholzer W, Fiedler E-M, Worm M, Weltrich R, Lochs H, Schmidt H, Ockenga J. Introducing genetic testing for adult-type hypolactasia. Digestion 2005; 71: 245–250.
47. Swallow DM. DNA test for hypolactasia premature. Gut 2006; 55: 131–132.

48. Swallow DM. Genetics of lactase persistence and lactose intolerance. Annu Rev Genet 2003; 37: 197–219.

49. Troelsen JT, Olsen J, Moller J, Sjostrom H. An upstream polymorphism associated with lactase persistence has increased enhancer activity. Gastroenterology 2003; 125: 1686–1694.

50. Suarez FL, Savaiano DA, Levitt MD. Review article: the treat- treatment of lactose intolerance. Aliment Pharmacol Ther 1995; 9: 589–597.

51. Di Stefano M, Veneto G, Malservisi S, Cecchetti L, Minguzzi L, Strocchi A, Corazza GR. Lactose malabsorption and intolerance and peak bone mass. Gastroenterology 2002; 122: 1793–1799.

52. Rask Pedersen E, Jensen BH, Jensen HJ, Keldsbo IL, Hylander Moller E, Norby Rasmussen S. Lactose malabsorption and tolerance of lactose-hydrolyzed milk. A double-blind controlled crossover study. Scand J Gastroenterol 1982; 17: 861–864.

53. Onwulata CI, Rao DR, Vankineni P. Relative efficiency of yogurt, sweet acidophilus milk, hydrolyzed-lactose milk, and a commercial lactase tablet in alleviating lactose maldigestion. Am J Clin Nutr 1989; 49: 1233–1237.

54. Reasoner J, Maculan TP, Rand AG, Thayer WR Jr. Clinical studies with low-lactose milk. Am J Clin Nutr 1981; 34: 54–60.

55. Nielsen OH, Schiotz PO, Rasmussen SN, Krasilnikoff PA. Calcium absorption and acceptance of low-lactose milk among children with primary lactase deficiency. J Pediatr Gastroenterol Nutr 1984; 3: 219–223.

56. Solomons NW, Guerrero AM, Torun B. Dietary manipulation of postprandial colonic lactose fermentation: II. Addition of exogenous, microbial beta-galactosidases at mealtime. Am J Clin Nutr 1985; 41: 209–221.

57. Barillas C, Solomons NW. Effective reduction of lactose maldigestion in preschool children by direct addition of betagalactosidases to milk at mealtime. Pediatrics 1987; 79: 766–772.

58. Lin MY, Dipalma JA, Martini MC, Gross CJ, Harlander SK, Savaiano DA. Comparative effects of exogenous lactase (betagalactosidase) preparations on in vivo lactose digestion. Dig Dis Sci 1993; 38: 2022–2027.

59. Montalto M, Nucera G, Santoro L, Curigliano V, Vastola M, Covino M, Cuoco L, Manna R, Gasbarrini A, Gasbarrini G. Effect of exogenous beta-galactosidase in patients with lactose malabsorption and intolerance: a crossover double-blind placebo-controlled study. Eur J Clin Nutr 2005; 59: 489–493.

60. Flood MT, Kondo M. Toxicity evaluation of a beta-galactosidase preparation produced by Penicillium multicolor. Regul Toxicol Pharmacol 2004; 40: 281–292.

61. DiPalma JA, Collins MS. Enzyme replacement for lactose malabsorption using a beta-D-galactosidase. J Clin Gastroenterol 1989; 11: 290–293.

62. Adolfsson O, Meydani SN, Russell RM. Yogurt and gut func- function. Am J Clin Nutr 2004; 80: 245–256.

63. Hove H, Norgaard H, Mortensen PB. Lactic acid bacteria and the human gastrointestinal tract. Eur J Clin Nutr 1999; 53: 339–350.

64. Bourlioux P, Pochart P. Nutritional and health properties of yogurt. World Rev Nutr Diet 1988; 56: 217–258.

65. McDonough FE, Hitchins AD, Wong NP, Wells P, Bodwell CE. Modification of sweet acidophilus milk to improve utilization by lactose-intolerant persons. Am J Clin Nutr 1987; 45: 570–574.

66. Savaiano DA, AbouElAnouar A, Smith DE, Levitt MD. Lac- Lactose malabsorption from yogurt, pasteurized yogurt, sweet acidophilus milk, and cultured milk in lactase-deficient individuals. Am J Clin Nutr 1984; 40: 1219–1223.

67. Onwulata CI, Rao DR, Vankineni P. Relative efficiency of yogurt, sweet acidophilus milk, hydrolyzed-lactose milk, and a commercial lactase tablet in alleviating lactose maldigestion. Am J Clin Nutr 1989; 49: 1233–1237.

68. de Vrese M, Stegelmann A, Richter B, Fenselau S, Laue C, Schrezenmeir J. Probiotics – compensation for lactase insufficiency. Am J Clin Nutr 2001; 73: 421S–429S.

69. Lin MY, Yen CL, Chen SH. Management of lactose maldigestion by consuming milk containing lactobacilli. Dig Dis Sci 1998; 43: 133–137.

70. Labayen I, Forga L, Gonzalez A, Lenoir-Wijnkoop I, Nutr R, Martinez JA. Relationship between lactose digestion, gastrointestinal transit time and symptoms in lactose malabsorbers after dairy consumption. Aliment Pharmacol Ther 2001; 15: 543–549.
71. Peuhkuri K, Vapaatalo H, Nevala R, Korpela R. Influence of the pharmacological modification of gastric emptying on lactose digestion and gastrointestinal symptoms. Aliment Pharmacol Ther 1999; 13: 81–86.
72. Szilagyi A, Salomon R, Seidman E. Influence of loperamide on lactose handling and oral-caecal transit time. Aliment Pharmacol Ther 1996; 10: 765–770.
73. Leichter J. Comparison of whole milk and skim milk with aqueous lactose solution in lactose tolerance testing. Am J Clin Nutr 1973; 26: 393–396.
74. Vesa TH, Marteau PR, Briet FB, Boutron-Ruault MC, Rambaud JC. Raising milk energy content retards gastric emptying of lactose in lactose-intolerant humans with little effect on lactose digestion. J Nutr 1997; 127: 2316–2320.
75. Johnson AO, Semenya JG, Buchowski MS, Enwonwu CO, Scrimshaw NS. Adaptation of lactose maldigesters to contin- continued milk intakes. Am J Clin Nutr 1993; 58: 879–881.
76. Hertzler SR, Savaiano DA. Colonic adaptation to daily lactose feeding in lactose maldigesters reduces lactose intolerance. Am J Clin Nutr 1996; 64: 232–236.
77. Hertzler SR, Savaiano DA, Levitt MD. Fecal hydrogen pro- production and consumption measurements. Response to daily lactose ingestion by lactose maldigesters. Dig Dis Sci 1997; 42: 348–353.
78. Hill MJ. Bacterial adaptation to lactase deficiency. Delmont J, ed. Milk intolerances and rejection. Basel, Switzerland: Karger, 1983: pp. 22–26.
79. Perman JA, Modler S, Olson AC. Role of pH in production of hydrogen from carbohydrates by colonic bacterial flora. Studies in vivo and in vitro. J Clin Invest 1981; 67: 643–650.
80. Briet F, Pochart P, Marteau P, Flourie B, Arrigoni E, Rambaud JC. Improved clinical tolerance to chronic lactose ingestion in subjects with lactose intolerance: a placebo effect? Gut 1997; 41: 632–635.
81. Montalto M, Curigliano V, Santoro L, Vastola M, Cammarota G, Manna R Gasbarrini A and Gasbarrini G. Management and treatment of lactose malabsorption. World J Gastroenterol 2006; 12: 187–191.
82. Kibbe AH, ed. Handbook of pharmaceutical excipients: American Pharmaceutical Association. London: Washington and the Pharmaceutical Press; 2000: pp. 276–285.
83. Lieb J, Kazienko DJ. Lactose filler as a cause of 'drug-induced' diarrhea. N Engl J Med 1978; 299: 314.
84. Brandstetter RD, Conetta R, Glazer B. Lactose intolerance associated with Intal capsules. N Eng J Med 1986; 315: 1613–1614.
85. Malen DG. Parnate formulation change. J Clin Psychiatry 1992; 53: 328–329.
86. Petrini L, Usai P, Caradonna A, Cabula R, Mariotti S. Lactose intolerance following antithyroid drug medications. J Endocrinol Invest 1997; 20: 569–570.
87. Honkanen R, Pulkkinen P, Jarvinen R, Kroger H, Lindstedt K, Tuppurainen M, Uusitupa M. Does lactose intolerance predispose to low bone density? A population based study of peri-menopausal Finnish women. Bone 1996; 19: 23–28.
88. Slemenda C, Christian J, Hui S, Fitzgerald J, Johnston C. No evidence for an effect of lactase deficiency on bone mass in pre-or postmenopausal women. J Bone Miner Res 1991; 6: 1367–1371.
89. Kudlacek S, Freudenthaler O, Weissboeck H, Schneider B, Willvonseder R. Lactose intolerance: a risk factor for reduced bone mineral density and vertebral fractures? J Gastroenterol 2002; 37: 1014–1019.
90. Rumessen JJ. Fructose and food related carbohydrates. Sources, intake, absorption, and clinical implications. Scand J Gastroenterol 1992; 27: 819–828.
91. Rumessen JJ, Gudmand-Hoyer E. Absorption capacity of fructose in healthy adults. Comparison with sucrose and its constituent monosaccharides. Gut 1986; 27: 1161–1168.
92. Mishkin D, Sablauskas L, Yalovsky M, Mishkin S. Fructose and sorbitol malabsorption in ambulatory patients with functional dyspepsia. Comparison with lactose maldigestion/malabsorption. Dig Dis Sci 1997; 42: 2591–2598.

93. Choi YK, Johlin FC Jr, Summers RW, Jackson M, Rao SS. Fructose intolerance: an under-recognized problem. Am J Gastroenterol 2003; 98: 1348–1353.
94. Truswell AS, Seach JM, Thorburn AW. Incomplete absorption of pure fructose in healthy subjects and the facilitating effect of glucose. Am J Clin Nutr 1988; 48: 1424–1430.
95. Fernandez-Banares F, Esteve-Pardo M, de Leon R, Humbert P, Cabre E, Llovet JM, Gassull MA. Sugar malabsorption in functional bowel disease: clinical implications. Am J Gastroenterol 1993; 88: 2044–2050.
96. Bueno L, de Ponti F, Fried M, Kullak-Ublick GA, Kwiatek MA, Pohl D, Quigley EM, Tack J, Talley NJ. Serotonergic and non-serotonergic targets in the pharmacotherapy of visceral hypersensitivity. Neurogastroenterol Motil 2007; 19: 89–119.
97. Wasserman D, Hoekstra JH, Tolia V, Taylor CJ, Kirschner BS, Takeda J, Bell GI, Taub R, Rand EB. Molecular analysis of the fructose transporter gene (GLUT5) in isolated fructose malabsorption. J Clin Invest 1996; 98: 2398–2402.
98. Burant CF, Saxena M. Rapid reversible substrate regulation of fructose transporter expression in rat small intestine and kidney. Am J Physiol 1994; 267: G71–G79.
99. Mesonero J, Matosin M, Cambier D, Rodriguez-Yoldi MJ, Brot-Laroche E. Sugar-dependent expression of the fructose transporter GLUT5 in Caco-2 cells. Biochem J 1995; 312: 757–762.
100. Gouyon F, Caillaud L, Carriere V, Klein C, Dalet V, Citadelle D, Kellett GL, Thorens B, Leturque A, Brot-Laroche E. Simple-sugar meals target GLUT2 at enterocyte apical membranes to improve sugar absorption: a study in GLUT2-null mice. J Physiol 2003; 552: 823–832.
101. Corpe CP, Bovelander FJ, Munoz CM, Hoekstra JH, Simpson IA, Kwon O, Levine M, Burant CF. Cloning and functional characterization of the mouse fructose transporter, GLUT5. Biochim Biophys Acta 2002; 1576: 191–197.
102. Hoekstra JH, van den Aker JH. Facilitating effect of amino acids on fructose and sorbitol absorption in children. J Pediatr Gastroenterol Nutr 1996; 23: 118–124.
103. Rumessen JJ, Gudmand-Hoyer E. Malabsorption of fructose-sorbitol mixtures. Interactions causing abdominal distress. Scand J Gastroenterol 1987; 22: 431–436.
104. Riby JE, Fujisawa T, Kretchmer N. Fructose absorption. Am J Clin Nutr 1993; 58: 748S–753S.
105. Shi X, Schedl HP, Summers RM, Lambert GP, Chang RT, Xia T, Gisolfi CV. Fructose transport mechanisms in humans. Gastroenterology 1997; 113: 1171–1179.
106. Fine KD, Santa Ana CA, Porter JL, Fordtran JS. Mechanism by which glucose stimulates the passive absorption of small solutes by the human jejunum in vivo. Gastroenterology 1994; 107: 389–395.
107. Elias E, Gibson GJ, Greenwood LF, Hunt JN, Tripp JH. The slowing of gastric emptying by monosaccharides and disaccharides in test meals. J Physiol 1968; 194: 317–326.
108. Hyams JS. Sorbitol intolerance: an unappreciated cause of functional gastrointestinal complaints. Gastroenterology 1983; 84: 30–33.
109. Summers RW, Johlin FC. Fructose intolerance is due to rapid orocecal transit and not small bowel bacterial overgrowth. Gastroenterology 2001; 120: A1369.
110. Romagnuolo J, Schiller D, Bailey RJ. Using breath tests wisely in a gastroenterology practice: an evidence-based review of indications and pitfalls in interpretation. Am J Gastroenterol 2002; 97: 1113–1126.
111. Doma S, Gaddipati K, Fernandez A, Friedenberg F, Bromer M, Parkman H. Results of the fructose breath test in healthy controls using different doses of fructose: which dose is best? Am J Gastroenterol 2003; 98: S265.
112. Skoog SM, Bharucha AE. Dietary fructose and gastrointestinal symptoms: a review. Am J Gastroenterol 2004; 99: 2046–2050.
113. Strocchi A, Levitt MD. Factors affecting hydrogen production and consumption by human fecal flora. The critical roles of hydrogen tension and methanogenesis. J Clin Invest 1992; 89: 1304–1311.
114. Shepherd SJ, Gibson PR. Fructose malabsorption and symptoms of irritable bowel syndrome: guidelines for effective dietary management. J Am Diet Assoc 2006; 106: 1631–1639.
115. Moshfegh AJ, Friday JE, Goldman JK, Ahuja JP. Presence of inulin and oligofructose in the diets of Americans. J Nutr 1999; 129: S1407–S1411.

Insect Sting Allergy in Adults

Anne K. Ellis and James H. Day

Introduction

Allergy to hymenoptera occurs world wide and is associated with significant morbidity and mortality. Most stings are associated with local reactions of various sizes, some being extensive, and characterized by pain, swelling, and redness. They usually last from a few hours to a few days and resolve with simple treatment measures. These reactions are mostly caused by the toxic components of venom and are usually limited in size and duration. However, widespread local reactions, often immunologic in nature, may extend from the sting site lasting up to 1 week, occur in approximately 10–15% of adults [1]. Systemic responses, mainly anaphylactic, occur in up to 0.8% of children and 3% of adults [1] and may be life-threatening.

The insects of the order Hymenoptera, which includes ants, bees, hornets, and wasps, have a stinging apparatus at the tail end of their abdominal segment and are capable of delivering between 100 ng (fire ants) [2] and 50 µg (bees and vespids) [3] of venom. Venoms have various peptide and protein components, some of which are capable of inducing toxic or vasoactive responses. A lethal dose of venom for a non-allergic adult weighing 70 kg could require up to 1500 stings [4]. Forty to fifty deaths a year in the U.S. are attributed to mostly single stings [5], and indicates the potential severity of a single sting occurring in persons with specific IgE antibodies already developed to various venom components either directly through previous stings or indirectly from insect product exposure such as bee dusts in honey producing settings [6].

A.K. Ellis
Assistant Professor, Division of Allergy and Immunology, Department of Medicine
and Department of Microbiology and Immunology, Queen's University Kingston, ON Canada

J.H. Day (✉)
Professor and Head, Division of Allergy and Immunology, Department of Medicine,
Queen's University, Kingston, ON, Canada
e-mail: dayj@kgh.kari.net

R. Pawankar et al. (eds.), *Allergy Frontiers: Clinical Manifestations*,
DOI: 10.1007/978-4-431-88317-3_28, © Springer 2009

After a systemic reaction to an apparent sting, the diagnosis of stinging insect hypersensitivity requires a detailed history as well as skin tests and/or *in vitro* tests for confirmation of reactivity and possible treatment with specific venom immunotherapy (VIT) [1,7,8].

Stinging Insects

Background

The insects of the order Hymenoptera responsible for clinical reactions include insects from the families of *Vespidae* (hornets, wasps), *Apidae* (bees), and *Formicidae* (fire ants – *Solenopsis* spp.).

Worldwide, yellow jackets are the most common stinging insect. These are urbanized insects usually encountered during yard work or gardening when nests are disturbed. Because of their predilection for human sourced food and drink, including garbage, they frequently come in contact with the general public in these settings. Such contact may include stings to the mouth, oropharynx, or esophagus, often resulting in life threatening acute swelling and airway obstruction, even in non-allergic persons.

Hornets mostly build papier-mâché nests in the vicinity of trees and shrubs, and attack if disturbed in the area surrounding their nest, usually resulting in multiple stings.

Wasps build honeycomb nests, some out of mud, that are several inches or more in diameter. The nests are usually located under the eaves of houses or barns, and occasionally in pipes on playgrounds or under patio furniture.

Domestic honeybees are found in commercial hives and on flowers. Wild honeybee nests can occasionally be found in tree hollows, old logs, and around buildings. Hives may contain thousands of bees. Honeybees are usually docile but may be aggressive around their hives, especially during cool damp weather. Beekeepers, their family members and employees in the bee-keeping industry are most likely to be stung by domestic honey bees. Africanized honeybees, which are especially aggressive, are hybrids resulting from interbreeding of domestic honeybees and African honeybees. Accidentally introduced in South America, they have expanded northward where they can be found in several of the Southern United States [1,7]. Occasionally Africanized queen bees have mistakenly been brought into the northern United States and Canada by the beekeeping industry, but are generally intolerant of winter. They are more aggressive than domestic/wild honeybees and their hives are often around buildings, which brings them in proximity to humans. Africanized honeybees are more likely to attack in swarms, and unlike non-Africanized bees will pursue and sting over long distances. Their venom, however, is antigenically similar to domestic honeybee venom, presenting no special allergic risk from their stings. A barbed stinger with attached venom sac in the skin at the sting site denotes a sting from a honey bee.

Bumblebees, another member of the apidae family, are generally slow-moving and non-aggressive, and rarely sting. They are thus only rarely responsible for hypersensitivity reactions, despite their use as pollinators of vegetables in commercial green houses [8].

The fire ant, which is endemic to Southeastern and Southcentral United States, is red or black in color, nests in mounds several inches high and up to two feet in diameter. They have also expanded northward into Virginia and beyond, and westward into California, facilitated by urbanization [9,10]. There are recent reports of building invasions leading to attacks inside [11]. Their presence may be identified by multiple ant mounds a few feet apart in vegetated areas. In sandy areas, the nests are flat and obscure. Fire ants are aggressive, particularly if their nests are disturbed, often leading to multiple stings. A sterile pseudopustule, surrounded by multiple sting sites, is a distinguishing feature of single fire ant attacks [12].

Geography plays an important role in determining the most likely insect causing the sting. Yellow jackets are the most common cause of allergic reactions in urban areas of North America and Europe [19], while *Polistes* wasps are especially common in the Gulf Coast states of the United States and in the Mediterranean countries of Europe [19]. Fire ants are perhaps the most likely cause of insect sting reactions in the southeast United States because of their abundance and high attack rate [13,14].

Other Hymenoptera insects which have caused allergic sting reactions include the sweat bee (Hymenoptera: *Halictidae*) as well as several types of ants, including *Rhytidoponera* (greenhead ant) [15] and *Myrmecia* (jumper and bull ants) [13] in Australia and *Pogonomyrmex* (harvester ant), in the United States [16].

At Risk Populations

Systemic reactions to hymenoptera venom can occur in any member of the general population given the ubiquitous presence of these insects; however, adult males are stung more frequently and consequently are at higher risk for reactions [17]. A recent epidemiologic study of the natural history of hymenoptera sensitivity in Spain showed that occasionally stung adult male agricultural workers were in particular at greater risk of having systemic reactions or large local reactions [18].

Beekeepers who are repeatedly stung on multiple occasions are at virtually no risk of developing systemic reactions to honeybees [7], a result of naturally developed desensitization to honey bee venom. Family members of professional beekeepers and beekeeper hobbyists have a significantly elevated risk of systemic reactivity (20%) as compared to the general population (3%), apparently due to sensitization produced by occasional stings beyond those sustained by the general population [7].

Systemic mastocytosis is over-represented in the Hymenoptera-allergic population and is associated with an increased risk of more severe reactions following field stings or sting challenges, increased side effects to VIT, as well as reduced efficacy of VIT [19]. Since these individuals may lack evidence of sensitization to venoms by skin test or radioallergosorbent test, the diagnosis of mastocytosis must be considered in patients with a history of allergic type systemic reactivity to hymenoptera sting but no evidence of venom-specific IgE.

Clinical Reactions to Insect Stings

Local Reactions

Most insect stings cause transient localized reactions that are usually of minimal medical consequence, and no specific treatment is usually required. These reactions are not IgE-mediated and patients are not at risk for future allergic reactions. However, when a sting occurs in the oropharnyx or esophagus due to accidental ingestion of a stinging insect, the resulting local reaction may lead to asphyxia from extensive swelling of the upper airway.

Fire ant stings are painful and typically cause sterile pseudopustules 24 h after the sting. The pain from a sting frequently persists up to 72 h. The vesicle consists of aseptic necrotic tissue, and should be left intact to avoid secondary infection [1].

Large Local Reactions

Some local reactions can expand from the site of the sting and consist of extensive erythematous swelling surrounding the sting site, and may involve the entire limb. These often continue to enlarge over 48 h before gradually resolving over a few days. Such reactions are usually painful and/or pruritic. Usually these are toxic responses to venom components but may represent IgE-mediated late phase reactivity [20,21]. Secondary large local reactions usually recur with future stings in these subjects, but are a slight risk factor (<10%) for anaphylaxis in subsequent stings [22]. Local reactions are usually manageable with supportive therapy, but secondary infection must always be considered when they occur.

Systemic Reactions

Systemic reactions may involve any or virtually all organ systems in the body. Anaphylaxis is the term used when more than one organ system is affected, and is the most severe expression of an allergic reaction, potentially with fatal consequences. As in all allergic responses, it results from immunologically induced mast cell or basophil mediator release after exposure to the specific venom antigen in previously sensitized persons [23].

An anaphylactic response usually develops within 30 min of antigen exposure, and is typically monophasic (i.e., one episode). Variants of the anaphylaxis syndrome do occur, including late-onset and protracted reactions [24]. Biphasic reactions also occur and have been well documented in the setting of insect sting hypersensitivity [25], resulting in a subsequent, potentially life-threatening reaction, even after stabilization and resolution of the first episode. Second-phase reactions occur in approximately 10–20% of patients, with asymptomatic windows of 1–38 h [26].

Severe systemic reactions to insect stings typically have a rapid onset. In a recent study, 45% of all reactions (including local ones) began within 5 min following a sting, indeed the majority of anaphylactic reactions with respiratory and/or cardiovascular symptoms or changes in consciousness were also evident early [13].

Regardless of the antigen source, symptoms of anaphylaxis can affect most organ systems. The most commonly affected are: cutaneous (urticaria, erythema, angioedema), respiratory (dyspnea, wheeze, deceased oxygen saturation), gastrointestinal (abdominal pain, nausea, vomiting) and cardiovascular (hypotension, tachycardia, syncope), often anteceded by a sense of impending doom (*angor*) [15].

Toxic reactions, sometimes indistinguishable from allergic reactions, may develop. These are responses to venom components that directly release mediators, many of which are produced in the course of allergic reactions as well. Such events typically occur in settings where individuals are multiply stung, and may lead to organ failure including the kidney [27,28].

Some unrecognized features of hymenoptera hypersensitivity have been described. Solley's 2004 paper observed that stings on the head or neck are not necessarily more likely to lead to life-threatening reactions nor do greater reactions typically follow lesser responses, but did confirm known observations that pre-existing asthma was a risk for severe asthmatic episodes; anaphylaxis is usually species-specific; and persons who receive numerous stings at one time may have true anaphylaxis and not just a "toxic" response. Anaphylaxis from other sources on the other hand is not a risk factor for hypersensitivity to insect stings or bites [13].

Other reported but rare complications of insect stings include serum sickness [29], vasculitis [20,30], neuritis [21], myasthenia gravis [21], cerebral infarction [21,31], Guillain-Barré syndrome [21], encephalitis [21,32,33], Reye-like syndrome [21], intravascular coagulation [34], optic neuropathy [35], hand-foot syndrome [36], acquired cold urticaria [37], oculopalatal syndrome [38], rhabdomyolysis [39,40], myocardial infarction [21], and cardiac arrhythmia [21,41].

Treament of Insect Sting Reactions

General

Most insect stings cause transient localized reactions that are usually of minimal concern, and symptomatic therapy is sufficient. However, when a sting occurs in the oropharynx or esophagus due to accidental ingestion of a stinging insect the resulting reaction may be life threatening even in the non-allergic individual.

Fire ant stings are invariably painful and typically cause sterile pseudopustules 24 h after the sting. The material in the vesicle consists of necrotic tissue and is not evidence of infection. The vesicle should be left intact to avoid secondary infection.

Large Local Reactions

Reactions may expand from the site of a sting and consist of extensive erythematous swelling surrounding the sting site, and may eventually affect an entire limb or other areas of the body. Most progress over 48 h before resolving in a few days, during which they are usually painful and/or pruritic [42]. They may result in a temporary loss of function, such as when the sting involves a foot or hand, or is near an eye. Secondary infections are rare, but can result from trauma to the affected site (e.g., rubbing). Progressive swelling lasting more than 2 days accompanied by fever and/or lymphadenitis suggests secondary infection [43].

Non-infected local reactions can usually be successfully managed with oral non-steroidal anti-inflammatory agents, antihistamines, and cold compresses. Topical antihistamines and corticosteroids may be added, with oral corticosteroids reserved for severe, extensive swelling. Secondary infection requires treatment with antibiotics that have efficacy against common skin organisms such as *Staphylcoccus aureus* and *Staphylococcus epidermis* (e.g., cephalexin, cloxacillin). Patients who manifest only local reactions should be reassured about their benign nature, and the unlikely progression to systemic reactions in future stings.

Systemic Reactions

Anaphylaxis is a medical emergency that requires immediate treatment. The management of acute anaphylaxis is summarized in Table 1. Parenteral epinephrine is the cornerstone of management [44]. The dosage for adults is 0.3–0.5 ml of a 1:1000 dilution, and recent research has established the intramuscular route to be superior to the subcutaneous route [45]. Epinephrine can be re-injected every 5–15 min until there is resolution of the anaphylaxis or signs of hyper-adrenalism (including palpitations, tremor, uncomfortable apprehension and anxiety) occur [24]. Intravenous epinephrine (1:10 000 dilution) should generally be reserved for severe hypotensive shock and administered by experienced personnel due to the risk of dosing errors with resulting epinephrine-induced tachyarrhythmias and/or myocardial infarction [46,47]. An adequate airway must be established and maintained, and supplemental oxygen given to all patients with anaphylactic reactions.

Other supplementary therapy for anaphylaxis includes the use of H_1 and H_2 antihistamines, for example, diphenhydramine, 25–50 mg intravenously, and

Table 1 Management of acute anaphylaxis

	Dose	Route	Frequency	Notes
First Line Treatment				
Epinephrine	0.3–0.5 cc of 1:1000 dil'n	IM	q 5–15 min prn after first dose	Repeat doses may be given until intolerable adrenergic side effects occur (tachycardia, etc.)
Supplemental Oxygen, Secure Airway, IV Access, Monitor, place patient in recumbent position and elevate legs if possible				
Intravenous fluids – Normal Saline or Ringer's Lactate: 500 ml bolus minimum, may require up to 4 or 5 l crystalloid to reverse hypotension				
Second Line, Ancillary Treatments				
Antihistamines				
e.g. diphenhydramine	50 mg	IV/PO	q 4 h prn	Diphenhydramine only H1 antagonist available in parenteral form, second generation agents such as cetirizine may be more effective with less sedation, longer duration of action
cetirizine	10 mg	PO	q 12 h prn (after first dose)	
Corticosteroids				
e.g. methylprednisolone	125 mg	IV	q 24 h prn (after first dose)	Given to prevent or minimize second phase reactivity, symptoms may still recur, however
prednisone	50 mg	PO		
H_2 receptor antagonists i.e. ranitidine	50 mg	IV	q 8 h prn	Combined H1 and H2 antagonism shown to provide better control of cutaneous symptoms than either alone
	150 mg	PO	q 12 h prn (after first dose)	
Beta-agonists e.g. salbutamol	5.0 mg	NEB	q 15 min prn	Wheezing, hypoxia in anaphylaxis often due to airway edema, not just bronchoconstriction, epinephrine required to reverse
Refractory Anaphylaxis				
Vasopressors				
e.g. epinephrine dopamine	0.1 mg	IV	q 15 min prn or start infusion	Arrange for transfer to ICU, look for sources of ongoing antigen exposure, evaluate for possible contributory medications (See below)
Due to concomitant Beta-blocker therapy				
Glucagon	1 mg	IV	q 10 min prn	Maximum safe dose is unclear

ranitidine, 50 mg intravenously or 150 mg orally. Current recommendations are to administer these agents in combination, because H_1 and H_2 blockade is more effective than H_1 blockade alone in preventing symptomatology of anaphylaxis in experimental models [48]. Inhaled β2-agonists (e.g., salbutamol) may be useful when bronchospasm is present, but not usually required. Corticosteroids (e.g., methylprednisolone, 125 mg intravenously, or prednisone, 50 mg orally; the intravenous route of administration is often used for more severe reactions) may help prevent or minimize second-phase reactions, however, biphasic reactions are well documented in patients who received corticosteroids as part of their initial management [49,50]. Hypotensive patients should receive intravenous fluid support with crystalloid or colloid, and severe cases may require vasopressor agents such as dopamine or high-dilution epinephrine (1:10 000). Individuals who use β-blockers (and possibly angiotensin-converting-enzyme inhibitors, although the evidence is incomplete) may not respond completely to epinephrine, in which case glucagon should be administered at a dose of 5–15 µg/min intravenously. Glucagon has inotropic, chronotropic and vasoactive effects that are independent of β-receptors, and it also releases endogenous catecholamines. Considering the reported incomplete prophylactic coverage of corticosteroids and the acknowledged benefit of histamine blockade in the prevention of anaphylactoid reactions e.g., to radiocontrast media [51], 4 days of prednisone (50 mg PO daily) and either diphenhydramine 50 mg PO q6h or cetirizine 10 mg PO daily should be prescribed upon discharge.

Post-treatment observation is required for all patients considering the possibility of second phase reaction. Although most of these reactions occur within 1–8 h, prolonged asymptomatic windows of up to 25 and 38 h have been reported [26,27,51]. A recent prospective study showed that 20% of patients with anaphylaxis went on to have a 2nd phase reaction, after a mean asymptomatic window of 10 h [26]. Given the above, close observation in a monitored setting for 24 h post anaphylaxis should be arranged with timely access to hospital for the ensuing 48 h. Patients should be discharged from the emergency department only under adequate supervision, and to environments with easy access to the emergency medical response system [23]. The efficacy and safety of epinephrine for the treatment of anaphylaxis has been clearly established, and must be the mainstay of treatment of anaphyaxis from any cause; indeed failure to provide epinephrine is associated with fatalities.

Epinephrine auto-injectors should be prescribed for any patient who has had an anaphylactic reaction to a hymenoptera sting. The instructions for use are printed on the side of each injector, but these should be reviewed with the patient when prescribing the medication. Patients should be educated to use epinephrine if signs or symptoms beyond a cutaneous reaction develop after a hymenoptera sting, and always to seek additional medical care after using an injector. Patients, caregivers and health care providers alike benefit from focused instruction and regular review of the optimal use of epinephrine in the first aid treatment of anaphylaxis [52,53]. In addition, some authors recommend that patients receive a tablet set containing a rapidly effective oral H_1-antihistamine (e.g., cetirizine $2 \times 10\,mg$) and corticosteroids (e.g., prednisone $2 \times 50\,mg$) [82].

Natural History of Stinging Insect Allergy

Local Reactions

If a large local reaction occurs in response to an insect sting, patients should be informed to expect a similar type of reactivity with future stings. There is a small but measurable increased risk (<10%) of anaphylaxis after future stings [14], but this is considered insufficient to warrant immunotherapy [1].

Since the pseudopustules formed in response to a fire ant sting contains necrotic tissue and is usually not infected, the vesicle should be left intact and should not be opened. If, however, it is accidentally opened, it should be cleansed with soap and water to prevent secondary infection. Secondary infection is an uncommon complication of fire ant stings, without which antibiotics are not indicated [54].

Systemic Reactions

Without appropriate medical intervention, individuals who have had an allergic reaction from an insect sting are at risk for a more severe allergic reaction if re-stung. VIT has been established as an effective means to prevent subsequent systemic reactions [1,8,55,56]. Specific venom extracts of honeybee, yellow jacket, white-faced hornet, yellow hornet, and wasp venom are available for skin testing and immunotherapy.

Adults with a history of systemic reactivity, even those with only mild cutaneous manifestations, who have demonstrable specific IgE antibodies either via a positive skin and/or *in vitro* test response, are at risk for subsequent life-threatening reactions if re-stung. VIT should be considered in such patients, and is discussed in detail in the ensuing section. Approximately 30–60% of untreated patients with a history of anaphylaxis from an insect sting and venom-specific IgE antibodies detectable by means of skin or *in vitro* testing will experience a systemic reaction when re-stung [1,8].

Less is known about the natural history of fire ant venom hypersensitivity and efficacy of immunotherapy, but fire ant whole body vaccine has been shown to contain relevant allergens [1,57,58]. Accumulating evidence supports the contention that immunotherapy with fire ant whole-body vaccine is protective [59,60]. Immunotherapy with fire ant whole-body vaccine should be initiated in patients with a history of systemic reactivity to fire ant stings and have a positive skin test response to whole-body extract or a positive *in vitro* assay [1,8].

Secondary Prevention

Based on the knowledge of the living conditions and habitat of hymenoptera, a series of recommendations have been formulated which should minimize the risk of field re-sting (Table 2).

Patients should be made aware that Hymenoptera insects sting in self-defense, and that any act which is perceived as a potential threat might result in a sting. Detailed information should be provided to subjects at risk: including favored nest sites, food attractants, clothing, etc. In the case of a honeybee sting, the stinger should be removed, usually by a finger nail, thereby limiting the quantity of venom injected [12].

Venom Immunotherapy

Specific VIT is very effective in reducing the risk of a subsequent systemic reaction from a future insect sting to less than 5%, and those who do experience reactions have milder symptoms.

Mechanisms

Though it is clear that tolerance to insect stings can be achieved through VIT, the mechanisms involved remain unclear. A rise in allergen-blocking IgG antibodies, particularly of the IgG4 class, the generation of IgE-modulating CD8+ T cells and a decrease in the release of mediators have been shown to be associated with successful immunotherapy [61,62]. Furthermore, specific immunotherapy is associated with a decrease in CD4+ T cells production of IL-4 and IL-5, and a shift towards increased IFN-γ production [63,64], although a full alteration of T-cell activity from a dominating Th2 type towards a Th1 type, is controversial [65,66]. Changes in the immune response to bee venom have been extensively investigated during VIT [51–55], phospholipase A peptide immunotherapy [67–69] and during natural excess allergen exposure in healthy bee keepers [70].

Table 2 Activities associated with increased risk for insect stings

Outdoor eating and drinking
Removing vespid nests from any site
Walking barefoot or with short pants, especially in long grass
Gardening (especially cutting pollinating flowers or hedges)
Picking fruit or vegetables, especially if over-ripe
Playing outdoor sports
Any activity in proximity to beehives when honey is collected

Successfully treated patients develop specific T-cell unresponsiveness against the entire phospholipase (PLA) allergen as well as T-cell epitope-containing peptides. The same anergic state of specific T cells has been observed in protected individuals such as bee keepers [56]. The anergic state of specific cells results from increased IL-10 secretion [55], the cellular origin of which has been demonstrated to be the antigen-specific T-cell population and activated CD4+CD25+ T cells as well as monocytes and B cells [56].

Another cellular player thought to play a central role in the mechanism of specific VIT is the Regulatory T cell (Treg). Treg cells are a population enriched within the CD4+CD25+ cells [71,72], and function in the suppression/regulation of immune responses [73,74]. They include Tr1 cells, which produce high levels of IL-10, and which likely play a pivotal role in the maintenance of peripheral tolerance [75], as well as Th3 cells, which are induced following oral administration of the antigen and secrete predominantly TGF-β. It has been shown that tolerance to aeroallergens is associated with the increased secretion of TGF-β [76], although this mechanism is likely not involved in VIT.

Differences in effect on T-cell reactivity are observed when VIT is administered using rapid versus conventional protocols. Although rapid immunotherapy, similarly to conventional immunotherapy, is associated with a shift from Th2 to Th1-type cytokine production by peripheral blood lymphocytes, the modulation of T-cell cytokines during conventional VIT takes much longer to develop [77]. Furthermore, in contrast to ultra-rush VIT inducing rapid T-cell anergy, conventional VIT involves a transient increase in T-cell proliferation in response to the allergen during the incremental phase of allergen administration followed by specific T-cell tolerance [66]. The implications of these observations in terms of clinical efficacy call for further investigation.

Most patients are already protected against bee stings at an early stage of VIT, which is not always paralleled by changes in antibody formation. It has been demonstrated that lower amounts of mediators of anaphylaxis (e.g., histamine or leukotrienes) are released *in vitro* from samples taken during specific IT [51,78,79]. These effects may be attributed to the direct suppressive effect of IL-10 on effector cells (mast cells, basophils) [80]. Anergic T cells, however, do not secrete the cytokines which are required for the priming, survival and activity of the effector cells [55].

Selection of Patients Requiring Venom Immunotherapy

VIT is indicated in adults with a history of systemic reaction, including cutaneous manifestations alone, and documented sensitization to the respective insect venoms with either skin tests and/or specific serum IgE tests.

VIT is especially indicated for those persons likely to receive future stings and/ or have a history of severe sting reactions [1,70,81]. Venom immunotherapy is only indicated when symptoms suggest systemic reactivity in the presence of supporting skin tests and/or serum specific IgE antibodies. VIT is not indicated for events such as vasculitis, nephrosis, fever, thrombocytopenia, etc. [82,83].

It is important to take the following specific points into consideration when starting VIT: Patients with insect sting allergy who are taking β-adrenergic blocking agents are generally thought to be at greater risk for more serious anaphylaxis to VIT or a sting [15,84–86]. Thus current recommendations are that patients who have stinging insect hypersensitivity should not be prescribed β-adrenergic blocking agents unless there is a clear requirement. If the patient who has stinging insect hypersensitivity cannot discontinue the β-adrenergic blocking agent, the decision to administer immunotherapy should be made on an individual basis after assessment of potential risks and benefits. Although there have been case reports that raised concern about the use of angiotensin-converting enzyme inhibitors as well [87,88] a recent study suggests that there is not an association between ACE-I use and increased frequency of SRs to venom immunotherapy [89]. Activities involving high-risk of re-sting should be stopped until the maintenance dose of VIT is reached.

Contraindications

Pregnancy is usually not considered a reason for disturbing an established and well tolerated VIT, but the treatment should not be initiated during pregnancy [90].

General contra-indications for VIT are the same as for immunotherapy with other allergens. In relation to the use of beta-blockers and ACE inhibitors, the decision must always consider the risk of discontinuing these treatments with the risk of a systemic reaction during VIT.

Selection of Venom to be Used in Immunotherapy

The stinging insect causing the reaction is rarely identified accurately by the patient, although careful questioning about locality and features of the event including a description of the insect can be helpful (e.g., honeybees leave their stinger behind). Thus, selecting which venoms to be used is not solely based on the identification of the species of Hymenopteran involved, but relies heavily on the result of specific venom tests and taking cross-reactivity between venoms into consideration [91].

Honey bee and bumblebee venoms share most antigens and have cross-reactivity. Venom immunotherapy with honeybee venom alone will be sufficient in nonprofessionally exposed bumblebee-allergic patients who most likely react on the basis of a cross-reactivity in the presence of primary sensitization to bee venom [92]. In heavily exposed green house workers who are frequently stung by bumble bees, it is recommended that bumblebee venom be used for VIT [93].

Pronounced cross-reactivity exists between the major venom components of several vespids, particularly between Vespula, Dolichovespula and Vespa venoms, but less so between Vespula and Polistes venoms [94]. In view of the relatively limited clinical importance of Polistes in temperate climates, treatment with Vespula venom alone is usually sufficient in vespid sensitive individuals in these areas.

Cross-reactivity is rare between Apidae and Vespidae. When present it is mainly due to hyaluronidase, an important component of the venoms. In the case of double-positive tests to honey bee and Vespula and where identification of the responsible insect is not possible, RAST-inhibition assays, if available, will help to distinguish between cross-reactivity and double sensitization [95,96]. In practical terms, however, when the patient cannot reliably discern the insect species, treatment is based on which species-specific IgE antibodies are demonstrated by skin testing and/or *in vitro* testing.

Venom Immunotherapy Treatment Protocols

Since the first immunotherapy with pure venom extract was carried out in 1974 [97], protocols of various durations have been devised in an effort to maximize protection, minimize side-effects and optimize patient convenience. The time required to reach the generally adequate maintenance dose of 100 µg with slow protocols is several weeks to months [98], whilst rush [99,100] and ultra-rush protocols [101,102] take several days or only a few hours respectively.

The recommended maintenance dose of Hymenoptera venom is 100 µg [1,103], equivalent to approximately two full bee stings and a greater number of Vespula stings. This dose is generally accepted as providing better protection than a 50 µg dose [104]. A dose of 200 µg is recommended when a systemic reaction follows a maintenance injection or an insect sting in spite of VIT with 100 µg [105]. A maintenance dose of 200 µg is also recommended by some authors in particularly exposed populations who are sensitive and liable to be stung [106].

The generally recommended interval for maintenance of VIT with 100 µg venom is 4 weeks [107]. Extending the maintenance interval between injections in the first year of treatment, however, from 4 to 6 weeks continued to give good clinical protection and maintained the immune response. Extending the maintenance interval to 8 weeks immediately upon reaching the full dose has led to declining levels of venom-specific IgG antibodies in the second year, and a 20% rate of systemic reaction to challenge stings [108]. These studies have helped to shape the consensus that the maintenance interval should be kept at 4 weeks for the first year, then extended to 6 weeks in the second year, and then to 8 weeks if VIT is continued over 5 years. In the past few years, however, some studies have emerged suggesting that patients who continue therapy might be safely maintained on 12-week maintenance intervals [109,110].

Efficacy of Venom Immunotherapy

The efficacy of VIT was analysed in three prospective, randomized, controlled trials [111–113], and a number of prospective uncontrolled studies with sting provocation tests during immunotherapy [91,114,115].

In the first single blind controlled trial [99], only 1 out of 18 venom-treated patients (5.5%) had a systemic reaction to a sting challenge compared to 64% of patients treated with whole body extract and 58% of placebo treated patients. Some of the reactions in the placebo- and whole body-extract-treated patients in this study were severe and required intensive care treatment.

In the second controlled study [100], 75% of the venom treated patients who were re-exposed to bee stings experienced allergic reactions; while the opposite was found in those treated with whole body extract. (i.e., 75% manifested mild to severe allergic symptoms, only 25% had no reaction).

Safety of Venom Immunotherapy

VIT aims to induce tolerance to hymenoptera stings but can be complicated by systemic reactions (SR) [116,117]. Reports in the literature reveal a high variation (0–46%) in the incidence of side effects attributable to VIT [86–90,118,119]. It is difficult to compare these reports on incidence of SR with different VIT protocols since the investigators used different classification systems for the severity of adverse reactions [79]. In a recent EAACI-multicentre study [105], 20% of patients had SR corresponding to 1.9% of injections during the dose-increase phase and 0.5% during the maintenance phase. Rapid dose increase (rush) regimens were associated with an increased risk of reactions. Other studies using rush protocols have suggested that they are at least as safe as slower protocols [88–90,107,120].

The issue of the higher incidence of adverse reactions with honeybee VIT has been addressed using different approaches devised to improve safety by changing protocols, through pretreatment with antihistamines [106,121–123], by administering beekeeper gamma-globulin [124,125] chemically modified honeybee venom [126–128] or recombinant hymenoptera venom allergens [129], all of which have proved successful to varying degrees. Pretreatment with antihistamines, must always be weighed against the possibility of masking reactivity potential to the VIT during the treatment period, and only reduces the number/severity of large local reactions and mild SR such as urticaria/angioedema. If used, they should be prescribed 1 or 2 days before VIT and be continued until the maintenance dose has been well tolerated at least three times.

Defining the risk factors for SR to VIT would be helpful in reducing their occurrence. In the previous mentioned EAACI-multicentre study [105], female sex, bee venom extract and rapid dose increase, but not the severity of insect sting reactions, increased the risk of a SR. In another recent study using ultra-rush VIT in a large number of patients [130], a few predictive risk factors were identified, which included bee VIT, dose-increase phase, and severity of the prior sting reaction. The size of positive skin test reactions, and elevated serum venom specific IgE concentrations were not risk factors.

In patients with underlying mast cell disease (elevated baseline serum tryptase and/or mastocytosis) VIT is well tolerated by the majority of affected patients [131,132]. Only a few patients with mastocytosis had repeated severe reactions during immunotherapy necessitating the early suspension of treatment [133,134].

Quality of Life

Anaphylactic reactions following insect stings can have a great impact on quality of life. A recent study has confirmed that in addition to conferring protection in the event of future stings, VIT, with information about the risks and benefits of the treatment, was shown to improve health related quality of life (HRQL) [135]. There were no patients whose HRQL was so severely impaired that they did not improve with VIT. Thus, patient education of these risks and benefits is important to achieve all therapeutic goals of venom immunotherapy.

Summary

Insect stings may occur in almost any environment and are usually limited to a painful swelling but in 3–5% of the population they may produce systemic manifestations with possible fatal consequences.

Localized responses no matter how severe are readily manageable and do not predict systemic reactivity. Venom specific skin tests and *in vitro* tests following systemic reactions indicate a threat of future reactivity to insect venoms and provide a basis for venom specific immunotherapy (VIT) which is highly efficacious. Yellow jackets and honey bees are the main source of stings in North America while fire ants present a special risk in warmer climates particularly south eastern United States.

Local reactions, no matter how extensive, usually need no special management or follow up.

Epinephrine by intramuscular injection is regarded as the treatment of choice for anaphylactic responses followed up by antihistamines alone or in combination with corticosteroids. Auto-injections of epinephrine should be prescribed and their use clearly demonstrated by trained medical personnel. There is a 10–20% incidence of a second phase anaphylactic reactivity occurring up to 30 h following the sting which may be severe.

Patients having systemic reactions should be referred for evaluation and, if indicated, VIT. VIT should be limited to 3 to 5 years but long term management may be considered in those with particularly severe reactions especially in settings where subsequent stings are likely. For persons at risk of re-sting reactions such as agricultural workers, those working in the bee industry and their family members while undergoing or completing VIT, emergency kits containing epinephrine auto-injectors should be readily available.

References

1. Moffitt JE, Golden DBK, Reisman RE, Lee R, Nicklas R, et al. Stinging insect hypersensitivity: a practice parameter update. J Allergy Clin Immunol. 2004 Oct; 114: 869–86.
2. Hoffman DR, Jacobson RS. Allergens in Hymenoptera venom. XII. How much protein in a sting? Ann Allergy 1984; 52: 276–78.

3. Guralnick MW, Benton AW. Entomological aspects of insect sting allergy. In: Levin MI, Lockey RF, eds. Monograph on insect allergy. 4th ed. Milwaukee, WI: American Academy of Allergy, Asthma and Immunology, 2003: pp. 11–26.

4. Goddard J. Physician's guide to arthropods of medical importance. 4th ed. Boca Raton, FL.: CRC Press, 2003: p. 4.

5. Barnard JH. Studies of 400 Hymenoptera sting deaths in the United States. J Allergy Clin Immunol 1973; 52: 259–64.

6. Day JH, Buckeridge DL, Welsh AC. Risk assessment in determining systemic reactivity to honeybee stings in sting-threatened individuals. J Allergy Clin Immunol 1994; 93: 691–705.

7. McKenna WR. Africanized honeybees. In: Levin MI, Lockey RF, eds. Monograph on insect allergy. 4th ed. Milwaukee, WI: American Academy of Allergy, Asthma and Immunology, 2003: pp. 27–36.

8. Hamilton, RG. Diagnosis of Hymenoptera venom sensitivity. Curr Opinion Allergy Immunol 2002; 2: 347–51.

9. Kemp SF. deShazo RD, Moffitt JE, et al. Expanding habitat of the imported fire ant (Solenopsis invicta): a public health concern. J Allergy Clin Immunol 2000; 105: 683–91.

10. Kemp SF, deShazo RD, Moffitt JE, Williams DF, Buhner WA 2nd. Expanding habitat of the imported fire ant (Solenopsis invicta): a public health concern. J Allergy Clin Immunol 2000; 105: 683–91.

11. deShazo RD, Williams DF, Moak ES. Fire ant attacks on residents in health care facilities: a report of two cases. Ann Intern Med 1999; 131: 424–9.

12. Ellis AK, Day JH. Allergy to insect bites and stings. Allergy 1996; 9(3): 18–22.

13. Tracy JM, Demain JG, Quinn J.M., et al. The natural history of exposure to the imported fire ant, J Allergy Clin Immunol 1995; 95: 824–828.

14. Caplan EL, Ford JL, Young PF, Ownby DR. Fire ants represent an important risk for anaphylaxis among residents of an endemic region. J Allergy Clin Immunol 2003; 111: 1274–7.

15. Solley GO. Stinging and biting insect allergy: an Australian experience. Ann Allergy Asthma Immunol 2004; 93: 532–37.

16. Yates AB, Moffitt JE, deShazo RD: Anaphylaxis to arthropod bites and stings. Immunol Allergy Clin North Am 2001; 21: 635–51.

17. Leveau P. Risk factors for allergy to hymenoptera stings Allerg Immunol (Paris) 1993; 25: 220, 224–6.

18. Fernandez J, Soriano V, Mayorga L, Mayor M. Natural history of Hymenoptera venom allergy in Eastern Spain. Clin Exp Allergy 2005; 35: 179–85.

19. Dubois AE. Mastocytosis and Hymenoptera allergy. Curr Opin Allergy Clin Immunol 2004; 4: 291–5.

20. Golden D. Insect allergy. In: Adkinson NF Jr, Yunginger JW, Busse WW, Bochner BS, Holgate ST, Simons FER, eds. Middleton's allergy: principles & practice. 4th ed. Vol. 2. Philadelphia, PA: Mosby, 2003: pp. 1475–86.

21. Golden DBK. Insect sting allergy and venom immunotherapy: a model and a mystery. J Allergy Clin Immunol 2005; 115: 439–47.

22. Mauriello PM, Barde SH, Georgitis JW, et al. Natural history of large local reactions from stinging insects. J Allergy Clin Immunol 1984; 74: 494–498.

23. Ellis AK, Day JH. Diagnosis and management of anaphylaxis. Can Med Assoc J 2003; 169(4): 307–12.

24. Stark BJ, Sullivan TJ. Biphasic and protracted anaphylaxis. J Allergy Clin Immunol 1986; 78: 76–83.

25. Ellis AK, Day JH. A prospective evaluation of 103 patients with biphasic anaphlyaxis. J Allergy Clin Immunol 2004; 113: S259 [Abs 935].

26. Ellis AK, Day JH. Incidence and characteristics of biphasic anaphylaxis: a prospective evaluation of 103 patients. Ann Allergy Asthma Immunol. 2007; 98: 64–9.

27. Gabriel DP, Rodrigues AG Jr, Barsante RC, dos Santos Silva V, Caramori JT, Martim LC, Barretti P, Balbi AL. Severe acute renal failure after massive attack of Africanized bees. Nephrol Dial Transplant. 2004; 19: 2680.

28. Daher Ede F, da Silva Junior GB, Bezerra GP, Pontes LB, Martins AM, Guimaraes JA. Acute renal failure after massive honeybee stings. Rev Inst Med Trop Sao Paulo. 2003; 45: 45–50.
29. Reisman R, Livingston A, Late onset allergic reactions including serum sickness after insect stings. J Allergy Clin Immunol 1989; 84: 331–7.
30. Moffitt JE. Allergic reactions to insect stings and bites. South Med J 2003; 96: 1073–9.
31. Chen DM, Lee PT, Chou KJ, Fang HC, Chung HM, Chen DM, Chang LK. Descending aortic thrombosis and cerebral infarction after massive wasp stings. Am J Med. 2004; 116: 567–9.
32. Boz C, Velioglu S, Ozmenoglu M. Acute disseminated encephalomyelitis after bee sting. Neurol Sci. 2003; 23: 313–5.
33. Likittanasombut P, Witoonpanich R, Viranuvatti K. Encephalomyeloradiculopathy associated with wasp sting. J Neurol Neurosurg Psychiatr 2003; 74: 134–135.
34. Gawlik R, Rymarczyk B, Rogala B. A rare case of intravascular coagulation after honey bee sting. J Investig Allergol Clin Immunol. 2004; 14: 250–2.
35. Sheth HG, Sullivan TJ. Optic neuropathy and orbital inflammatory mass after wasp stings. J R Soc Med 2004; 97: 436–7.
36. Carr ME. Hand-foot syndrome in a patient with multiple fire ant stings. South Med J. 2004; 97: 707–9.
37. Kalogeromitros D, Gregoriou S, Papaioannou D, Mousatou V, Makris M, Katsarou-Katsari A. Acquired primary cold contact urticaria after Hymenoptera sting. Clin Exp Dermatol. 2004; 29: 93–5.
38. Panagariya A, Sharma B, Garg A. Oculopalatal syndrome with ataxia following hymenoptera sting. J Assoc Physicians India 2003; 51: 1007–8.
39. Lin CC, Chang MY, Lin JL. Hornet sting induced systemic allergic reaction and large local reaction with bulle formation and rhabdomyolysis. J Toxicol Clin Toxicol 2003; 41: 1009–11.
40. Kim YO, Yoon SA, Kim KJ, Lee BO, Kim BS, Chang YS, Bang BK. Severe rhabdomyolysis and acute renal failure due to multiple wasp stings. Nephrol Dial Transplant. 2003; 18: 1235
41. Fisher BA, Antonios TF. Atrial flutter following a wasp sting. J Postgrad Med. 2003; 49: 254–5.
42. Mauriello PM, Barde SH, Georgitis JW, et al. Natural history of large local reactions from stinging insects. J Allergy Clin Immunol 1984; 74: 494–498.
43. Freeman TM. Hypersensitivity to Hymenoptera stings. New Engl J Med 2004; 351(19):1978–84.
44. Chamberlain D. Emergency medical treatment of anaphylactic reactions. Project Team of the Resuscitation Council (UK). J Accid Emerg Med 1999; 16(4): 243–7.
45. Simons FER, Gu X, Simons KJ. Epinephrine absorption in adults: intramuscular versus subcutaneous injection. J Allergy Clin Immunol 2001; 108(5): 871–3.
46. Anchor J, Settipane RA. Appropriate use of epinephrine in anaphylaxis. Am J Emerg Med 2004; 22: 488–90.
47. Shaver KJ, Adams C, Weiss SJ. Acute myocardial infarction after administration of low-dose intravenous epinephrine for anaphylaxis. CJEM. 2006; 8: 289–94.
48. Lieberman P. The use of antihistamines in the prevention and treatment of anaphylaxis and anaphylactoid reactions. J Allergy Clin Immunol 1990; 86(4 Pt 2): 684–6.
49. Stark BJ, Sullivan TJ. Biphasic and protracted anaphylaxis. J Allergy Clin Immunol 1986; 78 (1 Pt 1): 76–83.
50. Ellis AK, Day JH. Biphasic anaphylaxis with unusually late onset second phase: a case report. Can J Allergy Clin Immunol 1997; 2(3): 106–9.
51. Greenberger PA. Contrast media reactions. J Allergy Clin Immunol 1984; 74: 600–5.
52. Grouhi M, Alshehri M, Hummel D, Roifman CM. Anaphylaxis and epinephrine auto-injector training: who will teach the teachers? J Allergy Clin Immunol 1999; 104: 190–3.
53. Gold MS, Sainsbury R. First aid anaphylaxis management in children who were prescribed an epinephrine autoinjector device (Epipen). J Allergy Clin Immunol 2000; 106: 171–6.
54. DeShazo R, Butcher B, Banks W. Reactions to stings of the imported fire ant. N Engl J Med 1990; 323: 462–6.
55. Reisman R, Insect stings. N Engl J Med 1994; 331: 523–7.

56. Valentine M, Schuberth K, Kagey-Sobotka A. The value of immunotherapy with venom in children with allergy to insect stings. N Engl J Med 1990; 323: 1601–3.
57. Freeman TM, Hylander R, Ortiz A, Martin M, Imported fire ant immunotherapy: effectiveness of whole body extracts. J Allergy Clin Immunol 1992; 90: 210–5.
58. Tankersley MS, Walker RL, Butler WK, Hagan LL, et al. Safety and efficacy of an imported fire ant rush immunotherapy protocol with and without prophylactic treatment. J Allergy Clin Immunol 2002; 109: 556–62.
59. Freeman TM, Hylander R, Ortiz A, Martin M, Imported fire ant immunotherapy: effectiveness of whole body extracts. J Allergy Clin Immunol 1992; 90: 210–5.
60. Stafford C. Hypersensitivity to fire ant venom. Ann Allergy 1996; 77: 87–99.
61. Creticos PS, Franklin Adkinson N Jr, Kagey-Sabotka A, et al. Nasal challenge with ragweed in hay fever patients: effect of immunotherapy. J Clin Invest 1985; 76: 2247–53.
62. Jutel M, Müller UR, Fricker M, et al. Influence of bee venom immunotherapy on degranulation and leukotriene generation in human blood basophils. Clin Exp Allergy 1996; 26: 1112–8.
63. Bellinghausen I, Metz G, Enk AH, et al. Insect venom immunotherapy induces interleukin-10 production and a Th2-to-Th1 shift, and changes surface marker expression in venom-allergic subjects. Eur J Immunol 1997; 27: 1131–9.
64. Jutel M, Pichler WJ, Skrbic D, et al. Bee venom immunotherapy results in decrease of IL-4 and IL-5 and increase of IFN-γ secretion in specific allergen stimulated T cell cultures. J Immunol 1995; 154: 4178–94.
65. Akdis CA, Akdis M, Blesken T, et al. Epitope specific T cell tolerance to phospholipase A2 in bee venom immunotherapy and recovery by IL-2 and IL-15 in vitro. J Clin Invest 1996; 98: 1676–83.
66. Akdis CA, Blaser K. IL-10 induced anergy in peripheral T cell and reactivation by microenvironmental cytokines: two key steps in specific immunotherapy. FASEB J 1999; 13: 603–9.
67. Akdis CA, Blesken T, Wymann D, et al. Differential regulation of human T cell cytokine patterns and IgE and IgG4 responses by conformational antigen variants. Eur J Immunol 1998; 28: 914–25.
68. Müller UR, Akdis CA, Fricker M, et al. Successful immunotherapy with T cell epitope peptides of bee venom phospholipase A2 induces specific T cell anergy in bee sting allergic patients. J Allergy Clin Immunol 1998; 101: 747–54.
69. Carballido JM, Carballido-Perrig N, Kägi MK, et al. T cell epitope specificity in human allergic and non-allergic subjects to bee venom phospholipase A2. J Immunol 1993; 150: 3582–91.
70. Akdis CA, Blesken T, Akdis M, et al. Role of IL-10 in specific immunotherapy. J Clin Invest 1998; 102: 98–106.
71. Jonuleit H, Schmitt E, Stassen M, et al. Identification and functional characterization of human CD4+CD25+ T cells with regulatory properties isolated from peripheral blood. J Exp Med 2001; 193: 1285–90.
72. Suri-Payer E, Amar AZ, Thornton AM, Shevach EM. CD4+CD25+ T cells inhibit both the induction and effector function of autoreactive T cells and represent a unique lineage of immunoregulatory cells. J Immunol 1998; 160: 1212–18.
73. Thornton AM, Shevach EM. CD4+CD25+ immunoregulatory T cells suppress polyclonal T cell activation in vitro by inhibiting interleukin 2 production. J Exp Med 1998; 188: 287–96.
74. Read S, Mauze S, Asseman CF et al. CD38+CD45RB-low T cells: a population of T cells with immune regulatory activities in vitro. Eur J Immunol 1998; 28: 3435–47.
75. Read S, Powrie F. CD4(+) regulatory T cells. Curr Opin Immunol 2001; 13: 644.
76. Jutel M, Akdis M, Budak F, et al. IL-10 and TGF-β cooperate in the regulatory T cell response to mucosal allergens in normal immunity and specific immunotherapy. Eur J Immunol 2003; 33: 233–41.
77. Kammerer R, Chvatchko Y, Kettner A, Dufour N, Corradin G, Spertini F. Modulation of T-cell responses to phospholipase A2 and phospholipase A2-derived peptides by conventional Bee venom immunotherapy. J Allergy Clin Immunol 1997; 100: 96–103.

78. Bernstein DI, Mittman RJ, Kagen SL, et al. Clinical and immunologic studies of rapid immunotherapy in Hymenoptera sensitive patients. J Allergy Clin Immunol 1989; 84: 951–9.
79. Eberlein-Konig B, Ullmann S, Thomas P, Przybilla B. Tryptase and histamine release due to a sting challenge in bee venom allergic patients treated successfully or unsuccessfully with hyposensitisation. Clin Exp Allergy 1995; 25: 704–12.
80. Stephan V, Kuhr J, Urbanek R. Relevance of basophil histamine release changes during venom immunotherapy. Allergy 1989; 44: 453–9.
81. Bonifazi F, Jutel M, Biló BM, et al. Prevention and treatment of hymenoptera venom allergy: guidelines for clinical practice. Allergy 2005; 60(12): 1459–70.
82. Ellis AK, Day JH. Clinical reactivity to insect stings. Curr Opin Allergy Clin Immunol 2005; 5: 349–54.
83. Mauriello PM, Barde SH, Georgitis JW, Reisman RE. Natural history of large local reactions from stinging insects. J Allergy Clin Immunol 1984; 74: 494–8.
84. Hepner M, Ownby D, Anderson J. Risk of severe reactions in patients taking beta blocker drugs receiving allergen immunotherapy injections. J Allergy Clin Immunol, 1990; 86: 407–411.
85. Toogood JH. Risk of anaphylaxis in patients receiving beta-blocker drugs. J Allergy Clin Immunol 1988; 81: 1–5.
86. Alam MM, Alvarez del Real G, Hsieh FH. Cardiopulmonary resuscitation (CPR) in patients with acute anaphylaxis taking beta-blockers. J Allergy Clin Immunol 2005; 115 (Suppl 2): Abs 160.
87. Simon P, Potier J, Thebaud HE. Risk factors for acute hypersensitivity reactions in hemodialysis. Nephrologie 1996; 17: 163–70.
88. Hermann K, Ring J. The rennin-angiotensin in patients with repeated anaphylactic reactions during Hymenoptera venom hyposensitization and sting challenge. Int Arch Allergy Immunol 1997; 112: 251–6.
89. White KM, England RW. Safety of angiotensin-converting enzyme inhibitors while receiving venom immunotherapy. Ann Allergy Asthma Immunol. 2008; 101(4): 426–30.
90. Schwartz HJ, Golden DBK, Lockey RF. Venom immunotherapy in the Hymenoptera-allergic pregnant patient. J Allergy Clin Immunol 1990; 85: 709–12.
91. Müller U, Mosbech H. Position paper. Immunotherapy with Hymenoptera venoms. EAACI. Allergy 1993; 48: 36–46.
92. Bucher C, Korner P, Wüthrich B. Allergy to bumblebee venom. Curr Opin Allergy Immunol 2001; 1: 361–5.
93. Stern A, Mullner RG, Wüthrich B. Successful treatment of occupational allergy to bumblebee venom after failure with honeybee venom extract. Allergy 2000; 55: 88–91
94. Biló BM, Rueff F, Mosbech H, Bonifazi F, Oude-Elberink JNG, EAACI Interest Group on Insect Venom Hypersensitivity. Diagnosis of Hymenoptera venom allergy. Allergy 2005; 60: 1339–49.
95. Reisman RE, Müller UR, Wypych JI, Lazell MI. Studies of coexisting honeybee and vespid-venom sensitivity. J Allergy Clin Immunol 1984; 73: 246–52.
96. Straumann F, Bucher C, Wüthrich B. Double sensitization to honeybee and wasp venom: immunotherapy with one venom or with both venoms? Int Arch Immunol 2000; 123: 268–74.
97. Lichtenstein LM, Valentine MD, Sobotka AK. A case for venom treatment in anaphylactic sensitivity to Hymenoptera sting. N Engl J Med 1974; 290: 1223–7.
98. Golden DBK, Valentine MD, Kagey-Sobotka A, Lichtenstein LM. Regimens of Hymenoptera venom immunotherapy. Ann Intern Med 1980; 92: 620–4.
99. Yunginger JW, Paull BR, Jones RT, Santrach PJ. Rush venom immunotherapy program for honeybee sting sensitivity. J Allergy Clin Immunol 1979; 63: 340–7.
100. Laurent J, Smiejan JM, Bloch-Morot E, Herman D. Safety of Hymenoptera venom rush immunotherapy. Allergy 1997; 52: 94–6.
101. Bernstein AJ, Kagen SI, Bernstein DI. Rapid venom immunotherapy is safe routine in the treatment of patients with Hymenoptera anaphylaxis. Ann Allergy 1994; 73: 423–42.

102. Birnbaum J, Charpin D, Vervloet D. Rapid Hymenoptera venom immunotherapy: comparative safety of three protocols. Clin Exp Allergy 1993; 23: 226–30.

103. Golden DBK. Practical considerations in venom immunotherapy. Allergy Asthma Proc 1997; 18: 79–80.

104. Golden D, Kagey-Sobotka A, Valentine M, Lichtenstein L. Dose dependence of Hymenoptera venom immunotherapy. J Allergy Clin Immunol 1981; 67: 370–4.

105. Rueff F, Wenderoth A, Przybilla B. Patients still reacting to a sting challenge while receiving conventional Hymenoptera venom immunotherapy are protected by increased venom doses. J Allergy Clin Immunol 2001; 108: 1027–32.

106. Bousquet J, Menardo JL, Michel FB. Systemic reactions during maintenance immunotherapy in honeybee venom. Ann Allergy 1988; 61: 63–8.

107. Golden DBK, Kagey-Sobotka A, Valentine MD, Lichtenstein LM. Prolonged-maintenance interval in Hymenoptera venom immunotherapy. J Allergy Clin Immunol 1981; 67: 482–4.

108. Gadde J, Sobotka A, Valentine M, Lichtenstein L, Golden D. Intervals of six and eight weeks in maintenance venom immunotherapy. Ann Allergy 1985; 54: 348.

109. Confino-Cohen R, Goldberg A, Mekori YA. Deliberate bee sting challenge of patients receiving maintenance venom immunotherapy at a 3-months interval. J Allergy Clin Immunol 1993; 91: 189–94.

110. Kochuyt AM, Stevens EAM. Safety and efficacy of a 12-week maintenance interval in patients treated with Hymenoptera venom immunotherapy. Clin Exp Allergy 1994; 24: 35–41

111. Hunt KJ, Valentine MD, Sobotka AK, Benton AW, Amodio FJ, Lichtenstein LM. A controlled trial of immunotherapy in insect hypersensitivity. N Engl J Med 1978; 299: 157–61.

112. Müller U, Thurnheer U, Patrizzi R, Spiess J, Hoigne R. Immunotherapy in bee sting hypersensitivity. Bee venom versus wholebody extract. Allergy 1979; 34: 369–78.

113. Brown S, Wiese M, Blackman K, Heddle R. Ant venom immunotherapy: a double blind, placebo-controlled cross-over trial. Lancet 2003; 361: 1001–6.

114. Müller U, Helbling A, Berchtold E. Immunotherapy with honeybee venom and yellow jacket venom is different regarding efficacy and safety. J Allergy Clin Immunol 1992; 89: 529–35.

115. Mosbech H, Malling H, Biering I, Böwadt H, Sooborg M, Weeke B, Löwenstein H. Immunotherapy with yellow jacket venom. Allergy 1984; 39: 543–9.

116. Lockey RF, Turkeltaub PC, Olive ES, Hussard JM, Baird-Warren IA, Buckantz SC. The Hymenoptera venom study. III. Safety of venom immunotherapy. J Allergy Clin Immunol 1990; 86: 775–80.

117. Mosbech H, Müller U. Side-effects of insect venom immunotherapy: results from an EAACI multicenter study. Allergy 2000; 55: 1005–10.

118. Berchtold E, Maibach R, Müller U. Reduction of side effects from rush-immunotherapy with honey bee venom by pre-treatment with terfenadine. Clin Exp Allergy 1992; 22: 59–65.

119. Gillman SA, Cummins LH, Kozak PP, Hoffman DR. Venom immunotherapy: comparison of "rush" vs "conventional" schedules. Ann Allergy 1980; 45: 351–4.

120. Brehler R, Wolf H, Kutting B, Schnitker J, Luger T. Safety of a two-day ultrarush insect venom immunotherapy protocol in comparison with protocols of longer duration and involving a larger number of injections. J Allergy Clin Immunol 2000; 105: 1231–5.

121. Brockow K, Kiehn M, Riethu" C, Vieluf D, Berger J, Ring J. Efficacy of antihistamine pretreatment in the prevention of adverse reactions to Hymenoptera immunotherapy: a prospective, randomized placebo-controlled trial. J Allergy Clin Immunol 1997; 100: 458–63.

122. Müller U, Hari Y, Berchtold E. Premedication with antihistamines may enhance efficacy of specific-allergen immunotherapy. J Allergy Clin Immunol 2001; 107: 81–86.

123. Reimers RE, Hari Y, Müller U. Reduction of side-effects from ultrarush immunotherapy with honeybee venom by pretreatment with fexofenadine: a double-blind, placebo-controlled trial. Allergy 2000; 55: 484–8.

124. Przybilla B, Ring J, Galosi A, Geursen RG, Stickl HA. Bee venom immunoglobulin for prophylaxis of anaphylactic reactions during bee venom immunotherapy (rush hyposensitization). Immunol Allergy Pract 1986; 8: 107–11.

125. Jarisch R. Passive immunotherapy in bee venom allergic patients. Arch Dermatol Res 1981; 270: 230–5.
126. Quercia O, Rafanelli S, Puccinelli P, Stefanini GF. The safety of cluster immunotherapy with aluminium hydroxide-absorbed honeybee venom extract. J Investig Allergol Clin Immunol 2001; 11: 27–33.
127. Wyss M, Scheitlin T, Stadler BM, Wüthrich B. Immunotherapy with aluminium hydroxide absorbed insect venom extracts (Alutard SQ): immunologic and clinical results of a prospective study over 3 years. Allergy 1993; 48: 81–86.
128. Müller U, Rabson A, Bischof M, Lomnitzer R, Dreborg S, Lanner A. A double-blind study comparing monomethoxy polyethylene glycol modified honeybee venom and unmodified honeybee venom for immunotherapy. I. Clinical results. J Allergy Clin Immunol 1987; 80: 252–61.
129. Müller UR. Recombinant Hymenoptera venom allergens. Allergy 2002; 57: 570–6.
130. Birnbaum J, Ramadour M, Magnan A, Vervloet D. Hymenoptera ultra-rush venom immunotherapy (210 min): a safety study and risk factors. Clin Exp Allergy 2003; 33: 58–64.
131. Fricker M, Helbling A, Schwartz L, Müller U. Hymenoptera sting anaphylaxis and urticaria pigmentosa: clinical findings and results of venom immunotherapy in ten patients. J Allergy Clin Immunol 1997; 100: 11–15.
132. Haeberli G, Bronnimann M, Hunziker T, Müller U. Elevated basal serum tryptase and Hymenoptera venom allergy: relation to severity of sting reactions and to safety and efficacy of venom immunotherapy. Clin Exp Allergy 2003; 33: 1216–20.
133. Oude Elberink JNG, De Monchy JGR, Kors JW, Van Doormaal JJ, Dubois AEJ. Fatal anaphylaxis after a yellow jacket sting, despite venom immunotherapy, in two patients with mastocytosis. J Allergy Clin Immunol 1997; 99: 153–4.
134. Rueff F, Wenderoth A, Przybilla B. Patients still reacting to a sting challenge while receiving conventional Hymenoptera venom immunotherapy are protected by increased venom doses. J Allergy Clin Immunol 2001; 108: 1027–32.
135. Oude Elberink JN, Dubois AE. Quality of life in insect venom allergic patients. Curr Opin Allergy Clin Immunol 2003; 3: 287–93.

Fungal Allergy as Yet Unsolved

Robert K. Bush

Introduction

In the 1870s, Blackley [1] described allergic symptoms as a consequence of exposure to fungi. Often referred to as "molds," fungi belong to Kingdom Mycota, a biological kingdom separate from plants and are widely distributed around the world [2]. The classification of fungal species is in flux as new genetic techniques supplement the traditional identification of fungi based on their culture characteristics and microscopic spore morphology [3–5]. Some of the more common fungi that lead to allergic disease are listed in Table 1. This chapter will discuss the relevance of fungal exposure to various health effects, particularly with regard to immunologically-mediated conditions affecting the respiratory system.

Most fungal exposure occurs outdoors [2]. A number of fungal taxa have been found in atmospheric samples, some of which can only be identified by culture techniques due to the similarity in appearance of fungal spores, such as ascospores and basidiospores [2]. Surveys conducted in the U.S. show that ascospores, basidiospores and Cladosporium species comprise the majority of spores observed in outdoor samples [2]. Typically during wet weather, ascospores and basidiospores predominate, while during dry weather, Deuteromycetes (e.g., Alternaria, Cladosporium) are prominent [6]. Local concentrations of allergenically important taxa such as Alternaria, are common in various areas of the world [7]. The most well-known group of allergenic fungi are the Deuderomycetes (an artificial grouping) or Fungi Imperfecti (hypomycetes), which represent the asexual forms of ascomycetes [2]. New genetic techniques indicate that many fungi species exist in two stages – those that reproduce sexually (e.g., Ascomycetes) and those that reproduce asexually (e.g., Deuteromyces) [3–5]. Since these are stages of a single organism, allergen exposure attributed to one fungal species may occur from other forms of the same fungus. Depending on the sampling methodology, spore counts

R.K. Bush (✉)
Professor, Department of Medicine, Section of Allergy/Immunology, Pulmonary and Clinical Care Medicine, University of Wisconsin, Madison, WI, USA;
Chief of Allergy, Wm. S. Middleton VA Hospital, Madison, WI, USA;
K4/910 CSC, Box 9988, 600 Highland Avenue, Madison, WI 53792, USA

R. Pawankar et al. (eds.), *Allergy Frontiers: Clinical Manifestations*,
DOI: 10.1007/978-4-431-88317-3_29, © Springer 2009

Table 1 Frequently encountered allergenic fungi

Deuteromycetes (hypomycetes) or Fungi imperfecti
Alternaria esp. *Alternaria alternata*
Aspergillus species esp. *Fumigatus*
Cladosporium species esp. *herbarium* and *C. cladiosporoides*
Penicillium species *P. chrysogenum* (*notation*), and *P. citrinum*
Drechslera species
Epicoccum nigrum
Fusarium species
Curvularia lunata
Ulocladium species
Ascomycetes
Chaetomium species
Zygomycetes
Mucor species
Rhizopus nigricans
Basidiomycetes
Carpinus species
Ganoderma species
Psilocybe cubensis
Pleurotus ostreatus
Yeasts
Candida albicans

can vary tremendously in the sample. The use of impaction samplers such as RotoRod™ (Surveillance Data, Inc., Plymouth Meeting, PA) may miss capturing smaller spores and, therefore, falsely lower the actual concentration of certain spores in the atmosphere. Suction devices such as Burkard samples (Burkard Mfg, Rickmansworth, Herdfordshire, England, Hertfordshire, United Kingdom) and Allergenco (Allergenco MK-3 [formerly Samplair], Allergenco, San Antonio, TX) capture the smaller spores and give a better understanding of the range of concentrations of microscopically identifiable fungal spores [8]. Figure 1 shows the distribution of these in the United States. The terms "low, moderate, high and very high" spore counts simply represent historical data based on the observed concentrations of spores in the atmosphere [6], and, therefore, these concentrations do not necessarily predict the clinical response of a sensitized patient.

Certain genera of fungi, such as *Aspergillus* and *Penicillium*, often account for indoor exposures, although these may also be encountered in outdoor environments as well [9]. Sampling techniques in the indoor environment involve more than just airborne spore counts, but include culturing of materials with evident fungal growth [10]. Cellophane tape lifts of growing fungi may reveal spores that can be identified directly by microscopy [10]. Newer advances include measurement of fungal allergen concentrations from airborne or settled house dust samples [8, 11, 12]. One can also measure ergosterol, which is found in cell walls of fungi, but it is also found in other microbes [8]. Glucans found in fungal cell walls can be assayed, and they have been investigated in terms of their potential to create inflammatory airway changes [13, 14]) (as well as therapeutically altering Th2 responses)

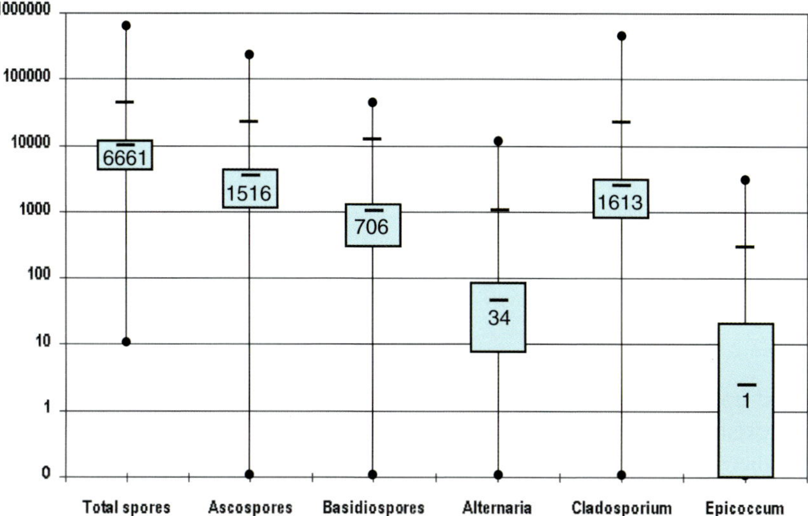

Fig. 1 Box plots of total spores, acrospores, basicdiospores, and three genera form National Allergy Bureau station as measured by Burkard samplers in the United Stated based on the 2000 Pollen and Spore Report (Used with permission from the National Allergy Bureau and all of its station American Academy of Allergy, Asthma and Immunology, November 2005)

[15, 16]. Mycotoxins can also be assayed which have particular relevance in the current climate of concern regarding their effect on health in individuals exposed to indoor fungi [17, 18].

Fungal Allergens

The advent of molecular biology approaches to identify and purify allergens has led to tremendous improvements in our understanding of biological role and relationship of allergens from a variety of sources. This has proven especially valuable in understanding fungal allergy [19–21]. Clearly, highly conserved functional protein in fungi can act as allergens and are distributed over a variety of fungal species (e.g., enolase, dehydrogenases, P_2 ribosomal proteins).

Table 2 lists some of the more important allergens that have been identified either by protein purification techniques or the newer molecular biological techniques. An extensive listing of reported fungal allergens can be obtained via the Allergome website (www.allergome.org). This valuable source of information lists purified fungal allergens, their biological characteristics, and studies on their use as diagnostic or therapeutic agents. The Allergenome database is updated monthly and, therefore, gives current information on virtually all purified and characterized fungal allergens. The molecular biology of fungal allergens has

Table 2 Some characterized fungal allergens

Species	IUIS description	Function
Alternaria alternata	Alt a 1	Unknown
	Alt a 11	Enolase
Aspergillus fumigatus	Asp f 1	Mitogillium (Ribotoxin)
	Asp f 13	Alkaline Serine protease
Penicillium chrysogenum	Pen ch 13	Alkaline Serine protease
Cladosporium herbarium	Cla h 1	Unknown
	Cla h 6	Enolase

opened up new horizons for research and classification of fungal species. Since fungi exist in more than one recognized form, genetic studies on fungi show that often there are similar proteins in other fungal and nonfungal sources [3, 4]. The full genomic sequencing of *Aspergillus fumigatus* has led to a better understanding of *Aspergillus* allergen gene sequences in the revision of gene databanks and fungal allergen nomenclature [4].

The identification, purification and characterization of allergens also allow for the production of monoclonal antibodies to these allergens, which are subsequently utilized to ascertain the concentration of allergens in diagnostic and therapeutic vaccines [22, 23]. Further, the development of immunoassays to quantitate allergen exposure either in air or dust samples from indoors have greatly expanded our knowledge about a variety of allergens, e.g., house dust mites, cat, cockroach, and mouse [24–27]. These techniques are utilized in assessing the concentration of fungal allergens from environmental samples as well [12]. However, work in this area has lagged behind that of other allergen sources. Studies from the U.S. utilizing rabbit antisera, instead of monoclonal antibodies, in immunoassays detected the presence of *Alternaria* allergens in the indoor environment in settled dust samples [11]. The detection of indoor *Alternaria* antigens in the samples correlated with the presence of asthma symptoms in individuals residing in such homes [28]. Of note is the fact that fungal allergens may not be detectable in nonviable spores. However, upon germination, major allergens such as Asp f 1 are readily secreted into the environment and detectable by these immunoassays [29]. Similar results have been demonstrated with *Alternaria* [30].

Health Effects of Fungal Exposure

The health effects related to fungal exposure include IgE-mediated sensitivity, which can elicit the symptoms of allergic rhinitis and allergic asthma [17]. Allergic fungal sinusitis (AFS) and allergic bronchopulmonary aspergillosis (ABPA) represent diseases in which fungi colonize (particularly Aspergillus) either in the sinuses or the bronchi where they produce allergens that induce both T and B cell responses [5]. Hypersensitivity pneumonitis may result from fungal exposure that induces

T-cell and B-cell pathogenic mechanisms that do not involve IgE [17]. Fungal infections primarily occur in immune-compromised individuals, but some organisms can infect normal, healthy individuals as well (e.g., blastomycosis).

Toxic effects of fungi may occur with high-level exposure to mycotoxin. (e.g., mycotoxicosis in silage workers). While a variety of health effects have been attributed to indoor fungal exposure (toxins), many are poorly characterized and represent a highly controversial area [31]. Idiopathic pulmonary hemorrhage/hemosiderosis occurring in infants has been attributed to exposure to *Stachybotrys*, although this also remains a controversial area [32, 33].

Fungi produce volatile organic compounds that are easily detected by their distinct odor. These compounds include alcohols and aldehydes that may produce irritant effects in the eyes and respiratory tract [34, 35]. Since fungi typically inhabit very moist environments, the musty smell of fungi also indicates that unseen, ubiquitous house dust mites may also be present.

The role of fungi sensitivity in allergic rhinitis is not as well investigated as it has been in asthma [7]. Clearly, in many patients who exhibit positive fungal allergen skin tests and experience rhinitis symptoms that persist past time of the first frost (in climates with distinct seasons), which may be in part due to exposure to fungal spores that prevail in the air until there is snow cover on the ground. Perennial symptoms may occur from indoor fungal exposure.

Allergic fungal sinusitis (AFS) represents a distinct entity (the diagnostic criteria are found in Table 3) [5]. Individuals with AFS develop sinus colonization with fungi frequently after being exposed to repeated courses of antibiotics. They are immunocompetent and often manifest nasal polyposis. The characteristic pathologic finding is "allergic" or eosinophilic mucin, which, with appropriate staining (Giemsa-Gomori silver staining) may reveal the presence of fungal hyphae. On computerized tomography, very radiodense areas (due to ferrous compound leposition) with the sinus cavity and bony erosions (due to the expansion of inspissated secretions) may be seen. Affected individuals may exhibit immediate positive skin tests to the responsible fungus (e.g., Aspergillus, Bipolaris). Treatment of AFS involves surgical drainage and courses of oral corticosteroids. It is not clear if oral antifungal therapy plays a significant role in the management of these patients [36, 37]. While subcutaneous immunotherapy has been touted to be beneficial [38], this modality has not been subjected to double-blind, placebo-controlled trials.

A syndrome termed "chronic rhinosinusitis" has been used to describe patients with typical chronic sinusitis (often associated with nasal polyposis) and have culturable fungi (e.g, *Alternaria*) in surgical specimens [39]. It has been postulated that the fungus induces mucosal inflammation by activating eosinophils

Table 3 Diagnostic criteria for Allergic fungal sinusitis

- Normal immune status (e.g., no HIV, B- or T-cell deficiency)
- Presence of nasal polyposis
- Characteristic computerized tomographic findings (e.g., bony erosions, radiodense areas in sinus)
- Eosinophilic mucin with fungal hyphae
- Demonstrable IgE sensitivity to implicated fungus (e.g., positive skin-prick test or *in vitro* test)

(via PAR-2 receptors) [39, 40] and that treatment with sinus-nasal irrigations continuing antifungal agents may be beneficial [41]. However, scrutiny of the controlled trials of the antifungal irrigations demonstrates limited benefit, and it is questionable whether such approaches can be generalized to all patients who have chronic sinusitis [42].

The Role of Fungi in Asthma

Recently, epidemiologic studies suggest that fungal sensitivity plays an important role in the development, persistence and severity of allergic asthma [7]. Many individuals throughout the world are sensitive to various fungi, particularly Deuderomyces species [5]. Testing for basidiomycete sensitivity has proved problematic since commercially-available extracts are not available, but research studies that employed basidiomycete skin test extracts demonstrated a significant rate of sensitization among individuals with allergic respiratory diseases [43]. Depending on the locale, approximately 25% of individuals appearing for evaluation of rhinitis or asthma have a positive skin test to one or more fungal species [43].

Sensitivity to *Alternaria alternate*, especially, appears to be associated with asthma [7]. Several studies indicate that it is a major sensitizer in children with asthma [7, 44–46]. Children who are sensitized early in life continue to have persistent asthma [44]. More importantly, several studies have shown near-fatal attacks of asthma being associated with sensitivity and exposure to this fungus [44, 47]. Urgent visits for acute asthma episodes have been correlated with *Alternaria* sensitivity and exposure to its spores in the atmosphere [48], and a recent publication demonstrated that fragmented *Alternaria* spores in the air and the presence of *Alternaria* sensitivity were highly correlated with acute emergency room visits for asthma during period of thunderstorms [49, 50]. Furthermore, other studies have linked the number of fungal spores in the atmosphere to asthma deaths [51]. Clearly, fungal sensitivity is a significant factor in asthma in many areas of the world.

The mechanisms by which fungi induce asthma are often IgE related. However, other mechanisms may also be important. There is evidence that proteases in fungal extracts are capable of causing direct effects on airway epithelium which generate production of inflammatory cytokines, such as IL-8 [52, 53]. Furthermore, proteases contained in many allergens (not limited to fungi) can activate eosinophils via the PAR-2 receptor [40]. Proteases have also been shown to act as Th-2-type adjuvants leading to enhanced eosinophilic inflammation and prolonged IgE responses in animal models [54]. This is a fertile area for further investigation.

Allergic Bronchopulmonary Aspergillosis

Allergic bronchopulmonary aspergillosis affects individuals with underlying cystic fibrosis or chronic asthma [55–57]. The exact etiology is not entirely clear; however, spores of *Aspergillus fumigatus* are felt to be trapped within the mucus secretions of the airways in these individuals where they germinate resulting in the secretion of *Aspergillus* allergens. There is a marked Th2-type response with elevations not only in serum-specific IgE to *Aspergillus fumigatus*, but in the total serum IgE level as well. Production of serum-specific IgG antibodies to *Aspergillus* also occurs. Serum *Aspergillus fumigatus* antibody titers can be measured by enzyme-linked immunoassays. Some individuals may have precipitating (IgG) antibodies to *Aspergillus* that is detected by radial immunodiffusion assays (Ouchterlony technique). Other fungi (e.g., Dreschlera) may produce a similar picture on occasion [55].

ABPA patients experience chronic wheezing but may also develop symptoms that include chest discomfort, cough with production of brown mucus plugs (containing fungal hyphae) and low-grade fever accompanied by peripheral blood eosinophilia. It is the presence of pulmonary infiltrates along with peripheral blood eosinophils that distinguishes this condition from the underlying asthma or CF. The differential diagnosis includes other syndromes known collectively as PIE (pulmonary infiltrates with eosinophilia) syndromes [55].

The diagnosis of ABPA is established in those individuals who have experienced pulmonary eosinophilia with infiltrates by the demonstration of sensitivity to *Aspergillus fumigatus* via a positive skin test and/or elevated serum-specific *Aspergillus fumigatus* IgE antibody titers (two times greater than that of an Aspergillus allergic and non-ABPA asthmatic) (Table 4). A subset of ABPA patients manifest proximal central saccular bronchiectasis (ABPA-CB) on chest computerized tomography (chest CT scanning), which is often considered a hallmark of the illness. However, some individuals with severe persistent asthma may also exhibit the serological manifestations of ABPA, yet do not have bronchiectasis (ABPA-S) [55]. A disease-staging system has been developed, e.g., stage 1, defined as the initial development of pulmonary infiltrates with eosinophilia to stage 5, defined by pulmonary fibrosis, a sequellae of repeat bouts of pulmonary infiltrates [57].

Table 4 Criteria for diagnosis of ABPA

Major
- Underlying asthma or cystic fibrosis
- Pulmonary infiltrates with peripheral blood eosinophilia
- Immediate hypersensitivity to *Aspergillus fumigatus* (elevated specific IgE to *A. fumigatus*, positive *A. fumigatus* skin test)

Minor
- Elevated total serum IgE
- Specific IgG to *Aspergillus fumigatus* (or presence of precipitating antibodies to *Aspergillus fumigatus*)

Subcategories of ABPA
- ABPA-CB
  - Presence of central (proximal) saccular bronchiectasis
- ABPA-S
  - Positive serologic assays without central bronchiectasis

Adapted from the Criteria of Greenberger PA. Allergic Bronchopulmonary Aspergillosis. In Adkinson NF Jr., Yunginger JW, Busse WW, Bochner BS, Simons FER, Holgate ST (eds.) Middleton's Allergy, Principles and Practices, 6th edition, Mosby, Philadelphia; 2003, p. 1355

Treatment of ABPA involves prolonged courses of oral corticosteroids and management of persistent asthma with appropriate therapy [56, 57]. Antifungals may be of some value in selected cases [58]. Allergen immunotherapy with *Aspergillus fumigatus* vaccines is generally avoided because of concerns regarding the potential development of immune complex disease [56]. However, this has not been systematically studied [55]. Omalizumab may be a treatment adjunct in the near future but has not been extensively studied.

Over the past several years, there has been growing concern about the health effects of indoor fungal exposure in public buildings and homes (references to go here). Indoor fungal growth is often the consequence of high-humidity levels due to leakage of moisture into the environment. Indoor fungal growth may potentially cause respiratory symptoms in individuals residing in these environments. Numerous epidemiological studies link home dampness to indoor fungal growth and, as a consequence, respiratory symptoms including cough and wheeze especially in children [59, 60]. Both pro and con studies have been reported [61–64].

Clearly, individuals with IgE-mediated sensitivity to the so-called "indoor fungi," *Aspergillus* and *Penicillium* species, among others, may experience rhinitis or asthma when these fungi are present in the environment [17, 65]. However, it should be noted that unless indoor airborne fungal spore levels exceed outdoor levels, exposure is typically far greater in the outdoor environment [2, 10]. Airborne samples containing levels of spores (esp. Aspergillus, Penicillium, or even Cladosporium) that exceed the simultaneously sampled outdoor level suggests an indoor "point" source.

Beyond their role as allergens, fungi produce volatile organic compounds (VOC) that are responsible for the "musty" smell associated with mold growth and can induce ocular and respiratory irritation as previously mentioned. The $(1\rightarrow3)$-beta-D-glucans, a component of fungal cell walls have been researched for a number of years. The effect of the $(1\rightarrow3)$-beta-D-glucans on respiratory health is somewhat controversial [14]. Some reports suggest they may elicit airway inflammation (through non-IgE-dependent mechanism, while other reports suggest that they may abrogate Th2 responses [15, 16].

Controversial Areas

The role of fungi in "illnesses" which does not involve infection or allergic reactions is controversial [17, 31]. The "Yeast Connection" or "Candidiasis Syndrome" is one example [66]. A variety of symptoms such as listless, headache, gastrointestinal and other nonspecific symptoms have been ascribed to "sensitivity" to *Candida albicans*, a ubiquitous, commensurate organism. Individuals diagnosed with this "condition" report exposures to antibiotics, mucosal yeast infections, and demonstrate delayed hypersensitivity to *Candida albicans*. Since delayed hypersensitivity to *Candida albicans* is a normal immune response, it is doubtful that the symptoms of the "Candidiasis Syndrome" can be attributed to an immune response to the organism.

Table 5 Some mycotoxins produced by fungi

Aflatoxin	*Aspergillus flavus, Aspergillus parastiticus*
Altenuic acid	*Alternaria alternata*
Alternariol	*Alternaria alternate*
Chaetoglobosin	*Chaetomium globosum*
Citrinin	*Aspergillus* spp., *Penicillium* spp.
Citreoviridin	*Aspergillus terreus, Penicillium citreoviride*
Cochliodinol	*Chaetomium cochliodes*
Cytochalasin E	*Aspergillus clavatus*
Deoxynivalenol (vomitoxin)	*Fusarium* spp.
Gliotoxin	*Alternaria, Penicillium, Aspergillus* spp.
Moniliformin	*Fusarium* spp.
Ochratoxin	*Aspergillus ochraceus, Penicillium viridictum*
Oxalic acid	*Aspergillus niger*
Patulin	*Aspergillus clavatus, Penicillium* spp.
Roridin E	*Myrothecium* spp., *Stachybotrys* spp.
Rubratoxin	*Pennicillium rubra*
Satratoxins F, G, H	*Stachybotrys chartarum*
Slaframine	*Rhizoctonia leguminicola*
Sterigmatocystin	*Aspergillus* spp., *Penicillium rugulosum*
T-1, T-2 toxins	*Fusarium* spp.
Tremorgens	*Aspergillus, Mucor, Rhizopus, Penicillium*
Tricothecenes	*Fusarium, Aspergillus, Stachybotrys* spp.
Trichoverrins, trichoverrols	*Stachybotrys chartarum*
Zearalenon	*Fusarium* spp.

Individuals with this diagnosis are often treated with nonabsorbed oral antifungal agents (nystatin), but no controlled trials have ever been conducted [66].

A list of potential mycotoxins produced by fungi is listed in Table 5. It is known that high-level exposure to mycotoxins can occur and may lead to the recognized "mycotoxicosis syndrome," chills, fever and pulmonary infiltrates, and the typical immunologic findings of hypersensitivity pneumonitis (HP) are not usually present in HP [67]. It should be noted that precipitating (IgG) antibodies to fungi in individuals is not specific for the diagnosis of HP, but reflects exposure to the fungus.

Another controversial "condition" is the "toxic mold syndrome" [68]. Individuals report living in environments where there is significant fungal growth that leads to headache, impaired cognition and "immune dysregulation" [17]. Many of these reports are anecdotal and do not employ case-controlled methodologies. The detection of the fungus, Stachybotrys ("black or toxic") which can produce mycotoxins under certain conditions does not necessarily indicate that the organism is indeed secreting mycotoxins into the environment [68–70]. It is questionable that the concentration of mycotoxins is sufficient to induce illness by the respiratory route [17] (ACOEM 2002). Position statements released by the American College of Occupational and Environmental Medicine (ACOEM 2002) and the American Academy of Allergy, Asthma and Immunology [17] recommend further research in this area will be necessary to fully understand whether indoor fungal exposure poses a significant health risk. Recent studies from flooded homes in the U.S. show that there is little effect of fungal exposure on respiratory function in children [71].

Diagnosis and Treatment of Fungal-Related Allergic Disease

Diagnostic Testing for Fungal Allergy

One of the limitations encountered by clinicians is the lack of standardized fungal allergenic extracts for diagnostic testing and therapy [22, 72, 73]. While a number of fungal allergens have been isolated, purified, and characterized, the standardization of diagnostic and therapeutic reagents for fungal allergy has not yet occurred. Commercially available fungal allergenic products for diagnostic and therapeutic testing vary in their allergenic composition and concentrations [23]. Unfortunately, attempts to develop an international reference of *Alternaria alternata* extract did not meet with success due to instability of the candidate reagent [74, 75].

Monoclonal antibody-based assays for quantifying fungals may lead to improved reagents for the clinician and researcher [22]. As newer technologies are developed, it is hoped that significant improvements can be made in *in vivo* and *in vitro* diagnostic tools

Treatment of Fungal Allergic Diseases

As with any allergen exposure, avoidance is the first principle of treatment. Exposure to fungal spores chiefly occurs in the outdoor environment [17]. Therefore, exposure avoidance is difficult at best. Individuals with fungal sensitivity can wear a dust-mite mask when performing activities in the outdoors, such as leaf-raking or working in composted materials to reduce high levels of exposure. Closing windows and using air conditioning may also reduce exposure to fungi from the outdoors [7].

Indoor exposure to fungi, which may be responsible for symptoms, is managed best by controlling the intrusion of moisture [17, 76]. Active fungal growth in materials can be mitigated by chlorine-containing bleach solutions with a detergent. Fungal growth that invades fabrics, wallpaper, woodwork may require removal and replacement. Air cleaners have been shown to remove fungal spores from circulating in the environment [77]. Ionic air cleaners are not recommended, since they may generate ozone, a respiratory irritant. There has been no data demonstrating whether the reduction in airborne spore levels in the indoor environment by air cleaners has any clinical benefit.

Immunotherapy for fungal allergens has had limited study [78]. However, it has been shown to reduce both allergic rhinitis and asthma symptoms in selected patients [79–81]. Subcutaneous immunotherapy has been the traditional method although more recently the employment of sublingual immunotherapy has gained interest, but there have been no well-controlled studies of its use in fungal allergy [82].

One would anticipate that the use of anti-IgE (omalizumab) during seasonal exposure to fungi may be helpful in reducing the risk of severe and fatal asthma, particularly in older children and young adults sensitive to *Alternaria*. No published papers have appeared at this time. In addition, anti-IgE therapy is being studied as an adjuvant in the treatment of ABPA, and a few preliminary reports have appeared [55]. Because the serum IgE level in ABPA by far exceeds the recommended level for therapy with anti-IgE, the use of this treatment will require further investigation.

Summary

It has been difficult to link fungal exposure with symptoms even in sensitized individuals [83]. Fungal-spore count is one marker that is utilized but since intact spores may not be actively producing allergen, the association between spore counts and allergic symptoms is problematic. Refined methods that include actual allergen exposure to the respiratory tract [30] may be more relevant. There are a number of controversial areas regarding fungal exposure and its health effects particularly as it relates to the indoor environment [17]. Advances in the identification of fungal allergens will lead to improvements in the diagnosis and treatment of fungal allergic disease. As the title of the chapter, "Fungal Allergies: As Yet Unsolved," indicates, the study of fungal exposure and its consequences on human health, including allergic respiratory diseases and their therapies, deserves further investigation.

References

1. Blackley C. Experimental Researches on the Causes of Catarrhus Aestivus (Hay Fever or Hay Asthma). London: Bailliere Tindal & Cox; 1873.
2. Esch RE, Bush RK. Aerobiology of outdoor allergens. In: Adkinson, editors. Middleton's Allergy: Principles and Practice. St. Louis, MO: Mosby; 2003.
3. Bowyer P, Fraczek M, Denning DW. Comparative genomics of fungal allergens and epitopes shows widespread distribution of closely related allergen and epitope orthologues. BMC Genomics 2006;7:251.
4. Bowyer P, Denning DW. Genomic analysis of allergen genes in Aspergillus spp: the relevance of genomics to everyday research. Med Mycol 2007;45:17–26.
5. Friedlander SL, Bush RK. Fungal allergy. In: Kurup, V, editors. Mold Allergy, Biology and Pathogenesis. Kerala, India: Research Signpost; 2005. pp. 1–15.
6. Portnoy J, Barnes C, Barnes CS. The National Allergy Bureau: pollen and spore reporting today. J Allergy Clin Immunol 2004;114:1235–8.
7. Bush RK, Prochnau JJ. Alternaria-induced asthma. J Allergy Clin Immunol 2004;113:227–34.
8. Portnoy JM, Barnes CS, Kennedy K. Sampling for indoor fungi. J Allergy Clin Immunol 2004;113:189–98.

9. Joint Task Force. Allergen immunotherapy: a practice parameter. Ann Allergy Asthma Immunol 2003;90:1–40.
10. Horner WE, Barnes C, Cohn RD, Levetin E. Guide for interpreting reports from inspections/ identifications of indoor molds. J Allergy Clin Immunol 2008; 121:592–97.
11. Salo PM, Arbes SJ Jr, Cohn RD, Burge HA, London SJ, Zeldin DC. Alternaria alternata antigens in US homes. J Allergy Clin Immunol 2006;117:473.
12. Barnes C, Portnoy J, Sever M, Arbes S Jr, Vaughn B, Zeldin DC. Comparison of enzyme immunoassay-based assays for environmental Alternaria alternata. Ann Allergy Asthma Immunol 2006;97:350–6.
13. Beijer L, Rylander R. (1 – > 3)-beta-D-glucan does not induce acute inflammation after nasal deposition. Mediators Inflamm 2005;2005(1):50–2.
14. Douwes J. (1 – > 3)-Beta-D-glucans and respiratory health: a review of the scientific evidence. Indoor Air 2005;15:160–9.
15. Yamada J, Hamuro J, Hatanaka H, Hamabata K, Kinoshita S. Alleviation of seasonal allergic symptoms with superfine beta-1,3-glucan: a randomized study. J Allergy Clin Immunol 2007;119:1119–26.
16. Iossifova YY, Reponen T, Bernstein DI, Levin L, Kalra H, Campo P, et al. House dust (1–3)-beta-D-glucan and wheezing in infants. Allergy 2007;62:504–13.
17. Bush RK, Portnoy JM, Saxon A, Terr AI, Wood RA. The medical effects of mold exposure. J Allergy Clin Immunol 2006;117:326–33.
18. Portnoy JM, Kennedy K, Barnes C. Sampling for indoor fungi: what the clinician needs to know. Curr Opin Otolaryngol Head Neck Surg 2005;13:165–70.
19. Kurup VP. Fungal allergens. Curr Allergy Asthma Rep 2003;3:416–23.
20. Vijay HM, Abebe M, Kurup VP. Alternaria and Cladosporium allergens and allergy. In: Kurup, VP (ed) Mold Allergy, Biology and Pathogenesis. Kerala, India: Research Signpost; 2005, pp. 51–68.
21. Singh BP, Kukreja N, Arora N. Clinically relevant allergens from fungi imperfecti and yeast. In: Kurup, VP (ed) Mold Allergy, Biology and Pathogenesis. Kerala, India: Research Signpost; 2005, pp. 77–92.
22. Esch RE. Manufacturing and standardizing fungal allergen products. J Allergy Clin Immunol 2004;113:210–5.
23. Vailes L, Sridhara S, Cromwell O, Weber B, Breitenbach M, Chapman M. Quantitation of the major fungal allergens, Alt a 1 and Asp f 1, in commercial allergenic products. J Allergy Clin Immunol 2001;107:641–6.
24. Huss K, Adkinson NF Jr, Eggleston PA, Dawson C, Van Natta ML, Hamilton RG. House dust mite and cockroach exposure are strong risk factors for positive allergy skin test responses in the Childhood Asthma Management Program. J Allergy Clin Immunol 2001;107:48–54.
25. Arbes SJ Jr, Cohn RD, Yin M, Muilenberg ML, Friedman W, Zeldin DC. Dog allergen (Can f 1) and cat allergen (Fel d 1) in US homes: results from the National Survey of Lead and Allergens in Housing. J Allergy Clin Immunol 2004;114:111–7.
26. Arbes SJ Jr, Sever M, Mehta J, Gore JC, Schal C, Vaughn B, et al. Abatement of cockroach allergens (Bla g 1 and Bla g 2) in low-income, urban housing: month 12 continuation results. J Allergy Clin Immunol 2004;113:109–14.
27. Chew GL, Higgins KM, Gold DR, Muilenberg ML, Burge HA. Monthly measurements of indoor allergens and the influence of housing type in a northeastern US city. Allergy 1999;54:1058–66.
28. Salo PM, Arbes SJ, Jr., Sever M, Jaramillo R, Cohn RD, London SJ, et al. Exposure to Alternaria alternata in US homes is associated with asthma symptoms. J Allergy Clin Immunol 2006;118:892–8.
29. Sporik RB, Arruda LK, Woodfolk J, Chapman MD, Platts-Mills TA. Environmental exposure to Aspergillus fumigatus allergen (Asp f I). Clin Exp Allergy 1993;23:326–31.
30. Green BJ, Yli-Panula E, Tovey ER. Halogen immunoassay, a new method for the detection of sensitization to fungal allergens; comparisons with conventional techniques. Allergol Int 2006;55:131–9.

31. Terr AI. Are indoor molds causing a new disease? J Allergy Clin Immunol 2004;113:221–6.
32. Update: pulmonary hemorrhage/hemosiderosis among infants – Cleveland, Ohio, 1993–1996. MMWR Morb Mortal Wkly Rep 2000;49:180–4.
33. Brown CM, Redd SC, Damon SA. Acute idiopathic pulmonary hemorrhage among infants. Recommendations from the Working Group for Investigation and Surveillance. MMWR Recomm Rep 2004;53:1–12.
34. Portnoy JM, Kennedy K, Barnes CS. Controversies regarding dampness and mold growth in homes. Allergy Asthma Proc 2007;28:257–8.
35. Hope AP, Simon RA. Excess dampness and mold growth in homes: an evidence-based review of the aeroirritant effect and its potential causes. Allergy Asthma Proc 2007;28:262–70.
36. Andes D, Proctor R, Bush RK, Pasic TR. Report of successful prolonged antifungal therapy for refractory allergic fungal sinusitis. Clin Infect Dis 2000;31:202–4.
37. Schubert MS. Allergic fungal sinusitis: pathogenesis and management strategies. Drugs 2004;64:363–74.
38. Marple BF, Gibbs SR, Newcomer MT, Mabry RL. Allergic fungal sinusitis-induced visual loss. Am J Rhinol 1999;13:191–5.
39. Shin SH, Ponikau JU, Sherris DA, Congdon D, Frigas E, Homburger HA, et al. Chronic rhinosinusitis: an enhanced immune response to ubiquitous airborne fungi. J Allergy Clin Immunol 2004;114:1369–75.
40. Inoue Y, Matsuwaki Y, Shin SH, Ponikau JU, Kita H. Nonpathogenic, environmental fungi induce activation and degranulation of human eosinophils. J Immunol 2005;175:5439–47.
41. Ponikau JU, Sherris DA, Weaver A, Kita H. Treatment of chronic rhinosinusitis with intranasal amphotericin B: a randomized, placebo-controlled, double-blind pilot trial. J Allergy Clin Immunol 2005;115:125–31.
42. Bush RK. Is topical antifungal therapy effective in the treatment of chronic rhinosinusitis? J Allergy Clin Immunol 2005;115:123–4.
43. Lehrer SB, Hughes JM, Altman LC, Bousquet J, Davies RJ, Gell L, et al. Prevalence of basidiomycete allergy in the USA and Europe and its relationship to allergic respiratory symptoms. Allergy 1994;49:460–5.
44. Halonen M, Stern DA, Wright AL, Taussig LM, Martinez FD. Alternaria as a major allergen for asthma in children raised in a desert environment. Am J Respir Crit Care Med 1997;155:1356–61.
45. Perzanowski MS, Sporik R, Squillace SP, Gelber LE, Call R, Carter M, et al. Association of sensitization to Alternaria allergens with asthma among school-age children. J Allergy Clin Immunol 1998;101:626–32.
46. Downs SH, Mitakakis TZ, Marks GB, Car NG, Belousova EG, Leuppi JD, et al. Clinical importance of Alternaria exposure in children. Am J Respir Crit Care Med 2001;164:455–9.
47. Black PN, Udy AA, Brodie SM. Sensitivity to fungal allergens is a risk factor for life-threatening asthma. Allergy 2000;55:501–4.
48. Dales RE, Cakmak S, Burnett RT, Judek S, Coates F, Brook JR. Influence of ambient fungal spores on emergency visits for asthma to a regional children's hospital. Am J Respir Crit Care Med 2000;162:2087–90.
49. Pulimood T, Corden J, Bryden C, Sharples L, Nasser S. Epidemic asthma and the role of the fungal mould Alternaria alternata. J Allergy Clin Immunol 2007:610–7.
50. Marks GB, Bush RK. It's blowing in the wind (editorial). J Allergy Clin Immunol 2007;120:530–2.
51. Targonski PV, Persky VW, Ramekrishnan V. Effect of environmental molds on risk of death from asthma during the pollen season. J Allergy Clin Immunol 1995;95:955–61.
52. Reed CE. Inflammatory effect of environmental proteases on airway mucosa. Current Allergy Reports 2007;7:368–374.
53. Kauffman HF, Tomee JF, van de Riet MA, Timmerman AJ, Borger P. Protease-dependent activation of epithelial cells by fungal allergens leads to morphologic changes and cytokine production. J Allergy Clin Immunol 2000;105:1185–93.

54. Kheradmand F, Kiss A, Xu J, Lee SH, Kolattukudy PE, Corry DB. A protease-activated pathway underlying Th cell type 2 activation and allergic lung disease. J Immunol 2002;169:5904–11.

55. Greenberger PA. Allergic bronchopulmonary Aspergillosis – clinical aspects. In: Kurup, VP (ed) Mold Allergy, Biology and Pathogenesis. Kerala, India: Research Signpost; 2005.

56. Virnig C, Bush RK. Allergic bronchopulmonary aspergillosis: a US perspective. Curr Opin Pulm Med 2007;13:67–71.

57. Greenberger PA. Allergic bronchopulmonary aspergillosis. J Allergy Clin Immunol 2002;110:685–92.

58. Stevens DA, Schwartz HJ, Lee JY, Moskovitz BL, Jerome DC, Catanzaro A, et al. A randomized trial of itraconazole in allergic bronchopulmonary aspergillosis. N Engl J Med 2000;342:756–62.

59. Peat JK, Dickerson J, Li J. Effects of damp and mould in the home on respiratory health: a review of the literature. Allergy 1998;53:120–8.

60. Verhoeff AP, Burge HA. Health risk assessment of fungi in home environments. Ann Allergy Asthma Immunol 1997;78:544–54.

61. Douwes J, Pearce N. Invited commentary: is indoor mold exposure a risk factor for asthma? Am J Epidemiol 2003;158:203–6.

62. Trout DB, Page EH. Fungal exposure and lower respiratory illness in children. Am J Respir Crit Care Med 2004;169:969–70.

63. Stark PC, Burge HA, Ryan LM, Milton DK, Gold DR. Fungal levels in the home and lower respiratory tract illnesses in the first year of life. Am J Respir Crit Care Med 2003;168:232–7.

64. Board of Health Promotion and Disease Prevention CoDISaH (2004) Damp indoor spaces and health. Washington, DC: Institute of Medicine of the National Academies.

65. Kim JL, Elfman L, Mi Y, Wieslander G, Smedje G, Norback D. Indoor molds, bacteria, microbial volatile organic compounds and plasticizers in schools – associations with asthma and respiratory symptoms in pupils. Indoor Air 2007;17:153–63.

66. Terr AI. Clinical ecology. J Allergy Clin Immunol 1987;79:423–6.

67. Emanuel DA, Wenzel FJ, Lawton BR. Pulmonary mycotoxicosis. Chest 1975;67:293–7.

68. Khalili B, Montanaro MT, Bardana EJ Jr. Inhalational mold toxicity: fact or fiction? A clinical review of 50 cases. Ann Allergy Asthma Immunol 2005;95:239–46.

69. Mahmoudi M, Gershwin ME. Sick building syndrome. III. Stachybotrys chartarum. J Asthma 2000;37:191–8.

70. Hossain MA, Ahmed MS, Ghannoum MA. Attributes of Stachybotrys chartarum and its association with human disease. J Allergy Clin Immunol 2004;113:200–8.

71. Rabito FA, Iqbal S, Kiernan MP, Hold E, Chew GL. Children's respiratory health and mold levels in New Orleans post-Katrina: a preliminary look. J Allergy Clin Immunol 2008;121(3):622–5. 72. Bush RK, Yunginger JW. Standardization of fungal allergens. Clin Rev Allergy 1987;5:3–21.

73. Bush RK. Fungal extracts in clinical practice. Allergy Proc 1993;14:385–90.

74. Helm RM, Squillace DL, Aukrust L, Borch SM, Baer H, Bush RK, et al. Production of an international reference standard alternaria extract. I. Testing of candidate extracts. Int Arch Allergy Appl Immunol 1987;82:178–89.

75. Helm RM, Squillace DL, Yunginger JW. Production of a proposed international reference standard Alternaria extract. II. Results of a collaborative trial. J Allergy Clin Immunol 1988;81:651–63.

76. Eggleston PA. Environmental control for fungal allergen exposure. Curr Allergy Asthma Rep 2003;3:424–9.

77. Maloney MJ, Wray BB, DuRant RH, Smith L, Smith L. Effect of an electronic air cleaner and negative ionizer on the population of indoor mold spores. Ann Allergy 1987;59:192–4.

78. Li JT, Pearlman DS, Nicklas RA, Lowenthal M, Rosenthal RR, Bernstein IL, et al. Algorithm for the diagnosis and management of asthma: a practice parameter update: Joint Task Force on Practice Parameters, representing the American Academy of Allergy, Asthma and Immunology, the American College of Allergy, Asthma and Immunology,

and the Joint Council of Allergy, Asthma and Immunology. Ann Allergy Asthma Immunol 1998;81:415–20.

79. Horst M, Hejjaoui A, Horst V, Michel FB, Bousquet J. Double-blind, placebo-controlled rush immunotherapy with a standardized Alternaria extract. J Allergy Clin Immunol 1990;85:460–72.

80. Dreborg S, Agrell B, Foucard T, Kjellman NI, Koivikko A, Nilsson S. A double-blind, multicenter immunotherapy trial in children, using a purified and standardized Cladosporium herbarum preparation. I. Clinical results. Allergy 1986;41:131–40.

81. Malling HJ, Dreborg S, Weeke B. Diagnosis and immunotherapy of mould allergy. V. Clinical efficacy and side effects of immunotherapy with Cladosporium herbarum. Allergy 1986;41:507–19.

82. Bernardis P, Agnoletto M, Puccinelli P, Parmiani S, Pozzan M. Injective versus sublingual immunotherapy in Alternaria tenuis allergic patients. J Investig Allergol Clin Immunol 1996;6:55–62.

83. Delfino RJ, Coate BD, Zeiger RS, Seltzer JM, Street DH, Koutrakis P. Daily asthma severity in relation to personal ozone exposure and outdoor fungal spores. Am J Respir Crit Care Med 1996;154:633–41.

Latex Allergy: Clinical Manifestations

Kevin J. Kelly and Brian T. Kelly

Introduction

The clinical manifestations of latex allergy are unique to certain risk groups and their multiple sources of environmental exposure to latex protein. During the 1980s and 1990s, a worldwide epidemic of latex allergy occurred. Multiple reasons have been speculated as the reason for this epidemic, but analysis of the best evidence available still suggests a deficit in our understanding of the contributing causes. A review of latex production, manufacturing, and use patterns of latex in the context of clinical symptoms is necessary.

Latex Production, Collection, and Manufacturing

Natural rubber latex (NRL or latex will be used in this chapter to denote the natural product) is produced in nearly 2,000 lactiferous plants and trees in the world. The commercial use of the polymer *cis*-1,4-polyisoprene found in NRL has been exploited for broad commercial use from the tree *Hevea brasiliensis*, but not from other lactiferous plants until recently [1]. Commercial use of latex from *H. brasiliensis* dates back to the nineteenth century although evidence of NRL materials found at archeological excavations reveal rubber materials to be abundant as far back as 1600 BC [2]. A British medical student, James Syme, discovered the first modern use of latex when he coated cloth to make the first

K.J. Kelly (✉)
Joyce C. Hall Distinguished Professor of Pediatrics, Chairman – Department of Pediatrics, Children's Mercy Hospitals & Clinics, Associate Dean – University of Missouri Kansas City School of Medicine, Kansas City, Missouri, USA
e-mail: kjkelly@cmh.edu

B.T. Kelly
University of Missouri, Kansas City School of Medicine, Kansas City, Missouri, USA

R. Pawankar et al. (eds.), *Allergy Frontiers: Clinical Manifestations*,   487
DOI: 10.1007/978-4-431-88317-3_30, © Springer 2009

raincoats in 1818. During the mid-nineteenth century, Charles Goodyear discovered a highly effective method of cross-linking the rubber polyisoprene known today as vulcanization. This process of heating rubber with sulfur retains elasticity while reducing the tackiness and sensitivity to temperature change of rubber. Common products made from NRL can be found in Table 1. Today, the majority of NRL are produced in Thailand, Indonesia, and Malaysia, and to a lesser extent in Central America and South America. This represents a dramatic shift in the last decade when Malaysia and India were the major producers of NRL. The plant seeds of *H. brasiliensis* were taken from Brazil in the late-nineteenth century, brought to England, germinated and then shipped to Asia to start numerous latex plantations [3]. The total amount of NRL consumption worldwide has increased dramatically even in the last decade with nearly 6 million tons/year produced in 1995 and over 8.79 million tons/year utilized in 2005 [4]. This increase in consumption is clearly due to China's spectacular growth, which has greatly increased the demand for the commodity while Japan, Europe, and North American demand has remained stable. Whether a new epidemic of latex allergy will emerge in China is unknown but is concerning.

The composition of fresh NRL can be seen in Table 2. Rubber hydrocarbon (*cis*-1,4-polyisoprene) makes up the majority of the latex suspensions while protein, carbohydrate, lipids, inorganic constituents, and amino acids are a minor percentage of the mix. Despite proteins being a minor portion of NRL, the retention of these proteins in finished products is the cause of IgE-mediated reactions in humans. During the manufacturing of latex products over 200 different chemicals have been utilized and fall into broad categories of accelerators of cross-linking,

Table 1 Common products made from natural rubber latex

Products made by dipping (more allergic)	Products made from coagulated latex (less allergic)
Balloons	Carpet pads
Barium enema retention catheter	Erasers
Bladder catheters	Hot-water bottles
Condoms	Molded toys
Dental dams	Multiple-dose medication bottles
Gloves – examination, household, surgeon	Tennis balls
Rubber bands	Tires

Table 2 Natural rubber latex composition

Component	Percentage
Rubber hydrocarbon	30–40
Water	55–65
Protein	1–2
Carbohydrate	1–2
Neutral and polar lipids	0.8–1.7
Inorganic constituents	0.5
Amino acids	<0.5

antioxidants, antiozonates, biocides, colorants, epoxies, and plasticizers. It is the accelerator class of chemicals, including thiurams, thiazoles, and carbamates, which most frequently cause type IV cell-mediated contact dermatitis of the skin from latex. Note that synthetic rubber materials and alternative medical glove materials may retain these same chemicals resulting in contact dermatitis as well. Gloves made of from either polyvinyl chloride, styrene butadiene rubber, or Tactylon® (styrene ethylene butylene styrene) do not contain these accelerators.

Collection of Latex

NRL flows through a circulation system in the bark of the tree and is collected when a slice of bark is shaved off just short of the cambium layer. Latex flow is directed from the cut in the bark to a spout that drains into a cup of glass, glazed earthenware, or a plastic bag. Within hours of tapping the tree, the latex is treated with a stabilizer such as sodium sulfite, formaldehyde, ammonia (0.05–0.2%), or ammonia with a 1:1 mixture of zinc oxide and tetramethylthiuram disulfide (TMTD). In order to enhance the yield of latex, a number of chemicals can be used to up regulate production. The effect of such chemicals on protein content and the type is not completely clear, but could enhance the quantity and distribution of allergenic proteins. For example, 2-chloroethylphosphonic acid (ethepon) was used frequently in the industry to enhance the production of latex. Pressure to produce more medical grade latex with the advent of standard precautions (aka universal precautions) in the 1980s resulted in more frequent tapping of trees and reduced storage time of latex. (Dr. Paul Caccioli, personal communication, 1998) What effect this had on the allergen content of latex is unclear. As many of the allergenic proteins in latex are defense proteins, production of these proteins would likely be enhanced. Failure to destroy proteins through reduced storage times may have enhanced the allergen content of finished products as well.

Approximately 88% or more of the world's harvested latex is prepared as dry raw rubber in sheets or crumbs of technically specified rubber. The latex is coagulated with either formic or acetic acid to a pH of 4.5. Sheets may be dried for up to a week at 60°C and crumbs dried at a higher temperature for up to 5 h. During preparation of dry rubber, the latex separates out into the three distinct layers: a bottom layer (B-fraction), a middle serum phase that contains many water-soluble proteins, and a latex portion that is found at the top of the admixture and easily separated from the other two layers. This is important since many inorganic materials and allergenic proteins can be removed resulting in the potential for lower allergen content. Good grade technically specified rubber still contains 2.2% protein, however. Allergic IgE-mediated reactions have been reported in very low frequency from this type of rubber although type IV cell-mediated reactions may be seen.

The other 10–12% of NRL is produced in a latex concentrate and makes products such as gloves and condoms from a dipping method. Most latex is concentrated in this form by centrifugation (although evaporation and creaming occasionally is used) to concentrate the latex to about 60% and is stabilized with a high concentration of ammonia (0.7%) or low ammonia (0.2%) with TMTD and zinc oxide. The concentrated latex is collected and bulked in storage tanks for at least 2–3 weeks and often longer before being shipped to consumers in bulk containers or steel drums. After shipping, the latex is prepared by the manufacturer with proprietary methods to prepare for dipping of molds with a surface coagulant into latex slurry. The latex adheres to the former and is wet leached, vulcanized, dried, and various methods are used to prevent the latex products from sticking to each other. In the past, the most common agent used was highly cross-linked cornstarch powder or talc. Because of the ability to act as a carrier of latex allergen, cornstarch powder has fallen out of favor. Talc was found to induce granulomatous inflammation and decrease wound healing and has mostly been abandoned in medical grade gloves. Halogenation or surface coating with a synthetic polymer has been useful in replacing donning powder.

Clinical Manifestations: Early Observations

In 1927, in the German literature, chronic urticaria from rubber prosthesis contact was observed in a single subject [5]. The spectrum of latex allergy was uncovered over the span of approximately 10 years starting with the first clear report of a case of immediate hypersensitivity to contact with latex. In 1979, a homemaker with atopic dermatitis presented with symptoms of intense pruritis from exposure to rubber gloves [6]. Confirmation of immediate hypersensitivity was accomplished by reproducing an urticaria reaction from a patch test and a prick test from a latex glove. This sentinel work was confirmed by another investigator in 1980 when a patient developed urticaria that was accompanied by rhinitis and ocular symptoms upon exposure to latex [7]. This appears to be the first time that respiratory epithelial response is noted in a subject with allergic symptoms from contact with latex. In fact, this is the first health care worker (HCW), a nurse, which can be found in the literature to react to latex. Also noteworthy is that this case occurs long before the advent of universal precautions for prevention of infection transmission from bodily fluids, a time after which a marked increase in latex exam glove use was observed in health care. A comprehensive review of available medical literature demonstrates a marked reporting of latex allergy soon after the introduction of these precautions. A plot of the number of scientific references to latex allergy by year since 1979 can be seen in Fig. 1. A number of important observations are readily apparent from this graphic. First, approximately 3–4 years after the introduction of universal precautions, the number of reports of latex allergy rapidly rises. This may be because of the awareness of the relatively few case reports of latex allergy that precede universal precautions and that the lag time to report and publish a clinical observation in the medical literature may be as long as 2 or more years. Second, the inflection point where latex allergy reports start to decline in 2002 may mark that the epidemic of latex allergy started to subside at the start of the millennium.

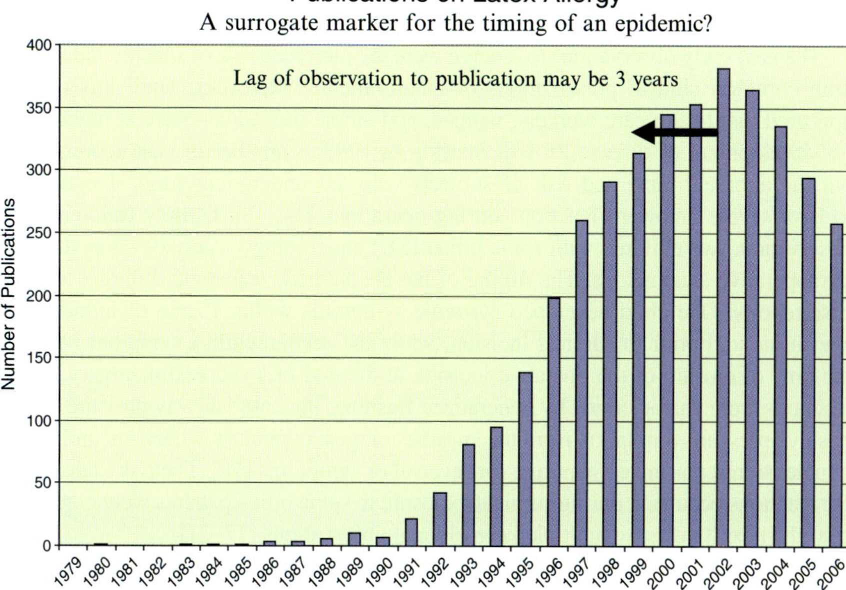

Fig. 1 This graph is a summary of the number of articles published on latex allergy yearly since 1979. A steady reduction in the number of articles has occurred since 2002

Alternatively, there may have been a significant decline in new information generated about latex allergy after that time.

A sentinel report appears in an abstract from Finland in 1984 where anaphylaxis from contact with a surgical latex glove is reported for the first time in patients undergoing surgical procedures [8]. This report again involves two nurses who were patients and later leads these investigators to perform the first prevalence study of latex allergy in health care workers. These two cases raise awareness that mucosal contact with latex may pose a significant risk in patients sensitized to latex as one reaction occurred after gynecologic surgery and the other after abdominal surgery. Published in 1987, a total of 15 of 512 (2.9%) hospital employees screened using a scratch chamber technique followed by prick test to latex extracted from a surgical glove and glove use test were confirmed to have latex allergy. The highest prevalence of latex allergy occurred in operating room personnel at 6.2%. Atopic subjects were more likely to develop latex allergy, being found in 10/15 (66.7%) latex allergic subjects [9]. Also in 1987, Axelsson reported systemic reactions in five individuals from NRL gloves but four fifths of these individuals were not working in the health care field [10].

In 1988, Seaton published the first case report of occupational asthma caused by latex gloves [11]. This was the first evidence that respiratory mucosal disease was likely airborne since the first rhinitis and ocular events could have been transferred from glove to nose or eye by direct inoculation. This important case report led to many further observations about the role of inhaled allergen in latex allergy.

The next early observations to emerge were the increased risk of specific individuals with common clinical presentations or environmental exposures. Until this time, it appeared that health care workers, women, and atopic individuals were at highest risk for development of disease [9–13]. Starting in 1989, a number of case reports point out the apparent increased risk of subjects who are undergoing surgical operations to have severe untoward reactions during operations [14, 15]. Closely following this observation, two children with spina bifida (SB) undergoing surgery developed severe intraoperative anaphylaxis. The timing of the anaphylaxis was quite different in these case reports. One child developed systemic symptoms within 15 min of induction of anesthesia and prior to surgical incision, while the second child's symptom began at the time of closure of the operative incision at the end of a successful surgery. These reactions were characterized by generalized flushing, increased airway pressure during positive pressure ventilation from the anesthesiologist, expiratory wheezing, and severe hypotension requiring epinephrine for reversal of symptoms [16]. The risky latex allergic reactions occurring during surgical exposure in spina bifida patients were confirmed over the next 3 years by multiple keen clinical observations [17–21].

Spina Bifida

Understanding the reasons that patients with spina bifida develop latex allergy at a high rate requires basic understanding of the cause and circumstances of medical care of these patients.

Neural tube defects (NTD) of spina bifida (SB) and anencephaly are relatively common birth defects that are preventable by folate-enriched dietary supplementation in pregnant females. In fact, all women who are able to become pregnant are encouraged to take 0.4 g/day and women at high risk of producing offspring with neural tube defects (previous delivery of a child with NTD) are offered 4 g/day of folate. Because of failure of selective use of folate to reduce the number of births of children with NTD, dietary enrichment of common foods with folate in the United States and other countries has led to a 25–30% reduction in births of children with NTD or approximately half of the number of cases presumed to be folate-responsive. This folate-neural tube defect is the only defect that is known to be preventable by such simple measures [22]. A definitive genetic cause to the development of NTD has proven elusive until a recent report where three mutations in the VANGL1 gene were characterized in the familial types [23].

In addition to the unique nature of NTD, patients with SB seem to be exceptionally capable of mounting an IgE allergic response to latex proteins. Early studies demonstrated that this group of patients was at the highest risk for developing latex allergy compared to other risk groups. In the early 1990s, the prevalence of latex allergy in SB as determined by medical history, skin prick testing, and serological assay was nearly 50% and when these subjects were selected for having surgery during the previous year prior to testing could be as high as 68% [24, 25]. Alarmingly, nearly one of every eight patients with spina bifida prior to the use of latex precautions in the operating room experienced anaphylaxis during induction of anesthesia. This rate is nearly 500-fold higher than the expected rates of anaphylactic reactions during general anesthesia and surgery [19]. There were two distinct times that anaphylaxis was observed during medical operations. Initial reports suggested that the time onset was between 40 and 220 min after the induction of anesthesia and surgery had commenced [20, 21]. A different case control series noted that all cases occurred within 30 min of anesthesia induction and before the surgeon made a first incision [19, 24]. The difference between these series is that an intravenous system that contained latex back-check valves in a buretrol and lumen of the tubing was used as a standard in the second case series to filter air from getting from the IV tubing to the patient [24]. It has been speculated that these patients' allergen was inadvertently injected intravenously when allergen was extracted into the intravenous fluid from the latex check valves. Indeed, no anaphylactic reactions were identified until after such a system had been introduced into the operating rooms at institution where a cluster of severe anaphylactic reactions occurred. The other case series of patients from Canada had mucosal surface contact by personnel wearing latex gloves and may explain the delay in symptom onset [21].

Why children with NTD develop latex allergy at a high rate has been speculated and only indirect proof has come by analysis of multiple studies. Because of the open spinal cord defect and accompanying Arnold Chiari malformations causing noncommunicating hydrocephalus, patients with NTD frequently undergo two surgeries in the first few weeks of life. The first surgery is to close the spinal defect followed by a second surgery to place a ventriculo-peritoneal shunt to relieve the hydrocephalus. It is common for these patients to require repeat shunt neurosurgeries, orthopedic surgeries on the lower extremities due to paraplegia complications, and urologic surgery due to neurogenic bladder and secondary kidney complications. Exposure to latex allergen from gloves and medical devices during these operations and general medical care are the most plausible explanations for such an allergy to occur. Indeed, a number of studies have identified that a common risk factor associated with the development of latex allergy in any patient is multiple surgeries [26, 27].

Specific risk factors associated with latex allergy in patients with spina bifida are consistent across multiple case and case-controlled series summarized in Table 3 [24, 26, 28–33]. The earliest case-controlled series appears in 1994 and NTD patients with >8 surgical operations, history of asthma, rubber contact-induced symptoms, rash from adhesive tape, elevated total IgE, elevated specific IgE to latex, nonwhite race, and daily rectal disimpaction were at highest risk for development of anaphylaxis during induction of anesthesia [24]. This case-controlled series is important because it is the first to characterize risk factors for patients with spina bifida, who are operated on who either develop or do not develop anaphylaxis during their operation. A second case-controlled series compares patients with spina bifida to atopic and non-atopic controls. Spina bifida patients developed specific IgE antibody at nearly four times the frequency of atopic children (40.5% vs. 11.4%) and >20 times the rate of healthy controls

Table 3 Risk factors associated with latex allergy in patients with spina bifida

Epidemiologic	Symptoms/tests
Atopy	Latex-specific IgE levels
History of asthma	Latex allergy symptoms with exposure
Nonwhite race	

Procedures	Food
>5 Surgeries	General food allergy
Bladder catheterization	Kiwi-/pear-/tomato-positive skin test
Daily rectal disimpaction	
Rash from adhesive tape	
Ventriculo-peritoneal shunt	

(40.5% vs. 1.9%) [30]. The prevalence of atopy in the spina bifida group was no different for those who were allergic to latex compared to those who were not. Surgical operations were found to be more frequent in spina bifida patients with latex allergy with >5 operations predicting the presence of latex allergy, while IgE antibody to banana proteins was identified more frequently as well in the latex allergic population.

Case series without control groups demonstrate the association of latex allergy with high total IgE (atopy), high specific anti-latex IgE antibody (>3.5 kU/L or class 3), positive skin test to fresh foods especially to kiwi, pear, or tomato, >5 or >8 operations, presence of a ventricular shunt, and symptoms upon contact with latex [29, 31–33]. Multivariate analysis demonstrates that atopy and >5 operations are the most important predictors of latex sensitization.

Latex Allergy in Patients with Neurologic or Urologic Defects

Since the development of latex allergy in spina bifida was so pervasive, it seemed logical to evaluate others who either had congenital anomalies of the urogenital tract or individuals who had bladder problems associated with neurological defects such as acquired paraplegia or quadriplegia. It became clear early that latex allergy may present as anaphylaxis in patients with urologic malformations such as cloacal anomalies and such anomalies represent a risk for sensitization [24, 30, 34, 35]. In addition, some children with chronic renal failure with or without anorectal or bladder malformations may develop latex allergy as well [36]. However, two studies published in the same year from separate institutions came to opposite conclusions about the risk of latex allergy or sensitization in patients with spinal cord injuries. Konz performed a cross-sectional study of 36 patients with spina bifida, 50 patients with spinal cord injury (SCI), 10 patients with cerebrovascular accidents (CVA), and 10 healthy controls. None of the SCI patients or CVA patients had any history of reactions to latex, while 72% of the SB patients had clinical histories suggestive of latex allergy [37]. All of the SB patients with positive histories had detectable anti-latex IgE in their sera, while only 4% of the SCI patients and none of the CVA or controls had detectable specific IgE. Given the size of the control and CVA groups, there was little difference between them and the SCI patients, but a marked difference from SB patients. Vogel studied 67 spinal cord injured patients with 10 patients found to have latex-specific IgE antibody in the serum [38]. Only two of these ten subjects had a history suggestive of latex allergic reactions, while the other eight subjects had no history of clinical reactions. Because different serologic assays were utilized in these studies, the differences may be explained by false positives and small sample sizes. Regardless, it appears that there are clear differences between neurologically injured patients and the congenital anomaly of spina bifida.

Health Care Workers

Clinical reactions in health care worker (HCW) to latex include nonimmunologic irritant contact reactions as well as immunologic reactions of which type IV cellular-mediated contact dermatitis and type I IgE-mediated reactions are subsets.

Irritant dermatitis is the most common reaction to latex seen in HCW. This is most often observed in individuals who frequently wear latex or non-latex gloves [9–11, 39–56]. Thirty percent or more of health care workers may report irritant reactions of the hands. Frequent hand washing, irritation from glove powder, multiple glove changes, and incomplete drying of the hands all contribute to this common dermatitis. Irritant dermatitis is recognized by the dry, cracked skin surface accompanied by itching and erythema without vesicles, blistering, or weeping. In addition, the dermatitis only appears in the area where contact with the latex product occurs since it is a nonimmune sensitizing reaction. This dermatitis may respond to cotton glove liners, reduction of powder use, thorough hand drying, nonpetroleum-based barrier creams that cause NRL to degrade, and topical skin moisturizers.

Contact dermatitis, a type IV immunologic reaction, may have a distinctly different presentation compared to irritant dermatitis [57]. The onset of clinical reaction occurs after hours of contact and is often accompanied by intense itching, erythema, blistering, or weeping skin that extends beyond the site of contact with the offending NRL product. (Fig. 2) The extension of dermatitis beyond the site of contact is due to sensitized lymphocytes and Langerhans cells that may home to remote sites away from the site of contact, but are activated upon contact with offending allergen. Chronic contact dermatitis, which may not be accompanied by the blistering and weeping of acute contact dermatitis, may be difficult to distinguish from irritant dermatitis at times. A diagnosis is confirmed with delayed hypersensitivity patch testing with chemicals retained in finished rubber products. Chemical ingredients of rubber, especially thiurams and mercaptobenzothiazoles are the most frequent cause of rubber contact dermatitis diagnosed by patch testing. As many as 11%

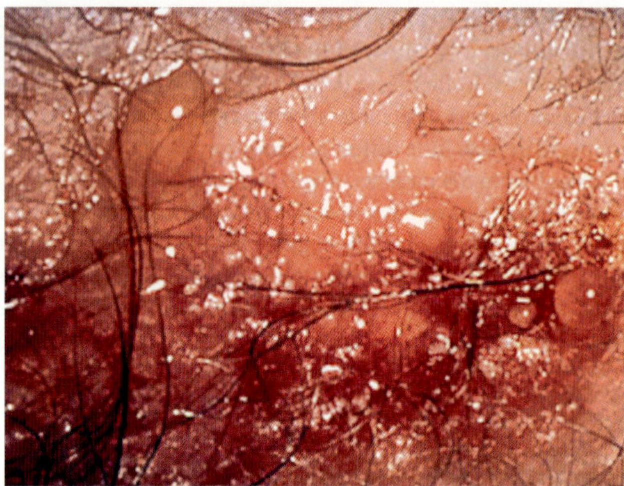

Fig. 2 Rubber contact dermatitis is most often caused by chemical additives retained in the finished product. The erythema, weeping, and vesicle formation should be noted in this picture (Reprinted from Kevin J. Kelly, Fireman's Atlas of Allergy 2006. With permission)

of health care workers presenting with hand dermatitis to an occupational health clinic have concurrent contact dermatitis to thiuram and contact urticaria to from immediate hypersensitivity to latex protein [58]. Recent studies suggest that some NRL proteins may be capable of inducing a type IV contact dermatitis in addition to their propensity to induce type I IgE-mediated reactions [59]. Murine data suggest that latex proteins themselves are capable of inducing contact dermatitis [60]. Complicating this problem is the presence of the same accelerators or antioxidants reside in some gloves made of non-latex material. If a patient has chemical-induced contact dermatitis and latex allergy, dermatitis may persist despite changing gloves to a different material.

Regardless of the etiology of the dermatitis, it often precedes and is a risk factor for the development of type I IgE-mediated NRL allergy to proteins in individuals who directly contact NRL in their daily activities or work (Fig. 3). Interestingly, dermatitis is rarely been reported or observed in other populations at high risk such as spina bifida patients. Although the mechanism for how the dermatitis may predispose to the development of NRL allergy is not confirmed, it is speculated that the dermatitis may enhance penetration of proteins through the epidermis resulting in access to the immune system and subsequent development of NRL-specific IgE. The contribution of this mechanism of disease in humans is not clear at this time.

The full spectrum of IgE-mediated disease has been reported in the literature in health care workers. These symptoms have included urticaria (local or generalized), flushing, angioedema, rhinitis, conjunctivitis, vaginitis, asthma (especially occupational asthma), and anaphylaxis. The prevalence of latex allergy in one Finnish

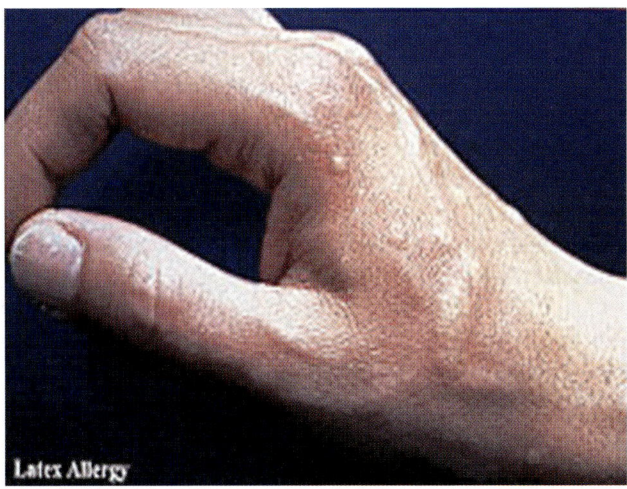

Fig. 3 IgE-mediated latex allergy is most often manifested as urticaria, angioedema, asthma, bronchospasm, and/or anaphylaxis (Reprinted from Kevin J. Kelly, Fireman's Atlas of Allergy 2006. With permission)

hospital found 3% of health care workers to be skin test-positive and symptomatic to contact with latex in 1987 [9]. There are subsequent reports of increasing prevalence of the disease in the rest of Europe and North America that rose to levels of 10–17% by 1994 [48, 51]. Unfortunately, many studies were unable to test all workers in a single setting, leading to difficult interpretation as to the true prevalence of latex allergy in the HCW population. A meta-analysis of 48 studies involving health care worker latex allergy prevalence studies concluded that latex allergy may not be higher in health care workers when compared to the general population [54]. This study was subjected to multiple criticisms [55] and was later followed up by an independent meta-analysis by the French National Regulatory Authority. That study clearly demonstrated that health care workers have an increased risk of sensitization and allergic symptoms to latex [56]. HCW exposed to latex have an increased risk of hand dermatitis (OR, 2.46), asthma or wheezing (OR, 1.55), rhinoconjunctivitis (OR, 2.73), and at least one generic symptom (OR, 1.27) by comparison with HCW who do not have latex exposure [56].

To date, there have been three prospective incident studies performed looking at sensitization rates to latex in HCW [47, 56, 57]. HCW seems to be sensitized at a rate of 1–2.5% yearly but a direct cause and effect from latex glove exposure could not completely be determined in any of the studies.

Occupational asthma became the most concerning manifestation of latex allergy in workers whose occupation placed them in an environment where latex allergen was airborne either directly from latex dust or from protein carried by lubricant cornstarch powder released from the surface of latex [55, 61–73]. Respiratory symptoms, asthma, and bronchial hyper responsiveness have been associated with contact with latex gloves and sensitivity to latex.

This was dramatically pointed out by Vandenplas in 1995 when respiratory assessment took place in 13 latex-sensitive health care workers. Twelve [12] of these workers agreed to undergo bronchial histamine challenge and all were found to be hyperresponsive. In addition, seven individuals responded with airway obstruction to latex inhalation challenge. Three of the seven individuals had a biphasic response with an early response only in four of the individuals [63]. As has been observed with other high-molecular weight allergens, Brugnami documented continued asthma in health care workers despite removal from an environment where airborne or skin exposure to latex occurred for up to 7 years [64]. Despite the multiple associations of latex with asthma, it is not always clear whether asthma in health care workers is a preexisting problem or acquired from exposure to latex allergen. Public information on surveillance of work-related asthma finds many health care professionals over-represented compared to other work types. Multiple reasons for this are possible but may not be related to specific work place exposures such as latex [74].

Several explanations have been offered for the increased prevalence of latex allergy in health care workers including standard precautions, powder resulting in airborne exposure, low-quality/high-allergen gloves flooding the market in the 1990s, reduced latex storage time prior to manufacturing, induction of higher yield of latex by chemicals that enhanced allergen production, and selective growth of high-yielding trees that contained more allergen in the latex [75].

Diagnosis of occupational asthma from latex, prevention, and treatment strategies are discussed in a separate chapter.

Latex Allergy in the General Population

Latex allergy has presented in multiple individuals who have had no apparent risk factors of exposure as seen in spina bifida, health care workers, and individuals who have required multiple surgeries. The symptoms manifested by these individuals are usually predictable by the route of exposure. Rhinitis, conjunctivitis, and asthma occur from inhalation, while anaphylaxis occurs from peritoneal surface or intravenous exposure. None has been more dramatic than the first cases of anaphylaxis seen after rectal mucosal surface exposure to latex balloons, latex glove, or condom materials. In the 1980s, air contrast barium enema procedures used a special catheter that was inflated to help retain the air and barium in the colon. Rectal manometry with a balloon catheter or coverage of a manometer by a latex finger from cut from a glove or condom was a common procedure also in the 1980s. Case series described severe anaphylaxis, including a death, associated with anaphylaxis and rectal mucosal surface contact with latex [76, 77]. Prior to widespread knowledge about latex allergy, anaphylaxis after barium enema was reported without conclusive causation defined [78]. Most of the patients who suffered anaphylactic reactions by this method were not workers from a job type that had frequent exposure to latex. Some of these had a prior history of atopy, including asthma, or surgical operations. Although one particular catheter was implicated in the problem with barium enema administration (E-Z-Em company) with as many as 148 episodes of anaphylaxis and 9 deaths, the concentration of mast cells and permeability of the rectal mucosa may be factors involved in these observations [79]. Since the majority of patients affected by these reactions were not from a high-risk industry, it naturally begs the question: Is the general population at significant risk of latex allergy?

Significant controversy has been raised over the actual prevalence of latex allergy in the general population. Two large studies from Finland and Italy demonstrate that 1.1% of the general population from a selected clinic population and 0.7% in an unselected population are sensitized to latex [80, 81]. This pointed out that the rates of sensitization in health care workers and spina bifida far exceeded these prevalence studies. These observations were called into question when blood donor samples found the presence of anti-latex IgE antibodies in over 4% of the samples in multiple studies [82–87]. One European study excluded HCW and found the prevalence of anti-latex IgE in the serum in 3% of the subjects [88]. The settings for these studies include presurgical patients, random blood donors, and emergency department patients. One weakness of these observations is that only a single testing method was used in each of the studies. Criticisms have also been stated that highly sensitive tests with low specificity in a population with a low prevalence of disease will result in the majority of tests being false-positive [89]. Two studies used either multiple labs or repeat assays to assure the accuracy of the assay [86, 87]. However, the lack of medical history, physical examination, and latex skin testing coupled with the serologic assays still raises significant questions. However, the presence of life-threatening reactions in the general population raises concerns that the prevalence of latex allergy may be higher than originally expected.

Fruit Allergy and Concurrent Latex Allergy

Shortly after the epidemic emergence of latex allergy in the 1980s, a number of reports were published over the next decade that noted multiple clinical reactions to foods in individuals with latex allergy. In addition, individuals with primary food allergy were found to have clinical reactions with latex but much less frequently than might have been expected from the initial frequency of cross-reactivity found in vitro. This syndrome has been termed the "latex-fruit syndrome" and was extended to the "latex vegetable syndrome" later when cross-reactions were found between a number of vegetables and latex proteins [90–125].

Multiple patients with primary latex allergy are found to have concurrent fruit allergy. M'Raihi was the first to identify the clinical cross-reaction between banana and latex in 1991 [90]. Over the next decade, multiple foods and mechanisms for this cross-reactivity were characterized. Up to 50% or more of the individuals may react to banana, avocado, mango, kiwi, chestnut, tomato, passion fruit, papaya, and stone fruits such as cherry or peaches. Some foods may only

Table 4 Foods that cross-react with *Hevea* latex

Common clinical cross-reacting foods with latex	Primary food allergies causing reactions to latex
Avocado	Banana
Banana	Melon
Chestnut	Peach
Kiwi	
Papaya	
Potato	

Foods with immunologic cross-reactivity in latex allergic patients but uncommon clinical allergy	
Apple	Passion fruit
Bell pepper	Peach
Cantaloupe	Pear
Celery	Pineapple
Cherry	Tomato
Fig	Turnip
Mango	Wheat
Melon	

have in vitro cross-reactivity with latex while others commonly cause clinical reactions. Table 4 includes a list of the common cross-reacting foods in patients who are latex allergic, as well as foods that cause primary allergy with secondary reactions to latex.

These episodes have been investigated thoroughly and can be linked to specific allergens from latex that cross-react with similar plant allergens [90–125]. Those allergens involved include Hev b 6 or hevein, which shares common tertiary structure with two banana proteins, avocado allergens, and chestnut allergens. Hev b 5 has significant homology with Kiwi and may cause cross-reactions. Hev b 7 is a patatin-like protein that may lead to symptoms from potato although the clinical relevance of this is small. Hev b 8 is a profilin-like protein and may cross-react with other plant profilins. Hev b 2 is a β-1,3-glucan, which is a pathogen-related protein that may cause clinical cross-reactions. Hev b 12 is a lipid transfer protein that has been a common protein type to cause reactions in vegetables and fruit in patients who are pollen reactive. These allergens are discussed in depth in the chapter on diagnosis and treatment of latex allergy [114].

In 1998, investigators from Spain looked at the issue of latex-fruit syndrome from the opposite point of view [110]. They investigated 57 individuals with primary fruit allergy who might be at risk of having latex allergy. A remarkable 49/57 (86%) of the subjects demonstrated IgE binding to latex allergen serologically and/or skin test. However, only 6/57 or 12.2% had prior symptoms from latex exposure and this was preceded by reactions to the offending fruit. Thus, patients with primary food allergy can have reactions to latex exposure, but it is a significantly lower rate than is seen in primary latex allergic patients reacting to ingested fruits.

Latex Protein as a Hidden Food Allergen

During the last 10 years when significant progress in our understanding of food allergen cross-reactivity was accomplished, three reports reminded us of the potential of latex protein to transfer allergen from gloves directly to food [126–128]. The first report of latex as a hidden allergen by Schwartz presented two cases of urticaria, angioedema, and dyspnea after ingestion of food handled by workers who prepared the food wearing latex gloves [126]. Beezhold and colleagues demonstrated by two methods of analysis, a modified western blot assay that was able to visualize a glove fingerprint containing latex protein directly on cheese and ELISA method after extraction of latex transferred by a latex glove to lettuce. This report included a case where a latex allergic subject developed anaphylaxis after eating at a salad bar where food preparation was performed by workers wearing latex gloves [127]. Bernardini in a double-blind food challenge reproduced an allergic reaction to latex that had transferred to a cream-filled doughnut handled by workers with a latex glove [128]. While one considers that a patient's symptoms are from food cross-reactivity to latex, it is imperative that the clinician pursue a history of potential contact by food handlers who wear latex gloves during the preparation. These reports all occurred from restaurants. It is not clear whether packaged foods sold in stores may also have latex allergen transferred to them and no industry standard exists precluding such use of gloves.

Diabetes and Latex Allergy

In 1995, a single case of systemic anaphylaxis during surgery from latex allergen in a medication admixture that contained a rubber stopper was reported in the anesthesia literature [129]. This is quickly followed by a series of case reports and a single prevalence study investigated the risk of latex allergy in patients with diabetes requiring insulin injections [130–135]. All of these cases resulting from insulin injection demonstrate that latex allergic reactions were observed when a needle used to draw up insulin was passed through a vial containing a latex top and subsequently used to inject the insulin into the patient. Removal of the latex top followed by drawing up the insulin directly into a syringe did not produce allergic reactions in any of these cases. Only localized reactions at the site of injection with no systemic symptoms were observed in all cases except one where anaphylaxis was observed [130]. These observations suggest that latex allergen may be present on the surface of the needle after it passes through latex in quantities high enough to cause allergic reactions. A report in the pharmacy literature asserts that no latex allergen can be found in medication in multiple-dose vials despite numerous needle penetrations [135]. However, the needle punctures of the latex vial may not elute allergen into the vial in quantities high enough to produce allergic reactions. A cross-sectional study of 112 serum samples from children with type I diabetes demonstrates that latex-specific IgE antibody occurs only in atopic children with diabetes and that rate of sensitization may be no higher than what is observed in atopic children without diabetes. In this study, 7/112 (6%) of subjects had IgE antibody while all 7/42 (17%) were atopic [132].

Summary

The clinical circumstances in patients who develop latex allergy are highly variable and require the clinician to be an astute historian and diagnostician. Since all industries where natural rubber products are produced or used may result in worker sensitization or patient reactions, a high index of suspicion must be always maintained by the clinician. Whether all patients who present with primary food reactions that are known to cross-react with latex should be screened for latex allergy is unclear. It would be prudent until a major organization of clinicians and scientists recommends such screening to consider each circumstance and patient individually. Patients who will need surgery or dental procedures would be the most likely patients to need such screening.

References

1. Subramaniam A. The chemistry of natural rubber latex. In: Immunology and Allergy Clinics of North America. Fink JN (ed) W.B. Saunders, Philadelphia, 1995;1–20
2. Hosler D, Burkett SL, Tarkanian JM. Prehistoric polymers: rubber processing in ancient Mesoamerica. Science 1999;284:1988–91
3. http://www.madehow.com/Volume-3/Latex.html (accession date 5/20/2007)
4. Burger K. The changing outlook for natural rubber. In: Natural Rubber (Newsletter of the Rubber Foundation Information Center for Natural Rubber) 2005;40(4): 1–2
5. Stern G. Überempfindlichkeit gegen Kautschuk als ursache von Urticaria und Quinckeschem Ödem. Klin Wochenschr 1927;6:1096–7
6. Nutter AF. Contact urticaria to rubber. Br J Dermatol 1979;101:597–8
7. Förström L. Contact urticaria from latex surgical gloves. Contact Dermat 1980;16:33–4
8. Turjanmaa K, Reunala T, Tuimala R, Karkkainen T. Severe IgE mediated allergy to surgical gloves [abstract]. Allergy 1984;39:S-2
9. Turjanmaa K. Incidence of immediate allergy to latex gloves in hospital personnel. Contact Dermat 1987 Nov; 17(5):270–5
10. Axelsson JG, Johansson SG, Wrangsjo K. IgE-mediated anaphylactoid reactions to rubber. Allergy. 1987 Jan; 42(1):46–50
11. Seaton A, Cherrie B, Turnbull J. Rubber glove asthma. BMJ 1988;42:604–11
12. Gaignon I, Veyckemans F, Gribomont BF. Latex allergy in a child: report of a case. Acta Anaesthesiol Belg 1991;42(4):219–23
13. Beuers U, Baur X, Schraudolph M, Richter WO. Anaphylactic shock after game of squash in atopic woman with latex allergy. Lancet 1990 May 5;335(8697):1095
14. Gerber AC, Jorg WZ, Zbinden S, Seger RA, Dangel PH. Severe intraoperative anaphylaxis to surgical gloves: latex allergy, an unfamiliar condition. Anesthesiology 1989 Nov; 71(5):800–2

15. Zenarola P. Rubber latex allergy: unusual complication during surgery. Contact Dermat 1989 Sept;21(3):197–8

16. Slater J. Rubber Anaphylaxis. N Engl J Med 1989;320(17):1126–30

17. Holzman R, Sethna N, Sockin S. Hypotension, Flushing and Bronchospasm in Myelodysplasia Patients. Anesthesiology1990:73(3A):A1122

18. Setlock M, Kelly KJ. Anaphylaxis on induction of anesthesia associated with latex allergy. Anesthesiology 1991;75(3A):A1043

19. Kelly KJ, Setlock M, Davis JP. Anaphylactic reactions during general anesthesia among pediatric patients. MMWR 1991;40(26):437

20. Swartz J, Braude B, Gilmour R, Shandling B, Gold M. Intraoperative anaphylaxis to latex. Can J Anaesth 1990:37(5):589–92

21. Gold M, Swartz J, Braude B, Dolovich J, Shandling B, Gilmour R. Intraoperative anaphylaxis: an association with latex sensitivity. J Allergy Clin Immunol 1991;87(3):662–6

22. Pitkin RM. Folate and neural tube defects. Am J Clin Nutr 2007 Jan;85(1):285S–288S

23. Kibar Z, Torban E, McDearmmid JR, Reynolds A, Berghout J, Mathieu M, et al. Mutations in VANGL1 associated with neural-tube defects. N Engl J Med 2007 Apr 5;356(14): 1432–7

24. Kelly KJ, Pearson ML, Kurup VP, Havens PL, Byrd RS, Setlock MA, et al. A cluster of anaphylactic reactions in children with spina bifida during general anesthesia: epidemiologic features, risk factors, and latex hypersensitivity. J Allergy Clin Immunol 1994;94(1):53–61

25. Kelly KJ, Kurup V, Zacharisen M, Resnick A, Fink JN. Skin and serologic testing in the diagnosis of latex allergy. J Allergy Clin Immunol 1993;91(6):1140–5

26. Bernardini R, Novembre E, Lombardi E, Pucci N, Monaco MG, Vierucci A, Marcucci F. Risk factor for latex allergy in 54 children with atopy and latex sensitization. J Allergy Clin Immunol 2003;111(1):199–200

27. Hourihane JO, Allard MN, Wade AM, McEwan AI, Strobel S. Impact of repeated surgical procedures on the incidence and prevalence of latex allergy: a prospective study of 1263 children. J Pediatr 2002;140(4):479–82

28. Michael T, Niggemann B, Moers A, Seidel U, Wahn U, Scheffner D. Risk factors for latex allergy in patients with spina bifida. Clin Exp Allergy 1996;26(8):934–9

29. Nieto A, Extornell F, Mazón A, Reig C, Nieto A, Garcia-Ibarra F. Allergy to latex in spina bifida: a multivariate study of associated factors in 100 consecutive patients. J Allergy Clin Immunol 1996;98(3):501–7

30. Cremer R, Hoppe A, Korsch E, Kleine-Diepenbruck U, Bläker F. Natural rubber latex allergy: prevalence and risk factors in patients with spina bifida compared with atopic children and controls. Eur J. Pediatr 1998;157(1):13–6

31. Niggemann B, Buck D, Michael T, Wahn U. Latex provocation tests in patients with spina bifida: who is at risk of becoming symptomatic? J Allergy Clin Immunol 1998;102(4 Pt 1): 665–70

32. Bernardini R, Novembre E, Lombardi E, Mezzetti P, Cianferoni A, Danti AD, Mercurella A, Vierucci A. Prevalence of and risk factors for latex sensitization in patients with spina bifida. J Urol 1998;160(5):1775–8

33. Bernardini R, Novembre E, Lombardi E, Mezzetti P, Cianferoni A, Danti DA, Mercurella A, Vierucci A. Risk factors for latex allergy in patients with spina bifida and latex sensitization. Clin Exp Allergy 1999;29(5):681–6

34. Moneret-Vautrin D, Beaudouin E, Widmer S, Mouton C, Kanny G, Prestat F, Kohler C, Feldmann L. Prospective study of risk factors in natural rubber latex hypersensitivity. J Allergy Clin Immunol 1993;92:668–77

35. Degenhardt P, Golla S, Wahn F, Niggemann B. Latex allergy in pediatric surgery is dependent on repeated operations in the first year of life. J Pediatr Surg 2001;36:1535–9

36. Sparta G, Kemper MJ, Gerber AC, Goetschel P, Neuhaus TJ. Latex allergy in children with urological malformation and chronic renal failure. J Urol 2004;171:1647–9

37. Konz KR, Chia JK, Kurup VP, Resnick A, Kelly KJ, Fink JN. Comparison of latex hypersensitivity among patients with neurologic defects. J Allergy Clin Immunol 1995;95:950–4

38. Vogel LC, Schrader T, Lubicky JP. Latex allergy in children and adolescents with spinal cord injuries. J Pediatr Orthop 1995;15:517–20
39. Katelaris CH, Widrner RP, Lazarus RM. Prevalence of latex allergy in a dental school. Med J Aust 1996;164:711–4
40. Safadi GS, Safadi TJ, Terezhalmy GT, Taylor JS, Battisto JR, Melton AL. Latex hypersensitivity: its prevalence among dental professionals. JADA 1996;127:83–8
41. Tarlo S, Sussman G, Holness D. Latex sensitivity in dental students and staff: a cross-sectional study. J Allergy Clin Immunol 1997;99:396–401
42. Kelly KJ, Walsh-Kelly CM. Latex allergy: a patient and health care system emergency. Ann Emerg Med 1998;32(6):723–9
43. Liss GM, Sussman GL, Deal K, Brown S, Cividino M, Siu S, et al. Latex allergy: epidemiological study of 1351 hospital workers. Occup Environ Med 1997;54:335–42
44. Safidi GS, Corey EC, Taylor JS, Wagner WO, Pien LC, Melton AL. Latex hypersensitivity in emergency medical service providers. Ann Allergy Asthma Immunol 1996;77:39–42
45. Mace S, Sussman G, Stark DF, Thompson R, Kelly KJ, Beezhold D. Latex allergy in operating room nurses. J Allergy Clin Immunol 1996;97:558
46. Hunt LW, Fransway AF, Reed CE, Miller LK, Jones RT, Swanson MC, Yunginger JW. An epidemic of occupational allergy to latex involving health care workers. J Occup Environ Med 1995;37(10):1204–9
47. Sussman GL, Liss GM, Deal K, et al. Incidence of latex sensitization among latex glove users. J Allergy Clin Immunol 1998;101(2)(1):171–8
48. Lagier F, Vervloet D, Lhermet I, Poyen D, Charpin D. Prevalence of latex allergy in operating room nurses. J Allergy Clin Immunol 1993;90(3):319–22
49. Brown RH, Schauble JF, Hamilton RG. Prevalence of latex allergy among anesthesiologists. Anesthesiology 1998;89(2):292–9
50. Yassin MS, Lierl MB, Fischer TJ, O'Brien K, Cross J, Steinmetz O. Latex allergy in hospital employees. Ann Allergy 1994;72:245–9
51. Allmers H, Brehler R, Chen Z, Raulf-Heimsoth M, Fels H, Baur X. Reduction of latex aeroallergens and latex-specific IgE antibodies in sensitized workers after removal of powdered natural latex gloves in a hospital. J Allergy Clin Immunol 1998;102:841–6
52. Amin A, Palenik CJ, Cheung SW, Burke FJT. Latex exposure and allergy: a survey of general dental practitioners and dental students. Int Dent J 1998;48:77–83
53. Garabrant DH, Schweitzer S. Epidemiology of latex sensitization and allergies in health care workers. J Allergy Clin Immunol 2002;110(2 Suppl):S82–95
54. Baur X. Letter to the editor. J Allergy Clin Immunol 2003;111(3):652
55. Bousquet J, Flahault A, Vandenplas O, Ameille J, Duron J, Pecquet C, Chevrie K, Annesi-Maesano I. Natural rubber latex allergy among health care workers: a systematic review of the evidence. J Allergy Clin Immunol 2006;118:447–54
56. Gautrin D, Ghezzo H, Infante-Rivard C, Malo JL. Incidence and determinants of IgE-mediated sensitization in apprentices. Am J Respir Crit Care Med 2000;162:1222–8
57. Jolanki R, Extlander T, Alanko K, Savela A. Incidence rates of occupational contact urticaria caused by natural rubber latex. Contact Dermat 1999;40:329–31
58. Holness DL, Mace SR. Results of evaluating health care workers with prick and patch testing. Am J Contact Dermat 2001;12(2): 88–92
59. Tanaka S, Yukiko N, Yoshinari M. Coexistence of immediate and delayed-type allergy to natural rubber latex. Contact Dermat 2000;42:177–8
60. Lehto M, Koivuluhta M, Wang G, et al. Epicutaneous natural rubber latex sensitization induces T helper 2-type dermatitis and strong prohevein-specific IgE response. J Invest Dermatol 2003; 120:633–640.
61. Orfan NA, Reed R, Dykewicz MS, Ganz M, Kolski GB. Occupational asthma in a latex doll manufacturing plant. J Allergy Clin Immunol 1994;94(5):826–30
62. Zaza S, Reeder JM, Charles LE, Jarvis WR. Latex sensitivity among perioperative nurses. AORN J 1994;60:806–12

63. Vandenplas O, Delwiche J, Evrard G, Aimont P, Van Der Brempt X, Jamart J, Delaunois L. Prevalence of occupational asthma due to latex among hospital personnel. Am J Respir Crit Care Med 1995;151:54–60
64. Brugnami G, Marabini A, Siracusa A, Abbritti G. Work-related late asthmatic response induced by latex allergy. J Allergy Clin Immunol 1995;96:457–64
65. Tarlo SM, Sussman GL, Holness DL. Latex sensitivity in dental students and staff: a cross-sectional study. J Allergy Clin Immunol 1997;99:396–401
66. Mace SR, Sussman GL, Liss G, Stark DF, Beezhold D, Thompson R, Kelly K. Latex allergy in operating room nurses. Ann Allergy Asthma Immunol 1998;80:252–6
67. Page EH, Esswein EJ, Petersen MR, Lewis DM, Bledsoe TA. Natural rubber latex: glove use, sensitization, and airborne and latent dust concentrations at a Denver hospital. J Occup Environ Med 2000;42:613–20
68. Archambault S, Malo JL, Infante-Rivard C, Ghezzo H, Gautrin D. Incidence of sensitization, symptoms, and probable occupational rhinoconjunctivitis and asthma in apprentices starting exposure to latex. J Allergy Clin Immunol 2001;107:921–3
69. Galobardes B, Quiliquini AM, Rux N, Taramarcaz P, Schira JC, Bernstein M, Morabia A, Hauser C. Influence of occupational exposure to latex on the prevalence of sensitization and allergy to latex in a Swiss hospital. Dermatology 2001;203(3):226–32
70. Holter G, Irgens A, Nyfors A, Aasen TB, Florvaag E, Overa KB, Elsayed S, Naerheim J. Self-reported skin and respiratory symptoms related to latex exposure among 5,087 hospital employees in Norway. Dermatology 2002;205:28–31
71. Verna N, Di Giampaolo L, Renzetti A, Balatsinou L, Di Sgtefano F, Di Gioacchino G, Di Rocco P, Schiavone C, Boscolo P, Di Gioacchino M. Prevalence and risk factors for latex-related diseases among healthcare workers in an Italian general hospital. Ann Clin Lab Sci 2003;33(2):184–91
72. Nettis E, Assennato G, Ferrannini A, Tursi A. Type I allergy to natural rubber latex and type IV allergy to rubber chemicals in health care workers with glove-related skin symptoms. Clin Exp Allergy 2002;32:441–7
73. Tomazic VJ, Shampaine EL, Lamanna A, Withrow TJ, Adlunson NF Jr., Hamilton RG. Cornstarch powder on latex products is an allergen carrier. J Allergy Clin Immunol 1994;93:751–8
74. http://www.cdc.gov/niosh/topics/asthma/#surv. The work-related lung disease surveillance report. Section 9, Asthma
75. Ownby DR. A history of latex allergy. J Allergy Clin Immunol 2002;110:S27–32
76. Ownby DR, Tomlanovich M, Sammons N, McCullough J. Anaphylaxis associated with latex allergy during barium enema examinations. Am J Radiol 1991;156:903–8
77. Sondheimer JM, Pearlman DS, Bailey WC. Systemic anaphylaxis during rectal manometry with a latex balloon. Am J Gastroenterol 1989;84(8):975–7
78. Schwartz EE, Glick SN, Foggs MB, Silverstein GS. Hypersensitivity reactions after barium enema examination. Am J Radiol 1984;143:103–4
79. Gelfand DW. Barium enemas, latex balloons, and anaphylactic reactions. Am J Radiolo 1991;156:1–2
80. Ylitalo L, Turjanmaa K, Palosuo T, Reunala T. Natural rubber latex allergy in children who had not undergone surgery and children who had undergone multiple operations. J Allergy Clin Immunol 1997;100(5):606–12
81. Bernardini R, Novembre E, Ingargiola A, Veltroni M, Mugnaini L, Cianferoni A, Lombardi E, Vierucci A. Prevalence and risk factors of latex sensitization in an unselected pediatric population. J Allergy Clin Immun 1998;101:621–5
82. Levenbom-Mansour MH, Oesterle JR, Ownby DR, et al. The incidence of latex sensitivity in ambulatory surgical patients: a correlation of historical factors with positive serum IgE levels. Anesth Analg 1997;85:44–9
83. Reinheimer G, Ownby DR. Prevalence of latex-specific IgE antibodies in patients being evaluated for allergy. Ann Allergy Asthma Immunol 1995;74:184–7

84. Ownby DR, Ownby HB, McCullough JA, et al. The prevalence of anti-latex IgE antibodies to natural rubber latex in 1000 volunteer blood donors. J Allergy Clin Immunol 1996;97:1188–92

85. Merrett TG, Merrett J, Kekwick R. The prevalence of immunolglobulin E antibodies to the proteins of rubber (Hevea brasiliensis) latex and grass (Phleum pretense) pollen in sera of British blood donors. Clin Exp Allergy 1999;29(11):1572–8

86. Saxon A, Ownby D, Huard T, Parsad R, Roth HD. Prevalence of IgE to natural rubber latex in unselected blood donors and performance characteristics of Ala STAT testing. Ann Allergy Asthma Immunol 2000;84(2):199–206

87. Grzybowski M, Ownby DR, Rivers EP, Ander D, Nowak RM. The prevalence of latex-specific IgE in patients presenting to an urban emergency department. Ann Emerg Med 2002;40:411–9

88. Senna GE, Crocco I, Roata C, et al. Prevalence of latex-specific IgE in blood donors: an Italian survey. Allergy 1999;54:80–1

89. Liss GM, Sussman GL. Latex sensitization: occupational versus general population prevalence rates. Am J Ind Med 1999;35(2):196–200

90. M'Raihi L, Charpin D, Pons A, Bongrand P, Wervloet D. Cross-reactivity between latex and banana. J Allergy Clin Immunol 1991;87:129–30

91. Rodriguez M, Vega F, Garcia MT, Panizo C, Laffond E, Montalvo A, Cuevas M. Hypersensitivity to latex, chestnut and banana. Ann Allergy 1993;70:31–4

92. Fernández de Corres L, Moneo I, Muñoz D, Bernaola G, Fernández E, audicana M, Urrutia I. Sensitization from chestnuts and bananas in patients with urticaria and anaphylaxis from contact with latex. Ann Allergy 1993;70:35–9

93. Dompmartin A, Szczurko C, Michel M, Castel B, Cornillet B, Guilloux L, Remond B, Dapogny C, Leroy D. 2 cases of urticaria following fruit ingestion, with cross-sensitivity to latex. Contact Dermat 1994;30:250–2

94. Mäkinen-Kiljunen Soili. Banana allergy in patients with immediate-type hypersensitivity to natural rubber latex: characterization of cross-reacting antibodies and allergens. J Allergy Clin Immunol 1994;93:990–6

95. Blanco C, Carrillo T, Castillo R, et al. Latex allergy: clinical features and cross reactivity with fruits. Ann Allergy 1994;73:309–14

96. Kurup VP, Kelly T, Elms N, Kelly KJ, Fink JN. Cross reactivity of food allergens in latex allergy. Allergy Proceedings 1994;15(4):211–6

97. Llátser R, Zambrano C, Guillaumet B. Anaphylaxis to natural rubber latex in a girl with food allergy. Pediatrics 1994;94(5):736–7

98. Vallier P, Balland S, Harf R, et al. Identification of profilin as an IgE-binding component in latex from Hevea brasiliensis: clinical implications. Clin Exp Allergy 1995;25:332–9

99. Lavaud F, Prevost A, Cossart C, et al. Allergy to latex avocado, pear, and banana: evidence for a 30 kd antigen in immunoblotting. J Allergy Clin Immunol 1995;95:557–64

100. Akasawa A, Hsieh L, Lin Y. Serum reactivities to latex proteins (Hevea brasiliensis). J Allergy Clin Immunol 1995;95:1196–205

101. Alroth M, Alenius H, Turjanmaa K, et al. Cross-reacting allergens in natural rubber latex and avocado. J Allergy Clin Immunol 1995;96:167–73

102. Alenius H, Mäkinen-Kiljunenen S, Ahlroth M, Turjanmaa K, Reunala T, Palosuo T. Crossreactivity between allergens in natural rubber latex and banana studied by immunoblot inhibition. Clin Exp Allergy 1996;26:341–8

103. Akasawa A, Hsieh LS, Martin BM, et al. A novel acidic allergen, Hev b 5, in latex Purification, cloning and characterization. J Biol Chem 1996;271:25389–93

104. Akasawa A, Hsieh L, Tanaka K, Lin Y, Iikura Y. Identification and characterization of avocado chitinase with cross-reactivity to a latex protein. J Allergy Clin Immunol 1996;97:321

105. Weiss SJ, Halsey JF. A nurse with anaphylaxis to stone fruits and latex sensitivity: potential diagnostic difficulties to consider. Ann Allergy Asthma Immunol 1996;77:504–8

106. Beezhold DH, Sussman GL, Liss GM, Chang NS. Latex allergy can induce clinical reactions to specific foods. Clin Exp Immunol 1996;26:416–22

107. Delbourg MF, Guillouz L, Moneret-Vautrin DA, Ville G. Hypersensitivity to banana in latex-allergic patients. Identification of two major banana allergens of 33 and 37 kD. Ann Allergy Asthma Immunol 1996;76:321–6

108. Brehler R, Theissen U, Mohr C, Luger T. "Latex-fruit syndrome." Frequency of cross-reacting IgE antibodies. Allergy 1997;52:404–10

109. Fuchs T, Spitzauer S, Vente C, Hevler J, Kapiotis S, Rumpold H, Kraft D, Valenta R. Natural latex, grass pollen, and weed pollen share IgE epitopes. J Allergy Clin Immunol 1997;100:356–64

110. Garcia Ortiz JC, Moyano JC, Alvarez M, Bellido J. Latex allergy in fruit-allergic patients. Allergy 1998;53:532–6

111. Chen Z, Posch A, Cremer R, Raulf-Heimsoth M, Baur X. Identification of Hevein (Hev b 6.02) in *Hevea* latex as a major cross-reacting allergen with avocado fruit in patients with latex allergy. J Allergy Clin Immunol 1998;102:476–81

112. Mikkola JH, Alenius H, Kalkkinen N, Turjanmaa K, Palosuo T, Reunala T. Hevein-like protein domains as a possible cause for allergen cross-reactivity between latex and banana. J Allergy Clin Immunol 1998;102:1005–12

113. Posch A, Wheeler CH, Chen Z, et al. Class I endochitinase containing a hevein domain is the causative allergen in latex-associated avocado allergy. Clin Exp Allergy 1999;29:667–72

114. Yagami T. defense-related proteins as families of cross-reactive plant allergens. Recent Res Dev Allergy Clin Immunol 2000;1:41–64

115. Reche M, Pascual CY, Vicente J, Caballero T, Martin-Muñoz, Sanchez S, Martin-Esteban M. Tomato allergy in children and young adults: cross-reactivity with latex and potato. Allergy 2001;56:1197–201

116. Schmidt MH, Raulf-Heimsoth M, Posch A. Evaluation of patatin as a major cross-reactive allergen in latex-induced potato allergy. Ann Allergy Asthma Immunol 2002;89(6):613–8

117. Isola S, Ricciardi L, Saitta S, Fedele R, Mazzeo L, Fogliani O, Gangemi S, Purello D'Ambrosio F. Latex allergy and gruit cross-reaction in subjects who are nonatopic. Allergy Asthma Proc 2003;24(3):193–7

118. Focke M, Hemmer W, Wöhrl S, Götz M, Jarisch R. Cross-reactivity between *Ficus benjamina* latex and fig fruit in patients with clinical fig allergy. Clin Exp Allergy 2003;33(7):971–7

119. Wagner S, Radauer C, Hafner C, Fuchs H, Jensen-Jarolim E, Wüthrich B, Scheiner O, Breiteneder H. Characterization of cross-reactive bell pepper allergens involved in the latex-fruit syndrome. Clin Exp Allergy 2004;34(11):1739–46

120. Karisola P, Kotovuori A, Poikonen S, Niskanen E, Kalkkinen N, Turjanmaa K, Palosuo T, Reunala T, Alenius H, Kulomaa MS. Isolated Hevein-like domains, but not 31-kd endochitinases are responsible for IgE-mediated in vitro and invivo reactions in latex-fruit syndrome. J Allergy Clin Immunol 2005;115(3): 598–605

121. Gamboa PM, Sanchez-Monge R, Diaz-Perales A, Salcedo G, Ansotegui J, Sanz ML. Latex-vegetable syndrome due to custard apple and aubergine: new variations of the hevein symphony. J Investig Allergol Clin Immunol 2005;15(4):308–11

122. Sanchez-Monge R, Blanco C, Lopez-Torrejon G, Cumplido J, Recas M, Figueroa J, Carrillo T, Salcedo G. Differential allergen sensitization patterns in chestnut allergy with or without associated latex-fruit syndrome. J Allergy Clin Immunol 2006;118(3):705–10

123. Rihs HP, Ruëff F, Lundberg M, Rozynek P, Barber D, Scheurer S, Cistero-Bahima A, Brüning T, Raulf-Heimsoth M. Relevance of the recombinant lipid transfer protein of *Hevea brasiliensis*: IgE-binding reactivity in fruit-allergic adults. Ann Allergy Asthma Immunol 2006;97(5):643–9

124. Pereira C, Tavares B, Loureiro G, Lundberg M, Chieira C. Turnip and zucchini: new foods in the latex-fruit syndrome. Allergy 2007;62(4):452–3

125. Conti A, Giuffrida MG, Hoffmann-Sommergruber K, Wagner S, Amato S, Mistrello G, Asero R. Identification of latex UDP glucose pyrophosphorylase (Hev b UDPGP) as a novel cause of latex fruit allergy syndrome. Allergy Immunol (Paris) 2007;39(4):116–8

126. Schwartz HJ. Latex: a potential hidden "food" allergen in fast food restaurants. J Allergy Clin Immunol 1995;95(1):139–40

127. Beezhold DH, Reschke JE, Allen JH, Kostyal DA, Sussman GL. Latex protein: a hidden "food" allergen. Allergy Asthma Proc 2000;21(5):301–6

128. Bernardini R, Novembre E, Lombardi E, Pucci N, Marcucci F, Vierucci A. Anaphylaxis to latex after ingestion of a cream-filled doughnut contaminated with latex. J Allergy Clin Immunol 2002;110(3):534–5

129. Vassallo SA, Thurston TA, Kim SH, Todres ID. Allergic Reaction to latex from stopper of a medication vial. Anesth Analg 1995;80:1057–8

130. Towse A, O'Brien M, Twarog FJ, Braimon J, Moses AC. Local reaction secondary to insulin injection. A potential role for latex antigens in insulin vials and syringes. Diabetes Care 1995;18(8):1195–7

131. MacCracken J, Stenger P, Jackson T. Latex allergy in diabetic patients: a call for latex-free insulin tops. Diabetes Care 1996;19(2):184

132. Danne T, Niggemann B, Weber B, Wahn U. Prevalence of latex-specific IgE antibodies in atopic and nonatopic children with type I diabetes. Diabetes Care 1997;20(4):476–8

133. Hoffman RP. Latex hypersensitivity in a child with diabetes. Arch Pediatr Adolesc Med 2000;154(3):281–2

134. Roest MA, Shaw S, Orton DI. Insulin-injection-site reactions associated with type I latex allergy. N Engl J Med 2003;348(3):265–6

135. Thomsen DJ, Burke TG. Lack of latex allergen contamination of solutions withdrawn from vials with natural rubber stoppers. Am J Health Syst Pharm 2000;57:44–7

Index